Advanced Concepts and Techniques of Cardiomyopathies

Advanced Concepts and Techniques of Cardiomyopathies

Edited by **Bernard Tyler**

FOSTER ACADEMICS

New Jersey

Published by Foster Academics,
61 Van Reypen Street,
Jersey City, NJ 07306, USA
www.fosteracademics.com

Advanced Concepts and Techniques of Cardiomyopathies
Edited by Bernard Tyler

International Standard Book Number: 978-1-63242-021-3 (Hardback)

Printed in China.

Contents

Preface

This book has been an outcome of determined endeavour from a group of educationists in the field. The primary objective was to involve a broad spectrum of professionals from diverse cultural background involved in the field for developing new researches. The book not only targets students but also scholars pursuing higher research for further enhancement of the theoretical and practical applications of the subject.

Cardiomyopathies are defined as myocardial diseases in which the heart muscle is functionally and structurally irregular. This book presents a complete, up to date analysis of the current information available regarding cardiomyopathies. It presents the complete cardiovascular system as a functional unit, and the various contributors to this book analyze pathophysiological mechanisms from diverse viewpoints including genetics, molecular biology, imaging techniques and surgical procedure. This book presents a comprehensive overview regarding cardiomyopathies which will be helpful for readers interested in this field.

It was an honour to edit such a profound book and also a challenging task to compile and examine all the relevant data for accuracy and originality. I wish to acknowledge the efforts of the contributors for submitting such brilliant and diverse chapters in the field and for endlessly working for the completion of the book. Last, but not the least; I thank my family for being a constant source of support in all my research endeavours.

Editor

Part 1

Cardiomyopathies and Imaging Methods

1

Role of Advanced Cardiac Magnetic Resonance Imaging in Atypical Cardiomyopathies such as Stress-Induced Cardiomyopathies and Left-Ventricular Non-Compaction Cardiomyopathy

Oliver Strohm[1,2], Abdullah Shehab[3] and Anwer Qureshi[4]
[1]*University of Calgary,*
[2]*Center for Cardiology and Pediatric Cardiology Baden-Baden,*
[3]*UAE University,*
[4]*Tawam Hospital, Al Ain,*
[1]*Canada*
[2]*Germany*
[3,4]*United Arab Emirates*

1. Introduction

Magnetic Resonance Imaging (MRI) is a medical imaging technique that has been in clinical use since the 1980's, and has advanced significantly in the last decade.

MRI scans are usually performed at magnetic field strengths of 1.5 to 3.0 Tesla. Such a magnetic field is at least 25,000 times stronger than that of the earth and is required to align and modify the behaviour of unevenly charged protons in the patient's body. Brief radio frequency pulses with specific properties are applied, which change the axis of rotation (precession) in the protons. The protons rapidly resume their original precession angle and emit a small signal, which is used to compute images. Importantly, the behaviour of resuming their previous state is strongly dependent on the molecular environment; in other words: different tissue composition creates different image contrasts (14-16)

The main advantages of MRI techniques include their completely non-invasive nature, lack of any harmful radiation or radioactivity, and the lack of need for Iodine-based contrast agents. It is considered to be free of any harm to patients, but - since metal is affected in a magnetic field - it may not be performed if the patient carries certain magnetic material such as specific electronic devices or some metallic implants. The most commonly performed MRI scans are of the head, brain, spine, large joints and abdomen (15).

Cardiac applications of MRI have been applied since the late 1980's and have evolved into a robust, clinically valid application due to recent advances in both hardware and software. CMR provides a variety of valuable diagnostic information including anatomy and function of the heart, flow of blood, and perfusion and viability of the myocardium. Its most unique advantage is the ability to visualize tissue characteristics selectively based on molecular environments, adding a new and valuable piece of information to medical testing

Contrast-enhanced cardiac magnetic resonance imaging (CMR) allows for a non-invasive assessment of the tissue composition using contrast-free (T2, e.g. STIR) and contrast-enhanced techniques (early and late Gadolinium enhancement). Together with a functional assessment, it can be used to determine the acuity of e.g. inflammatory diseases and provide a non-invasive follow-up tool.

1.1 CMR techniques used

Functional imaging with high-resolution sequences such as SSFP cines allow to assess the whole left and right ventricles and calculate volumes, ejection fraction and mass. Myocardial wall stress can be calculated from these.

Assessment of valvular function is needed and may require additional flow studies for the calculation of regurgitation fraction of aortic and mitral valve. Assessment of the pericardium can be done on the functional images, too.

T2-weighted images with fat suppression allow assessing myocardial water content, thus allowing to assess the stage of disease. To provide an "internal standard", skeletal muscle is used as control; an SI-ratio of more than 2.0 is considered abnormal.

T1-weighted images allow to demonstrate acute inflammatory changes including increased extracellular volume and membrane integrity. As in T2-weighted imaging a skeletal muscle is used as "internal standard"; an enhancement - ratio (myocardial enhancement / muscle enhancement) of more than 4.0 is considered abnormal. The body-coil is used to obtain homogenous SI through the images, short axis or axial images are selected to optimize image quality.

Newer sequences may improve image quality and allow for the use of multi-element coils.

Late Gadolinium enhancement allows to non-invasively diagnose irreversible damage in the myocardium (e.g. fibrosis, infarcts). Due to the specific location in ischemic damages (starts at the subendocardial layer), it is easy to distinguish non-ischemic damages (as in myocarditis) from ischemic problems. Combining T2-information, early and late enhancement, CMR is able to safely assess the acuity and reversibility of the disease process in non-ischemic Cardiomyopathies and inflammatory processes (16).

2. Left ventricular non-compaction

2.1 Introduction

Left ventricular non-compaction (LVNC) is a distinct cardiomyopathy resulting from arrest of fetal development of the heart (1). This leads to altered myocardial architecture that is seen as a two layered myocardium with a thin, compacted epicardial layer and a thick, non-compacted endocardial region. The non-compacted myocardial region is comprised of prominent trabeculations and deep intertrabecular recesses that directly communicate with the left ventricular cavity (2, 3) .The condition may present without any associated cardiac malformation and is then labelled isolated left ventricular non compaction (LVNC). Non compacted myocardium is also seen in conjunction with other cardiac abnormalities including cyanotic congenital heart disease, Ebstein's anomaly and other cardiomyopathies. Clinical presentation in LVNC is seen with congestive heart failure, ventricular arrhythmia and systemic thromboembolism. The condition is listed as an unclassified cardiomyopathy in the WHO and European Society of Cardiology classification of cardiomyopathies (4, 5) and as a primary genetic cardiomyopathy in the American Heart Association classification (6).

2.2 Pathophysiology

Early intrauterine myocardial perfusion is through direct diffusion of nutrients from the left ventricular (LV) cavity to the myocardium. The presence of deep trabecular recesses filled with blood facilitates this process. Development of coronary circulation in the second trimester provides direct blood supply to the myocardium with consequent compaction of extensive intrauterine trabeculations of the myocardial wall. Failure in this process results in a non-compacted myocardium (1). The exact mechanism for this is not known.

2.3 Inheritance

Both sporadic and familial forms are described. In the latter an autosomal dominant or X-linked inheritance with genetic heterogeneity is reported. Mutations in *MYH7* encoding β-myosin heavy chain is seen in patients with Ebstein's anomaly and LVNC (7). In X-linked inheritance mutation of G4.5 TAZ gene with abnormality of tafazzin is reported (8, 9). This can be seen with or without Barth syndrome.

2.4 Prevalence

The presence of significant non compaction is estimated at 1:2.000 in the general population (10). The condition is, however, more prevalent in heart failure patients. More frequent use of cardiac imaging in clinical practice has increased recognition of this condition.

2.5 Clinical presentation

This is variable from asymptomatic individuals to those with severe disease presenting with heart failure, ventricular arrhythmia and systemic thromboembolism (9, 11-13). Non cardiac features may include facial dysmorphism and neuromuscular disorders.

2.6 Diagnostic criteria

Trabeculation in the LV wall is seen even in healthy volunteers. To separate benign LV trabeculation from pathological LVNC following diagnostic criteria is proposed.

- Echo: ratio of non-compacted to compacted myocardium in end-systole of > 2:1 (14)
- Cardiac MRI: ratio of non-compacted to compacted myocardium in end-diastole of > 2.3:1 (15)

2.7 Cardiac MRI in the diagnosis of LVNC

Cardiovascular imaging is central to the diagnosis of left ventricular non compaction. Compared to echocardiography better resolution of cardiac MRI makes it a preferred imaging modality particularly in those with limited echo windows. Additionally, non-compacted segment may be confined to the LV apex where echo has inherent imaging problems. Cardiac MRI is also reliable in distinguishing LVNC from other causes of LV apical deformity including apical variant of hypertrophic cardiomyopathy, endomyocardial fibrosis and apical thrombus.

2.8 Cardiac MRI imaging protocol

LV morphology and function is evaluated with cine images using a steady-state free precession (SSFP) technique. Images are usually displayed in three to six long axes and in contiguous short axis projections.

After baseline imaging post Gadolinium delayed enhancement (LGE) is performed to assess myocardial fibrosis.

2.9 Myocardial morphology on cardiac MRI

Besides pathological LVNC myocardial trabeculation is also seen in normal healthy individuals as well as in patients with hypertrophic and dilated cardiomyopathies. In LVNC distribution of non-compacted myocardium can be accurately assessed by MRI. There is involvement of the LV apex along with more frequent non compaction of the mid and apical segments of inferior and lateral wall. Non-compaction of the right ventricular wall is seen in some of these individuals. However, it is the severity of non-compaction rather than the distribution that distinguishes pathological LVNC from other disorders (15). A ratio of non-compacted to compacted myocardium of > 2.3 in diastole has as a sensitivity of 86% with a very high specificity of 99% and positive and negative predictive values of 75% and 99% respectively.

In contrast to echocardiography where systolic frame images are used to measure the relationship of non-compacted to compacted myocardium, diastolic frame images are used in MRI. This is possible because of improved spatial resolution of MRI. In systole, thickening of compacted myocardium may account for the altered relationship of compacted and non-compacted myocardium and this may explain the lower ratio of non-compacted to compacted myocardium of > 2:1 used in echocardiography (15).

Others have suggested that a trabeculated LV mass of > 20% of the total LV mass separates LVNC from other causes of LV trabeculation both benign and that seen in dilated and hypertrophic cardiomyopathy with a sensitivity and specificity of > 90%(16).

2.10 Myocardial kinetics and function

Cine short-axis images are used for calculation of ejection fraction (EF) using Simpson's method by tracing end diastolic and end systolic volumes in all imaging planes.

The spectrum of myocardial function may range from normal to severe systolic dysfunction. Quantitative assessment of left ventricular function by cardiac MRI is the current reference standard and can be compared longitudinally. However, in patients with LVNC interobserver and intraobserver reproducibility may be affected, depending on whether the inner contour (interface between the LV cavity and non-compacted myocardium) or outer contour (interface between the compacted and non-compacted myocardium) are used to calculate LV volumes. Latter may have the effect of increasing left ventricular end-diastolic volume and falsely overestimating volumetric EF (17). Therefore, additional qualitative information of LV function from review of myocardial kinetics on cine images is suggested.

2.11 Tissue characterization-late gadolinium enhancement

Late Gadolinium enhancement (LGE), a marker of myocardial fibrosis, was seen in 23 out of 42 patients (55%) in a study conducted by Nucifora, et al. The degree of LGE in their study correlated with clinical symptoms, LV systolic dysfunction and arrhythmia (18). In another study Dodd et al. demonstrated a correlation between trabecular LGE and LV dysfunction (19).

2.12 Clinical management

This is largely supportive with standard heart failure therapy. Heart transplantation remains an option in patients with advanced disease. Ventricular arrhythmia is not directly related to severity of LV dysfunction and a prophylactic ICD is recommended. Anticoagulation to prevent thromboembolic complications is recommended, particularly in patients with severe contractile dysfunction. Family members of affected individual should be screened and counseled.

2.13 Summary

Left ventricular non-compaction is a rare cardiomyopathy arising from developmental arrest of the left ventricular myocardium. It has distinct morphometric appearance with a two layer myocardium-a compacted and a non-compacted zone. Sporadic and familial forms are described. The triad of heart failure, arrhythmia and systemic thromboembolism are feared complications. In milder forms the patient may be completely asymptomatic. Increased awareness of this disorder and improvement in cardiovascular imaging has contributed to greater recognition of this condition. Cardiac MRI with its improved spatial resolution can conclusively establish the diagnosis and the unique property of LGE on cardiac MRI can identify severe forms of this disorder which may have both therapeutic and prognostic implications.

3. Stress-induced or "Tako-Tsubo" cardiomyopathy

3.1 Introduction

This cardiomyopathy is a transient and reversible cardiomyopathy that was first reported in Japan by Dote, et al., in 1991 (1). Clinical presentation may be indistinguishable from acute coronary syndrome, invariably necessitating coronary angiography for exclusion of obstructive coronary artery disease. Prevalence is in 1-2% of patients undergoing coronary angiography for acute coronary syndrome. Complimentary imaging modalities including echocardiography and cardiac MRI are helpful in diagnosis and in monitoring clinical recovery. Absence of delayed hyperenhancement on cardiac MRI is particularly important in differentiating this condition from ischemic and other types of non-ischemic cardiomyopathy and acute myocarditis (2). Based on morphologic features of the left ventricle, presumed causative role of stress and catecholamine excess and transient nature of the contractile dysfunction, other nomenclature used to describe this cardiomyopathy include ampulla cardiomyopathy, stress cardiomyopathy or catecholamine cardiotoxicity and transient left ventricular apical ballooning syndrome.

3.2 Pathophysiology

Distinct pattern of contractile abnormality is noted in the left ventricle. In the typical case the LV apex is dyskinetic and expanded and may be associated with hyperdynamic contractility of the basal LV segments. The shape of left ventricle in systole resembles a Japanese octopus trap (Takotusbo), which has a narrow neck and a wide base (1).

The condition is associated with markedly elevated circulating catecholamine, which is assumed to be central in the pathophysiology of this condition though exact mechanism at the cellular level is not fully understood. In a report by Wittstein, et al., two to three times higher plasma catecholamine concentrations were found in 13 patients with transient LV apical ballooning syndrome compared with 7 controls hospitalized for acute MI with Killip class III heart failure (3). Other proposed mechanisms include neurogenic stunned myocardium, coronary vasospasm, microvasculature dysfunction and altered cellular metabolism (4, 8-11). Preponderance of females afflicted by this condition is unclear. Estrogen deficiency in the post-menopausal state may play a role. Of particular interest, in other conditions with elevated catecholamine levels like subarachnoid hemorrhage, segmental wall motion abnormality is also predominantly seen in women (12). A reverse pattern of contractile abnormality with apical sparing has also been reported (13).

3.3 Clinical features

The presentation is typically following intense emotional or physical stress. The condition is predominantly seen in post-menopausal female with more than 80% of patients being female and more than 90% above the age of 50 years. Presentation may be clinically indistinguishable from ACS including ST segment elevation on ECG and rise in cardiac biomarkers. Chest pain and mild dyspnea are most common features encountered in more than 70% of patients. More significant heart failure and some degree of LVOT tract obstruction from hyperdynamic contraction of basal LV segments may be encountered in 15-20% of patients. Complications including cardiogenic shock may complicate the clinical course in up to 5% of patients. This may be secondary to either severe LV systolic dysfunction or obstruction of LVOT or both. Systemic thromboembolism from apical LV thrombus is reported. Ventricular arrhythmia is seen in 1-2% of patients (1-14).

Although presentation is typically encountered in the setting of profound emotional or physical stress, this characteristic trigger can be absent in up to a third of patients (14). Right ventricular involvement in takotsubo is seen in 25-30% of patients and is associated with a more complicated clinical course (15). It is encountered in patients with more severe LV involvement (16). However, isolated right ventricular takotsubo has been reported (17).

3.4 Diagnosis

History of intense emotional or physical stress and a typical pattern of left ventricular contractile dysfunction on cardiac imaging are suggestive of the diagnosis. Invariably, however, coronary angiography is required in the acute setting to exclude obstructive coronary artery disease. Both echocardiography and cardiac MRI provide information on the distinct morphologic and contractile dysfunction of takotsubo cardiomyopathy. However, cardiac MRI is instrumental in conclusively distinguishing takotsubo cardiomyopathy from other conditions.

3.5 Cardiac MRI in the diagnosis of Takotsubo cardiomyopathy

3.5.1 Assessment of myocardial morphology and contractility

Imaging sequence includes Standard TrueFISP (fast imaging with steady-state precession) cine images acquisition in 3 long-axis slices and 11 to 15 short-axis slices, 7 mm in thickness with a 3-mm interslice gap, achieving full ventricular coverage. Apical ballooning with or without mid myocardial contractile dysfunction and with basal sparing can be easily appreciated. In addition hyperdynamic contraction of basal segments with LVOT obstruction can be identified. The above-described pattern of contractile dysfunction in takotsubo cardiomyopathy does not fit a coronary artery distribution and is helpful in differentiating this condition from acute coronary syndrome. Left ventricular apical thrombus, which can complicate the clinical course, can be diagnosed using the long axis cine projections and LGE images.

Right ventricular involvement is seen in some patients. Because of the difficulty in assessing RV morphology and function by echocardiography, cardiac MRI is a preferred modality for identification of right ventricular involvement (15-17) and in quantification of RV dysfunction. However, cautious interpretation of RV dysfunction by MRI is advised in view of some degree of projection dependent contractile dysfunction seen even in normal subjects (18-19).
Sequential cardiac imaging study will show normalization of contractile dysfunction within a few days to weeks.

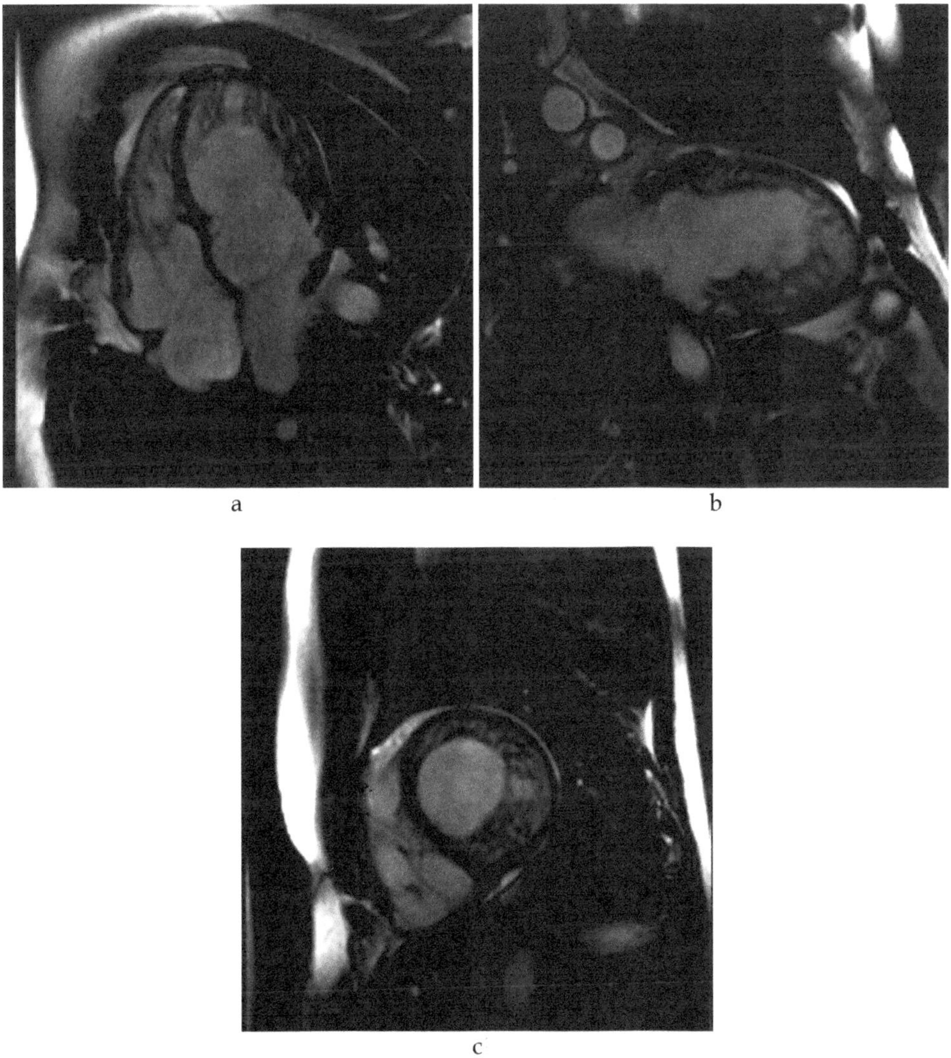

Fig. 1. Long axis and short axis SSFP images in diastole (a: 4-chamber view long axis; b: 2-chamber view long axis; c: short axis at mid ventricular level) in a patient with genetically proven non-compaction cardiomyopathy. Note increased end-diastolic volume and increased

3.5.2 First pass myocardial perfusion

In contrast to apical myocardial infarction rest first-pass contrast enhanced myocardial perfusion on cardiac MRI is usually normal in takotsubo cardiomyopathy providing another feature to distinguish between the two conditions.

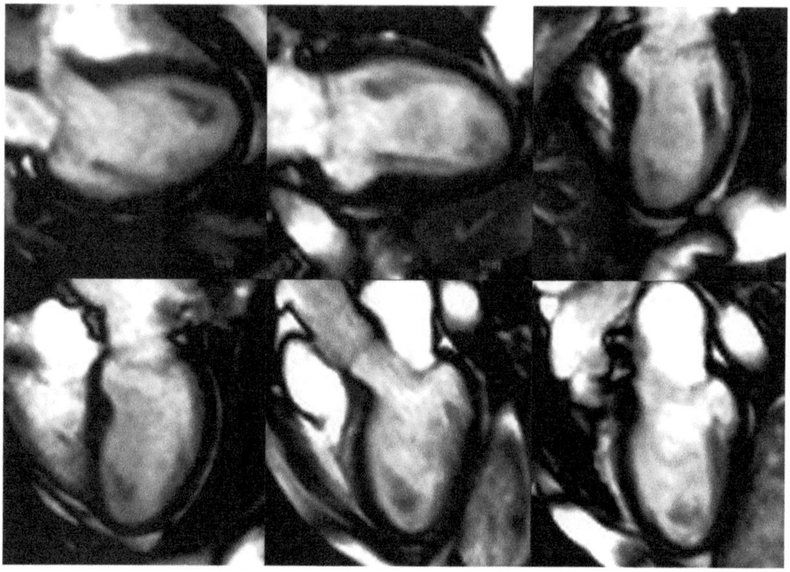

a

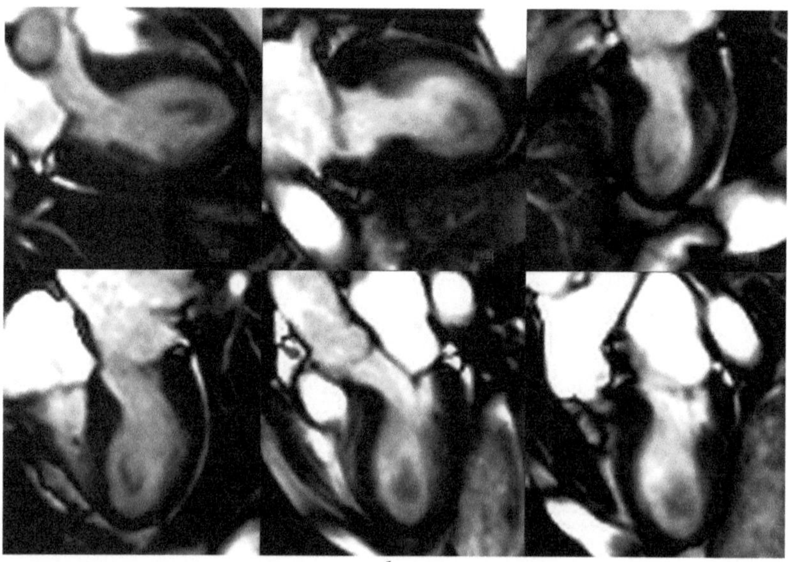

b

Fig. 2. Set of mulitple long axis SSFP cines in diastole (2-a) and systole (2-b). Note hypo- to akinetic mid ventricular and apical segments in this apical ballooning syndrome.

3.5.3 Tissue characterization – Myocardial edema on t2-weighted images

Myocardial edema following myocardial injury, ischemic or non-ischemic, can be detected using T2-weighted short tau inversion recovery (T2-STIR) images obtained in basal, mid, and apical short-axis, vertical long-axis, 3-chamber, and horizontal long-axis planes (20). Elevated T2- signal consistent with myocardial edema is seen in patients with takotsubo cardiomyopathy. T2 signal is highest in myocardium with the most impaired function and resolves over time (21-22). Myocardial edema on T2-STIR sequence is also a hallmark of ischemic myocardium prior to irreversible myocardial injury (23). In contrast to ischemic myocardium, myocardial edema in patients with takotsubo cardiomyopathy may represent catecholamine-induced myocardial stunning due to microvascular dysfunction (2).

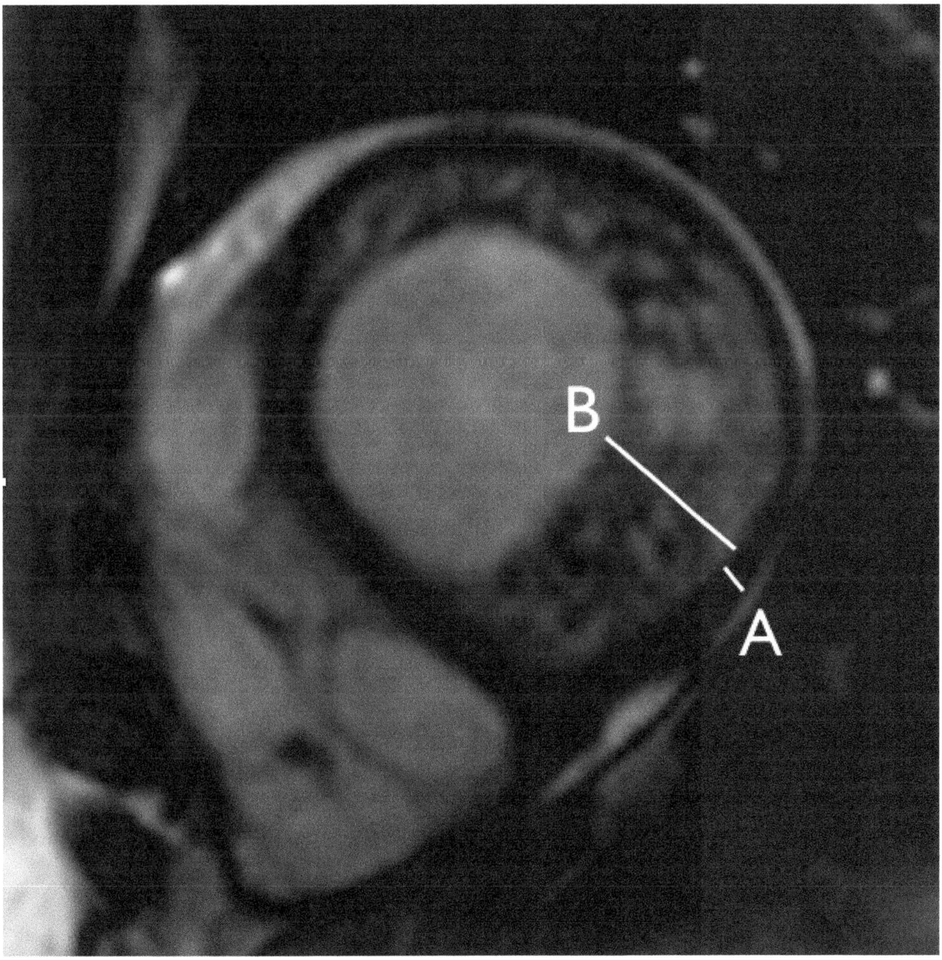

Fig. 3. Short axis SSFP cine image in diastole in a patient with non-compaction cardiomyopathy. Line A denotes the thickness of the compacted myocardium, line B denotes the non-compacted myocardium.

3.5.4 Tissue characterization – Late gadolinium enhancement (LGE) on T1-weighted Images

Gadolinium concentrates in region of damaged myocardium and appears bright on T1-weighted images (24). Cine images using a segmented gradient-echo sequence (6-mm slice thickness) is obtained in multiple short-axis views every 10 mm covering the whole left ventricle (LV). Ten to 15 min after injection of a Gadolinium-based contrast agent, images are acquired in the same orientation as the cine images using a segmented inversion-recovery gradient-echo pulse sequence. Abnormal myocardium is usually bright on T1-weighted images. LGE is absent in patients with takotsubo cardiomyopathy (2, 3, 5, 25). This indicates viable myocardium and is particularly useful in distinguishing it from myocardial infarction, other types of non-ischemic cardiomyopathy and myocarditis.

In a prospective study using CMR conducted by Eitel, et al., 6.100 patients presenting with ACS underwent coronary angiography and left ventriculography. In 59 patients with normal coronary angiography and typical contractile pattern of takotsubo cardiomyopathy, cardiac MRI was performed. Using strict criteria of absence of any late Gadolinium enhancement, takotsubo cardiomyopathy was diagnosed in 38. In the remaining 21 patients, based on the pattern of delayed hyperenhancement, a diagnosis of ischemic heart disease was made in 13 and of myocarditis in 8 patients (2). However, in a study of 15 patients with takotsubo cardiomyopathy, low intensity, patchy, mid-myocardial LGE was seen in 5 out of 15 patients. Increase in extracellular collagen was reported to be a plausible mechanism for this finding (26).

3.5.5 Coronary magnetic resonance angiography (MRA)

Coronary MRA though quite helpful in delineating the course of proximal coronary arteries (27), is not feasible for assessment of obstructive coronary artery disease and hence cannot be substituted for invasive or CT angiography (28).

3.6 Management

Treatment is supportive. ß-blockers are the mainstay in blunting catecholamine cardiotoxicity. This should be used cautiously to avoid worsening of heart failure. In patients with cardiogenic shock inotropic and IABP support may be required. However, the possibility of exacerbating LVOT obstruction with these measures requires careful monitoring and appropriate adjustment of therapy including discontinuation of inotropes and IABP support (29). ACE-I are beneficial and warfarin is recommended till left ventricular recovery is complete. In addition to these therapeutic measures, emotional or physical precipitating factors should be addressed. Prognosis is usually very good with complete or near complete recovery of LV contractile dysfunction. For prevention of rare recurrent episodes of takotsubo even after removal of initial trigger, indefinite neurohormonal modulation with ß-blockers and ACE-I merits consideration (30).

3.7 Summary

Takotsubo cardiomyopathy presents with clinical features that can be indistinguishable from acute coronary syndrome. However, distinct myocardial contractile dysfunction on echocardiography or cardiac MRI, absence of obstructive CAD on invasive angiography and exposure to an emotional or physical stressor is helpful in initially distinguishing it from ACS. Furthermore, cardiac MRI with normal first-pass contrast enhanced rest myocardial perfusion, reversible myocardial edema in regions of contractile dysfunction and absence of late gadolinium enhancement is strongly indicative of the diagnosis of takotsubo cardiomyopathy. Resolution of contractile dysfunction, days to weeks after initial presentation, is confirmatory of the diagnosis.

4. References

4.1 Part one references

[1] Sedmera D, Pexieder T, Vuillemin M, Thompson RP,Anderson RH. Developmental patterning of the myocardium. *Anat Rec* 2000; 258: 319–337.

[2] Chin TK, Perloff JK, Williams RG, Jue K, Mohrmann R. Isolated noncompaction of left ventricular myocardium. A study of eight cases. Circulation 1990;82:507-513.

[3] Dusek J, Ostadal B, Duskova M. Postnatal persistence of spongy myocardium with embryonic blood supply. Arch Pathol 1975;99:312-317.

[4] *Richardson P, McKenna W, Bristow M, Maisch B, Mautner B, O'Connell J, Olsen E, Thiene G, Goodwin J.*Report of the 1995 World Health Organisation/International Society and Federation of Cardiology Task Force on the definition and classification of cardiomoypathies. Circulation 1996; 93:841–842.

[5] Perry Elliott, Bert Andersson, Eloisa Arbustini, Zofia Bilinska, Franco Cecchi, Philippe Charron, Olivier Dubourg, Uwe Kühl, Bernhard Maisch, William J. McKenna, Lorenzo Monserrat, Sabine Pankuweit, Claudio Rapezzi, Petar Seferovic, Luigi Tavazzi, Andre Keren. Classification of the cardiomyopathies: a position statement from the European society of cardiology working group on myocardial and pericardial diseases. *Eur Heart J* (2008) 29 (2): 270-276

[6] Barry J. Maron, MD, Chair; Jeffrey A. Towbin, MD, FAHA; Gaetano Thiene, MD; Charles Antzelevitch, PhD, FAHA; Domenico Corrado, MD, PhD; Donna Arnett, PhD, FAHA; Arthur J. Moss, MD, FAHA; Christine E. Seidman, MD, FAHA; James B. Young, MD, FAHA. Contemporary Definitions and Classification of the Cardiomyopathies. An American Heart Association Scientific Statement from the Council on Clinical Cardiology, Heart Failure and Transplantation Committee; Quality of Care and Outcomes Research and Functional Genomics and Translational Biology Interdisciplinary Working Groups; and Council on Epidemiology and Prevention. *Circulation.* 2006;113:1807-1816.

[7] Mutations in the Sarcomere Gene *MYH7* in Ebstein Anomaly / Clinical Perspective.Alex V. Postma, Klaartje van Engelen, Judith van de Meerakker, Thahira Rahman, Susanne Probst, Marieke J.H. Baars, Ulrike Bauer, Thomas Pickardt, Silke R. Sperling, Felix Berger, Antoon F.M. Moorman, Barbara J.M. Mulder, Ludwig Thierfelder, Bernard Keavney, Judith Goodship, and Sabine Klaassen. Circ Cardiovasc Genet. *2011;4:43-50*

[8] Ichida F, Tsubata S, Bowles KR, Haneda N, Uese K, Miyawaki T, Dreyer WJ, Messina J, Li H, Bowles NE, Towbin JA. Novel Gene Mutations in Patients with Left Ventricular Noncompaction or Barth Syndrome. Circulation 2001;103;1256-1263.

[9] Pignatelli RH, McMahon CJ, Dreyer WJ, Denfield SW, Price J, Belmont JW, et al. Clinical characterization of left ventricular noncompaction in children: a relatively common form of cardiomyopathy. Circulation 2003;108:2672–8

[10] Ritter M, Oechslin E, Sutsch G, Attenhofer C, Schneider J, Jenni R. Isolated noncompaction of the myocardium in adults. Mayo Clin Proc 1997;72:26-31.

[11] Oechslin EN, Attenhofer Jost CH, Rojas JR, Kaufmann PA, Jenni R. Long-term follow-up of 34 adults with isolated left ventricular noncompaction: a distinct cardiomyopathy with poor prognosis. *J Am Coll Cardiol* 2000; 36: 493–500.

[12] Ichida F, Hamamichi Y, Miyawaki T, Ono Y, Kamiya T, Akagi T, et al., Clinical features of isolated noncompaction of the ventricular myocardium. *J Am Coll Cardiol* 1999; 34: 233–240.

[13] Murphy RT, Thaman R, Blanes JG, Ward D, Sevdalis E, Papra E, Kiotsekolglou A, Tome MT, Pellerin D, McKenna WJ, Elliott PM. Natural history and familial characteristics of isolated left ventricular non-compaction. European Heart Journal (2005) 26, 187–192.

[14] Jenni R, Oechslin E, Schneider J,Attenhofer Jost C, Kaufmann PA. Echocardiographic and pathoanatomical characteristics of isolated left ventricular non-compaction: a step towards classification as a distinct cardiomyopathy. Heart 2001;86:666-671.

[15] Petersen SE, Selvanayagam JB, Wiesmann F, Robson, MD, Francis JM, Anderson RH, Watkins H, Neubauer S. Left ventricular non-compaction: insights from cardiovascular magnetic resonance imaging J Am Coll Cardiol 2005;46:101-105

[16] Jacquier A, Thuny F, Jop B, Giorgi R, Cohen F, Gaubert J, Vidal V, Bartoli JM, Habib G, Moulin G. Measurement of trabeculated left ventricular mass using cardiac magnetic resonance imaging in the diagnosis of left ventricular non-compaction. *Eur Heart J* (2010) 31 (9): 1098-1104.

[17] Papavassiliu T, Kuhl HP, Schroder M, Suselbeck T, Bondarenko O, Bohm CK, Beek A, Hofman MM, van Rossum AC. Effect of endocardial trabeculae on left ventricular measurements and measurement reproducibility at cardiovascular MR imaging. Radiology 2005;236:57–64.

[18] Nucifora G, Aquaro GD, Pingitore A, Masci PG, Lombardi M: Myocardial fibrosis in isolated left ventricular non-compaction and its relation to disease severity. *Eur J Heart Fail* (2011) 13 (2): 170-176.

[19] Dodd JD, Holmvang G, Hoffmann U, et al. Quantification of left ventricular noncompaction and trabecular delayed hyperenhancement with cardiac MRI: correlation with clinical severity. Am J Roentgenol 2007;189:974-980.

4.2 Part two references

[1] Dote K, Sato H, Tateishi H, Uchida T, Ishihara M. Myocardial stunning due to simultaneous multivessel coronary spasms: a review of 5 cases. J Cardiol 1991;21: 203–214.

[2] Eitel I, Behrendt F, Schindler K, Kivelitz D, Gutberlet M, Schuler G, Thiele H. Differential diagnosis of suspected apical ballooning syndrome using contrast-enhanced magnetic resonance imaging. Eur Heart J (2008) 29 (21): 2651-2659.

[3] Wittstein IS, Thiemann DR, Lima JA, Baughman KL, Schulman SP, Gerstenblith G, et al. Neurohumoral features of myocardial stunning due to sudden emotional stress. N Engl J Med. 2005;352:539–548.

[4] Abe Y, Kondo M, Matsuoka R, Araki M, Dohyama K, Tanio H. Assessment of clinical features in transient left ventricular apical ballooning. J Am Coll Cardiol. 2003;41:737–742.

[5] Sharkey SW, Lesser JR, Zenovich AG, Maron MS, Lindberg J, Longe TF, Maron BJ. Acute and Reversible Cardiomyopathy Provoked by Stress in Women From the United States. Circulation 2005;111:472-479.

[6] Bybee KA, Prasad A. Stress-related cardiomyopathy syndromes Circulation 2008;118:397-40.

[7] Sharkey SW, Windenburg DC, Lesser JR, Maron MS, Hauser RG, Lesser JN, Haas TS, Hodges JS, Maron BJ. Natural History and Expansive Clinical Profile of Stress (Tako-Tsubo) Cardiomyopathy. J. Am. Coll. Cardiol., January 26, 2010; 55(4): 333 - 341.

[8] Bybee KA, Prasad A, Barsness GW, et al. Clinical characteristics and thrombolysis in myocardial infarction frame counts in women with transient left ventricular apical ballooning syndrome. Am J Cardiol 2004;94:343-346.

[9] Sansen V, Holvoet G. Takotsubo cardiomyopathy presenting as multivessel coronary spasm syndrome: case report and review of the literature. Acta Cardiol 2007;62:507-511.

[10] Afonso L, Bachour K, Awad K, Sandidge G. Takotsubo cardiomyopathy: pathogenetic insights and myocardial perfusion kinetics using myocardial contrast echocardiography Eur J Echocardiogr 2008;9:849-854

[11] Kurisu S, Inoue I, Kawagoe T, Ishihara M, Shimatani Y, Nishioka K, Umemura T, Nakamura S, Yoshida M, Sato H. Myocardial perfusion and fatty acid metabolism in patients with tako-tsubo-like left ventricular dysfunction. J Am Coll Cardiol. 2003 Mar 5;41(5):743-8.

[12] Mayer SA, Lin J, Homma S, et al. Myocardial injury and left ventricular performance after subarachnoid hemorrhage Stroke 1999;30:780-786.

[13] Hurst RT, Prasad A, Askew III JW, Sengupta PP, Tajik AJ. Takotsubo Cardiomyopathy: A Unique Cardiomyopathy with Variable Ventricular Morphology. J. Am. Coll. Cardiol. Img., June 1, 2010; 3(6): 641 - 649.

[14] Gianni M, Dentali F, Grandi AM, Sumner G, Hiralal R, Lonn E. Apical ballooning syndrome or takotsubo cardiomyopathy: a systematic review. European Heart Journal (2006) 27, 1523–1529.

[15] Elesber AA, Prasad A, Bybee KA, Valeti U, Motiei A, Lerman A, Chandrasekaran K, Rihal CS, Transient Cardiac Apical Ballooning Syndrome: Prevalence and Clinical Implications of Right Ventricular Involvement. J Am Coll Cardiol, 2006; 47:1082-1083.

[16] Haghi D, Athanasiadis A, Papavassiliu T, Suselbeck T, Fluechter S, Mahrholdt H, Borggrefe M, Sechtem U. Right ventricular involvement in Takotsubo Cardiomyopathy. Eur Heart J (2006) 27, 2433–2439.

[17] Mrdovic I, Kostic J, Perunicic J, Asanin A, Vasiljevic Z, and Ostojic M. Right Ventricular Takotsubo Cardiomyopathy. J. Am. Coll. Cardiol., April 20, 2010; 55(16): 1751 - 1751.

[18] Sievers B, Addo M, Franken U, Trappe HJ. Right ventricular wall motion abnormalities found in healthy subjects by cardiovascular magnetic resonance imaging and characterized with a new segmental model. J Cardiovasc Magn Reson 2004;6:601–608.

[19] Fritz J, Solaiyappan M, Tandri H, MD, Bomma C, Genc A, Claus D. Claussen CD, Lima JAC, Bluemke DA.Right Ventricle Shape and Contraction Patterns and Relation to Magnetic Resonance Imaging Findings. J Comput Assist Tomogr 2005;29:725–733.

[20] Simonetti OP, Finn JP, White RD, Laub G, Henry DA. 'Black blood' T2-weighted inversion-recovery MR imaging of the heart. Radiology 1996;199:49–57.

[21] Abdel-Aty H, Cocker M, Friedrich MG. Myocardial edema is a feature of Tako-Tsubo cardiomyopathy and is related to the severity of systolic dysfunction: Insights from T2-weighted cardiovascular magnetic resonance. Int J Cardiol. 2009 Feb 20;132(2):291-3.

[22] Joshi SB, Chow T, Herzka DA, Zeman PR, Cooper HA, Lindsay J, Fuisz AR. Cardiovascular magnetic resonance T2 signal abnormalities in left ventricular ballooning syndrome. Int J Cardiovasc Imaging: Vol. 26, No. 2, 227-232.

[23] Abdel-Aty H, Cocker M, Meek C, Tyberg JV, Friedrich MG. Edema as a very early marker for acute myocardial ischemia: a cardiovascular magnetic resonance study J Am Coll Cardiol 2009;53:1194-120.

[24] Saeed M, Wendland MF, Yu KK, Lauerma K, Li HT, Derugin N, Cavagna FM, Higgins CB. Identification of myocardial reperfusion with echoplanar magnetic resonance imaging: discrimination between occlusive and reperfused infarction. Circulation 1994; 90:1492–1501.

[25] Teraoka K, Kiuchi S, Takada N, Hirano M, Yamashina A. Images in cardiovascular medicine. No delayed enhancement on contrast magnetic resonance imaging with Takotsubo cardiomyopathy. Circulation. 2005;111:e261–e262

[26] Rolf A, Nef HM, Mollmann H, et al. Immunohistological basis of the late gadolinium enhancement phenomenon in tako-tsubo cardiomyopathy. *Eur Heart J.* 2009;30:1635-1642.

[27] Taylor AM, Thorne SA, Rubens MB, Jhooti P, Keegan J, Gatehouse PD,Wiesmann F, Grothues F, Somerville J, Pennell DJ. Coronary artery imaging in grown up congenital heart disease: complementary role of magnetic resonance and x-ray coronary angiography. *Circulation.* 2000;101:1670 -1678.

[28] Bluemke DA, Achenbach S, Budoff M, Gerber TC, Gersh B, Hillis LD, Hundley WG, Manning WJ, Printz BF, Stuber M, Woodard PK. Noninvasive coronary artery imaging: magnetic resonance angiography and multidetector computed tomography angiography: a scientific statement from the American Heart Association Committee on Cardiovascular Imaging and Intervention of the Council on Cardiovascular Radiology and Intervention, and the Councils on Clinical Cardiology and Cardiovascular Disease in the Young. *Circulation.* 2008;118:586–606.

[29] Echocardiographic Guidance in Treatment of Cardiogenic Shock Complicating Transient Left Ventricular Apical Ballooning Syndrome. Good CW, Hubbard CR, Harrison TA, Qureshi A: J Am Coll Cardiol Img 2009 March 2; (3):372-374.

[30] Dec, GW. Recognition of the Apical Ballooning Syndrome in the United States. Circulation: 2005;111:388-390.

2

The Use of Contrast-Enhancement Cardiovascular Magnetic Resonance Imaging in Cardiomyopathies

Marlon A.G.M. Olimulder, Michel A. Galjee, Jan van Es, Lodewijk J. Wagenaar and Clemens von Birgelen
Medisch Spectrum Twente
The Netherlands

1. Introduction

The clinical applications of cardiovascular magnetic resonance imaging (CMR), are expanding as the result of the development in hardware, pulse sequence and the ability of post-processing techniques. As the result of the flexibility of CMR to use different pulse-sequences, with or without the use of Gadolinium, CMR has developed as a powerful tool for clinical relevant tissue characterization. CMR in combination with the contrast-enhancement (CE) technique was initially developed to distinguish viable from non-viable myocardium following myocardial infarction. Nowadays, CE-CMR is increasingly used for tissue characterization in ischemic as well as non-ischemic cardiomyopathies to determine the exact etiology, guide proper treatment, and predict outcome and prognosis. In this chapter, we would like to discuss and illustrate the value of CE-CMR imaging in various cardiomyopathies.

2. Utility of different CMR acquisition modes in cardiomyopathy

CMR imaging includes several techniques that can be used in various combinations to assess left ventricular functional parameters, morphology, as well as myocardial disorders (such as edema, scar/fibrosis, microvascular obstruction, myocardial salvage) within one examination. Therefore, it is increasingly used in clinical practice for the diagnosis and management of cardiac diseases. In this respect, recent reviews concerning this aspect have been published (Marcu et al., 2007; Olimulder et al. 2011; Vogel-Claussen et al. 2006; Vohringer 2007; Weinsaft et al. 2007). Some technical aspect of cine - and CE imaging but also T2-weighted imaging (increasingly used when CE imaging is applied) are shortly discussed below.

2.1 Cine CMR for quantitative assessment of ventricular dimension, function and mass

By application of ECG-gated, breath-holding, cine-bright blood sequences, a stack of contiguous left ventricular short-axis slices (5-10 mm thick) are made from basal to apical (figure 1a) (Marcu et al. 2006). CMR is a tomographic technique that uses volumetric quantification based on Simpson's rule. Each separate slice is distributed approximately in 30 phases (simplified in figure 1b; from 1 separate slice, 8 phases from end-diastolic to end-systolic are shown); the endocardium is traced manually in the end-diastolic and end-systolic phase. Left ventricular end-diastolic and end-systolic volume is then calculated by summation of the endocardial surfaces and multiplication by the slice thickness of each separate slice.

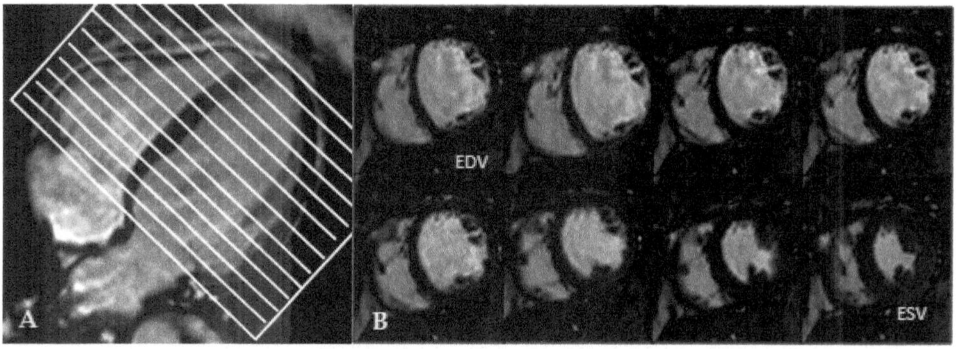

Fig. 1. Schematic figure for A: multiple short axis slices from basal to apical are made from a four chamber view, B: from 1 separate short axis slice, phases from end-diastolic to end-systolic are illustrated.

Left ventricular ejection fraction is calculated by the formula: ((end-diastolic volume - end-systolic volume)/end-diastolic volume) × 100%.
Left ventricular mass can be calculated by 1. tracing the epicardium in the end-diastolic phase in each separate slice; 2. obtaining a myocardial volume by summation of the surfaces between the epicardial and endocardial lines and multiplication by the slice thicknesses; and 3. multiplication of the myocardial volume with weight density (1.05 g/cm^3) of muscle.

2.2 CE-CMR imaging for assessment of damaged myocardium

The technique of CE-CMR imaging involves an intravenous injection of a contrast agent (e.g., gadolinium at a preferred dose of 0.2 mmol/kg body weight) followed by an ECG-gated T1-weight pulse sequence 10-15 minutes after injection (5 minutes after injection if microvascular obstruction is assessed). (Jackson et al. 2007) The timing of the image acquisition is of paramount importance, as too early image acquisition reduces the difference in contrast between normal and damaged myocardium (such as scar or fibrosis) because of an insufficient washout of contrast medium from the normal myocardium; too late image acquisition, on the other hand, may result in an excessive washout from damaged myocardial tissue that leads to an inferior signal-to-noise ratio. (Vogel-Claussen et al. 2006) The typical pulse sequence for CE-CMR imaging is a segmented T1-weighted inversion-recovery-prepared fast gradient-echo sequence. An inversion-recovery pulse is used to null the signal of normal myocardium in order to optimize the difference between normal and damaged myocardial areas (which still contain contrast medium) (Figure 2).

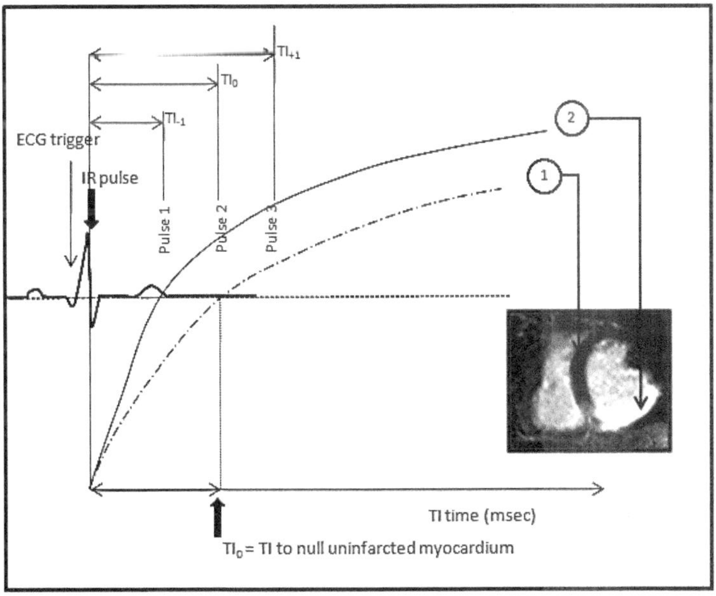

Fig. 2. Schematic figure for inversion time (TI) mapping. Following the ECG trigger, an inversion recovery (IR) pulse is applied. Before image acquisition, low-resolution TI scout images at mid-ventricular level with increasing TI (interval TI 30 msec) are performed. The optimal time to inversion (TI_0) is defined visually as the inversion time at which the uninfarcted myocardium (1) is nulled. (2) = infarcted myocardium.

The optimal inversion time depends on the contrast clearance from the normal myocardium which may show considerable inter-patient variability, depending on several factors such as the patient weight, left ventricular or renal function. Therefore, just before image acquisition, the inversion time is optimized on a per-patient basis using low-resolution scout images at mid-ventricular level with increasing inversion times at intervals of 30ms, from which the optimal inversion time can be derived (Jackson et al. 2007). The process is synchronized to the *R*-wave of the ECG and mid-diastolic images are acquired every other heart beat during breath-hold (Marcu et al. 2007).

2.3 T2-weighted CMR imaging for assessment of myocardial edema

T2-weighted CMR imaging is a pulse sequence sensitive to regional or global increases of myocardial water (a substantial feature of inflammatory responses) (Zagrosek et al. 2008; bdel-Aty et al. 2005). Therefore very useful in the (sub) acute phase of myocardial infarction and myocarditis. The long T2 relaxation times of water-bound protons are used to generate a water-specific contrast when applying T2-weighted sequences resulting in a high signal intensity of edematous tissue. Standard T2-weighted imaging of myocardial edema typically utilizes turbo spin-echo readouts with or without fat saturation pulses (to separate fat from water), mostly combined with dark-blood preparation (Eitel et al. 2011). An alternative acquisition mode can be the T2-prepared steady state free precession technique, which may be more reliable in imaging edema as it provides fewer artifacts and has better diagnostic accuracy than conventional darkblood acquisitions (Kellman et al. 2007).

3. CE-CMR findings in the different cardiomyopathies

3.1 CE-CMR after myocardial infarction

Myocardial infarction occurs after coronary occlusion of at least 20-30 minutes (without sufficient collateral blood supply to the affected myocardium) (Edelman, 2004). In the early phase of myocardial infarction, cellular degradation in the infarcted myocardium results in an increase in the permeability and enlargement of the extravascular space (edema), and thus, an increased distribution volume for the CMR contrast agent. Later on, due to different wash-in and wash-out kinetics, myocardial scars retain contrast agents longer than normal myocardium. The net result of both mechanisms is that infarcted myocardium appears bright on CE-T1-weighted images.

CE in patients with MI generally shows a typical pattern that is related to the perfusion area of the culprit vessel. Myocardial changes (and thus CE) of the subendocardium can generally be found which may extend to a transmural distribution in cases with prolonged coronary occlusion (Figure 3a,b).

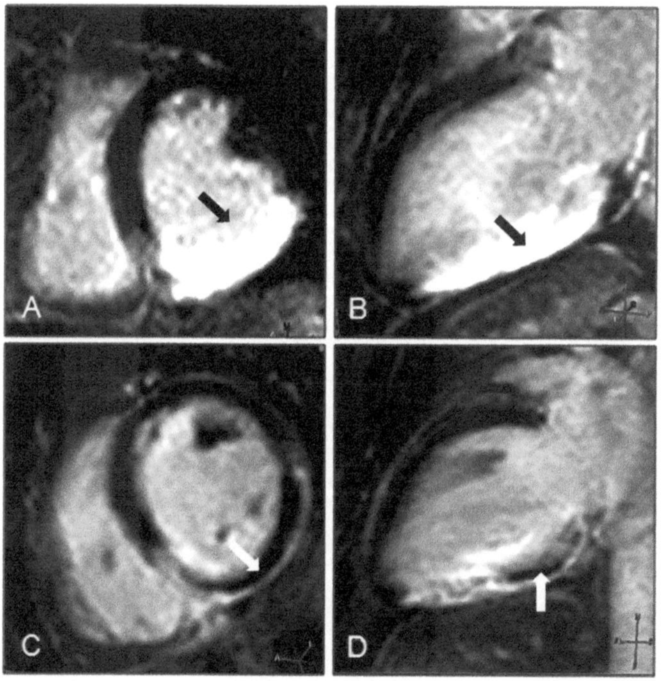

Fig. 3. CE-CMR patterns post myocardial infarction. A,B: CE short axis and long axis view showing transmural inferior infarction (black arrow). C,D: Short axis and long axis view showing an inferior infarction with microvascular obstruction (white arrow).

In patients after MI, the assessment of myocardial viability can provide clinically important information to guide further treatment because only viable myocardium may benefit from revascularization (Kim et al., 2005). Generally, a standardized 17 myocardial segment-model is used to report the results of viability assessment by CE-CMR (Figure 4) (Cerquira et al., 2002).

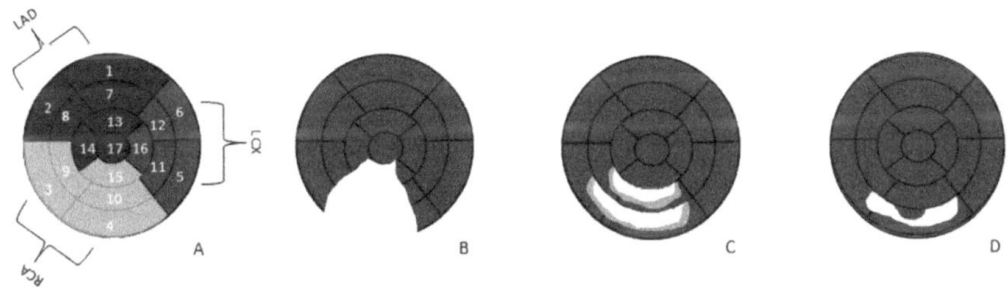

Fig. 4. Bulls eye scheme according to the 17 segmental model, demonstrating CE characteristics post myocardial infarction. A: assignment of the 17 segments to one of the 3 major coronary arteries, with segment 1, 2, 7,8, 13, 14, and 17 corresponding to the left anterior descending coronary artery ; segments 3, 4, 9, 10 and 15 corresponding to the right coronary artery when it is dominant; and segments 5, 6, 11, 12, and 16 are assigned to the left circumflex artery. B: Transmural inferior MI. C: Inferoseptal MI with a core zone (white area) and a peri infarction zone (gray area). D: Inferior MI with microvascular obstruction (black area in myocardial infarction area).

In addition, quantification of infarcted tissue helps to prognosticate left ventricular remodeling (Orn et al., 2007). In this respect, the transmural extent of infarcted tissue as determined by CE-CMR has been shown to be a powerful predictor of the contractile response to both medical therapy and myocardial revascularization (Weinsaft et al., 2007).

Primary coronary intervention with stent implantation is meanwhile the standard for treatment of all acute ST-segment elevation myocardial infarctions, even in cases with a very challenging anatomy (Basalus et al., 2009). The early intervention rapidly restores the patency of the epicardial coronary vessels and often improves the prognosis, as is early indicated by ST-segment resolution on the electrocardiogram (van der Zwaan et al., 2010). Nowadays, aspiration of thrombi is often performed prior to stent implantation in thrombus-containing lesions in order to minimize distal embolization (Hermens et al. 2010; Stoel et al., 2009) that contributes to the development of left ventricular dysfunction after MI. In our recent CMR study, we also found that left ventricular wall motion abnormalities were significantly better in patients who underwent successful early revascularization for acute myocardial infarction (Olimulder et al., 2011).

Increasing interest is also laid on the assessment of characteristics of infarcted myocardial tissue as potential predictor of life-threatening ventricular arrhythmias. Recently, a highly significant relation between inferior MI and ventricular arrhythmias has been observed (Pascale et al. 2009). Multivariate analysis of data from 91 patients suggested that the heterogeneity of infarcted tissue (also called peri infarct zone or border zone), can be an important predictor of spontaneous ventricular arrhythmias (Roes et al., 2009).

The area of CE tends to be larger during the acute phase of MI (first week) and progressively decreases in size during the healing phase (1-4 weeks), until it reaches the state of a healed myocardial infarction (after 4 weeks) (Thygesen et al. 2007). These observations are consistent with the established pathological understanding of remodeling after MI: during the acute phase, there is myocardial edema which subsequently regresses while the necrotic myocardium is replaced by scar tissue (Marcu et al., 2007). Experimental studies have revealed that final MI size is strongly influenced by the extent of the edema in the acute phase, which is also called *area at risk*. By combining T2-weighted images to visualize myocardial edema (and thus the area at risk) and CE-CMR imaging to visualize scar (the *final infarct size*), a *myocardial salvage index* can be calculated by subtracting the infarct size from the area at risk (Aletras et al.,

2006). The myocardial salvage index has recently shown to be independently associated with adverse left ventricular remodeling and early ST-segment resolution, and may represent an interesting parameter for the assessment of novel reperfusion strategies in patients with myocardial infarction (trial registration number: NL19151.044.07).

In addition, some patients develop microvascular obstruction within the ischemic myocardial region in the acute phase of a myocardial infarction (Masci et al. 2010). Microvascular obstruction is represented by a dark zone within the infarcted region, usually located in the subendocardium because the contrast medium does not reach this area (Figure 3c,d). Its presence is associated with greater left ventricular remodeling and inferior clinical outcome. (Nijveldt et al. 2008).

3.2 CE-CMR in nonischemic cardiomyopathies

3.2.1 Hypertrophic cardiomyopathy

Hypertrophic cardiomyopathy is a primary myocardial disease characterized by focal (mostly septal) or diffuse left ventricular wall thickening (with or without left ventricular outflow obstruction). Myofibrillar hypertrophy and disarray and myocardial fibrosis have been described histologically. Inadequate capillary density and intimal hyperplasia of intramural coronary arteries, which were also seen in such patients, may contribute to myocardial ischemia (Marcu et al., 2007). There are predilection patterns of CE in patients with hypertrophic cardiomyopathies: more than 80% of patients exhibit patchy fibrosis at the right ventricular insertion points and in the anteroseptal wall in the region of characteristic septal thickening (Figure 5ab; Figure 6a) (Moon et al., 2003; Choudhury et al., 2002).

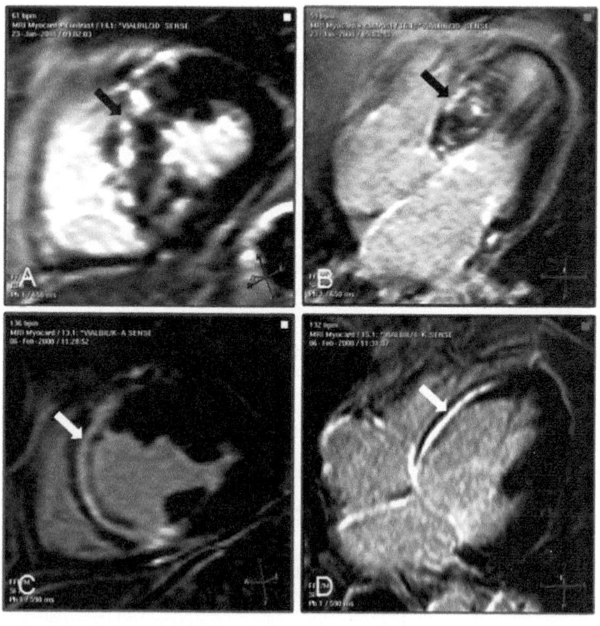

Fig. 5. CE-CMR patterns in nonischemic cardiomyopathies. A,B: CE short axis and long axis view showing hypertrophic cardiomyopathy with patchy CE septal and in the right ventricular insertion points. (black arrow). C,D: Short axis and long axis view showing dilated cardiomyopathy with CE having septal midwall predominance (white arrow).

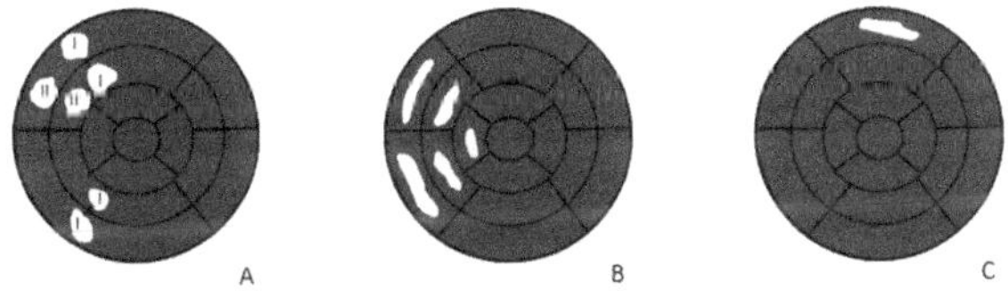

Fig. 6. Bulls eye scheme according to the 17 segmental model, demonstrating typical CE patterns in nonischemic cardiomyopathies. A: Hypertrophic cardiomyopathy with predilection CE (i.e., fibrosis) pattern at the right ventricular insertion points (I) and anteroseptal (II). Myocardial fibrosis is also located in non-hypertrophic segments. B: Idiopathic dilated cardiomyopathy with CE predominantly located in the midwall with septal predominance. C: Arrhythmogenic right ventricular cardiomyopathy with midwall CE found in the basal anterior region. CE is also found in the right ventricular outflow tract.

Myocardial fibrosis, however, is also located in non-hypertrophic segments (Bohl et al., 2008). As the amount of CE in hypertrophic cardiomyopathies often corresponds with functional parameters and the frequency of cardiac events, CE-CMR may potentially be useful for risk stratification and selection for implantable cardioverter defibrillator implantation (Rubinstein et al., 2010). Presence and extent of CE following percutaneous alcohol septal ablation for the treatment of significant left ventricular outflow tract obstruction indicates the location and extent of therapeutic myocardial tissue destruction. (Sievers et al., 2002).

3.2.2 Idiopathic dilated cardiomyopathy

Idiopathic dilated cardomyopathy is characterized by dilation and impaired contractility of the left ventricle or both ventricles in the absence of abnormal loading conditions (e.g., arterial hypertension; valvular disease), and/or a cardiomyopathy with a distinct cause (e.g., ischemic heart disease; peripartum cardiomyopathy; toxin, chemotherapy or tachycardia induced cardiomyopathy; certain endocrinopathies) (Mueller & Attili, 2008). Histology is nonspecific and a variety of myocardial tissue alterations may occur or coexist, including myocyte hypertrophy and segmental or diffuse interstitial fibrosis. Current CE-CMR techniques are unlikely to detect diffuse fibrosis due to limited voxel resolution (Vohringer et al., 2006). Myocardial fibrosis in idiopathic dilated cardiomyopathy is mostly seen in the left ventricular midwall with septal predominance and a linear pattern (Figure 5c,d; Figure 6b); however, it has occasionally been described at subendocardial and subepicardial locations with a more patchy pattern. (Bohl et al., 2008). Of note, in various studies the prevalence of myocardial fibrosis varied from 13% to 62% (Yokokawa et al., 2009; Isbell et al., 2006). It has been suggested that the degree of CE may correlate with functional impairment of the left ventricle (Koito et al., 1996). There are preliminary data demonstrating that the presence of CE is associated with an unfavorable clinical outcome and may be a predictor of sudden death in patients with idiopathic dilated cardiomyopathy (Yokokawa et al., 2009, 2009; Assomull et al., 2009).

3.2.3 Arrhythmogenic right ventricular cardiomyopathy

The arrhythmogenic right ventricular cardiomyopathy is characterized by structural and functional abnormalities, with progressive fibrous and fatty infiltration involving variable regions of the right and left ventricular myocardium. This process finally leads to progressive right ventricular failure and ventricular tachyarrhythmia (Bohl et al., 2008). Diagnosis of this condition remains a challenge, with nonspecific abnormalities on echocardiographic and angiographic examinations. Endomyocardial biopsy has a low sensitivity, as samples are usually taken from the septum, a region that is infrequently involved (Bohl et al., 2008). Further, endomyocardial biopsy is potential a dangerous procedure.

Information from CE-CMR may help to guide targeted endomyocardial biopsies. Predilection patterns with midwall CE are found in the basal anterior region (Figure 6c) and/or the right ventricular outflow tract. These patterns of fibrosis correlate with fibro-fatty replacement of the myocardium at histologic assessment and predict induction of ventricular tachycardia during electrophysiological studies. As the presence of arrhythmogenic right ventricular cardiomyopathy cannot be ruled out based on CMR findings alone, standardized guidelines have been proposed which define major and minor criteria, including morphological, histological, electrocardiographic, functional, and genetic characteristics (McKenna et al., 1994).

3.3 CE-CMR in myocarditis

3.3.1 Myocarditis

Myocarditis is an acute or chronic inflammatory disease of the myocardium, which can be caused by viruses or initiated by post-infectious immune or primarily organ-specific autoimmune responses. (Caforio et al., 2002). Patients generally recover or infrequently develop dilated cardiomyopathy, sometimes even with life-threatening complications including severe heart failure and malignant arrhythmias (Zagrosek et al., 2008). Diagnosis of myocarditis is challenging because of a diverse clinical presentation and a limited sensitivity of endomyocardial biopsies, but may be facilitated by use of CE-CMR or myocardial global relative enhancement CMR (bdel-Aty et al., 2005; Gutberlet et al., 2008). Diagnosis of acute myocarditis is more important nowadays because of the therapeutic medical options in selected patients. (Corsten et al., 2010). Presence of CE has been reported in 44-95% of patients with myocarditis, (Mahrholdt et al., 2004, 2006) indicating areas of myocardial damage with a sensitivity of 100% and a specificity of 90% (compared to histopathology) (Mahrholdt et al., 2004). In acute myocarditis, CE is frequently located in the lateral wall, originating from the epicardium. The subendocardium is generally not involved, with the exception of eosinophilic myocarditis, which frequently involves the endomyocardium (Figure 7a). (Bohl et al., 2008; Deb et al., 2008).

In chronic myocarditis, besides an increased edema on T2-weighted imaging, an increased global relative enhancement is a common finding as confirmed in immunohistological analyses. (Gutberlet et al., 2008). CE-CMR identified areas of myocardial damage in 70% of patients with biopsy-proven chronic myocarditis and showed a predilection pattern (left ventricular midwall and/or subepicardial). In myocarditis, CE may provide additional information that could help to differentiate between viral origins, as in the majority of parvovirus B19 patients, CE is found in the lateral free wall, while in patients with human herpes virus 6 myocarditis CE frequently involves the interventricular septal midwall (Yelgec et al;2007). In addition, we recently studied a limited number of patients with chronic fatigue syndrome and concomitant ebstein barr virus or cytomegalovirus myocarditis who showed in the presence of CE a certain predilection of the septal region. Inflammatory activity on T2-weighted imaging and myocardial fibrosis on CE-CMR may have relevant prognostic implications in acute and chronic myocarditis and may ultimatively serve as a tool to triage patients. In addition, cardiac function and regression of myocardial changes can be well observed with CMR.

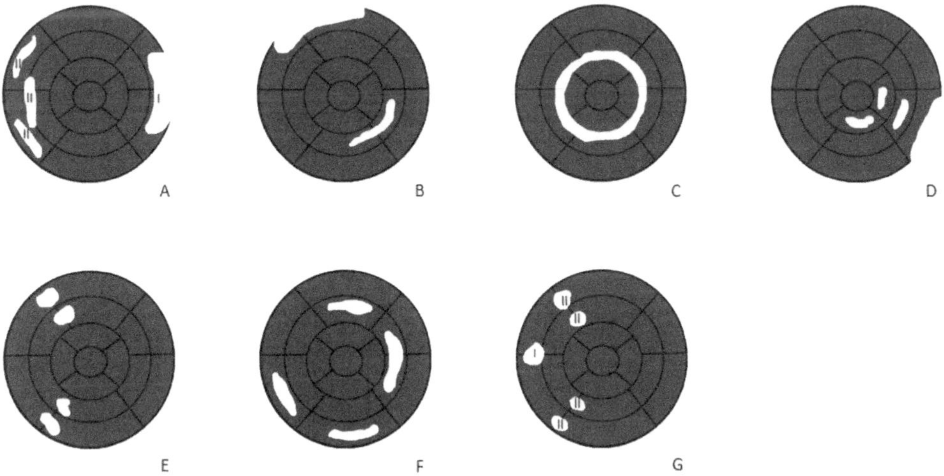

Fig. 7. Bulls eye scheme according to the 17 segmental model, demonstrating typical CE patterns in myocarditis and cardiac involvement of other diseases.
A: Myocarditis with CE frequently located in the lateral wall originating from the epicardium (I). CE patterns in myocarditis differ according to viral origin, with parvovirus B19 having CE in the lateral free wall (I), HHV6 having CE frequently in the interventricular septal midwall (II), and chronic fatigue syndrome myocarditis having CE anteroseptal and inferoseptal (III). B: Sarcoidosis with CE midwall or epicardial; however subendocardial or transmural CE may be observed. C: Amyloidosis , usually with a global diffuse CE pattern, frequently involving the subendocardium. D: Chagas' disease with CE epicardial or midwall, with a predilection pattern inferolateral. E. Pulmonary hypertension with CE involving the right ventricular insertion points and the interventricular septum. F: Muscular dystrophy with CE observed in the midwall. G: Chloroquine induced cardiomyopathy with hypertrophy and accompanying CE in the basal septum (I) and the right ventricular insertion points (I).

3.4 CE-CMR in systemic diseases inducing cardiomyopathy

3.4.1 Sarcoidosis

Cardiac involvement in sarcoidosis, a multisystem granulomatous disorder of unknown etiology, is clinically often asymptomatic (95%) while autopsy revealed cardiac manifestation in up to 60% (Patel et al., 2009). *Advanced* sarcoidosis leads to septal thinning, systolic and diastolic dysfunction, and pericardial effusion which can be detected with echocardiography (Jackson et al., 2007). *Early* sarcoidosis, however, is more challenging to diagnose, and CMR can be very useful in this context. During the acute stage of this disease, regions of active inflammation and edema are visible on T2-weighted images as areas of increased signal intensity. During the chronic stage, CE will typically appear as a midwall or epicardial nonischemic pattern (Figure 7b; figure 8).

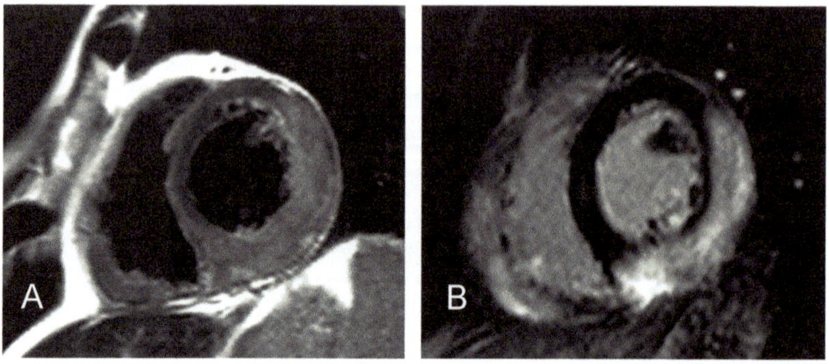

Fig. 8. CMR in a patient with sarcoidosis. A: T2 weighted imaging shorta axix view showing Figure 8 hyperenhancement epicardial inferior, inferolateral and anterolateral.
B: Short axis view showing CE epicardial inferior, inferolateral and anterolateral.

But occasionally subendocardial or transmural CE may be observed, mimicking a pattern of post-MI. CE has been found in 50% of all patients diagnosed with sarcoidosis (Shimada et al., 2001). CE-CMR may also be useful to evaluate the response to therapy. In a CMR study of patients with sarcoidosis, CE was markedly diminished 1 month after the initiation of steroid therapy (Shimada et al., 2001). CE in sarcoidosis patients may be associated with future adverse events (including cardiac death) but confirmation in larger patient cohorts is required (Patel et al., 2009).

3.4.2 Amyloidosis

Both primary and secondary amyloidosis are characterized by extracellular deposition of fibrillar proteins (Mueller et al, 2008), which may lead to restrictive cardiomyopathy with an initially preserved systolic left ventricular function (Wynne et al., 2005). In cardiac amyloidosis, CE is commonly found as a result of the expansion of interstitial space and some endomyocardial fibrosis (Maceira et al., 2008), leading to a usually global and diffuse CE pattern (Jackson et al., 2007). Although the subendocardium is commonly involved (as in ischemic heart disease), the distribution of CE is not related to a particular coronary perfusion area (Figure 7c; figure 9) (Jackson et al., 2007).

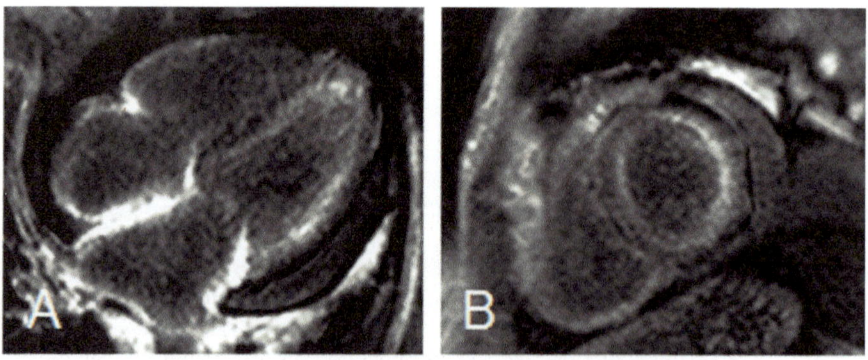

Fig. 9. CMR in a patient with amyloidosis.
A,B: four chamber and short axis view showing diffuse subendocardial CE.

3.4.3 Chagas' disease

The parasitic protozoan Trypanosoma cruzi causes Chagas' disaese, which is endemic in the Latin American region (Jackson et al., 2007). During chronic disease, the heart is the most frequently affected organ, and patients present with refractory heart failure, disorders of the conduction system, or ventricular tachycardia (Marcu et al., 2007; Rochitte et al., 2005). The fundamental pathological processes include an inflammatory response, cellular damage with a broad variation of intensity (minimal alterations up to extensive necrosis), and fibrosis (Rochitte et al., 2007). Early cardiac involvement may be detected by CE-CMR before the onset of symptoms (Rochitte et al., 2003). CE is often located epicardial or in the left ventricle midwall with a inferolateral predilection pattern (Figure 7d), but other regions - including the apex - may also sometimes be affected (Jackson et al., 2007).

3.4.4 Pulmonary hypertension

Pulmonary arterial hypertension, both primary and secondary, is characterized by an increased pulmonary vascular resistance that results in pressure overload on the right ventricle (Kovacs et al., 2008). Cine CMR permits accurate assessment of right ventricular mass and volumes which is often difficult to accomplish with other imaging modalities (Marcu et al., 2007). Myocardial CE is frequently observed in patients with severe symptomatic pulmonary artery hypertension with predilection patterns involving both right ventricular septal insertion points and the interventricular septum (Figure 7e). CE in the interventricular septum was found to be associated with septal bowing (on cine CMR), and the extent of CE correlated inversely with right ventricular systolic function (Blyth et al., 2005).

3.4.5 Muscular dystrophy

Both Becker and Duchenne muscular dystrophies are progressive X chromosome-linked recessive neuromuscular diseases with myocardial involvement in up to 72% of patients showing a mildly reduced left ventricular function up to severe left ventricular impairment and dilated cardiomyopathy. Cardiac myocyte dystrophin deficiency leads to necrosis causing replacement of damaged myocardium by connective tissue and fat in both ventricles. On CE-CMR, hyperenhancement is predominantly seen in left ventricular midwall (Figure 7f) and has been described in 73-100% of patients (Yilmaz et al., 2008). Early diagnosis of myocardial involvement as assessed with CE-CMR may permit an earlier treatment of heart failure which could increase life expectancy.

3.4.6 Chloroquine-induced cardiomyopathy

Chloroquine-induced cardiomyopathy is a rare iatrogenic disease that is associated with long-term intake of chloroquine, which is most frequently prescribed for treatment of rheumatoid arthritis and malaria prophylaxis (Reffelman et al., 2006). This cardiomyopathy is characterized by ineffective lysosomal metabolism because of an increase in pH that leads to accumulation of lysosomal glycosphingolipids and finally thickening of cardiac walls (Pieroni et al., 2007). The time interval between the start of chloroquine therapy and disease manifestation varies greatly, ranging from several months to more than 20 years (Reffelman et al., 2006). CMR may demonstrate the presence of left ventricular hypertrophy with accompanying areas of CE in the basal septum and at the insertion point of the right ventricle (Figure 7g).

Fabry disease, an X chromosome-linked lysosomal storage disease caused by a deficient activity of the enzyme α-galactosidase A, can also result in the accumulation of glycosphingolipids in multiple organs, including the heart (Pieroni et al., 2007; Gange et al.,2009). Fabry disease cardiomypathy should therefore always be considered in the differential diagnosis of "idiopathic" left ventricular hypertrophy (in the absence of arterial hypertension or valvular disease).

3.5 CE-CMR in other diseases inducing cardiomyopathy

3.5.1 Tsako Tsubo cardiomyopathy

This relatively 'novel' cardiomyopathy is characterized by acute but rapidly reversible distinctive regional left ventricular dysfunction, in the absence of significant coronary artery disease. Japanese investigators were intrigued by the unusual end-systolic shape of the left ventricle, resembling the original Japanese octupus trap (figure 10a) (Sharkey et al., 2011).

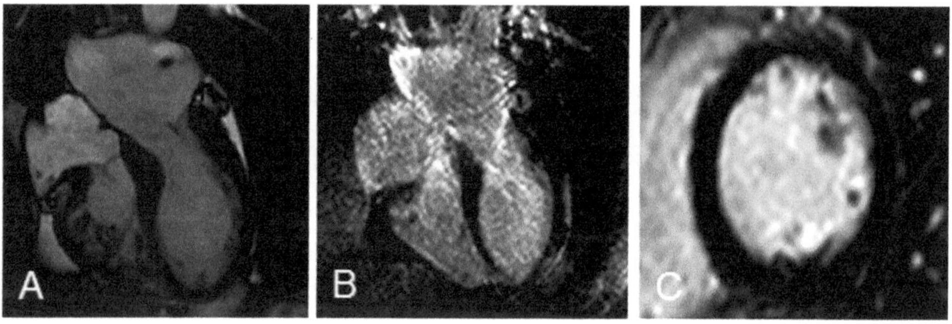

Fig. 10. CMR of a patient with tsako tsubo. A: cine four chamber view with characteristic end-systolic apical ballooning. B,C: four chamber and short axis view with no presence of CE in the myocardium.

Consequently, the term tsako tsubo cardiomyopathy was introduced in 1990. Several pathofysiological mechanisms have been proposed, including multivessel coronary spasm, catecholamine induced myocardial stunning, coronary emboli with spontaneous fibrinolysis, and myocardial inflammation (Eitel et al., 2010). Recently, variant forms are described, including inverted tako-tsubo and mid-ventricular ballooning cardiomyopathy (Marti et al., 2009; Yasu et al., 2006).

In the setting of tako tsubo cardiomyopathy, CMR may identify increased myocardial mass and myocardial edema (using T2-weighted imaging) as well as the normalization of these parameters as the left ventricular dysfunction improves. (Stensaeth et al. 2011). Of important note, (with only a few exceptions, reported in literature) (Koeth et al. 2008) no CE is present in this disease, consistent with preserved myocardial viability, as reflected by the transient nature of left ventricular dysfunction (figure10b) (Eitel et al, 2010; Deetjen et al., 2006) .At follow up, there is complete normalization of left ventricular function, in the absence of CE, edema and pericardial effusion (Eitel et al., 2010; Koeth et al., 2008). The lack of CE (initial and follow up) allows thus for distinction between different causative aetiologies including MI, infiltrative diseases and cases of myocarditis.

Therefore, CMR in combination with T2 weighted imaging and CE may provide valuable additional information for the differential diagnoses and therapeutic decision-making in patients with suspected tako tsubo cardiomyopathy.

3.5.2 Noncompaction cardiomyopathy

Left ventricular noncompaction cardiomyopathy is characterized by a thin, compacted epicardial layer and a thick endocardial layer with prominent trabeculation and deep recessesm (figure 11) (Jacuier et al,).

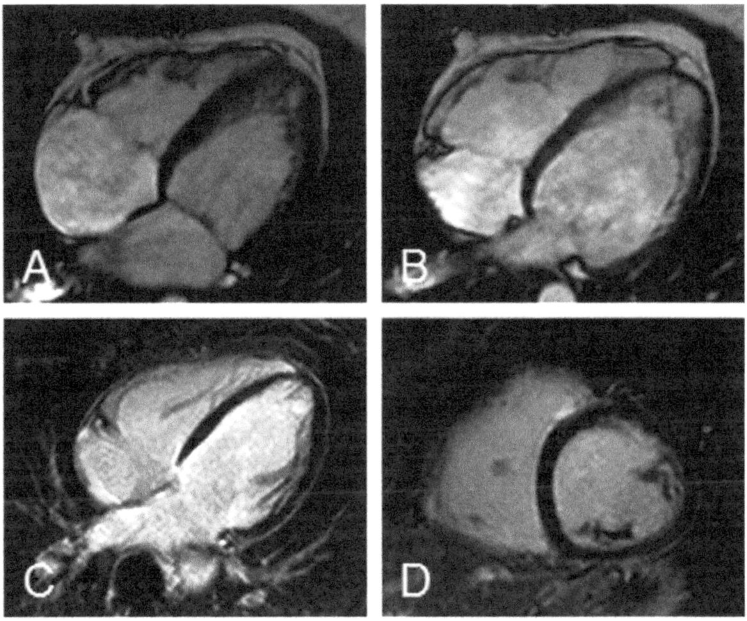

Fig. 11. Patient with noncompaction cardiomyopathy. A,B: end-systolic and end-diastolic four chamber view with characteristic prominent trabeculation and deep recessesm. C,D: four chamber and short axis view with no presence of CE.

It can occur isolated or in association with numerous congenital cardiac malformations, including atrial and ventricular septal defects, aortic stenosis, and aortic calcification. It is usually diagnosed in pediatric age. Accurate diagnostic criteria are clinically important as it is associated with severe left ventricular dysfunction, thrombo-embolism, and ventricular arrhythmia. According to Jacuier et al., a CMR-assessed trabeculated left ventricular mass above 20% of the global left ventricular mass is highly sensitive and specific for the diagnosis of left ventricular noncompaction. Right ventricular noncompaction which can be easily assessed with CMR, is reported in up to 60% op patients (Dursun et al., 2010). Recently, Dursun et al. found that presence of CE (fibrosis) was found in 70% of the investigated patients with left ventricular noncompaction. Dodd et al, showed that the amount of CE in patients with left ventricular noncompaction is inversely related with left ventricular ejection fraction (Dodd et al., 2007). The presence of CE is thus probably of bad prognosis in this disease (Jacquier et al., 2010).

3.5.3 CE-CMR imaging in chemotherapy induced cardiomyopathy

Several chemotherapeutic therapies in the setting of malignant diseases have been associated with the development of cardiac failure. Chemotherapies with a high incidence of cardiac failure are anthracyclines (doxorubicin) 3-26%, and monoclonal antibodies (trastuzumab) 2-28% (Yeh et al., 2009). The cumulative dose (especially doxorubicin; cumulative dose 550 mg/m^2), the administration schedule, concomitant use of other cardiotoxic therapies, and a history of cardiovascular disease, determines the likelihood of inducing cardiomyopathy.
Little is known about the utility of CE-CMR in the assessment of chemotherapy induced cardiomyopathy. Fallah-Rad et al. reported in 10 out of 160 breast cancer patients with trastuzumab induced cardiomyopahty (left ventricular ejection fraction < 40%), presence of epicardial CE. Recently, Kirthy et al. studied (using CE-CMR) 12 breast cancer patients with adjuvant trastuzumab; whereas left ventricular dysfunction was observed, no evidence of necrosis or fibrosis was found in any of the patients (Kirthy et al., 2011). Data on other chemotherapy induced cardiomypathy assessed with CE-CMR are scarce (Lightfoot et al., 2010; Wassmuth et al., 2001; Wu et al., 2009). Therefore, further studies are needed to validate the usefulness of CE-CMR as a marker for (irreversible) left ventricular dysfunction and development as well as prevention of cardiac failure when chemotherapy is given.

4. Guided endomyocardial biopsy

CE patterns on CMR imaging may also help to guide endomyocardial biopsies as scar/fibrosis patterns on CE-CMR may serve as a map for the exact location to accomplish endomyocardial biopsies if necessary; thus enhancing the diagnostic accuracy. A small study has indeed confirmed that the diagnostic performance of endomyocardial biopsies is increased when biopsies are obtained from the region of CE in the case of myocarditis (Mahrholdt et al., 2004, 2006). However, according to Yilmaz et al. who where unable to confirm the value of CE-CMR for guiding endomyocardial biopsies, endomyocardial biopsies exactly obtained from the region of CE may sometimes be impracticle as the area of CE may be small and as a consequence cannot exactly be reached by the bioptome because of the limited steerability of the bioptome (Yilmaz et al., 2010).

5. Screening for cardiomyopathy

Cardiomyopathy can occur as part of inherited syndromes. In the case of hypertrophic cardiomyopathy, over 900 gene mutations have been linked. The gene mutations predominantly encode for contractile proteins, such as cardiac myosin-binding protein C (MYBPC3) and beta-myosin heavy chain (MYH7) (thick filament of the sarcomere), and troponin T and troponin I (encoding for thin filament of the sarcomere; accounting for ≈ 6% of the hypertrophic cardiomyopathy-causing mutations). Next to sarcomeric mutations, several metabolic disorders are linked to the hypertrophic cardiomyopathy phenotype, such as Fabry disease (as mentioned above), an X chromosome-linked lysosomal storage disease (Brouwer et al., 2011). Thus, there is currently no consensus of a definitive screening test based on genetic studies for hypertrophic cardiomyopathy. Additionally, genetic screening can not differentiate between gene carriers who express the disease and those who do not (Devlin et al., 2000). As a consequence, the heterogeneous expression includes patients suffering from severe symptomatic hypertrophic cardiomyopathy (diminished left ventricular function and fibrosis of the myocardium) as well as asymptomatic individuals.

CE-CMR imaging is able to provide accurate assessment of functional parameters and myocardial disorders in one single examination. Therefore, familial screening (especially in autosomal dominant disorders) with CE-CMR may be of utmost importance as individual findings may have significant therapeutic consequences.
As an example, in our tertiary centre, an 18 year old female patient was diagnosed with familiar hypertrophic cardiomyopathy (cardiac myosin-binding protein C). CE-CMR imaging revealed assymmetrical septal hypertrophy (septal thickness 38 mm) and presence of fibrosis (figure 12).

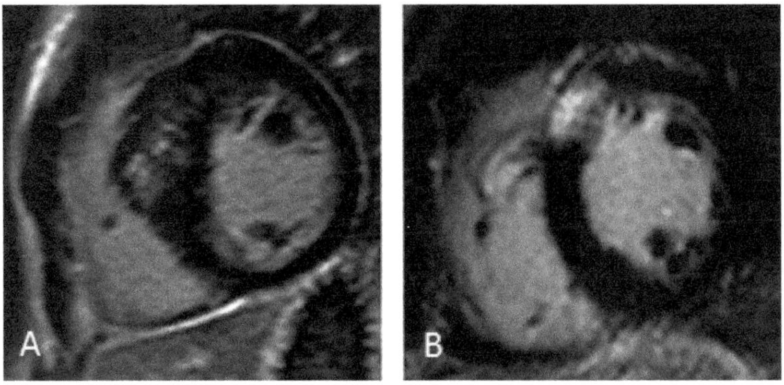

Fig. 12. Screening a relative for cardiomyopathy A. 18 year old female patient with genetic disorder cardiac myosin-binding protein C. Short axis view showing assymetrical septal hypertrophy with CE anteroseptal. B. 56 year old male patient (father) with the same genetic disorder. Short axis view showing identical CE anteroseptal.

Following the guidelines (septal thickness >30 mm) in addition with a medical history of a collapse, she was selected for implantable cardioverter defibrillator therapy (Maron et al., 2003). Her father, (familiar screened and having the same genetic disorder) showed the same pattern of assymetrical septal hypertrophy (septal thickness 24 mm) and presence of fibrosis with CE-CMR imaging, following the guidelines not an indication for implantable cardioverter defibrillator therapy. As mentioned earlier, the amount of CE in hypertrophic cardiomyopathies often corresponds with functional parameters and the frequency of cardiac events, therefore CE-CMR may potentially be useful for risk stratification and selection for implantable cardioverter defibrillator implantation.

6. Future developments

Several new strategies for the treatment of the various forms of cardiomypathy are currently subject of research, including the transplantation of primitive cell types (e.g., stem cells or myoblasts) into damaged myocardium in an attempt to promote trans-differentiation into functional myocardial cells. CE-CMR imaging can be used to monitor such studies and to evaluate the results of novel therapeutic strategies such as direct injection of primitive cell types into segments with transmural infarction. (Orlic et al., 2002). In animal models, mesenchymal stem cells have been labeled with iron-based contrast agents to examine the process of "homing" of such cells in the myocardium (Hill et al., 2003; Kraitchman et al., 2003; Garot et al., 2003).

Recently, 3.0 T CMR imaging with a 3D inversion-recovery gradient-echo sequence was compared to standard 2D imaging. The 3D technique showed superior spatial image resolution, shorter image acquisition time, preserved contrast-to-noise ratio, and similar intra and interobserver variabilities (compared to the 2D approach), which could improve the clinical utility of CE-CMR in the future (Bauner et al., 2009). At higher heart rates, though, motion artifacts can be seen.

7. Conclusion

CE-CMR is increasingly used to establish the etiology, monitor therapeutic strategies (follow up), and obtain prognostic information in a variety of cardiomyopathies. While CE-CMR can provide valuable information, there is considerable overlap in CE patterns. For that reason, CE-CMR findings should always be considered in the light of the clinical history and presentation as well as findings obtained from other diagnostic modalities. Development in CMR hardware and software are required for the ability to perform tissue characterization which fully corresponds with histopathological findings.

8. References

Aletras, AH.; Tilak, GS.; Natanzon, A.; Hsu, LY.; Gonzalez, FM.; Hoyt, RF. & Arai AE. (2006). Retrospective determination of the area at risk for reperfused acute myocardial infarction with T2-weighted cardiac magnetic resonance imaging: histopathological and displacement encoding with stimulated echoes (DENSE) functional validations. *Circulation*, Vol.113, No.15, (April 2006), pp. 1865-1870.

Amado, LC.; Gerber, BL.; Gupta, SN.; Rettman, DW.; Szarf, G.; Schock, B.; Nasir K.; Kraitchman, DL.; & Lima, JA. (2004). Accurate and objective infarct sizing by contrast-enhanced magnetic resonance imaging in a canine myocardial infarction model. *J Am Coll Cardiol* , Vol.44, No.12, (December 2004), pp.2383-2389.

Assomull ,RG.; Prasad, SK.; Lyne, J.; Smith, G.; Burman, ED.; Khan, M.; Sheppard MN.; Poole-Wilson, PA. & Pennell DJ. (2006). Cardiovascular magnetic resonance, fibrosis, and prognosis in dilated cardiomyopathy. *J Am Coll Cardiol*, Vol.48, No10, (November 2006), pp. 1977-1985.

Basalus, M.; Louwerenburg, JW.; van Houwelingen, KG.; Stoel, MG. & von Birgelen, C. (2009). Primary percutaneous coronary intervention in the left main stem of a monocoronary artery. *Neth Heart J* , Vol.17 No.7-8, (Augustus 2009), pp. 274-276.

Bauner, KU.; Muehling, O.; Theisen, D.; Hayes, C.; Wintersperger, BJ.; Reiser, MF. & Huber, AM. (2009). Assessment of Myocardial Viability with 3D MRI at 3 T. AJR *Am J Roentgenol*, Vol.192, No.6, (Juny 2009), pp. 1645-1650.bdel-Aty, H.; Boye, P.; Zagrosek, A.; Wassmuth, R.; Kumar, A.; Messroghli, D.; Bock, P.;

Dietz, R.; Friedrich, MG. & Schulz-Menger J. (2005). Diagnostic performance of cardiovascular magnetic resonance in patients with suspected acute myocarditis: comparison of different approaches. *J Am Coll Cardiol*, Vol.45, No11, (Juny 2005), pp. 1815-1822.

Bello, D.; Fieno, DS.; Kim, RJ.; Pereles, FS.; Passman, R.; Song, G.; Kadish, AH. & Goldberger, JJ. (2005). Infarct morphology identifies patients with substrate for sustained ventricular tachycardia. *J Am Coll Cardiol* , Vol.45, No7, (April 2005), pp. 1104-1108.

Blyth, KG.; Groenning, BA.; Martin, TN.; Foster, JE.; Mark, PB.; Dargie, HJ. & Peacock, AJ. (2005). Contrast enhanced-cardiovascular magnetic resonance imaging in patients with pulmonary hypertension. *Eur Heart J*, Vol.26, No.19, (Oktober 2005), pp. 1993-1999.

Bohl, S.; Wassmuth, R.; bdel-Aty, H.; Rudolph, A.; Messroghli, D.; Dietz, R. & Schulz-Menger, J. (2008). Delayed enhancement cardiac magnetic resonance imaging reveals typical patterns of myocardial injury in patients with various forms of non-ischemic heart disease. *Int J Cardiovasc Imaging*, Vol.24, No.6, (Augustus 2008), pp. 597-607.

Brouwer, WP.; van Dijk, SJ.; Stienen, GJ.; van Rossum, AC.; van der Velden, J. & Germans T. (2011). The development of familial hypertrophic cardiomyopathy: from mutation to bedside. *Eur J Clin Invest*, Vol.41, No.5, (May 2011), pp. 568-578.

Caforio, AL.; Mahon, NJ.; Tona, F. & McKenna, WJ. (2002). Circulating cardiac autoantibodies in dilated cardiomyopathy and myocarditis: pathogenetic and clinical significance. *Eur J Heart Fail*, Vol.4, No.4 (Augustus 2002), pp. 411-417.

Cerqueira, MD.; Weissman, NJ.; Dilsizian, V.; Jacobs, AK.; Kaul, S.; Laskey, WK.; Pennell, DJ.; Rumberger, JA.; Ryan, T. & Verani MS. (2002). Standardized myocardial segmentation and nomenclature for tomographic imaging of the heart: a statement for healthcare professionals from the Cardiac Imaging Committee of the Council on Clinical Cardiology of the American Heart Association. *Circulation*, Vol.105, No.4, (January 2002), pp. 539-542.

Choudhury, L.; Mahrholdt, H.; Wagner, A.; Choi, KM.; Elliott, MD.; Klocke, FJ.; Bonow, RO.; Judd, RM. & Kim, RJ. (2002). Myocardial scarring in asymptomatic or mildly symptomatic patients with hypertrophic cardiomyopathy. *J Am Coll Cardiol*, Vol.40, No.12 (December 2002), pp. 2156-2164.

Corsten, MF.; Dennert, R.; Jochems, S.; Kuznetsova, T.; Devaux, Y.; Hofstra, L.; Wagner, DR.; Staessen, JA.; Heymans, S. & Schroen B. (2010). Circulating MicroRNA-208b and MicroRNA-499 reflect myocardial damage in cardiovascular disease. *Circ Cardiovasc Genet*, Vol.3, No.6 (December 2010), pp. 499-506.

Deb, K.; Djavidani, B.; Buchner, S.; Poschenrieder, F.; Heinicke, N.; Feuerbach, S.; Riegger, G. & Luchner A. (2008). Time course of eosinophilic myocarditis visualized by CMR. *J Cardiovasc Magn Reson*, Vol.10, No.1, (2008), pp. 21.

Deetjen, AG.; Conradi, G.; Mollmann, S.; Rad, A.; Hamm, CW. & Dill T. (2006). Value of gadolinium-enhanced magnetic resonance imaging in patients with Tako-Tsubo-like left ventricular dysfunction. *J Cardiovasc Magn Reson*, Vol.8, No.2, (2006), pp. 367-372.

Devlin, AM. & Ostman-Smith, I. (2000). Diagnosis of hypertrophic cardiomyopathy and screening for the phenotype suggestive of gene carriage in familial disease: a simple echocardiographic procedure. *J Med Screen 2000*, Vol.7, No.2, (2000), pp. 82-90.

Dodd, JD.; Holmvang, G.; Hoffmann Ferencik, M.; Abbara, S.; Brady, TJ. & Cury RC. (2007). Quantification of left ventricular noncompaction and trabecular delayed hyperenhancement with cardiac MRI: correlation with clinical severity. *AJR Am J Roentgenol* , Vol.189, No.4, (Oktober 2007), pp. 974-980.

Dursun, M.; Agayev, A.; Nisli, K.; Ertugrul, T.; Onur, I.; Oflaz, H. & Yekeler E. (2010). MR imaging features of ventricular noncompaction: emphasis on distribution and pattern of fibrosis. *Eur J Radiol* 2010, Vol.74, No.1, (April 2010), pp. 147-151.

Edelman, RR. (2004) Contrast-enhanced MR imaging of the heart: overview of the literature. *Radiology*, Vol.232, No.3, (September 2004), pp. 653-668.

Eitel, I.; Lucke, C.; Grothoff, M.; Sareban, M.; Schuler, G.; Thiele, H. & Gutberlet M. (2010). Inflammation in takotsubo cardiomyopathy: insights from cardiovascular magnetic resonance imaging. *Eur Radiol*, Vol.20, No.2 (February 2010), pp. 422-431.

Eitel, I. & Friedrich, MG. (2011) T2-weighted cardiovascular magnetic resonance in acute cardiac disease. *J Cardiovasc Magn Reson*, Vol.13, (2011), pp. 13.

Gange, CA.; Link, MS. & Maron MS. (2009). Utility of cardiovascular magnetic resonance in the diagnosis of Anderson-Fabry disease. *Circulation*, Vol.120, No.13, (September 2009), pp. 96-97.

Garot, J.; Unterseeh, T.; Teiger, E.; Champagne, S.; Chazaud, B.; Gherardi, R.; Hittinger, L.; Gueret, P. & Rahmouni A. (2003). Magnetic resonance imaging of targeted catheter-based implantation of myogenic precursor cells into infarcted left ventricular myocardium. *J Am Coll Cardiol*, Vol.41, No.10, (May 2003), pp. 1841-1846.

Gutberlet, M.; Spors, B.; Thoma, T.; Bertram, H.; Denecke, T.; Felix, R.; Noutsias, M.; Schultheiss, HP. & Kuhl U. (2008). Suspected chronic myocarditis at cardiac MR: diagnostic accuracy and association with immunohistologically detected inflammation and viral persistence. *Radiology*, Vol.246, No.2, (February 2008), pp. 401-409.

Hermens, JA.; van Houwelingen, GK.; de Man, FH.; Louwerenburg, HW. & von Birgelen C. (2010). Thrombus aspiration in a series of patients with stable or unstable angina pectoris and lesion-site thrombus formation. *Neth Heart J*, Vol. 18, No.9 (September 2010), pp. 423-429.

Hill, JM.; Dick, AJ.; Raman, VK.; Thompson, RB.; Yu, ZX.; Hinds, KA.; Pessanha, BS.; Guttman, MA.; Varney, TR.; Martin, BJ.; Dubar, CE.; McVeigh, ER. & Lederman RJ. (2003). Serial cardiac magnetic resonance imaging of injected mesenchymal stem cells. *Circulation*, Vol.108, No.8, (Augustus 2003), pp. 1009-1014.

Hsu, LY.; Natanzon, A.; Kellman, P.; Hirsch, GA.; Aletras, AH. & Arai AE. (2006). Quantitative myocardial infarction on delayed enhancement MRI. Part I: Animal validation of an automated feature analysis and combined thresholding infarct sizing algorithm. *J Magn Reson Imaging*, Vol.23, No.3 (March 2006), pp. 298-308.

Isbell, DC. & Kramer, CM. (2006). The evolving role of cardiovascular magnetic resonance imaging in nonischemic cardiomyopathy. *Semin Ultrasound CT MR*, Vol.27, No.1 (February 2006), pp. 20-31.

Jackson, E. Bellenger, N.; Seddon, M.; Harden, S. & Peebles C. (2007). Ischaemic and non-ischaemic cardiomyopathies--cardiac MRI appearances with delayed enhancement. *Clin Radiol*, Vol.62, No.5 (May 2007), pp. 395-403.

Jacquier, A.; Thuny, F.; Jop, B.; Giorgi, R.; Cohen, F.; Gaubert, JY.; Vidal, V.; Bartoli, JM.; Habib, G. & Moulin G. (2010). Measurement of trabeculated left ventricular mass using cardiac magnetic resonance imaging in the diagnosis of left ventricular non-compaction. *Eur Heart J*, Vol.31, No.9, (May 2010), pp. 1098-1104.

Kellman, P.; Aletras, AH.; Mancini, C.; McVeigh, ER. & Arai, AE. (2007) T2-prepared SSFP improves diagnostic confidence in edema imaging in acute myocardial infarction compared to turbo spin echo. *Magn Reson Med*, Vol.57, No.5, (May 2007), pp.891-897.

Kim, RJ.; Wu, E.; Rafael, A.; Chen, EL.; Parker, MA.; Simonetti, O.; Klocke, FJ.; Bonow, RO. & Judd, RM. (2000). The use of contrast-enhanced magnetic resonance imaging to identify reversible myocardial dysfunction. *N Engl J*, Vol.343, No.20, (November 2000), pp. 1445-1453.

Kirthy, V.; Schultz, C. & Davies S. (2011). Cardiac Imaging of trastuzumab-induced cardiomyopathy. *European Journal of Heart Failure Supplements*, Vol.10, (2011) Koeth,

O.; Mark, B.; Kilkowski, A.; Layer, G.; Cornelius, B.; Kouraki, K.; Bauer, T.; Zahn, R.;

Senges, J. & Zeymer U. (2008). Clinical, angiographic and cardiovascular magnetic resonance findings in consecutive patients with Takotsubo cardiomyopathy. *Clin Res Cardiol*, Vol.97, No.9, (September 2008), pp. 623-627.

Koito, H.; Suzuki, J.; Ohkubo, N.; Ishiguro, Y.; Iwasaka, T. & Inada M. (1996). Gadolinium-diethylenetriamine pentaacetic acid enhanced magnetic resonance imaging of dilated cardiomyopathy: clinical significance of abnormally high signal intensity of left ventricular myocardium. *J Cardiol*, Vol.28, No1. (July 1996), pp. 41-49.

Kovacs, G.; Reiter, G.; Reiter, U.; Rienmuller, R.; Peacock, A. & Olschewski H. (2008). The emerging role of magnetic resonance imaging in the diagnosis and management of pulmonary hypertension. *Respiration*, Vol.76, No.4, (2008), pp. 458-470.

Kraitchman, DL.; Heldman, AW.; Atalar, E.; Amado, LC.; Martin, BJ.; Pittenger, MF.; Hare, JM. & Bulte JW. (2003). In vivo magnetic resonance imaging of mesenchymal stem cells in myocardial infarction. *Circulation*, Vol.107, No.18, (May 2003), pp. 2290-2293.

Lightfoot, JC.; D'Agostino, RB.; Jr., Hamilton, CA.; Jordan, J.; Torti, FM.; Kock, ND.; Jordan, J.; Workman, S. & Hundley WG. (2010). Novel approach to early detection of doxorubicin cardiotoxicity by gadolinium-enhanced cardiovascular magnetic resonance imaging in an experimental model. *Circ Cardiovasc Imaging* 2010, Vol.3, No.5, (September 2010), pp. 550-558.

Maceira, AM.; Prasad, SK.; Hawkins, PN.; Roughton, M. & Pennell DJ. (2008). Cardiovascular magnetic resonance and prognosis in cardiac amyloidosis. *J Cardiovasc Magn Reson*, Vol.10, No.1, (2008), pp. 54.

Mahrholdt, H.; Goedecke, C.; Wagner, A.; Meinhardt, G.; Athanasiadis, A.; Vogelsberg, H.; Fritz, P.; Klingel, K.; Kandolf, R. & Sechtem U. (2004). Cardiovascular magnetic resonance assessment of human myocarditis: a comparison to histology and molecular pathology. *Circulation*, Vol.109, No.10, (March 2004), pp. 1250-1258.

Mahrholdt, H.; Wagner, A.; Deluigi, CC.; Kispert, E.; Hager, S.; Meinhardt, G.; Vogelsberg, H.; Fritz, P.; Dippon, J.; Bock, CT.; Klingel, K.; Kandolf, R. & Sechtem U. (2004). Presentation, patterns of myocardial damage, and clinical course of viral myocarditis. *Circulation*, Vol.114, No.15, (Oktober 2006), pp. 1581-1590.

Marcu, CB.; Beek, AM. & van Rossum, AC. (2006). Clinical applications of cardiovascular magnetic resonance imaging. *CMAJ*, Vol.175,No.8, (Oktober 2006), pp. 911-917.

Marcu, CB.; Nijveldt, R.; Beek, AM. & van Rossum, AC. (2007). Delayed contrast enhancement magnetic resonance imaging for the assessment of cardiac disease. *Heart Lung Circ*, Vol.16, No.2, (April 2007), pp70-78

Maron, BJ.; McKenna, WJ.; Danielson, GK.; Kappenberger, LJ.; Kuhn, HJ.; Seidman, CE.; Shah, PM.; Spencer. WH.; Spirito, P.; Ten Cate, FJ. & Wigle ED. (2002). American College of Cardiology/European Society of Cardiology clinical expert consensus document on hypertrophic cardiomyopathy. A report of the American College of Cardiology Foundation Task Force on Clinical Expert Consensus Documents and the European Society of Cardiology Committee for Practice Guidelines. *J am Coll Cardiol*, Vol.42, No.9, (March 2003), pp. 1687-1713

Orlic, D.; Hill, JM. & Arai AE. (2002). Stem cells for myocardial regeneration. *Circ Res*, Vol.91, No.12, (December 2002), pp. 1092-1102.

Marti, V.; Carreras, F.; Pujadas, S. & De Rozas JM. (2009). Transient left ventricular basal ballooning-"inverted" Tako-tsubo. *Clin Cardiol*, Vol.32. No.7, (September 2009), pp. 20-21.

Masci, PG.; Ganame, J.; Strata, E.; Desmet, W.; Aquaro, GD.; Dymarkowski, S.; Valenti, V.; Janssens, S.; Lombardi, M.; Van de Werf.; L'Abbate, A. & Bogaert J. (2010). Myocardial salvage by CMR correlates with LV remodeling and early ST-segment resolution in acute myocardial infarction. *JACC Cardiovasc Imaging* , Vol.3, No.1, (January 2010), pp. 45-51.

McKenna, WJ.; Thiene, G.; Nava, A.; Fontaliran, F.; Blomstrom-Lundqvist, C.; Fontaine, G. & Camerini F. (1994). Diagnosis of arrhythmogenic right ventricular dysplasia/cardiomyopathy. Task Force of the Working Group Myocardial and Pericardial Disease of the European Society of Cardiology and of the Scientific Council on Cardiomyopathies of the International Society and Federation of Cardiology. *Br Heart J* , Vol.71, No.3, (March 1994), pp. 215-218.

Moon, JC.; McKenna, WJ.; McCrohon, JA.; Elliott, PM.; Smith, GC,. & Pennell DJ. (2003). Toward clinical risk assessment in hypertrophic cardiomyopathy with gadolinium cardiovascular magnetic resonance. *J Am Coll Cardiol*, Vol.41, No.9 (May 2003), pp. 1561-1567.

Mueller, GC. & Attili A. Cardiomyopathy: magnetic resonance imaging evaluation. *Semin Roentgenol* , Vol.43, No.3, (July 2008), pp. 204-222.

Nijveldt, R.; Beek, AM.; Hirsch, A.; Stoel, MG.; Hofman, MB.; Umans, VA.; Algra, PR.; Twisk, JW. & van Rossum AC. (2008). Functional recovery after acute myocardial infarction: comparison between angiography, electrocardiography, and cardiovascular magnetic resonance measures of microvascular injury. *J Am Coll Cardiol*, Vol.52, No3. (July 2008), pp. 181-189.

Olimulder, MA.; Galjee, MA.; van Es, J.; Wagenaar, LJ.; von Birgelen, C. (2011). Contrast-enhancement cardiac magnetic resonance imaging beyond the scope of viability. *Neth Heart J*, Vol.19, No.5 (May 2011), pp. 236-245.

Olimulder, MA.; Kraaier, K.; Galjee, MA.; Scholten, MF.; van Es, J.; Wagenaar, LJ.; van der Palen, J. & von Birgelen, C. (2011). Infarct tissue characteristics of patients with versus without early revascularization for acute myocardial infarction: a contrast-enhancement cardiovascular magnetic resonance imaging study. *Heart Vessels*, (May 2011).

Orn, S.; Manhenke, C.; Anand, IS.; Squire, I.; Nagel, E.; Edvardsen, T. & Dickstein K. (2007). Effect of left ventricular scar size, location, and transmurality on left ventricular remodeling with healed myocardial infarction. *Am J Cardiol*, Vol.99, No.8 (April 2007), pp. 1109-1114.

Pascale, P.; Schlaepfer, J.; Oddo, M.; Schaller, MD.; Vogt, P. & Fromer M. (2009). Ventricular arrhythmia in coronary artery disease: limits of a risk stratification strategy based on the ejection fraction alone and impact of infarct localization. *Europace*, Vol.11, No.12, (December 2009), pp. 1639-1646.

Patel, MR.; Cawley, PJ.; Heitner, JF.; Klem, I.; Parker, MA.; Jaroudi, WA.; Meine, TJ.; White', JB.; Elliott, MD.; Kim, HW.; Judd, RM. & Kim RJ. (2009). Detection of myocardial damage in patients with sarcoidosis. *Circulation*, Vol.120, No.20, (November 2009), pp. 1969-1977.

Pieroni, M.; Bellocci, F. & Crea F. (2007). Letter by Pieroni et al regarding article, "Contrast-enhanced magnetic resonance imaging of a patient with chloroquine-induced cardiomyopathy confirmed by endomyocardial biopsy". *Circulation*, Vol.115, No.5 (February 2007), pp. 67.

Reffelmann, T.; Naami, A.; Spuentrup, E. & Kuhl HP. (2006). Images in cardiovascular medicine. Contrast-enhanced magnetic resonance imaging of a patient with chloroquine-induced cardiomyopathy confirmed by endomyocardial biopsy. *Circulation*, Vol.114, No.8 (Augustus 2006), pp. 357-358.

Rochitte, CE.; Oliveira, PF.; Andrade, JM.; Ianni, BM.; Parga, JR.; Avila, LF.; Kalil-Filho, R.; Mady, C.; Meneghetti, JC.; Lima, JA. & Ramires, JA. (2005). Myocardial delayed enhancement by magnetic resonance imaging in patients with Chagas' disease: a marker of disease severity. *J Am Coll Cardiol*, Vol.46, No.8, (Oktober 2005), pp. 1553-1558.

Rochitte, CE.; Nacif, MS.; de Oliveira Junior, AC.; Siqueira-Batista, R.; Marchiori, E.; Uellendahl, M. & de Lourdes HM. (2007). Cardiac magnetic resonance in Chagas' disease. *Artif Organs*, Vol.31, No.4 (April 2007) pp. 259-267.

Rochitte, CE.; Olivera, PF. & Joalbo M. (2003). Chagas disease is characterised by specific pattern and location of myocardial delayed enhancement MRI. *J Cardiovasc Magn Reson*, Vol. 5 (2003), pp. 113

Roes, SD.; Borleffs, C.; van der Geest, RJ.; Westenberg, JJM.; Marsan, NA.; Kaandorp, TAM.; Reiber, JHC.; Zeppenfeld, K.; Lamb, HJ. & de Roos. (2009). Infarct Tissue Heterogeneity Assessed With Contrast-Enhanced MRI Predicts Spontaneous Ventricular Arrhythmia in Patients With Ischemic Cardiomyopathy and Implantable Cardioverter-Defibrillator. *Circulation: Cardiovascular imaging*, Vol.2, No.3, (2009), pp.183

Thygesen, K.; Alpert, JS. & White HD. (2007). Universal definition of myocardial infarction. *Eur Heart J*, Vol.28, No.20, (Oktober 2007), pp. 2525-2538.

Rubinshtein, R.; Glockner, JF.; Ommen, SR.; Araoz, PA.; Ackerman, MJ.; Sorajja, P.; Bos, JM.; Tajik. AJ.; Valeti, US.; Nishimura, A. & Gersh BJ. (2010). Characteristics and clinical significance of late gadolinium enhancement by contrast-enhanced magnetic resonance imaging in patients with hypertrophic cardiomyopathy. *Circ Heart Fail*, Vol.3, No.1, (January 2010), pp. 51-58.

Sharkey, SW.; Lesser, JR.; Maron, MS. &Maron BJ. (2011). Why not just call it tako-tsubo cardiomyopathy: a discussion of nomenclature. *J Am Coll Cardiol*, Vol.57, No.13 (March 2011), pp. 1496-1497.

Shimada, T.; Shimada, K.; Sakane, T.; Ochiai, K.; Tsukihashi, H.; Fukui, M.; Inoue, S.; Katoh, H.; Murakami, Y.; Ishibashi, Y. & Maruyama, R. (2001). Diagnosis of cardiac sarcoidosis and evaluation of the effects of steroid therapy by gadolinium-DTPA-enhanced magnetic resonance imaging. *Am J Med*, Vol.110, No.7 (May 2001), pp. 520-527.

Sievers, B.; Moon, JC. & Pennell DJ. (2002). Images in cardiovascular Medicine. Magnetic resonance contrast enhancement of iatrogenic septal myocardial infarction in hypertrophic cardiomyopathy. *Circulation* , Vol. 105, No.8, (February 2002), pp. 1018.

Stensaeth, KH.; Fossum, E.; Hoffmann, P.; Mangschau, A.; Skretteberg, PT. & Klow, NE. (2011).Takotsubo cardiomyopathy in acute coronary syndrome; clinical features and contribution of cardiac magnetic resonance during the acute and convalescent phase. *Scand Cardiovasc J*, Vol.45, No.2, (April 2011), pp. 77-85.

Stoel, MG.; von Birgelen, C. & Zijlstra F. (2009). Aspiration of embolized thrombus during primary percutaneous coronary intervention. *Catheter Cardiovasc Interv*, Vol.73. No.6 (May 2009), pp. 781-786.

Van der Zwaan, HB.; Stoel, MG.; Roos-Hesselink, JW.; Veen, G.; Boersma, E. & von Birgelen C. (2010). Early versus late ST-segment resolution and clinical outcomes after percutaneous coronary intervention for acute myocardial infarction. *Neth Heart J*, Vol.18. No.9 (September 2010), pp. 416-422.

Vogel-Claussen, J.; Rochitte, CE.; Wu, KC.; Kamel, IR.; Foo, TK, Lima, JA.; Bluemke, DA. (2006). Delayed enhancement MR imaging: utility in myocardial assessment. *Radiographics, Vol.26, No.3 (May* 2006) pp. 795-810.

Vohringer, M.; Mahrholdt, H.; Yilmaz, A. & Sechtem U. (2007) Significance of late gadolinium enhancement in cardiovascular magnetic resonance imaging (CMR). *Herz* Vol. 32, No.2, (March 2007), pp. 129-137.

Wassmuth, R.; Lentzsch, S.; Erdbruegger, U.; Schulz-Menger, J.; Doerken, B.; Dietz, R. & Friedrich MG. (2001). Subclinical cardiotoxic effects of anthracyclines as assessed by magnetic resonance imaging-a pilot study. *Am Heart J*, Vol.141, No.6, (Juny 2001), pp. 1007-1013.

Weinsaft, JW.; Klem, I. & Judd RM. (2007). MRI for the assessment of myocardial viability. *Cardiol Clin*, Vol.25, No.1 (February 2007), pp. 35-56.

Wu, CF.; Chuang, WP.; Li, AH. & Hsiao CH. (2009). Cardiac magnetic resonance imaging in sunitinib malate-related cardiomyopathy: no late gadolinium enhancement. *J Chin Med Assoc*, Vol.72, No.6, (Juny 2009), pp. 323-327.

Wynne, J. & Braunwald E. (2005). Restrictive and infiltrative cardiomyopathies. In: Zipes, DP.; Libby, P.; Bonow, RO. & Braunwald E, editors. *Braunwald's heart disease: a textbook of cardiovascular medicine*. p. 1682-1692. Elsevier Saunders, Pilalphia, Pennsylvania.

Yasu, T.; Tone, K.; Kubo, N. & Saito M. (2009). Transient mid-ventricular ballooning cardiomyopathy: a new entity of Takotsubo cardiomyopathy. *Int J Cardiol*, Vol.110, No.1, (Juny 2006), pp. 100-101.

Yeh, ET. & Bickford CL. (2009). Cardiovascular complications of cancer therapy: incidence, pathogenesis, diagnosis, and management. *J Am Coll Cardiol*, Vol.53, No.24, (Juny 2009), pp. 2231-2247.

Yelgec, NS.; Dymarkowski, S.; Ganame, J. & Bogaert J. (2007). Value of MRI in patients with a clinical suspicion of acute myocarditis. *Eur Radiol*, Vol.17, No.9, (September 2007), pp. 2211-2217.

Yilmaz, A.; Gdynia, HJ.; Baccouche, H.; Mahrholdt, H.; Meinhardt, G.; Basso, C.; Thiene, G.; Sperfeld, AD.; Ludolph, AC. & Sechtem U. (2008). Cardiac involvement in patients with Becker muscular dystrophy: new diagnostic and pathophysiological insights by a CMR approach. *J Cardiovasc Magn Reson*, Vol.10, No.1, (2008), pp. 50.

Yilmaz, A.; Kindermann, I.; Kindermann, M.; Mahfoud, F.; Ukena, C.; Athanasiadis, A.; Hill, S.; Mahrholdt, H.; Voehringer, M.; Schieber, M.; Klingel, K.; Kandolf, R.; Bohm, M. & Sechtem U. (2010). Comparative evaluation of left and right ventricular endomyocardial biopsy: differences in complication rate and diagnostic performance. *Circulation*, Vol.122, No.9, (Augustus 2010), pp. 900-909.

Yokokawa, M.; Tada, H.; Koyama, K.; Ino, T.; Hiramatsu, S.; Kaseno, K.; Naito, S.; Oshima, S. & Taniguchi, K. (2009). The characteristics and distribution of the scar tissue predict ventricular tachycardia in patients with advanced heart failure. *Pacing Clin Electrophysiol*, Vol.32, No.3, (March 2009), pp. 314-322.

Yokokawa, M.; Tada, H.; Koyama, K.; Naito, S.; Oshima, S. & Taniguchi, K. (2009). Nontransmural scar detected by magnetic resonance imaging and origin of ventricular tachycardia in structural heart disease. *Pacing Clin Electrophysiol*, Vol.32, No1. (March 2009), pp. 52-56.

Zagrosek, A.; Wassmuth, R.; bdel-Aty, H.; Rudolph, A.; Dietz, R. & Schulz-Menger, J. (2008). Relation between myocardial edema and myocardial mass during the acute and convalescent phase of myocarditis--a CMR study. *J Cardiovasc Magn Reson*, Vol.10, No.1, (2008), pp. 19.

Part 2

Metabolic and Drug-Induced Cardiomyopathies

3

Diabetic Cardiomyopathy: Cardiac Changes, Pathophysiological Mechanisms, Biologic Markers, and the Available Therapeutic Armamentarium

Michael F. Hill
Department of Medicine, Division of Cardiovascular Medicine, Vanderbilt University Medical Center, Nashville, Tennessee United States of America

1. Introduction

Patients with diabetes mellitus (DM) exhibit greatly increased cardiovascular morbidity and mortality. The increased mortality of patients with DM stems from the more frequent development of heart failure (HF) (Bell, 2003a; Jaffe et al., 1984; Kamalesh, 2007; Marwick, 2006; Solomon et al., 2002). In the past, the high incidence and poor prognosis of HF in diabetic patients was attributed to the concurrent presence of hypertension and/or myocardial ischemia. However, follow-up studies have shown that the increased risk for developing HF persists in DM patients even after adjusting for concomitant risks such as coronary artery disease and blood pressure (Ho et al., 1993; Kannel & McGee, 1979). It is now well established that DM increases the risk of cardiovascular morbidity and mortality by promoting cardiomyopathy, a distinct entity independent of coronary artery disease, hypertension or other known cardiac risk factors with origins in diabetic cardiac muscle (Bell, 1995; Cohen, 1995; Hamby et al., 1974; Regan et al., 1977; Spector, 1998).
According to a new study commissioned by the Centers for Disease Control and Prevention, 25.8 million children and adults in the United States, or 8.3% of the population, have DM, with about 1.9 million new cases of DM being diagnosed annually (Centers for Disease Control and Prevention, 2011). Worldwide, the number of people with DM has more than doubled since 1980 to 347 million (Danaei et al., 2011). With the global burden of DM rising, it is likely that the incidence of diabetes-induced cardiomyopathy and subsequent HF will continue to increase in this high-risk population. The goal of this chapter is to review the structural and functional changes in the diabetic heart and the pathophysiological mechanisms involved in the development of diabetic cardiomyopathy, taking into account the most recent developments in basic and clinical research. An overview of the latest advances in therapeutic approaches to treat diabetic cardiomyopathy will also be presented. Particular attention is given to the role of oxidative stress in the pathogenesis of diabetic cardiomyopathy and the potential of anti-oxidative therapy. The value of newly identified candidate biomarker proteins in assessing disease presence and progression, prognosis, and efficacy of therapies in the setting of diabetic cardiomyopathy will also be discussed.

2. Cardiomyopathy in diabetes

Sustained DM leads to a deterioration of heart function that is independent of any of the known concomitant risk factors and pathologies that are frequently seen in DM patients such as dyslipidemia, coronary artery disease, thrombosis, myocardial infarction (MI), and hypertension. The clinical presentation of cardiac dysfunction in DM patients without evidence of any of these other risk factors was first reported by Rubler et al. in 1972 (Rubler et al., 1972) based on postmortem findings of HF in diabetic patients free of coronary disease. These and similar findings have been reported in numerous other clinical studies (Bell, 2003a; Boyer et al., 2004; Devereux et al., 2000; Fang et al., 2003, 2005; Galderisi et al., 1991; Hamby et al., 1974; Kannel et al., 1974; Regan et al., 1977; Zabalgoitia et al., 2001) and animal models (Borges et al., 2006; Hamblin et al., 2007a; Kaul et al., 1995, 1996; Kralik et al., 2005; Loganathan et al., 2006; Mihm et al., 2001; Shen et al., 2005, 2006). This has led to the increased recognition that DM produces damage to cardiac muscle without depending on the co-existence of other cardiovascular risk factors. This unique form of heart disease in the absence of clinically detectable atherosclerosis and/or coronary artery disease has been termed "diabetic cardiomyopathy". This diabetes-related cardiomyopathy affects the myocardium secondary to DM and is accompanied by a prolonged decline in cardiac function. This unique cardiac phenomenon has been documented to progress to HF in both type 1 and type 2 DM patients.

2.1 Contemporary clinical epidemiology of diabetic cardiomyopathy

Older cardiovascular epidemiological studies showed that 30% of diabetic subjects without overt cardiac disease had LV dysfunction (Beljic & Miric, 1994; Di Bonito et al., 1996; Nicolino et al., 1995). However, this prevalence was based on standard echocardiography testing which frequently was not able to detect mild and early diastolic dysfunction (Bell, 2003b). Contemporary assessments of the epidemiology of diabetic cardiomyopathy using more rigorous Doppler methods demonstrate that the prevalence of diabetic cardiomyopathy is much higher than was previously believed, and in addition, emphasize the ominous impact of DM on myocardial function by highlighting the high prevalence of pre-clinical diabetic cardiomyopathy in the diabetic population and its strong association with an adverse prognosis (Kiencke et al., 2010; Van Den Hurk et al., 2010). In an ambulatory clinic-based sample of middle-aged, overweight-to-obese individuals with prevalent DM for an average duration of over 10 years, diabetic cardiomyopathy was present in 48% of patients as assessed by Doppler echocardiography (Kiencke et al., 2010). Of note, diastolic function was abnormal in 38% of the DM patients studied (Kiencke et al., 2010). The use of flow and tissue Doppler techniques suggests an even higher prevalence of diastolic dysfunction (as high as 40% to 60%) in individuals with type 1 and type 2 DM without discernable coronary heart disease (Boudina & Abel, 2007; Di Bonito et al., 2005; Poirier et al., 2001; Shivalkar et al., 2006). The high incidence of such diastolic dysfunction and its association with HF and with mortality (From et al., 2010) underscore the existence of diabetic cardiomyopathy as a very serious clinical condition.

2.2 Diagnostic indices

Cardiomyopathy in type 1 or type 2 DM is associated with a cluster of common cardiac abnormalities (Table 1). The most frequent and earliest detectable functional abnormality in diabetic cardiomyopathy is impaired diastolic function (Fang et al., 2003, 2005; Karamitsos et al., 2007), owing to reduced elasticity of the diabetic myocardium as a result of interstitial collagen deposition. The reduced diastolic function early in the time course of DM is followed by late decreases in systolic performance (Devereux et al., 2000; Fang et al, 2003; Mildenberger et al., 1984; Raev, 1994; Von Bibra et al., 2005). Diabetic cardiomyopathy in humans is also manifested by left ventricular hypertrophy (LVH) (Devereux et al., 2000; Kannel et al., 1974; Ozasa et al., 2008). Although no single diagnostic test for diabetic cardiomyopathy exists, the use of different imaging modalities (echocardiography, cardiac MRI) makes it possible to detect the phenotypic features of this condition (Asghar et al., 2009). Echocardiography is the diagnostic method that can achieve early detection of diabetic cardiomyopathy since it can detect structural myocardial changes (LVH and increased cardiac mass) in addition to evaluation of diastolic and systolic heart dysfunction (Mytas et al., 2009). As a result, echocardiography based methods currently stand as the preferred diagnostic approach for diabetic cardiomyopathy in clinical practice (Maya & Villarreal, 2010).

Abnormality	Manifestation (Stage of Disease)
Diastolic Dysfunction	Early
Systolic Dysfunction	Late
Left Ventricular Hypertrophy	Late
Myocardial Fibrosis	Late

Table 1. Diagnosis of Diabetic Cardiomyopathy

Although brain natriuretic peptide (BNP), a hormone secreted by the ventricles of the heart in response to ventricular volume and pressure overload, is both sensitive and specific for HF, research has shown that BNP is of limited diagnostic utility for diagnosing diabetic cardiomyopathy (Fang et al., 2005; Valle et al., 2006). This is due in part to the fact that BNP cannot reliably distinguish between systolic and diastolic HF, which limits its use in diabetic cardiomyopathy (Asghar et al., 2009; Fang et al., 2005; Maisel et al., 2003). Furthermore, the triggers for BNP secretion (increased intraventricular volume and pressure) does not occur in patients with subclinical, asymptomatic diabetic cardiomyopathy (Mytas et al., 2009; Stevanovic et al., 2006). In light of these findings, it is recommended that BNP not be used in isolation to diagnose or exclude diabetic cardiomyopathy (Fang et al., 2005; Kamalesh, 2007).

3. Cardiac changes

3.1 Structural remodeling

3.1.1 LVH

Data from the Framingham Heart Study (Kannel et al., 1974) as well as the Strong Heart Study (Devereux et al., 2000) indicated a disproportionate increase in LV mass and wall thickness among DM patients as compared to non-DM patients, even after adjusting for other cardiac risk factors (Devereux et al., 2000). In a recent multi-ethnic population study, the presence of type 2 DM, independent of body size, was associated with a 1.5-fold increase in risk of having LV mass >75th percentile of the general population (Eguchi et al., 2008). While LVH has consistently been linked to the increased incidence of cardiovascular events in a variety of high-risk patient groups, several studies have demonstrated that this cardiovascular risk is further enhanced by the presence of DM and thereby portends an especially poor prognosis (Boner et al., 2005; Struthers & Morris, 2002; Valensi et al., 1997). Emerging evidence has implicated the diabetic milieu of hyperinsulinemia, insulin resistance, hyperglycemia, and increased non-esterified fatty acids in the pathophysiology of LVH in DM patients. In addition, higher circulating levels of the hormone leptin have been linked to the development of LVH in obese diabetic humans. Disruption of downstream leptin signaling leading to leptin excess and resistance has been implicated as a novel pathophysiological mechanism by which leptin contributes to adverse remodeling. The consistency of results demonstrate a clear impact of DM *per se* on increased LV mass that encompasses the development of diabetes-related LVH.

3.1.2 Increased connective tissue collagen deposition and fibrosis

Diabetic cardiomyopathy has been documented to be characterized by myocardial fibrosis. A significant increase in collagen deposition has frequently been observed in heart biopsy samples from DM patients without significant coronary artery disease (Regan et al., 1977; Shimizu et al., 1993; Van Heerebeek et al., 2008). Similar to humans, increased cardiac collagen deposition has also been observed in animal models of DM (Bhimji et al., 1986; Spiro & Crowley, 1993). In addition, an increase in the formation of advanced glycation end products (AGEs) has also been reported to occur in the myocardium of DM patients (Van Heerebeek et al., 2008) which cross-link with collagen and increase its tensile strength. The excess deposition of collagen as well as AGE cross-linking of collagen induced by DM has been shown to augment LV stiffness of the failing diabetic heart in the absence of coronary artery disease (Van Heerebeek et al., 2008). Because excessive LV stiffness of the diabetic heart is an important contributor to worsening HF in patients with DM, increased myocardial collagen and AGEs are thought to be important therapeutic targets for modulating the development of diabetic cardiomyopathy and subsequent HF.

3.2 Functional alterations

3.2.1 Diastolic dysfunction

LV diastolic dysfunction has been reported to be the earliest detectable functional defect in diabetic cardiomyopathy (Fang et al., 2003, 2005; Karamitsos et al., 2007; Valle et al., 2006) and is characterized by increased LV end-diastolic pressure and a decreased LV end-diastolic volume (Hamblin et al, 2007a; Regan et al., 1977). The higher filling pressures are a result of reduced diastolic ventricular compliance which thereby alters diastolic filling and HF ensues. Diastolic dysfunction is a common functional abnormality in diabetic cardiomyopathy that has been related to myocardial fibrosis occurring in response to hyperglycemia. The early reductions in diastolic performance have been found to be followed by progressive reductions in systolic function during the later stages of diabetic cardiomyopathy. Therefore, diastolic dysfunction may not necessarily exist in isolation in the setting of diabetic cardiomyopathy.

3.2.2 Systolic dysfunction

In both human and animal models of type 1 and type 2 DM, systolic functional disorders have been shown to be associated with a reduction in ejection fraction (EF), fractional shortening (FS), and cardiac output (CO) (Mihm et al., 2001; Mildenberger et al., 1984; Mytas et al., 2009). *In vivo* animal studies using invasive catheterization have revealed load-dependent and -independent indices of systolic dysfunction in diabetic hearts (Hamblin et al., 2007a; Van Den Bergh et al., 2006). Comparative investigation of cardiac dysfunction in rodent models of type 1 and type 2 DM suggest that systolic dysfunction may be more pronounced in type 1 diabetic cardiomyopathy (Radovits et al., 2009).

4. Mechanisms of diabetes-induced cardiomyopathy

4.1 Derangements in cardiac energy metabolism

The primary metabolic defect observed in diabetic hearts is an exaggerated reliance on fatty acid metabolism due to reduced insulin production or insulin resistance. As a result, cardiac glucose uptake and utilization declines while free fatty acid use and oxidation by the diabetic heart increases. The augmented fatty acid metabolism of the diabetic heart leads to intracellular lipid accumulation, energy deprivation and ultimately cardiomyopathy (An & Rodrigues, 2006). Accumulation of lipids can result in increased non-oxidative production of toxic lipid products that precipitate cell death and decrease myocardial contractile dysfunction, thereby inducing myocardial lipotoxicity. In addition, the metabolic switch to increased usage of free fatty acids impairs cardiac energy efficiency in the diabetic heart due partly to the fact that glucose utilization is about 10% more efficient at generating ATP per O_2 consumed (2.58 vs. 2.33 ATP/ oxygen atom) (Wang et al., 2006a).

We and others have shown that type 1 DM alters the protein composition of cardiac mitochondria to accommodate the increased oxidation of fatty acids (Hamblin et al., 2007a; Shen et al., 2004). In-depth mining of the type 1 diabetic myocardial proteome by proteomic analysis revealed that half of the altered proteins were localized to the mitochondria (Hamblin et al., 2007a; Shen et al., 2004). Most of the cardiac protein changes were due to increased content of enzymes required for fatty acid metabolism and oxidation (e.g. acyl coenzyme A thioester hydrolase, acyl CoA dehydrogenase) (Hamblin et al., 2007a; Shen et al., 2004). These findings identify a specific 'type 1 diabetic' pattern of cardiac proteome changes indicative of diabetic cardiomyopathy and its attendant altered metabolic phenotype of enhanced fatty acid utilization.

4.2 Advanced Glycation End products (AGEs)

AGEs are a heterogeneous group of molecules formed from the non-enzymatic reaction of reducing sugars with free amino groups of proteins, lipids, and nucleic acids (Peppa et al., 2003). The formation of these sugar-derived substances is markedly accelerated in DM because of the increased availability of glucose (Peppa et al., 2003). A common consequence of their formation is covalent cross-link formation with proteins such as collagen which decrease the compliance of the extracellular matrix (ECM) (Brownlee, 2000; Singh et al., 2001). In the myocardium, this may lead to ventricular stiffness (Bell, 1995; Spiro & Crowley, 1993) with resultant impaired diastolic function. Increased activation of the diacylglycerol (DAG)-protein kinase C (PKC) signal transduction pathway has been shown in hearts of streptozotocin (STZ)-diabetic animals (Inoguchi et al., 1992) and activation of this pathway has been documented as a mechanism linking AGEs to diabetic complications (Mamputu & Renier, 2002; Way et al., 2001).

AGEs are not only directly damaging through covalent modification of proteins but they also contribute to the increased production of reactive oxygen species (ROS) by binding to the receptor for advanced glycation end products, RAGE (Wang et al., 2006a). The resulting RAGE activation by AGEs has been shown to lead to an increased generation of intracellular ROS (Brownlee, 2001).

4.3 Renin-Angiotensin-Aldosterone System (RAAS)

It is well recognized that DM is characterized by enhanced up-regulation of the local and systemic RAAS. Although the basis for dysfunction of the RAAS system in the setting of DM remains incompletely understood, its activation during DM has been demonstrated to be associated with increased oxidative damage which in turn activates the death pathways implicated in myocardial cell apoptosis and necrosis (Frustaci et al., 2000; Privratsky et al., 2003). These myocyte and non-myocyte alterations in diabetic hearts resulting from increased activation of RAAS induces impairment of ventricular function. The benefits of RAAS blockade in preventing and reversing diabetic cardiomyopathy in DM patients (Asghar et al., 2009) underscore the importance of dysregulated RAAS in the pathogenesis of diabetic cardiomyopathy.

4.4 Mitochondrial dysfunction

Abnormalities in myocardial mitochondrial function have been reported in human as well as animal models of DM. Morphological study of diabetic cardiomyopathy in OVE26 mice, a chronic model of type 1 DM, revealed a significant increase in mitochondrial area and number as well as focal regions with severe damage to mitochondria (Shen et al., 2004). Mitochondria isolated from these OVE26 diabetic hearts exhibited a reduced respiratory control ratio due to lower state 3 respiration (Shen et al., 2004), indicating impaired mitochondrial function. Similar observations have also been reported in STZ and other animal models of DM (Kuo et al., 1983; Pierce & Dhalla, 1985; Tomita et al., 1996). Impairment in mitochondrial respiratory capacity has also been shown to occur in diabetic human hearts. The most comprehensive and direct evidence to date for the presence of myocardial mitochondrial dysfunction in human diabetes comes from a recent study examining mitochondrial respiration in the atrium of type 2 diabetic human myocardium (Anderson et al., 2009). This study demonstrated decreased mitochondrial respiratory capacity with palmitoyl-carnitine and glutamate in atrial tissue of type 2 DM individuals. Collectively, these findings provide solid evidence of impairment of mitochondrial function in both type 1 and type 2 diabetic hearts which may contribute to or amplify derangements in cardiac energetics that have been linked to contractile dysfunction in diabetic cardiomyopathy over time.

4.5 Myocardial fibrosis

Interstitial and perivascular fibrosis has been described in the myocardia of patients and animals with DM. Most of this has been documented to be composed of collagen fibers (Shimizu et al., 1993). In that regard, the percentage of type III collagen in the perimysium and perivascular region has been reported to be significantly higher in the hearts of patients with DM, indicating the occurrence of collagen remodeling (Shimizu et al., 1993). It has been suggested that although collagen is a major determinant of ventricular stiffness, alterations in collagen phenotype may play an important role in the impaired LV diastolic filling that is typical of diabetic cardiomyopathy (Shimizu et al., 1993).
As indicated earlier in this chapter, it has been demonstrated that collagen is particularly susceptible to AGE cross-linking (Susic et al., 2004). The cross-linking of collagen molecules to each other not only leads to loss of elasticity but also impairment of collagen degradation, leading to further collagen accumulation or fibrosis (Wang et al., 2006a). As a result, the cross-linking of collagen molecules due to accelerated AGEs formation in the diabetic heart

is thought to be an important mechanism that contributes to the myocardial fibrosis and resulting decreased myocardial compliance characteristic of diabetic cardiomyopathy.

4.6 Myocardial oxidative stress: A key contributor to diabetic cardiomyopathy

Oxidative stress is defined as an imbalance between the generation of free oxygen radicals (FORs) and the antioxidant defense system. In the simplest of terms, a free radical is any atom or molecule that has an unpaired electron in their outer orbit making that atom or molecule a highly reactive species. Free radical production occurs via the addition of an electron or by its removal in a reduction/oxidation reaction. Due to its unique diradical configuration, oxygen is a major intracellular source of radical species. A sequential univalent reduction of oxygen gives rise to reactive intermediate products (Kaul et al., 1993; Singal et al., 1988). A single electron reduction of oxygen gives rise to superoxide anion (O_2^-), which can act as both a reducing and an oxidizing agent. The relatively short half life of superoxide anion limits its diffusion away from the site of its generation. The divalent reduction of oxygen yields the nonradical species, hydrogen peroxide (H_2O_2). H_2O_2 has a relatively long half life and therefore can travel significant distances, causing damage at sites distant from its origin. A three electron reduction of oxygen yields the hydroxyl radical (OH^-), which is the most reactive and potent of all the FORs. Addition of a fourth electron results in the formation of water.

FORs are neutralized by various cellular defense mechanisms consisting of enzymatic [(superoxide dismutase (SOD), catalase (CAT), and glutathione peroxidase (GSHPx)] and non-enzymatic (vitamin E, β-carotene, vitamin C) antioxidants (Palace et al., 1999). However, during pathological conditions, the delicate balance between FOR production and the protective antioxidant defense system may shift in favor of a relative increase in free-radical production and resultant FOR-induced tissue injury via lipid peroxidation of polyunsaturated fatty acids located in the cell membrane. Hyperglycemia can elevate levels of FORs by increasing mitochondrial superoxide anion production or by the process of glucose auto-oxidation (Eriksson & Borg, 1993; Nishikawa et al., 2000).

Early experimental evidence implicating myocardial oxidative stress in diabetic cardiomyopathy was mainly derived from reports evaluating the rate of lipid peroxidation. Increased cardiac levels of thiobarbituric acid reactive substances (TBARS) and lipid peroxides were observed in rats with STZ-induced diabetic cardiomyopathy (Jain & Levine, 1995; Kaul et al., 1996; Nishio et al., 1998). More recently, F_2-isoprostanes (F_2-IsoPs), a novel class of prostaglandin F_2-like compounds formed *in vivo* by non-enzymatic free radical-catalyzed peroxidation of arachidonic acid (Montuschi et al., 2004; Morrow et al., 1990), have emerged as one of the most reliable approaches to assess oxidative stress status *in vivo* (Montuschi et al., 2004). Of these, 8-*iso*-prostaglandin $F_{2\alpha}$ (8-*iso* $PGF_{2\alpha}$) has recently been shown to be a specific and sensitive quantitative index of oxidative stress *in vivo* (Delanty et al., 1997). We and others have found that in STZ rats with type 1 diabetic cardiomyopathy, LV levels of 8-*iso* $PGF_{2\alpha}$ were significantly increased *in vivo* (Hamblin et al. 2007a, 2007b; Xia et al., 2007). Collectively, these experimental animal studies demonstrate that diabetic cardiomyopathy is associated with greater myocardial oxidative stress burden.

Intermediates in the pathway of formation of IsoPs are endoperoxides, which are reduced to form F_2-IsoPs but also undergo rearrangement to form isomeric ketoaldehydes termed isoketals (IsoKs) (Roberts et al., 1999). IsoKs are remarkably reactive compounds that adduct almost instantaneously and irreversibly with lysine (Lys) residues on proteins and cross-link proteins (Iyer et al., 1989; Jirousek et al., 1990; Salomon et al., 1987) and as such, would be expected to profoundly alter protein function. Because myocardial ischemia can induce oxidative stress and the high incidence and poor prognosis of post-MI HF in DM patients has been linked in part to the presence of an underlying diabetic cardiomyopathy, we have recently performed a preliminary study in which we measured the levels of IsoK-lysyl-lactam adducts in STZ-diabetic post-MI rat hearts at 4 weeks after induction of MI using liquid chromatography electrospray tandem mass spectrometry (LC/MS) methods (Fukuda et al., 2005). Levels of IsoK-lysyl-lactam adduct were increased strikingly in the viable LV myocardium of diabetic infarcted rats compared with the same LV region in non-diabetic infarcted hearts (Fig. 1). These results clearly demonstrate that IsoK adducts are selectively increased in diabetic post-MI hearts. Protection of diabetic hearts from the downstream effects of these novel products formed via the IsoP pathway of free radical-mediated lipid peroxidation deserves evaluation as a new therapeutic approach for the prevention and treatment of oxidative-dependent cardiac complications of DM, including cardiomyopathy.

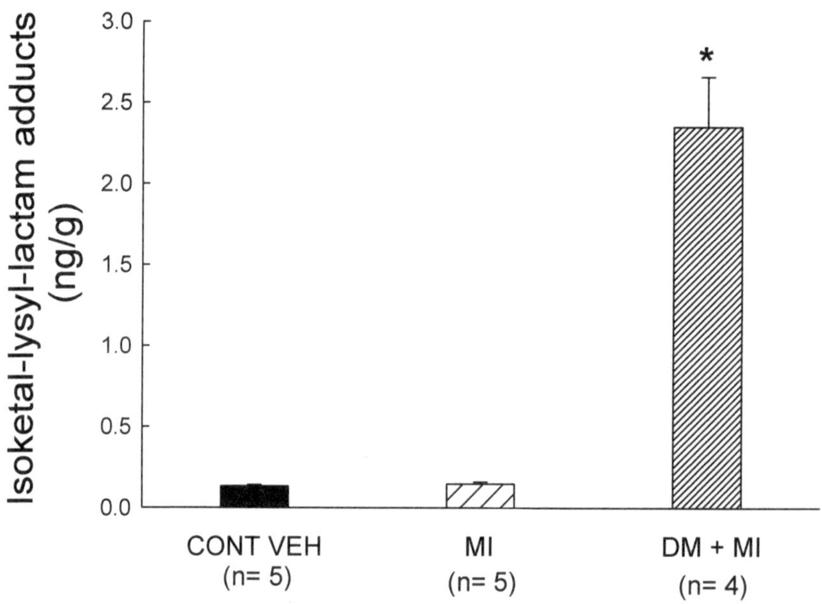

Fig. 1. Myocardial isoketal-lysyl-lactam adducts increase in DM + MI.

Myocardial isoketal-lysyl-lactam adducts in control vehicle (CONT VEH), MI, and DM + MI rats at 4 weeks post-MI. The levels of isoketal-lysyl-lactam adducts were measured in the surviving myocardium remote from the site of infarction. *Significantly different ($P<0.05$) from CONT VEH and MI groups.

Increased FOR production has also been shown to be involved in triggering cardiomyocyte apoptosis associated with diabetic cardiomyopathy (Cai et al., 2002). In addition, recent investigations have suggested that DM induces an inflammatory response by oxidative mechanisms, which may contribute to the development of diabetic cardiomyopathy (Garcia-Bailo et al., 2011). These synergistic impacts of myocardial oxidative stress in the presence of DM suggest that it is a major player in the pathogenesis of diabetic cardiomyopathy.

5. Candidate cardiac-specific biologic markers of diabetic cardiomyopathy

Proteomics (the concept of characterizing global alterations in protein expression of cells, tissues, and organs in health and disease) has become a powerful tool in the search for clinically useful biomarkers of disease and treatment response. Since the sum of the temporal alterations in proteins ultimately promotes or reflects the particular disease state, proteins represent an array of potential disease-specific markers and drug targets (Chaurand et al., 2004). Until recently, information concerning alterations that occur in the diabetic myocardial proteome and in the cardiac proteome of hearts with diabetic cardiomyopathy was lacking because proteomics had not been used to examine global cardiac protein changes that occur in diabetic cardiac complications. In an effort to bridge this gap, we recently performed proteomic analysis of diabetic cardiomyopathy utilizing two-dimensional difference gel electrophoresis and mass spectrometry (DIGE/MS) techniques (Hamblin et al., 2007a). Employing this technology, we established a specific 'type 1 diabetic' pattern of cardiac proteome changes indicative of diabetic cardiomyopathy (Hamblin et al., 2007a). We found that a high proportion (50%) of the altered proteins that could be identified by MS were localized to the mitochondria, many of which were up-regulated and involved in fatty acid metabolism. Specifically, protein expression levels for acyl coenzyme A thioester hydrolase and acyl CoA dehydrogenase, both of which are involved in fatty acid oxidation (J.J. Kim & Battaile, 2002), were found to be elevated 2-to 2.5-fold in the LV myocardium of rats with STZ-induced diabetic cardiomyopathy (Hamblin et al., 2007a). Our finding by proteomic analysis that these fatty acid utilization proteins are significantly more abundant in type 1 diabetic cardiomyopathy has been confirmed in proteomics-based studies of diabetic cardiomyopathy in OVE26 mice (Shen et al., 2004). Taken together, these consistent proteomic results show that elevated cardiac fatty acid utilization proteins are associated with diabetic cardiomyopathy and, hence, could serve as candidate markers and indicators of diabetic cardiomyopathy. As such, these results represent a starting point for the identification and development of a panel of cardiac biomarkers able to delineate diabetic cardiomyopathy. Continued proteomics-based studies of diabetic cardiomyopathy are essential to rapidly expand the range of biomarkers that is required for the emergence of new and successful protein diagnostics of diabetic cardiomyopathy.

6. Therapeutic strategies for the treatment of diabetic cardiomyopathy

6.1 Glycemic control

Until recently, clinical trials examining the effectiveness of good glycemic control in reducing cardiovascular events in diabetics has produced mixed results. The publication of 2 randomized intervention trials, Action in Diabetes and Vascular Disease: Preterax and Diamicron Modified Release Controlled Evaluation (ADVANCE) trial and the Action to Control Cardiovascular Risk in Diabetes Study Group (ACCORD) trial, showed that lowering of blood glucose in type 2 diabetics to near-normal levels did not significantly reduce cardiovascular events and actually increased mortality (Gerstein et al., 2008; Patel et al., 2008). However, these results were obtained from middle-aged and older patients with a long duration of DM and a high risk of cardiovascular disease. A recent epidemiologic analysis of the cardiovascular effect of glucose lowering in patients with type 2 DM revealed that patients with high levels of co-morbidity may receive diminished cardiovascular benefit from intensive blood glucose control (Greenfield et al., 2009). Furthermore, the ACCORD trial was not designed to test whether patients with HbA_{1c} levels below 7.5% receive greater benefit from intensive glucose lowering (Gerstein et al., 2008). Examination of the hazard ratios for the primary outcome and death from any cause in relation to glycated hemoglobin levels at baseline in the ACCORD trial showed a fewer number of events in type 2 DM patients with HbA_{1c} levels at baseline < 8%, suggesting a better response to therapy than patients with higher HbA_{1c} levels. This hypothesis is supported by a recent epidemiologic analysis of the cardiovascular effect of glucose lowering in type 2 DM patients whereby HbA_{1c} levels of 7.0% or less at baseline was associated with a lower 5-year incidence of cardiovascular events (Greenfield et al., 2009).

A series of recent reports have also established that improved glycemic control reduces the subsequent risk of any cardiovascular disease event in type 1 DM. The most convincing clinical evidence in support of this paradigm stems from the Diabetes Control and Complications Trial (DCCT) in which the DCCT randomly assigned 1441 patients with type 1 DM to receive either intensive diabetes therapy (three or more daily injections of insulin or insulin treatment with an external pump) or conventional diabetes therapy (one or two daily injections of insulin) for a mean of 6.5 years (DCCT, 1993). After treating them for a mean of 6.5 years, mean HbA_{1c} was 7.2% in the intensive therapy arm and 9.0% in the conventional treatment arm. Although a reduction in the risk for macrovascular events was observed in the intensive diabetes therapy arm, it did not achieve statistical significance (DCCT, 1993). After completion of this component of the DCCT, ninety-three percent of the 1441 patients were continued to be followed up as part of an ongoing observational study (Epidemiology of Diabetes Interventions and Complications [EDIC] study). After a mean follow-up of 17 years, intensive diabetes therapy, as compared to conventional therapy, reduced the risk of a cardiovascular event by 42% (Nathan et al., 2005). These beneficial effects were observed despite non-significant differences in mean HbA_{1c} concentrations between the previous intensive and conventional therapy groups at year 11 of the EDIC study, indicating intensive diabetes therapy has long-term, sustained beneficial effects on the risk of cardiovascular disease in patients with type 1 DM (Nathan et al., 2005).

The recent publication of an observational study involving type 1 DM patients has demonstrated the benefits of optimum glycemic control in reducing specifically the risk of HF in type 1 DM (Lind et al., 2011). The positive association between glycated hemoglobin and risk of HF in fairly young patients with type 1 DM together with the finding that tight control of glycemia in type 1 diabetes can prevent HF besides other aspects of cardiovascular disease (Lind et al., 2011) indicates a potential for prevention of HF with improved glycemic control. Given that patients with poorly controlled type 1 DM, as in those included in this recent observational study, have a high probability of diabetic cardiomyopathy, these results suggest that intensive glucose control be initiated as early as possible in people with type 1 DM to reduce the risk of cardiovascular complications, including cardiomyopathy and HF. In that regard, evidence that diabetic cardiomyopathy does not develop in patients with tightly controlled type 1 DM (Konduracka et al., 2007) supports the use of anti-hyperglycemic agents as part of the treatment regime for diabetic cardiomyopathy.

6.1.1 Sulfonylureas

Sulfonylureas are agents that act to increase insulin release from the beta cells in the pancreas and thus are almost exclusively used in the management of type 2 DM. Clinical studies examining the use of sulfonylureas in diabetic HF are rather limited but have produced conflicting results due in large part to the fact that the subjects included in these studies either had pre-existing cardiovascular disease or were at high risk of cardiovascular events (Simpson et al., 2006). In animal models of STZ-induced diabetic cardiomyopathy that are devoid of cardiovascular co-morbidities, chronic treatment with glyburide, the most widely used sulfonylurea, ameliorated the decline in myocardial function associated with diabetic cardiomyopathy (Mozaffari et al., 1989). Clearly, further studies are needed to determine the benefits of these drugs in patients with DM and HF.

6.1.2 Metformin

Metformin is a member of the insulin-sensitizing drugs that was previously contraindicated in patients with HF due to concerns over lactic acidosis. Although its use is still strongly cautioned, recent evidence from three cohort studies in which metformin therapy was compared with other anti-hyperglycemic agents demonstrated that metformin treatment was associated with a lower risk of all-cause mortality and all-cause hospital admissions (Eurich et al., 2007). In addition, metformin therapy has been reported to improve outcomes in older patients with DM and HF (Masoudi et al., 2005). Metformin has also been demonstrated to have favorable actions on the development of diabetic cardiomyopathy in Zucker diabetic rats (ZDF) (Forcheron et al., 2009).

6.1.3 Thiazolidinediones (TZDs)

The TZDs [PPARγ (peroxisome-proliferator-activated receptor γ) receptor agonists] are primarily insulin-sensitizing agents that have been shown to exert beneficial effects on the myocardium. However, due to their propensity for fluid retention, their use is limited to patients in New York Heart Association (NYHA) functional class I-II HF. The PROspective pioglitAzone Clinical Trial In macroVascular Events (PROactive) is currently the only completed cardiovascular (CV) outcomes study with a thiazolidinedione and remains the only large-scale, prospective, secondary prevention trial carried out entirely in patients with type 2 DM (Betteridge et al., 2008). The results from this study demonstrated that the TZD pioglitazone does not increase the risk of macrovascular events or worsen outcomes in those who develop signs of heart failure in a high-risk population with type 2 DM with macrovascular disease (Betteridge et al., 2008). Even when the increased incidence of signs of HF (with a normal ejection fraction) was taken into account, the overall CV benefit of pioglitazone remained (Betteridge et al., 2008). These results suggest that from a safety perspective, the favorable cardiovascular effects of pioglitazone treatment outweigh any inherent risks (Betteridge et al., 2008).

6.1.4 Incretins: A new line of therapy

Incretins are hormones produced by the gastrointestinal tract in response to nutrient entry that act to regulate postprandial glucose homeostasis. Among several incretin hormones, glucagon-like peptide-1 (GLP-1) stimulates insulin secretion in a glucose dependent fashion. As a result, an important safety advantage of incretin-based therapy is the abolishment of risk for hypoglycemia. Currently, there are two types of incretin-based drugs that have been developed to improve the effects of glucagon-like peptide-1 (GLP-1): incretin mimetics such as GLP-1 receptor agonists and the dipeptidyl peptidase-4 (DPP-4) inhibitors, which potentiate the incretin hormones by inhibiting the enzyme responsible for their degradation.

The GLP-1 receptor agonists mimic the actions of endogenous GLP-1 and are currently marketed as exenatide and liraglutide. Clinical trials of GLP-1 analogues have demonstrated improved LV function in patients with LV dysfunction after acute MI (Nikolaidis et al., 2004) and in patients with chronic advanced HF (Sokos et al., 2006). In an observational study involving patients with DM and HF, administration of GLP-1 over a period of three days improved the glycemic state and caused a trend towards improvement of parameters expressing LV function in DM patients with stable HF (Thrainsdottir et al., 2004). The beneficial actions on cardiac function reported so far with GLP-1 analogues provide a rationale for their use in DM patients with cardiomyopathy (Jax, 2009).

The DPP-4 inhibitors are newer drugs and currently marketed products include sitagliptin, saxagliptin, and vildagliptin. Cardiovascular outcomes as well as safety trials using this class of incretin-based drugs in patients with DM is underway to determine their efficacy and safety.

6.2 RAAS blockade

6.2.1 Renin inhibitors

The discovery that the binding of prorenin or renin to the prorenin/renin or (pro)renin receptor results in the augmented formation of angiotensin I has led to the development of direct renin inhibitors. Cardiac (pro)renin receptor expression has recently been documented to be increased in experimental diabetic cardiomyopathy (Connelly et al., 2011). Blockade of RAAS via administration of the direct renin inhibitor, aliskiren (10 mg/kg per day for 6 weeks duration), reduced cardiac over-expression of both (pro)renin mRNA and protein in diabetic TGR (mRen2)-27 rats, a transgenic rodent model that following the induction of STZ-diabetes develops diabetic cardiomyopathy (Connelly et al., 2011). Just as importantly, the reduced cardiac pro(renin) receptor expression with aliskiren treatment was associated with improved cardiac structure/function (Connelly et al., 2011). Given these exciting findings, direct renin inhibitors, particularly aliskiren, are ripe for further evaluation as novel therapeutics to modulate/prevent diabetic cardiomyopathy.

6.2.2 Angiotensin Converting Enzyme (ACE) inhibitors

Treatment with ACE inhibitors has been shown to exert an ameliorative effect on diabetic cardiomyopathy in both diabetic animals and diabetic patients. Administration of ramipril (2.5 mg/day) for 3 months to asymptomatic type 2 DM patients with echocardiographic indices of early diabetic cardiomyopathy improved echocardiographic indices of LV diastolic function in these patients (Symeonides et al., 2007). The reversal of indices of diabetic cardiomyopathy in these type 2 DM patients with ramipril was accompanied by a reduction of plasma BNP levels (Symeonides et al., 2007). In an experimental rat model of diabetic cardiomyopathy, administration of captropril (13 mg/kg) for 8 weeks in rats with clear cardiomyopathy improved the myocardial structure and cardiac function (C.H. Zhang et al., 2008). Taken together, these results suggest that treatment with ACE inhibitors can exert a beneficial effect on the development of diabetic cardiomyopathy.

6.2.3 Angiotensin Receptor Blockers (ARBs)

ARBs have emerged as a promising treatment modality for diabetic cardiomyopathy. Damage to the myocardial ultrastructure of rats with diabetic cardiomyopathy has been shown to be reduced by the type 1 angiotensin II receptor blocker (AT_1RB) valsartan (C.H. Zhang et al., 2008). In DM patients with cardiomyopathy as assessed by Doppler echocardiography, the administration of the ARB telmisartan resulted in improved echocardiographic and biochemical indices of diabetic cardiomyopathy (Symeonides et al., 2007). Since a majority of patients develop dry cough with ACE inhibitors, the cardioprotection afforded by ARBs offer the distinct advantage of having better compliance.

6.3 β-blockers

Until recently, patients with DM were less likely to be prescribed β-blockers due in part over fears of worsening insulin resistance and lipid metabolism. However, the realization of the importance of the sympathetic nervous system in the release of vasoactive substances (Murarka & Movahed, 2010) and the demonstrated benefit of β-blockers in other forms of HF has led to β-blockers being accepted as a mainstay in the treatment of DM patients with HF. The utility of β-blockade has also been demonstrated in experimental models of diabetic cardiomyopathy. Chronic treatment with the β-blocker metoprolol (β1-selective inverse agonist) has been shown to improve cardiac function in STZ-induced diabetic cardiomyopathy in rats as evidenced by significant increases in cardiac output (Sharma et al., 2008). Treatment with bisoprolol (β1-selective antagonist) for 3 months reversed myocardial hypertrophy and changes in diabetic cardiomyopathy rats (J.N. Zhang et al., 2003). Clinical trials to evaluate β-blocker intervention in patients specifically with diabetic cardiomyopathy are lacking and should be conducted to exploit this recent experimental data.

6.4 Antioxidants

As the pathogenesis of diabetic cardiomyopathy involves oxidative stress, antioxidants have received considerable interest as a therapeutic strategy. Several different approaches, such as dietary supplementation, administration of pharmacological agents with antioxidant properties, and over-expression of antioxidant enzymes to augment antioxidant defense mechanisms, have proven to be effective in reversing diabetic cardiomyopathy in animal models of both type 1 and type 2 DM.

Vitamin E, a lipid-soluble and potent antioxidant, has been shown in diabetic rats to evoke cardioprotective effects against diabetic cardiomyopathy. We have previously reported that dietary supplementation with vitamin E (2000 IU of tocopherol acetate/kg of feed) beginning early after the onset of type 1 DM in rats and continuing for a period of 8 weeks improved LV function as evidenced by a significant improvement in LVSP, LVEDP, and +dP/dt compared with un-supplemented DM rats (Hamblin et al., 2007b). The improved LV hemodynamic function of type 1 diabetic cardiomyopathy rats supplemented with vitamin E was accompanied by significantly reduced levels of myocardial oxidative stress (Hamblin et al., 2007b). Specifically, vitamin E blunted the diabetes-induced amplification of myocardial 8-*iso* $PGF_{2\alpha}$ and oxidized glutathione (GSSG) formation (Hamblin et al., 2007b). Vitamin E administration has also been documented to be associated with a significant decline in apoptosis, lipid peroxidation, protein oxidation, and enhancement of the antioxidant defense system, suggesting that this antioxidant may promote a convalescing effect on diabetic cardiomyopathy through the attenuation of oxidative stress and abrogation of apoptotic signals (Shirpoor et al., 2009). These findings demonstrate the usefulness of vitamin E as a protective anti-oxidative agent against cardiac sequel of DM involving cardiomyopathy.

Resveratrol, the principal effector constituent of red wine, has been shown to improve cardiac function in diabetic cardiomyopathy (Huang et al., 2010; Sulaiman et al., 2010). Oral administration of resveratrol (2.5 mg/kg body wt/day) to STZ-diabetic rats for 15 days has been shown to result in a direct cardioprotective effect on the diabetic myocardium (Thirunavukkarasu et al. 2007). Resveratrol treatment of chronic diabetic mice resulted in a tremendous improvement of all functional parameters to the extent that cardiac function was comparable to age-matched controls (Sulaiman et al., 2010). These data demonstrate that resveratrol can prevent diabetes-induced decline in cardiac function and resultant cardiomyopathy. Studies have revealed that resveratrol treatment improves cardiac dysfunction of diabetic myocardium in part via modulation of oxidative stress proteins (Dekkers et al., 2008). The recognition that resveratrol treatment up-regulates the protein expression of the antioxidant enzyme catalase in diabetic hearts (Dekkers et al., 2008) is further evidence of its ability to increase protection against oxidative stress.

Tempol is a membrane-permeable SOD mimetic that has been shown to attenuate the effects of FORs (Thiemermann et al., 2001). *In vivo* treatment with the antioxidant tempol (1 mmol/l in drinking water) for a period of 4-weeks to mice rendered insulin-resistant by deficiency of the insulin-sensitive GLUT4 transporter significantly and potently attenuated cardiac hypertrophy in concert with tempol up-regulated ventricular expression of thioredoxin-2 (confirming an antioxidant action) (Ritchie et al., 2007). Since the pre-diabetic insulin-resistant heart exhibits many features of diabetic cardiomyopathy, including both left ventricular dysfunction and structural abnormalities such as cardiac hypertrophy and fibrosis (Ritchie et al., 2007), these results indicate that tempol should be considered for preventing oxidative stress and cardiomyopathy in the diabetic heart.

Metallothionein (MT), a cysteine-rich protein, is a potent antioxidant owing to its high thiol content. Using a cardiac-specific, MT-overexpressing transgenic (MT-TG) mouse model, MT has been shown to be effective in preventing diabetic cardiomyopathy through the suppression of oxidative damage (Cai et al., 2005, 2006; Liang et al., 2002). Supplementation with Zinc (Zn), a potent inducer of MT, prevented the increases in cardiac morphological impairment, fibrosis, and dysfunction observed in diabetic mice without Zn supplementation (Wang et al., 2006b). Silencing of MT expression with small-interfering RNA abolished the prevention of diabetic cardiomyopathy by Zn supplementation (Wang et al., 2006b). These results demonstrate that Zn supplementation protects against diabetic cardiomyopathy via cardiac MT induction and suggest Zn supplementation, with cardiac MT induction, as a potential therapeutic approach to prevent diabetic cardiomyopathy.

Targeted over-expression of the antioxidant proteins SOD and catalase to the heart has been shown to be effective in reducing diabetic cardiomyopathy (Shen et al., 2006; Ye et al., 2004). Chronic over-expression of catalase has been documented to eliminate excess FOR production in diabetic cardiomyocytes concomitant with preservation of normal cardiac morphology and contractile function (Ye et al., 2004). Over-expression of the mitochondrial antioxidant protein manganese SOD (Mn SOD) has been reported to protect against the formation of exogenous oxidants and also completely normalize contractile function in both type 1 and type 2 models of diabetic cardiomyopathy (Shen et al., 2006).

Although a number of previous large randomized placebo-controlled clinical trials have failed to show any beneficial effects of antioxidants (in particular vitamin E) on cardiovascular events, recently published literature suggests that these clinical trials of antioxidants and cardiovascular diseases may be fatally flawed (Blumberg & Frei, 2007; Roberts et al., 2007; Traber et al., 2008). Implicit in the majority of randomized placebo-controlled clinical trials that have previously explored the benefits of antioxidants is that the antioxidants tested effectively suppressed oxidative stress status but this was never determined (Roberts et al., 2007). Furthermore, not including elevated oxidative stress in patient eligibility criteria substantially reduces statistical power to detect antioxidant or cardiovascular effects (Block et al., 2008; Roberts et al., 2009). To that end, it has recently been reported that *"the negative evidence regarding vitamin E supplements from previous randomized clinical trials is more a reflection of inadequate study design and methods of analysis than proof of failure of vitamin E in primary prevention"*(Blumberg & Frei, 2007). Data obtained in experimental animals must obviously be extrapolated to the clinical arena with caution. Nevertheless, the present findings suggest that vitamin E and other antioxidants may confer cardiovascular benefit in select patients who are diabetic and in greater oxidative stress. Indeed, support for this paradigm has recently been demonstrated in a retrospective analysis of the Heart Outcomes Prevention Evaluation (HOPE) trial where vitamin E administration to diabetic individuals homozygous for the haptoglobin (Hp) 2 allele, which confers markedly less antioxidant protection against hemoglobin-induced oxidation, was shown to result in a 50% reduction in non-fatal MI and cardiovascular death (Levy et al., 2004). The validity of these findings have subsequently been confirmed in Hp 2-2 DM individuals in a prospective, double-blind, placebo-controlled trial of vitamin E (Milman et al., 2008). These positive results impel future clinical trials to study the efficacy of antioxidants specifically in patients with diabetic cardiomyopathy.

6.5 Cell transplantation

Transplantation of stem cells has emerged as an alternative therapeutic approach to improve cardiac function in the post-MI setting as well as in ischemic cardiomyopathic hearts. However, until recently, stem cell therapy studies had not been evaluated in the diabetic heart. In the past few years, cell transplantation has begun to be examined in the setting of diabetic cardiomyopathy. Transplantation of bone marrow mesenchymal stem cells (MSCs) into the hearts of STZ-diabetic rats via injection into the femoral vein has been shown to improve the cardiac function of diabetic cardiomyopathy through increased angiogenesis and attenuation of cardiac remodeling (N. Zhang et al., 2008). Bone marrow MSC transplantation has also been reported to improve cardiac function in the rat diabetic cardiomyopathy model through an anti-apoptotic effect (Li et al., 2008). Treatment combining smooth muscle cell (SMC) transplantation via intramyocardial injection and insulin therapy has been shown to result in the preservation of heart function in STZ-diabetic rats with cardiomyopathy as assessed by echocardiographic and hemodynamic techniques (B.O. Kim et al., 2008). Although the clinical significance of these studies will require further testing and confirmation in other animal models of DM, cell transplantation holds great promise for the treatment of diabetic cardiomyopathy.

7. Conclusions and future directions

The full spectrum of diabetic cardiomyopathy encompasses a progression from subclinical LV diastolic and systolic dysfunction to clinically overt symptomatic HF. Recognition and treatment of diabetes-induced myocardial dysfunction in its infancy is paramount for the prophylaxis of ensuing cardiomyopathy and HF. Thus, there is an eminent need for early detection of this clinical entity. In that regard, the knowledge that structural and functional alterations of a particular disease state are preceded by changes in proteins has led to the recent application of proteomics to the field of DM. The use of proteomic technologies, such as mass spectrometry, provides an ideal vehicle into this arena. Analysis of protein expression profiles in serum and tissues from diabetic animals and humans is now underway and will increase our power to identify early and subtle abnormalities of cardiac dysfunction in DM. One can also foresee the use of this technology to help establish biomarkers that are predictive for risk of developing diabetic cardiomyopathy. The potential capability of proteomics to elucidate protein changes occurring in response to pharmacological therapeutics is a particularly exciting application of this technology. Studies of drug-induced proteomic changes will be required to determine the ability of this molecular technology to correlate changes in protein expression with efficacy of established and novel therapies for cardiomyopathy in DM. The recent development of more sensitive and sophisticated echocardiographic techniques such as tissue Doppler, strain, strain rate, and ultrasonic tissue characterization appears helpful in identifying early myocardial dysfunction in asymptomatic patients with DM. Integration of proteomics with sensitive diagnostic imaging modalities holds tremendous potential for the comprehensive detection of preclinical cardiac dysfunction in patients with DM and thus should facilitate earlier therapeutic intervention to prevent cardiomyopathy and subsequent HF in this high-risk patient population.

8. Acknowledgments

Supported by National Heart, Lung, and Blood Institute grant 5 R01 HL089385-02 (to M.F. Hill). I gratefully acknowledge Salisha Hill, B.Sc., for expert consultation on proteomic technologies and proteomics approaches.

9. References

An, D. & Rodrigues, B. (2006). Role of changes in cardiac metabolism in development of diabetic cardiomyopathy. *Am J Physiol Heart Circ Physiol*, 291:H1489-1506.

Anderson, E.J., Kypson, A.P., Rodriguez, E., Anderson, C.A., Lehr, E.J., & Neufer, P.D. (2009). Substrate-specific derangements in mitochondrial metabolism and redox balance in the atrium of the type 2 diabetic human heart. *J Am Coll Cardiol*, 54:1891-1898.

Asghar, O., Al-Sunni, A., Khavandi, K., Khavandi, A., Withers, S., Greenstein, A., Heagerty, A.M., & Malik, R.A. (2009). Diabetic cardiomyopathy. *Clin Sci*, 116:741-760.

Beljic, T. & Miric, M. (1994). Improved metabolic control does not reverse left ventricular filling abnormalities in newly diagnosed non-insulin-dependent diabetes patients. *Acta Diabetol*, 31:147-150.

Bell, D.S. (1995). Diabetic cardiomyopathy. A unique entity or a complication of coronary artery disease? *Diabetes Care*, 18:708-714.

Bell, D.S. (2003a). Heart failure: the frequent, forgotten, and often fatal complication of diabetes. *Diabetes Care*, 26:2433-2441.

Bell, D.S. (2003b).Diabetic cardiomyopathy. *Diabetes Care*, 26:2949-2951.

Betteridge, D.J., DeFronzo, R.A., & Chilton, R.J. (2008). PROactive: time for a critical appraisal. *Eur Heart J*, 29:969-983.

Bhimji, S., Godin, D.V., & McNeill, J.H. (1986). Insulin reversal of biochemical changes in hearts from diabetic rats. *Am J Physiol*, 251:H670-H675.

Block, G., Jensen, C.D., Morrow, J.D., Holland, N., Norkus, E.P., Milne, G.L., Hudes, M., Dalvi, T.B., Crawford, P.B., Fung, E.B., Schumacher, L., & Harmatz, P. (2008). The effect of vitamins C and E on biomarkers of oxidative stress depends on baseline level. *Free Radic Biol Med*, 45:377-384.

Blumberg, J.B. & Frei, B. (2007). Why clinical trials of vitamin E and cardiovascular diseases may be fatally flawed. Commentary on "The relationship between dose of vitamin E and suppression of oxidative stress in humans". *Free Radic Biol Med*, 43:1374-1376.

Boner, G., Cooper, M.E., McCarroll, K., Brenner, B.M., de Zeeuw, D., Kowey, P.R., Shahinfar, S., Dickson, T., Crow, R.S., & Parving, H.H.; RENAAL Investigators. (2005). Adverse effects of left ventricular hypertrophy in the reduction of endpoints in NIDDM with the angiotensin II antagonist losartan (RENAAL) study. *Diabetologia*, 48:1980-1987.

Borges, G.R., de Oliveira, M., Salgado, H.C., & Fazan, R. Jr. (2006). Myocardial performance in conscious streptozotocin diabetic rats. *Cardiovasc Diabetol*, 5:26.

Boudina, S. & Abel, E.D. (2007). Diabetic cardiomyopathy revisited. *Circulation*, 115:3213-3223.

Boyer, J.K., Thanigaraj, S., Schechtman, K.B., & Pérez, J.E. (2004). Prevalence of ventricular diastolic dysfunction in asymptomatic, normotensive patients with diabetes mellitus. *Am J Cardiol*, 93:870-875.

Brownlee, M. (2000). Negative consequences of glycation. *Metabolism*, 49:9-13.

Brownlee, M. (2001). Biochemistry and molecular cell biology of diabetic complications. *Nature*, 414:813-820.

Cai, L., Li, W., Wang, G., Guo, L., Jiang, Y., & Kang, Y.J. (2002). Hyperglycemia-induced apoptosis in mouse myocardium: mitochondrial cytochrome C-mediated caspase-3 activation pathway. *Diabetes*, 51:1938-1948.

Cai, L., Wang, J., Li, Y., Sun, X., Wang, L., Zhou, Z., & Kang, Y.J. (2005). Inhibition of superoxide generation and associated nitrosative damage is involved in metallothionein prevention of diabetic cardiomyopathy. *Diabetes*, 54:1829-1837.

Cai, L., Wang, Y., Zhou, G., Chen, T., Song, Y., Li, X., & Kang, Y.J. (2006). Attenuation by metallothionein of early cardiac cell death via suppression of mitochondrial oxidative stress results in a prevention of diabetic cardiomyopathy. *J Am Coll Cardiol*, 48:1688-1697.

Centers for Disease Control and Prevention. National diabetes fact sheet: national estimates and general information on diabetes and prediabetes in the United States, 2011. Atlanta, GA: U.S. Department of Health and Human Services, Centers for Disease Control and Prevention.

Chaurand, P., Sanders, M.E., Jensen, R.A., & Caprioli, R.M. (2004). Proteomics in diagnostic pathology: profiling and imaging proteins directly in tissue sections. *Am J Pathol*, 165:1057-1068.

Cohen, A. (1995). Diabetic cardiomyopathy. *Arch Mal Coeur Vaiss*, 88:479-486.

Connelly, K.A., Advani, A., Kim, S., Advani, S.L., Zhang, M., White, K.E., Kim, Y.M., Parker, C., Thai, K., Krum, H., Kelly, D.J., & Gilbert, R.E. (2011). The cardiac (pro)renin receptor is primarily expressed in myocyte transverse tubules and is increased in experimental diabetic cardiomyopathy. *J Hypertens*, 29:1175-1184.

Danaei, G., Finucane, M.M., Lu, Y., Singh, G.M., Cowan, M.J., Paciorek, C.J., Lin, J.K., Farzadfar, F., Khang, Y-H., Stevens, G.A., Rao, M., Ali, M.K., Riley, L.M., Robinson, C.A., & Ezzati, M., on behalf of the Global Burden of Metabolic Risk Factors of Chronic Diseases Collaborating Group (Blood Glucose). (2011). National, regional, and global trends in fasting plasma glucose and diabetes prevalence since 1980: systematic analysis of health examination surveys and epidemiological studies with 370 country-years and 2·7 million participants. *Lancet*, 378:31-40.

Dekkers, D.H., Bezstarosti, K., Gurusamy, N., Luijk, K., Verhoeven, A.J., Rijkers, E.J., Demmers, J.A., Lamers, J.M., Maulik, N., & Das, D.K. (2008). Identification by a differential proteomic approach of the induced stress and redox proteins by resveratrol in the normal and diabetic rat heart. *J Cell Mol Med*, 12:1677-1689.

Delanty, N., Reilly, M.P., Pratico, D., Lawson, J.A., McCarthy, J.F., Wood, A.E., Ohnishi, S.T., Fitzgerald, D.J., & FitzGerald, G.A. (1997). 8-epi PGF2 alpha generation during coronary reperfusion. A potential quantitative marker of oxidant stress in vivo. *Circulation*, 95:2492- 2499.

Devereux ,R.B., Roman, M.J., Paranicas, M., O'Grady, M.J., Lee, E.T., Welty, T.K., Fabsitz, R.R., Robbinsm, D., Rhoades, E.R., & Howard, B.V. (2000). Impact of diabetes on cardiac structure and function: the strong heart study. *Circulation*, 101:2271-2276.

Di Bonito, P., Cuomo, S., Moio, N., Sibilio, G., Sabatini, D., Quattrin, S., & Capaldo, B. (1996). Diastolic dysfunction in patients with non-insulin-dependent diabetes mellitus of short duration. *Diabet Med*, 13:321-324.

Di Bonito, P., Moio, N., Cavuto, L., Covino, G., Murena, E., Scilla, C., Turco, S., Capaldo, B., & Sibilio, G. (2005). Early detection of diabetic cardiomyopathy: usefulness of tissue Doppler imaging. *Diabet Med*, 22:1720-1725.

Eguchi, K., Boden-Albala, B., Jin, Z., Rundek, T., Sacco, R.L, Homma, S., & Di Tullio, M.R. (2008). Association between diabetes mellitus and left ventricular hypertrophy in a multiethnic population. *Am J Cardiol*, 101:1787-1791.

Eriksson, U.J. & Borg, L.A. (1993). Diabetes and embryonic malformations. Role of substrate-induced free-oxygen radical production for dysmorphogenesis in cultured rat embryos. *Diabetes*, 42:411-419.

Eurich, D.T., McAlister, F.A., Blackburn, D.F., Majumdar, S.R., Tsuyuki, R.T., Varney, J., & Johnson, J.A. (2007). Benefits and harms of antidiabetic agents in patients with diabetes and heart failure: systematic review. *BMJ*, 335:497.

Fang, Z.Y., Yuda, S., Anderson, V., Short, L., Case, C., & Marwick, T.H. (2003). Echocardiographic detection of early diabetic myocardial disease. *J Am Coll Cardiol*, 41:611-617.

Fang, Z.Y., Schull-Meade, R., Leano, R., Mottram, P.M., Prins, J.B., & Marwick, T.H. (2005). Screening for heart disease in diabetic subjects. *Am Heart J*, 149:349-354.

Forcheron, F., Basset, A., Abdallah, P., Del Carmine, P., Gadot, N., & Beylot, M. (2009). Diabetic cardiomyopathy: effects of fenofibrate and metformin in an experimental model- the Zucker diabetic rat. *Cardiovasc Diabetol*, 8:16.

From, A.M., Scott, C.G., & Chen, H.H. (2010). The development of heart failure in patients with diabetes mellitus and pre-clinical diastolic dysfunction a population-based study. *J Am Coll Cardiol*, 55:300-305.

Frustaci, A., Kajstura, J., Chimenti, C., Jakoniuk, I., Leri, A., Maseri, A., Nadal-Ginard, B., & Anversa, P. (2000). Myocardial cell death in human diabetes. *Circ Res*, 87:1123-1132.

Fukuda, K., Davies, S.S., Nakajima, T., Ong, B.H., Kupershmidt, S., Fessel, J., Amarnath, V., Anderson, M.E., Boyden, P.A., Viswanathan, P.C., Roberts, L.J. 2nd, & Balser, J.R. (2005). Oxidative mediated lipid peroxidation recapitulates proarrhythmic effects on cardiac sodium channels. *Circ Res*, 97:1262-1269.

Galderisi, M., Anderson, K.M., Wilson, P.W., & Levy, D. (1991). Echocardiographic evidence for the existence of a distinct diabetic cardiomyopathy (the Framingham Heart Study). *Am J Cardiol*, 68:85-89.

Garcia-Bailo, B., El-Sohemy, A., Haddad, P.S., Arora, P., Benzaied, F., Karmali, M., & Badawi, A. (2011). Vitamins D, C, and E in the prevention of type 2 diabetes mellitus: modulation of inflammation and oxidative stress. *Biologics*, 5:7-19.

Gerstein, H.C., Miller, M.E., Byington, R.P., Goff, D.C. Jr., Bigger, J.T., Buse, J.B., Cushman, W.C., Genuth, S., Ismail-Beigi, F., Grimm, R.H. Jr., Probstfield, J.L., Simons-Morton, D.G., & Friedewald, W.T. (2008). Action to Control Cardiovascular Risk in Diabetes Study Group. Effects of intensive glucose lowering in type 2 diabetes. *N Engl J Med*, 358:2545- 2559.

Greenfield, S., Billimek, J., Pellegrini, F., Franciosi, M., De Berardis, G., Nicolucci, A., & Kaplan, S.H. (2009). Comorbidity affects the relationship between glycemic control and cardiovascular outcomes in diabetes: a cohort study. *Ann Intern Med*, 151:854-860.

Hamblin, M., Friedman, D.B., Hill, S., Caprioli, R.M., Smith, H.M., & Hill, M.F. (2007a). Alterations in the diabetic myocardial proteome coupled with increased myocardial oxidative stress underlies diabetic cardiomyopathy. *J Mol Cell Cardiol*, 42:884-895.

Hamblin, M., Smith, H.M., & Hill, M.F. (2007b). Dietary supplementation with vitamin E ameliorates cardiac failure in type I diabetic cardiomyopathy by suppressing myocardial generation of 8-iso-prostaglandin F2alpha and oxidized glutathione. *J Card Fail*, 13:884- 892.

Hamby, R.I., Zoneraich, S., & Sherman, L. (1974). Diabetic cardiomyopathy. *JAMA*, 23:1749-1754.

Ho, K.K., Pinsky, J.L., Kannel, W.B., & Levy, D. (1993). The epidemiology of heart failure: the Framingham Study. *J Am Coll Cardiol*, 22(4 Suppl A):6A-13A.

Huang, J.P., Huang, S.S., Deng, J.Y., Chang, C.C., Day, Y.J., & Hung, L.M. (2010). Insulin and resveratrol act synergistically, preventing cardiac dysfunction in diabetes, but the advantage of resveratrol in diabetics with acute heart attack is antagonized by insulin. *Free Radic Biol Med*, 49:1710-1721.

Inoguchi, T., Battan, R., Handler, E., Sportsman, J.R., Heath, W., & King, G.L. (1992). Preferential elevation of protein kinase C isoform beta II and diacylglycerol levels in the aorta and heart of diabetic rats: differential reversibility to glycemic control by islet cell transplantation. *Proc Natl Acad Sci U S A*, 89:11059-11063.

Iyer, R.S., Ghosh, S., & Salomon, R.G. (1989). Levuglandin E2 crosslinks proteins. *Prostaglandins*, 37:471-480, 1989.

Jaffe, A.S., Spadaro, J.J., Schechtman, K., Roberts, R., Geltman, E.M., & Sobel, B.E. (1984). Increased congestive heart failure after myocardial infarction of modest extent in patients with diabetes mellitus. *Am Heart J*, 108:31-37.

Jain, S.K. & Levine, S.N. (1995). Elevated lipid peroxidation and vitamin E-quinone levels in heart ventricles of streptozotocin-treated diabetic rats. *Free Radic Biol Med*, 18:337-341.

Jax, T. (2009). Treatment of patients with diabetes with GLP-1 analogues or DPP-4-inhibitors: a hot topic for cardiologists? *Clin Res Cardiol*, 98:75-79.

Jirousek, M.R., Murthi, K.K., & Salomon, R.G. (1990). Electrophilic levuglandin E2-protein adducts bind glycine: a model for protein crosslinking. *Prostaglandins*, 40:187-203.

Kamalesh, M. (2007). Heart failure in diabetes and related conditions. *J Card Fail*, 13:861-873.

Kannel, W.B., Hjortland, M., & Castelli ,W.P. (1974). Role of diabetes in congestive heart failure: the Framingham study. *Am J Cardiol*, 34:29-34.

Kannel, W.B. & McGee, DL. (1979). Diabetes and cardiovascular disease. The Framingham study. *JAMA*, 11:2035-2038.

Karamitsos, T.D., Karvounis, H.I., Dalamanga, E.G., Papadopoulos, C.E., Didangellos, T.P., Karamitsos, D.T., Parharidis, G.E., & Louridas, G.E. (2007). Early diastolic impairment of diabetic heart: the significance of right ventricle. *Int J Cardiol*, 114:218-223.

Kaul, N., Siveski-Iliskovic, N., Hill, M., Slezak, J., & Singal, P.K. (1993). Free radicals and the heart. *J Pharmacol Toxicol Methods*, 30:55-67.

Kaul, N., Siveski-Iliskovic, N., Thomas, T.P., Hill, M., Khaper, N., & Singal, P.K. (1995). Probucol improves antioxidant activity and modulates development of diabetic cardiomyopathy. *Nutrition*, 11:551-554.

Kaul, N., Siveski-Iliskovic, N., Hill, M., Khaper, N., Seneviratne, C., & Singal P.K. (1996). Probucol treatment reverses antioxidant and functional deficit in diabetic cardiomyopathy. *Mol. Cell. Biochem*, 160/161: 283-288.

Kiencke, S., Handschin, R., von Dahlen, R., Muser, J., Brunner-Larocca, H.P., Schumann ,J., Felix, B., Berneis, K., & Rickenbacher, P. (2010). Pre-clinical diabetic cardiomyopathy: prevalence, screening, and outcome. *Eur J Heart Fail*, 12:951-957.

Kim, B.O., Verma, S., Weisel, R.D., Fazel, S., Jia, Z.Q., Mizuno, T., & Li, R.K. (2008). Preservation of heart function in diabetic rats by the combined effects of muscle cell implantation and insulin therapy. *Eur J Heart Fail*, 10:14-21.

Kim, J.J. & Battaile, K.P. (2002). Burning fat: the structural basis of fatty acid beta-oxidation. *Curr Opin Struct Biol*, 12:721-728.

Konduracka, E., Gackowski, A., Rostoff, P., Galicka-Latala, D., Frasik, W., & Piwowarska, W. (2007). Diabetes-specific cardiomyopathy in type 1 diabetes mellitus: no evidence for its occurrence in the era of intensive insulin therapy. *Eur Heart J*, 28:2465-2471.

Kralik, P.M., Ye, G., Metreveli, N.S., Shen, X., & Epstein, P.N. (2005). Cardiomyocyte dysfunction in models of type 1 and type 2 diabetes. *Cardiovasc Toxicol*, 5:285-292.

Kuo, T.H., Moore, K.H., Giacomelli, F., & Wiener, J. (1983). Defective oxidative metabolism of heart mitochondria from genetically diabetic mice. *Diabetes*, 32:781-787.

Levy, A.P., Gerstein, H.C., Miller-Lotan, R., Ratner, R., McQueen, M., Lonn, E, & Pogue, J. (2004). The effect of vitamin E supplementation on cardiovascular risk in diabetic individuals with different haptoglobin phenotypes. *Diabetes Care*, 27:2767.

Li, J.H., Zhang, N., & Wang, J.A. (2008). Improved anti-apoptotic and anti-remodeling potency of bone marrow mesenchymal stem cells by anoxic pre-conditioning in diabetic cardiomyopathy. *Endocrinol Invest*, 31:103-110.

Liang, Q., Carlson, E.C., Donthi, R.V., Kralik, P.M., Shen, X., & Epstein, P.N. (2002). Overexpression of metallothionein reduces diabetic cardiomyopathy. *Diabetes*, 51:171 181.

Lind, M., Bounias, I., Olsson, M., Gudbjörnsdottir, S., Svensson, A-M., & Rosengren, A. (2011). Glycaemic control and incidence of heart failure in 20 985 patients with type 1 diabetes: an observational study. *Lancet*, 378: 140–146.

Loganathan, R., Bilgen, M., Al-Hafez, B., Alenezy, M.D., & Smirnova, I.V. (2006). Cardiac dysfunction in the diabetic rat: quantitative evaluation using high resolution magnetic resonance imaging. *Cardiovasc Diabetol*, 5:7.

Maisel, A.S., McCord, J., Nowak, R.M., Hollander, J.E., Wu, A.H., Duc, P., Omland, T., Storrow, A.B., Krishnaswamy, P., Abraham, W.T., Clopton, P., Steg, G., Aumont, M.C., Westheim, A., Knudsen, C.W., Perez, A., Kamin, R., Kazanegra, R., Herrmann, H.C., & McCullough, P.A.; Breathing Not Properly Multinational Study Investigators. (2003). Bedside B-Type natriuretic peptide in the emergency diagnosis of heart failure with reduced or preserved ejection fraction. Results from the Breathing Not Properly Multinational Study. *J Am Coll Cardiol*, 41:2010-2017.

Mamputu, J.C. & Renier, G. (2002). Advanced glycation end products increase, through a protein kinase C-dependent pathway, vascular endothelial growth factor expression in retinal endothelial cells. Inhibitory effect of gliclazide. *J Diabetes Complications*, 16:284-293.

Marwick, T.H. (2006). Diabetic heart disease. *Heart*, 92:296-300.

Masoudi, F.A., Inzucchi, S.E., Wang, Y., Havranek, E.P., Foody, J.M., & Krumholz, H.M. (2005). Thiazolidinediones, metformin, and outcomes in older patients with diabetes and heart failure: an observational study. *Circulation*, 111:583-590.

Maya, L. & Villarreal, F.J. (2010). Diagnostic approaches for diabetic cardiomyopathy and myocardial fibrosis. *J Mol Cell Cardiol*, 48:524-529.

Mihm, M.J., Seifert, J.L., Coyle, C.M., & Bauer, J.A. (2001). Diabetes related cardiomyopathy time dependent echocardiographic evaluation in an experimental rat model. *Life Sci*, 69:527-542.

Mildenberger, R.R., Bar-Shlomo, B., Druck, M.N., Jablonsky, G., Morch, J.E., Hilton, J.D., Kenshole, A.B., Forbath, N., & McLaughlin, P.R. (1984). Clinically unrecognized ventricular dysfunction in young diabetic patients. *J Am Coll Cardiol*, 4:234-238.

Milman, U., Blum, S., Shapira, C., Aronson, D., Miller-Lotan, R., Anbinder, Y., Alshiek, J., Bennett, L., Kostenko, M., Landau, M., Keidar, S., Levy, Y., Khemlin, A., Radan, A., & Levy, A.P. (2008). Vitamin E supplementation reduces cardiovascular events in a subgroup of middle-aged individuals with both type 2 diabetes mellitus and the haptoglobin 2-2 genotype: a prospective double-blinded clinical trial. *Arterioscler Thromb Vasc Biol*, 28:341-347.

Montuschi, P., Barnes, P.J., & Roberts, L.J. 2nd. (2004). Isoprostanes: markers and mediators of oxidative stress. *FASEB J*, 18:1791-1800.

Morrow, J.D., Hill, K.E., Burk, R.F., Nammour, T.M., Badr, K.F., & Roberts, L.J. 2nd. (1990). A series of prostaglandin F2-like compounds are produced in vivo in humans by a non- cyclooxygenase, free radical-catalyzed mechanism. *Proc Natl Acad Sci U S A*, 87:9383- 9387.

Mozaffari, M.S., Allo, S., & Schaffer, S.W. (1989). The effect of sulfonylurea therapy on defective calcium movement associated with diabetic cardiomyopathy. *Can J Physiol Pharmacol*, 67:1431-1436.

Murarka, S. & Movahed, M.R. (2010). Diabetic cardiomyopathy. *J Card Fail*, 16:971-979.

Mytas, D.Z., Stougiannos, P.N., Zairis, M.N., Foussas, S.G., Pyrgakis, V.N., & Kyriazis, I.A. (2009). Diabetic myocardial disease: pathophysiology, early diagnosis and therapeutic options. *Diabetes Complications*, 23:273-282.

Nathan, D.M., Cleary, P.A., Backlund, J.Y., Genuth, S.M., Lachin, J.M., Orchard, T.J., Raskin, P., & Zinman B; Diabetes Control and Complications Trial/Epidemiology of Diabetes Interventions and Complications (DCCT/EDIC) Study Research Group. (2005). Intensive diabetes treatment and cardiovascular disease in patients with type 1 diabetes. *N Engl J Med*, 353:2643-2653.

Nicolino, A., Longobardi, G., Furgi, G., Rossi, M., Zoccolillo, N., Ferrara, N., & Rengo, F. (1995). Left ventricular diastolic filling in diabetes mellitus with and without hypertension. *Am J Hypertens*, 8:382-389.

Nikolaidis, L.A., Mankad, S., Sokos, G.G., Miske, G., Shah, A., Elahi, D., & Shannon, R.P. (2004). Effects of glucagon-like peptide-1 in patients with acute myocardial infarction and left ventricular dysfunction after successful reperfusion. *Circulation*, 109:962-965.

Nishikawa, T., Edelstein, D., Du, X.L., Yamagishi, S., Matsumura, T., Kaneda, Y., Yorek, M.A., Beebe, D., Oates, P.J., Hammes, H.P., Giardino, I., & Brownlee, M. (2000). Normalizing mitochondrial superoxide production blocks three pathways of hyperglycemic damage. *Nature*, 404:787-790.

Nishio, Y., Kashiwagi, A., Taki, H., Shinozaki, K., Maeno, Y., Kojima, H., Maegawa, H., Haneda, M., Hidaka, H., Yasuda, H., Horiike, K., & Kikkawa, R. (1998). Altered activities of transcription factors and their related gene expression in cardiac tissues of diabetic rats. *Diabetes*, 47:1318-1325.

Ozasa, N., Furukawa, Y., Morimoto, T., Tadamura, E., Kita, T., & Kimura, T. (2008). Relation among left ventricular mass, insulin resistance, and hemodynamic parameters in type 2 diabetes. *Hypertens Res*, 31:425-432.

Palace, V., Kumar, D., Hill, M.F., Khaper, N., & Singal, P.K. (1999). Regional differences in non-enzymatic antioxidants in the heart under control and oxidative stress conditions. *J Mol Cell Cardiol*, 31:193-202.

Patel, A., MacMahon, S., Chalmers, J., Neal, B., Billot, L., Woodward, M., Marre, M., Cooper, M., Glasziou, P., Grobbee, D., Hamet, P., Harrap, S., Heller, S., Liu, L., Mancia, G., Mogensen, C.E., Pan, C., Poulter, N., Rodgers, A., Williams, B., Bompoint, S., de Galan, B.E., Joshi, R., & Travert, F. (2008). ADVANCE Collaborative Group. Intensive blood glucose control and vascular outcomes in patients with type 2 diabetes. *N Engl J Med*, 358:2560-2572.

Peppa, J., Uribarri, J., & Vlassara, H. (2003). Glucose, advanced glycation end products, and diabetes complications: what is new and what works. *Clin Diabetes*, 21: 186–187.

Pierce, G.N. & Dhalla, N.S. (1985). Heart mitochondrial function in chronic experimental diabetes in rats. *Can J Cardiol*, 1:48-54.

Poirier, P., Bogaty, P., Garneau, C., Marois, L., & Dumesnil, J.G. (2001). Diastolic dysfunction in normotensive men with well-controlled type 2 diabetes: importance of maneuvers in echocardiographic screening for preclinical diabetic cardiomyopathy. *Diabetes Care*, 24:5- 10.

Privratsky, J.R., Wold, L.E., Sowers, J.R., Quinn, M.T., & Ren, J. (2003). AT1 blockade prevents glucose-induced cardiac dysfunction in ventricular myocytes: role of the AT1 receptor and NADPH oxidase. *Hypertension*, 42:206-212.

Radovits, T., Korkmaz, S., Loganathan, S., Barnucz, E., Bömicke, T., Arif, R., Karck, M., & Szabó, G. (2009). Comparative investigation of the left ventricular pressure-volume relationship in rat models of type 1 and type 2 diabetes mellitus. *Am J Physiol Heart Circ Physiol*, 297:H125-H133.

Raev, D.C. (1994). Which left ventricular function is impaired earlier in the evolution of diabetic cardiomyopathy? An echocardiographic study of young type I diabetic patients. *Diabetes Care*, 17:633-639.

Regan ,T.J., Lyons, M.M., Ahmed, S.S., Levinson, G.E., Oldewurtel, H.A., Ahmad, M.R., & Haider, B. (1977). Evidence for cardiomyopathy in familial diabetes mellitus. *J Clin Invest*, 60:884-899.

Ritchie, R.H., Quinn, J.M., Cao, A.H., Drummond, G.R., Kaye, D.M., Favaloro, J.M., Proietto, J., & Delbridge, L.M. (2007). The antioxidant tempol inhibits cardiac hypertrophy in the insulin-resistant GLUT4-deficient mouse in vivo. *J Mol Cell Cardiol*, 42:1119-1128.

Roberts, L.J. 2nd, Salomon, R.G., Morrow, J.D., & Brame, C.J. (1999). New developments in the isoprostane pathway: identification of novel highly reactive gamma-ketoaldehydes (isolevuglandins) and characterization of their protein adducts. *FASEB J*, 13:1157-1168.

Roberts, L.J. 2nd, Oates, J.A., Linton, M.F., Fazio, S., Meador, B.P., Gross, M.D., Shyr, Y., & Morrow, J.D. (2007). The relationship between dose of vitamin E and suppression of oxidative stress in humans. *Free Radic Biol Med*, 43:1388-1393.

Roberts, L.J. 2nd, Traber, M.G., & Frei, B. (2009). Vitamins E and C in the Prevention of Cardiovascular Disease and Cancer in Men. *Free Radic Biol Med*, 46:1558.

Rubler, S., Dlugash, J., Yuceoglu, Y.Z., Kumral, T., Branwood, A.W., & Grishman, A. (1972). New type of cardiomyopathy associated with diabetic glomerulosclerosis. *Am J Cardiol*, 30:595-602.

Salomon, R.G., Jirousek, M.R., Ghosh, S., & Sharma, R.B. (1987). Prostaglandin endoperoxides 21. Covalent binding of levuglandin E2 with proteins. *Prostaglandins*, 34:643-656.

Sharma, V., Dhillon, P., Wambolt, R., Parsons, H., Brownsey, R., Allard, M.F., & McNeill, J.H. (2008). Metoprolol improves cardiac function and modulates cardiac metabolism in the streptozotocin-diabetic rat. *Am J Physiol Heart Circ Physiol*, 294:H1609-H1620.

Shen, X., Zheng, S., Thongboonkerd, V., Xu, M., Pierce, W.M. Jr., Klein, J.B., & Epstein, P.N. (2004). Cardiac mitochondrial damage and biogenesis in a chronic model of type 1 diabetes. *Am J Physiol Endocrinol Metab*, 287:E896-E905.

Shen, X., Ye, G., Metreveli, N.S., & Epstein, P.N. (2005). Cardiomyocyte defects in diabetic models and protection with cardiac-targeted transgenes. *Methods Mol Med* ,112:379-388.

Shen, X., Zheng, S., Metreveli, N.S., & Epstein, P.N. (2006). Protection of cardiac mitochondria by overexpression of MnSOD reduces diabetic cardiomyopathy. *Diabetes*, 55:798-805.

Shimizu, M., Umeda, K., Sugihara, N., Yoshio, H., Ino, H., Takeda, R., Okada, Y., & Nakanishi, I. (1993). Collagen remodelling in myocardia of patients with diabetes. *J Clin Pathol*, 46:32-36.

Shirpoor, A., Salami, S., Khadem-Ansari, M.H., Ilkhanizadeh, B., Pakdel, F.G., & Khademvatani, K. (2009). Cardioprotective effect of vitamin E: rescues of diabetes-induced cardiac malfunction, oxidative stress, and apoptosis in rat. *Diabetes Complications*, 23:310-316.

Shivalkar, B., Dhondt, D., Goovaerts, I., Van Gaal, L., Bartunek, J., Van Crombrugge, P., & Vrints, C. (2006). Flow mediated dilatation and cardiac function in type 1 diabetes mellitus. *Am J Cardiol*, 97:77-82.

Simpson, S.H., Majumdar, S.R., Tsuyuki, R.T., Eurich, D.T., & Johnson, J.A. (2006). Dose-response relation between sulfonylurea drugs and mortality in type 2 diabetes mellitus: a population-based cohort study. *CMAJ*, 174:169-174.

Singal, P.K., Petkau, A., Gerrard, J.M., Hrushovetz, S., & Foerster, J. (1988). Free radicals in health and disease. *Mol Cell Biochem*, 84:121-122.

Singh, R., Barden, A., Mori, T., & Beilin, L. (2001). Advanced glycation end-products: a review. *Diabetologia*, 44:129-146.

Sokos, G.G., Nikolaidis, L.A., Mankad, S., Elahi, D., & Shannon RP. (2006). Glucagon-like peptide-1 infusion improves left ventricular ejection fraction and functional status in patients with chronic heart failure. *J Card Fail*,12:694-699.

Solomon, S.D., St John Sutton, M., Lamas, G.A., Plappert, T., Rouleau, J.L., Skali, H., Moyé, L., Braunwald, E., & Pfeffer, M.A.; Survival And Ventricular Enlargement (SAVE) Investigators. (2002). Ventricular remodeling does not accompany the development of heart failure in diabetic patients after myocardial infarction. *Circulation*, 106, 1251-1255.

Spector, K.S. (1998). Diabetic cardiomyopathy. *Clin Cardiol*, 21:885-887.

Spiro, M.J. & Crowley, T.J. (1993). Increased rat myocardial type VI collagen in diabetes mellitus and hypertension. *Diabetologia*, 36:93-98.

Stevanovic,A., Dekleva, M., Andric, V., Sevic, L.J.,Pencic, B., Podnar, G., & Davidovic, N. (2006). Brain natriuretic peptide level could predict the late progression of left ventricular diastolic dysfunction in diabetic patients; one year follow up. *European Journal of Echocardiography*, 7 (Suppl 1):S26.

Struthers, A.D. & Morris, A.D. (2002). Screening for and treating left-ventricular abnormalities in diabetes mellitus: a new way of reducing cardiac deaths. *Lancet*, 359:1430-1432.

Sulaiman, M., Matta, M.J., Sunderesan, N.R., Gupta, M.P., Periasamy, M., & Gupta, M. (2010). Resveratrol, an activator of SIRT1, upregulates sarcoplasmic calcium ATPase and improves cardiac function in diabetic cardiomyopathy. *Am J Physiol Heart Circ Physiol*, 298:H833-H843.

Susic, D., Varagic, J., Ahn, J., & Frohlich, E.D. (2004). Collagen cross-link breakers: a beginning of a new era in the treatment of cardiovascular changes associated with aging, diabetes, and hypertension. *Curr Drug Targets Cardiovasc Haematol Disord*, 4:97-101.

Symeonides, P., Koulouris, S., Vratsista, E., Triantafyllou, K., Ioannidis, G., Thalassinos, N., & Katritsis, D. (2007).Both ramipril and telmisartan reverse indices of early diabetic cardiomyopathy: a comparative study. *Eur J Echocardiogr*, 8:480-486.

The Diabetes Control and Complications Trial Research Group. (1993). The effect of intensive treatment of diabetes on the development and progression of long-term complications in insulin-dependent diabetes mellitus. *N Engl J Med*, 329:977-986.

Thiemermann, C., McDonald, M.C., & Cuzzocrea, S. (2001). The stable nitroxide, tempol, attenuates the effects of peroxynitrite and oxygen-derived free radicals. *Crit Care Med*, 29:223-224.

Thirunavukkarasu, M., Penumathsa, S.V., Koneru, S., Juhasz, B., Zhan, L., Otani, H., Bagchi, D., Das, D.K., & Maulik, N. (2007). Resveratrol alleviates cardiac dysfunction in streptozotocin-induced diabetes: Role of nitric oxide, thioredoxin, and heme oxygenase. *Free Radic Biol Med*, 43:720-729.

Thrainsdottir, I., Malmberg, K., Olsson, A., Gutniak, M., & Rydén, L. (2004). Initial experience with GLP-1 treatment on metabolic control and myocardial function in patients with type 2 diabetes mellitus and heart failure. *Diab Vasc Dis Res*, 1:40-43.

Tomita, M., Mukae, S., Geshi, E., Umetsu, K., Nakatani, M., & Katagiri, T. (1996). Mitochondrial respiratory impairment in streptozotocin-induced diabetic rat heart. *Jpn Circ J*, 60:673-682.

Traber, M.G., Frei, B., & Beckman, J.S. (2008). Vitamin E revisited: do new data validate benefits for chronic disease prevention? *Curr Opin Lipidol*, 19:30-38.

Valensi, P., Sachs, R.N., Lormeau, B., Taupin, J.M., Ouzan, J., Blasco, A., Nitenberg, A., Metz, D., Paries, J., Talvard, O., Leutenegger, M., & Attali, J.R. (1997). Silent myocardial ischaemia and left ventricle hypertrophy in diabetic patients. *Diabetes Metab*, 23:409-416.

Valle, R., Bagolin, E., Canali, C., Giovinazzo, P., Barro, S., Aspromonte, N., Carbonieri, E., & Milani, L. (2006). The BNP assay does not identify mild left ventricular diastolic dysfunction in asymptomatic diabetic patients. *Eur J Echocardiogr*, 7:40-44.

Van Den Bergh, A., Flameng, W., & Herijgers, P. (2006). Type II diabetic mice exhibit contractile dysfunction but maintain cardiac output by favourable loading conditions. *Eur J Heart Fail*, 8:777-783.

Van Den Hurk, K., Alssema, M., Kamp, O., Henry, R.M., Stehouwer, .C.D, Diamant, M., Boomsma, F., Heine, R.J., Nijpels, G., Paulus, W.J., & Dekker, J.M. (2010). Slightly elevated B-type natriuretic peptide levels in a non-heart failure range indicate a worse left ventricular diastolic function in individuals with, as compared with individuals without, type 2 diabetes: the Hoorn Study. *Eur J Heart Fail*, 12:958-965.

Van Heerebeek, L., Hamdani, N., Handoko, M.L., Falcao-Pires, I., Musters, R.J., Kupreishvili, K., Ijsselmuiden, A.J., Schalkwijk, C.G., Bronzwaer, J.G., Diamant, M., Borbély, A., van der Velden, J., Stienen, G.J., Laarman, G.J., Niessen, H.W., & Paulus, W.J. (2008). Diastolic stiffness of the failing diabetic heart: importance of fibrosis, advanced glycation end products, and myocyte resting tension. *Circulation*, 117:43-51.

Von Bibra, H., Thrainsdottir, I.S., Hansen, A., Dounis, V., Malmberg, K., & Rydén, L. (2005). Tissue Doppler imaging for the detection and quantitation of myocardial dysfunction in patients with type 2 diabetes mellitus. *Diab Vasc Dis Res*, 2:24-30.

Wang, J., Song, Y., Wang, Q., Kralik, P.M., & Epstein, P.N. (2006a). Causes and characteristics of diabetic cardiomyopathy. *Rev Diabet Stud*, 3:108-117.

Wang, J., Song, Y., Elsherif, L., Song, Z., Zhou, G., Prabhu, S.D., Saari, J.T., & Cai, L. (2006b). Cardiac metallothionein induction plays the major role in the prevention of diabetic cardiomyopathy by zinc supplementation. *Circulation*, 113:544-554.

Way, K.J., Katai, N., & King, G.L. (2001). Protein kinase C and the development of diabetic vascular complications. *Diabet Med*, 18:945-959.

Xia, Z., Kuo, K.H., Nagareddy, P.R., Wang, F., Guo, Z., Guo, T., Jiang, J., & McNeill, J.H. (2007). N-acetylcysteine attenuates PKCbeta2 overexpression and myocardial hypertrophy in streptozotocin-induced diabetic rats. *Cardiovasc Res*, 73:770-782.

Ye, G., Metreveli, N.S., Donthi, R.V., Xia, S., Xu, M., Carlson, E.C., & Epstein, P.N. (2004). Catalase protects cardiomyocyte function in models of type 1 and type 2 diabetes. *Diabetes*, 53:1336-1343.

Zabalgoitia, M., Ismaeil, M.F., Anderson, L., & Maklady, F.A. (2001). Prevalence of diastolic dysfunction in normotensive, asymptomatic patients with well-controlled type 2 diabetes mellitus. *Am J Cardiol*, 87:320-323.

Zhang, C.H., Lu, J., Yu, X.J., Sun, L., & Zang, W.J. (2008). Ameliorative effect of Captopril and Valsartan on an animal model of diabetic cardiomyopathy. *Biol Pharm Bull*, 31:2045-2049.

Zhang, J.N., Geng, Q., Chen, X.J., Fang, W.W., Wu, X.H., & Yang, D. (2003). Alteration of endothelin system and calcium handling protein in left ventricles following drug treatment in dilated cardiomyopathy rats. *Acta Pharmacol Sin*, 24:1099-1102.

Zhang, N., Li, J., Luo, R., Jiang, J., & Wang, J.A. (2008). Bone marrow mesenchymal stem cells induce angiogenesis and attenuate the remodeling of diabetic cardiomyopathy. *Exp Clin Endocrinol Diabetes*, 116:104-111.

4

The Evolving Face of Heart Failure Associated with Elevated Cardio-Metabolic Risk Factors

Chaitanya Dutt, Vijay Chauthaiwale, Anookh Mohanan,
Kumar Prafull Chandra, Shital Kumar Zambad,
Ram Gupta and Siralee Parikh
Torrent Pharmaceuticals Limited
India

1. Introduction

1.1 Evolving profile of heart failure

There have been many definitions of Heart Failure and yet the most recent definitions rely heavily on clinical manifestations: dyspnoea or undue fatigue on exertion, along with the evidence of fluid retention, supported by objective evidence of structural or functional abnormalities of the heart at rest. A more recent classification also recognizes and emphasizes the need for the above signs and symptoms for both the development and progression of heart failure (Dickstein et al., 2008). The 2009 update of the AHA guideline identifies patients at higher risk of developing or progressing more rapidly to heart failure as traditionally defined. Table 1.

The presence of cardio-metabolic risk factors (hypertension, diabetes, obesity and metabolic syndrome) in addition to atherosclerotic disease puts the patient at twice greater risk of developing and/or progressing to heart failure as currently defined i.e. with structural or functional heart disease at rest. Studies across the world, particularly in India, China and Latin America suggest that overweight, metabolically challenged individuals are at greater risk of heart failure at a younger age and are also twice as likely to have heart failure linked events such as hospitalization or mortality (Clarke et al., 2010).

Echocardiography and Doppler imaging of the heart are the current gold standards for identification of structural and to extent also functional abnormalities. Advances in Echocardiography and Doppler imaging have enabled the identification of an under-diagnosed entity described as diastolic dysfunction, an additional handicap for a failing heart. Prognosis of patients with predominant diastolic dysfunction (Heart Failure with Preserved Ejection Fraction: HFPEF) has been reported to be similar to those who have predominant systolic dysfunction. In some population surveys, up to 50% of patients fall in this category (Paulus, 1998). Many have co-morbidities identified as risk factors in Stage A of the AHA classification. It is therefore pertinent to understand why and how these additional risk factors influence the development and progression of heart failure as different from and often in addition to Atherosclerotic Coronary Artery Disease.

Diabetes, hypertension, dyslipidemia and thyroid dysfunction affecting heart are often considered as factors contributing to coronary artery disease. However, there is evidence to suggest that diabetes and hypertension may affect myocardial function largely independent of significant epicardial coronary artery disease. The main objective of this chapter is to explain holistic effects of cardio-metabolic risk factors on heart failure. We urge the reader to consider factors beyond the myocardium, such as vascular responsiveness, neuroendocrine maladaptation and renal function and correlate it with clinical manifestations. This chapter elucidates and correlates recent advances in understanding of etiological factors affecting the myocardial function, the mechanisms which could be influencing overall progression and presentation of heart failure, current diagnostic approaches, their limitations and emerging concepts, current medical therapies, their limitations and newer emerging therapeutic approaches.

Subjects at Risk for Heart Failure

STAGE A	STAGE B
High risk for HF Non symptomatic No structural defects	Non symptomatic Structural defects present
PATIENTS WITH – Hypertension – Atherosclerotic disease – Diabetes – Obesity – Metabolic syndrome or – Using cardiotoxins – With FHx CM	**PATIENTS WITH** – Previous MI – LV remodeling including LVH & low EF – Asymptomatic valvular disease
THERAPY ***Goals*** • Treat hypertension • Encourage smoking cessation • Treat lipid disorder • Encourage regular exercise • Discourage alcohol intake • Control metabolic syndrome ***Drugs*** • ACEI or ARB in appropriate patients for vascular disease or diabetes	**THERAPY** ***Goals*** • All measures under stage A ***Drugs*** • ACEI or ARB • β blockers ***Devices*** • In selected patients: Implantable defibrillators

Table 1. Stages in the development of heart failure and recommended therapy by stage. ACEI, angiotensin-converting enzyme inhibitors; ARB, angiotensin II receptor blocker; EF, ejection fraction; FHx CM, family history of cardiomyopathy; HF, heart failure; LVH, left ventricular hypertrophy; and MI, myocardial infarction. Modified from Jessup M, Abraham WT, Casey DE et al. 2009 focused update: ACCF/AHA guidelines for the diagnosis and management of heart failure in adults (Jessup et al., 2009).

2. Cardio-Metabolic Cardiomyopathy (CMCM)

The etiology of cardiomyopathy associated with diabetes is widely debated. While hyperglycemia is regarded as a sole culprit in causation of diabetic cardiomyopathy, there is a cluster of associated risk factors - obesity, hyperlipidemia, prothrombotic state, hypertension, activation of multiple hormone and cytokine systems etc, which are commonly seen in most patients presenting with diabetes of more than five years and these in turn have intricate effects in causation of cardiomyopathy. More and more researchers are now focusing on the overall impact of diabetes and cluster of these observable conditions on altered metabolism and energetics at cellular level of the target end organs, which are known to be most vulnerable to such altered conditions. Increasing evidence are now available which suggest that altered myocyte functioning is more a function of altered cellular metabolism. It is seen that simultaneous over-activation of renin-angiotensin-aldosterone system (RAAS), increased oxidative stress and compromised endothelial function, contributed by each individual component adds to overall dysfunction of myocardium. Effect on peripheral vasculature adds on to the already stressed myocardium and predispose to an early compromise in over all cardiovascular functions.

Many of the changes described occur in predisposed individuals even before the onset of diabetes, often at the stage when they may be diagnosed as having pre-hypertension or impaired glucose tolerance. There is therefore a need for holistic terminology which could represent contribution of not only of diabetes and associated hyperglycemia but equally of other factors - obesity, dyslipidemia, hypertension, in the pathogenesis of cardiomyopathy, for which the term "Cardio-metabolic Cardiomyopathy (CMCM)" seems appropriate (Fig. 1). The terminology CMCM is based on available evidence of altered

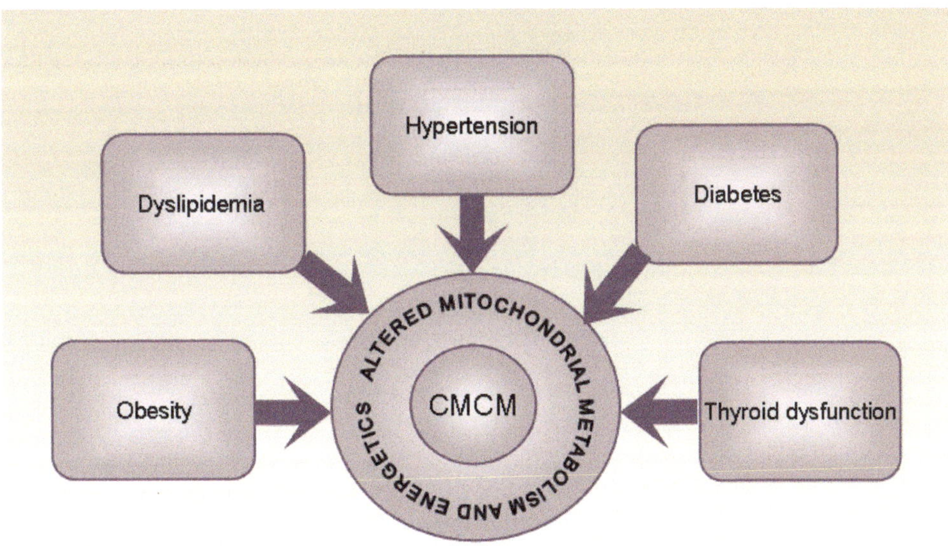

Fig. 1. Various possible risk factors that could contribute to the development of Cardio-metabolic Cardiomyopathy (CMCM).

myocytes metabolism and energetics leading to cardiomyopathy. This would need further support from ongoing and future research to consolidate itself as a new class of cardiomyopathy representing cluster of metabolic derangement and altered energetics of myocytes with a common underlying derangement - diminishing flexibility to use the appropriate fuel to provide adequate energy, resulting in dysfunctional mitochondria.

2.1 Mechanisms of CMCM

2.1.1 Myocardial metabolism in normal heart

A normal healthy heart uses free fatty acid (FFA) as its preferred fuel source and to a lesser extent, circulating glucose (Fig 2). In case of severe starvation it can also utilize lactate,

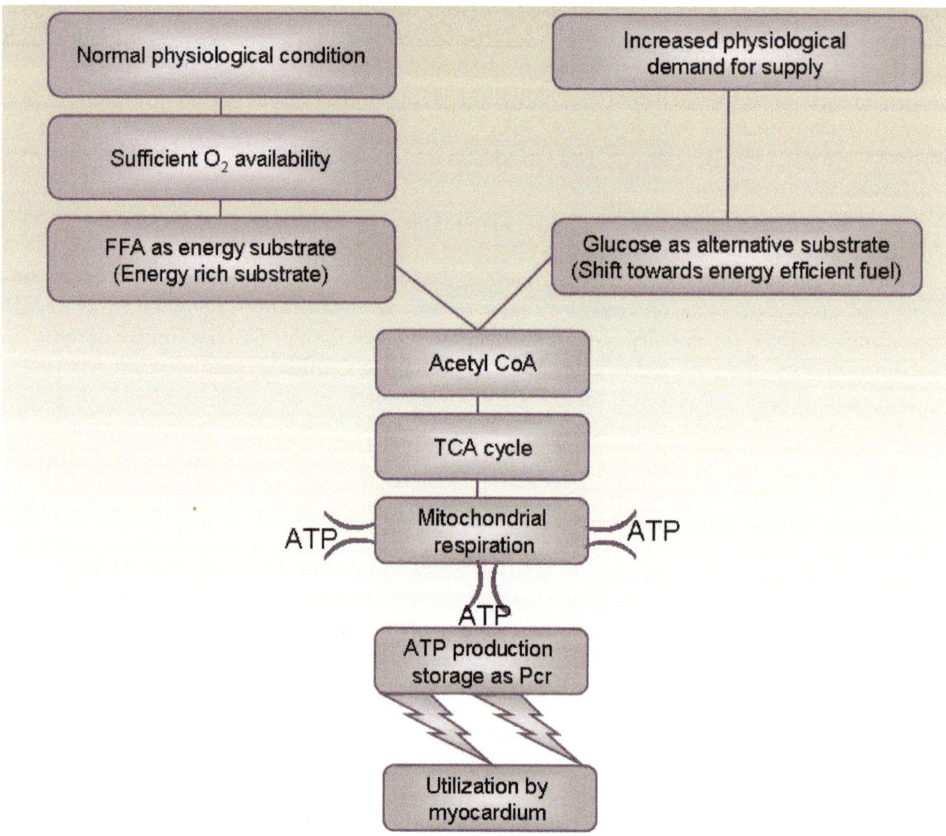

Fig. 2. Myocardial metabolism in normal heart. Normal myocardium at resting state uses FFA as a preferred fuel source, which is energy rich substrate but yield less ATP per mol of O_2. While in the state of increased peripheral physiological demand (e.g. exercise) myocardium uses glucose as energy source which is more efficient energy source and yield more ATP per mol of O_2.. ATP, Adenosine triphosphate; FFA, Free fatty acid; O_2, oxygen; Pcr, Phospho creatinine.

ketone bodies and amino acids. The regulation of myocardial metabolism is dependent on the availability and abundance of substrate, hormone levels, coronary blood flow and oxygenation and inotropic state of the tissue. With ageing, relative contribution of glucose as myocardial substrate increases as seen in elderly. The levels of FFA determine its uptake by myocytes. Following uptake and conjugation with acetyl CoA (FA-CoA), FA-CoA enters the mitochondria, via the carnitine acyl transferase shuttle (CPT-1 and CPT-2). CPT-1 is subject to allosteric regulation by malonyl CoA and effective transfer to the mitochondria requires adequate amounts of carnitine (Abel & Doenst, 2011). Upon entering the mitochondrial matrix, FA-CoA undergoes β-oxidation. Post prandial, higher levels of insulin in blood increases muscle glucose uptake by increasing glucose transporters (GLUT-1 and GLUT-4) translocation and by suppressing FFA release from adipose tissues thereby removing FFA mediated inhibition of glycolysis and pyruvate oxidation.

2.1.2 Metabolic disturbances in cardio-metabolic cardiomyopathy (CMCM)

There are many factors considered as initiators to the functional and structural alterations which contribute to the development and progression of CMCM. Most of these evidence are from animal experimental studies. Though development of CMCM is multi-factorial, metabolic disturbance is the major culprit.

2.1.2.1 Altered fuel supply and altered substrate utilization

Increasing evidence suggests that altered substrate supply and utilization by cardiac myocytes could be the initial trigger in the pathogenesis of CMCM. Under deranged metabolic milieu, inclusive of diabetes, heart use relatively more fat than normal heart (Herrero et al., 2006; Carley & Severson, 2005). The shift towards increased fatty acids and decreased glucose utilization is linked to elevated circulating levels of FFA and triglycerides as a consequence of enhanced adipose tissue lipolysis, increased FFA uptake as well as high tissue FFAs caused by hydrolysis of augmented myocardial triglyceride stores. Animal studies in db/db mice, (a model of type II diabetes with obesity and hyperglycemia), have shown increased cell membrane fatty acid (FA) transporters (FAT/CD36) and FA binding proteins leading to increased FA uptake in db/db mice hearts (Carley & Severson, 2008). To handle this increased FA, there is upregulation of mitochondrial enzymes involved in fat metabolism.

The reduced glucose utilization seen in such condition is partly accounted for by the slow rate of glucose transport across the sarco-lemmal membrane into the myocardium, which is probably due to the cellular depletion/reduced translocation of GLUT-4 caused by insulin resistance (Garvey et al., 1993). High circulating FFA and increased FA oxidation inhibits pyruvate dehydrogenase complex thereby reducing glucose oxidation.

Exercise influences myocardial glucose utilization, perhaps independent of insulin levels. Graded exercise in all cases of heart failure has been documented to be beneficial. It is likely that exercise has a beneficial effect in maintaining the substrate flexibility of the myocardium.

2.1.2.2 Lipotoxicity associated with excessive accumulation of intracellular lipids

When FA uptake exceeds FA oxidation capabilities, lipid accumulation occurs resulting in lipotoxicity. This is evident in diabetics and obese patients but not seen in non-obese. High circulating and cellular FFA necessitates abnormal higher oxygen demand during FFA metabolism in addition to enhancing peripheral insulin resistance. This results in accumulation of toxic intermediates of FFA metabolism leading to impaired functional performance. Fuel surplus is likely to activate peroxisome proliferators-activated receptor (PPAR-α) with subsequent increase in FA oxidation. Accumulation of palmitate results in increased free radical production and endoplasmic reticular stress which leads to apoptosis (Borradaile et al., 2006). Palmitate accumulation can also promote denovo ceramide production which is also an inducer of apoptosis. Carnitine, an essential substrate for myocardial FFA metabolism is reduced along with abnormal appearing mitochondria (Ashrafian et al., 2007).

Thus, impaired substrate flexibility and inefficient adenosine triphosphate (ATP) generation, resulting in inability in fulfillment of myocardial energy demand, initially on exertion, progressing to inadequacy at rest, is the hallmark of CMCM.

2.1.2.3 Increased generation of advanced glycation and lipoxidation end products along with reactive oxygen species affecting heart in altered metabolic conditions

Advanced glycation end products (AGEs) and advanced lipoxidation end products (ALEs) are formed when carbohydrate- or lipid-derived intermediates react with the amino group of proteins to form covalently modified, stable protein adducts. AGEs/ALEs formation results from a combination of hyperglycemia, hyperlipidemia, oxidative/carbonyl stress and/or decreased renal clearance (Miyata et al., 2001). These modifications may be a single change on the peptide chain or multiple modifications that can produce crosslinks within or between proteins. Long-lived proteins like collagen and elastin are highly vulnerable for crosslink formation with AGEs and ALEs. These modifications lead to impaired collagen degradation and thereby increased collagen accumulation and subsequent fibrosis.

AGEs accumulation exert their detrimental effect on cardiac structure and function by different mechanisms. Firstly, structural modification/crosslinkage of myocardial proteins involved in cardiac contraction or relaxation may occur, resulting in impaired systolic or diastolic function and structural alteration. By disrupting intra- and inter-domain tertiary structures of Sarcoplasmic/endoplasmic reticulum Ca2+-ATPase (SERCA2a), AGE complexes have shown to compromise structural movements required for translocating calcium ions from the cytosol to the lumen of the sarcoplasmic reticulum. Secondly, AGEs promote trans-differentiation of epithelial cells to myofibroblasts via their specific receptors (e.g., RAGE). Finally, activation of RAGE promotes inflammation and oxidative stress, which can decrease the bioavailability of nitric oxide. This may result in further increased oxidative stress and attenuated contribution of nitric oxide during myocardial relaxation (Goldin et al., 2006). Thus, AGE-RAGE interaction can have a direct functional impact on myocardial relaxation. There is also increased free radical generation and oxidative stress with subsequent activation of many deleterious pathways which lead to apoptosis and cell death. Effects of AGEs leading to increased stiffness of connective tissue, increased permeability and pro-coagulant state due to effects on endothelial functions, increased vascular matrix through mononuclear cell activation and defective vascular relaxation due to decreased nitrous oxide (NO) release, run hand in hand, with direct effects on heart and contribute to overall patho-physiology of CMCM.

Although many studies have not been reported with ALEs, yet, recent evidence suggests that ALEs induce inflammatory pathways and network similar to AGEs leading to vascular complications (Shanmugam et al., 2008). ALEs and AGEs go hand in hand from their generation to effect on different end organs and are not limited to diabetes. Effects of ALEs on myocardium in isolation, could be similar to AGEs, however, need further studies for better understanding.

2.1.3 Dysfunctional calcium homeostasis

Calcium, essential for the process of excitation-contraction, is the primary ionic regulator in the heart. In Type 2 rodent models of diabetes, altered expression, activity and function of many regulatory and contractile proteins/transporters involved in excitation-contraction coupling; SERCA, Na^+/Ca^{2+} exchange (NCX), ryanodine receptors (RyR) and plasma membrane Ca^{2+}-ATPase (PMCA), as well as dysfunctional intracellular calcium signaling, have been reported (Pereira et al., 2006; Vetter et al., 2002). These alterations have been attributed to accumulation of toxic molecules such as long-chain acylcarnitines, free radicals and abnormal membrane lipid content as well as to AGEs altering the structure and function of several proteins described above. The consequences of these changes include alterations to the calcium sensitivity of regulatory proteins involved in the regulation of the cardiac actomyosin system, possibly due to phosphorylation of sarcomeric protein troponin I. The diminished calcium sensitivity and altered activity of regulatory and contractile proteins may all contribute to impaired left ventricular (LV) function.

2.1.4 Altered thyroid hormone status

Recent evidence indicates that heart failure can lead to down-regulation of the thyroid hormone signaling system in the heart. In the failing heart, there is decrease in thyroid hormone receptor expression; in addition, serum levels of T4 and T3 are decreased with heart failure in the frame of the non-thyroidal illness syndrome (Kinugawa et al., 2001). Thyroid hormone levels have a profound impact on mitochondria, the organelles responsible for the majority of cellular ATP production. The hypermetabolic effects of thyroid hormones are partially due to an increased demand for ATP and partially due to increased uncoupling. In addition, thyroid hormones are potent activators of mitochondriogenesis. Key events in thyroid-hormone-induced mitochondriogenesis include the increased expression of the mitochondrial transcription factors, nuclear respiratory factor-1 (NRF-1) and peroxisome-proliferator-activated receptor gamma co-activator-1a (PGC-1a). In addition, transcriptional and post-transcriptional mechanisms are important for the effects of T3, for example, in the synthesis of cytochrome c oxidase subunits. Thus, thyroid hormones are key regulator of mitochondrial energetics. In animal models, it has been shown that in pressure overload-induced cardiac hypertrophy a decrease of thyroid hormone receptor level occurs. The decrease in T3 serves as an indicator for a bad prognosis in the heart failure patient being linked to increased mortality (Dillmann, 2010).

2.1.5 Up regulated renin-angiotensin-aldosterone and sympathetic system

RAAS and sympathetic system are profoundly dysregulated in metabolic deranged conditions and adipose tissue has a full local renin-angiotensin system that is active at local and systemic level (Sarzani et al., 2008). RAAS is considered to have a prime role in hypertensive cardiomyopathy even though several growth factors influence initiation and maintenance of myocardial hypertrophy. Both angiotensin II and aldosterone are shown to contribute to myocardial fibrosis (Sopel et al., 2011; Struthers & Unger, 2011). Correlation between circulating renin-angiotensin levels and left ventricular mass have long been established and same has been proved by the study showing regression of hypertensive left ventricular hypertrophy upon targeting RAAS (Solomon et al., 2009). Though synergistic effects of angiotensin II and aldosterone are well established with regard to perivascular and interstitial fibrosis of the ventricle; angiotensin-independent effect of aldosterone on myocardial fibrosis has also been demonstrated. Current evidence shows that aldosterone has some role in the transition of left ventricular hypertrophy to cardiac failure. In addition, aldosterone also has a role in fluid retention. Altered RAAS has implication in chronic kidney disease and impaired kidney function resulting in volume overload which results in exacerbation of symptoms of heart failure and disease progression.

In addition to high RAAS drive, sympathetic hyperactivity present in patients with deranged metabolic profile contributes not only to high blood pressure, but seems to have further adverse metabolic effects also, such as insulin resistance, hyperinsulinaemia and hyperlipidaemia. Experimental evidence has indicated that heightened sympathetic nervous system activity facilitates the development of myocardial hypertrophy in animals and humans. Antihypertensive vasodilators (hydralazine and minoxidil) which are known to have some stimulating effect on sympathetic nervous system fail to reduce left ventricular hypertrophy despite their well-documented antihypertensive effects (Elliott et al., 2008). Thus, if such a relationship between RAAS, sympathetic activation and left ventricular hypertrophy exists, there are all possibilities that cardiomyopathy in hypertensive patients may be resultant of this interaction. This becomes more evident especially since neuroendocrine activation is found in hypertensive cardiomyopathy, with activation of the RAAS and the sympathetic system. All these components are hypothesized to be constituent part of CMCM as both RAAS and sympathetic systems are up-regulated in them.

2.1.6 Diastolic dysfunction, systolic dysfunction and ventricular hypertrophy in CMCM

Ventricular diastolic function is dependent on an active relaxation process in conjunction with passive elastic properties of the myocardium. In diastolic dysfunction, there is impairment in ventricular relaxation and passive filling. About 75% of diabetics show this dysfunction which is more pronounced when other metabolic abnormalities co-exist. In diastolic heart failure, though the ejection fraction may be normal, there is diastolic dysfunction along with elevated end diastolic pressure.

Functional abnormalities occur as a result of structural remodeling. In diastolic dysfunction a moderate increase in left ventricular mass and an elevated ventricular wall thickness to chamber radius is seen (Ozasa et al., 2008). The end diastolic volume is nearly normal. Increase in AGE crosslinks of cardiac SERCA impairs the ability or capacity of SERCA to translocate calcium and thus slows the rate of cardiac relaxation. The reduction in elasticity of the myocardium is due to myocardial collagen deposition and AGE crosslinks with elastin (Van et al., 2008). This early cardiac dysfunction, along with other exacerbating risk factors accelerates the decline in cardiac function.

Under conditions of hyperinsulinemia, a basic component of increased cardio-metabolic risks, insulin stimulates hypertrophy in cardiomyocytes by several pathways, mainly by activation of Akt and ERK. Increased circulating angiotensin II induces cardiomyocyte hypertrophy and interstitial fibrosis (He et al., 2005). Angiotensin II is also reported to increase reactive oxygen species (ROS) production and excess ROS produces cardiomyocyte death and results in replacement fibrosis. Sympathetic activation, in addition to effects on blood pressure, seems to have adverse metabolic effects. Hence, the interstitial fibrosis, protein glycosylation and myocyte hypertrophy are likely factors contributing to reduced diastolic compliance and ventricular hypertrophy in CMCM patients.

In the presence of predominant diastolic dysfunction, supervening reduced systolic reserve is often overlooked by diagnostic imaging at rest. Increased intracellular fatty acids and its metabolites are toxic to the mitochondria and induce apoptosis and damage the contractile apparatus. Many studies have demonstrated that the inhibitory cardiac troponin-I (cTnI) expression is markedly raised in the heart of diabetic rats and in cardiac hypertrophy. GATA binding protein 4 (GATA-4) binding site in the proximal region of cTnI gene is necessary for the transcriptional activation of this gene. GATA-4 found in cardiac myocytes regulates many other cardiac-specific gene expressions, like angiotensin II (AT_{1A}) and endothelin-1 (ET_A) receptors, atrial natriuretic factor (ANF), beta-type natriuretic peptide (BNP), myosin heavy chain (MHC) etc. Studies have shown that activation of MEK/ERK pathway by hyperglycemia-induced ROS or by direct adrenergic stimulation, increase GATA-4 phosphorylation and nuclear translocation, in addition MEK/ERK activation also causes GSK3β phosphorylation, thereby lowering the export of GATA-4 from nucleus, leading to GATA-4 preservation in the nucleus, which finally leads to an increase in the expression level of cTnI resulting in reduced cardiac contractility (Ku et al., 2011).
The longitudinal fibres responsible for long-axis contraction lie in the sub-endocardium and are particularly susceptible to the effects of fibrosis, ischemia or hypertrophy. Initially the long-axis systolic dysfunction is associated with a compensatory increase in radial thickening and mass, thus preserving left ventricular ejection fraction (LVEF). The preservation of ejection fraction is directly related to the presence of LV hypertrophy and the effect of increased muscle mass. However, reserve systolic functions are reduced and these patients show enhanced systolic functional abnormalities only during stress or exercise. Clinical studies have demonstrated that diabetic patients have an increased end-systolic diameter and volume, a diminished ejection fraction and a decreased minor axis shortening and velocity of circumferential fiber shortening in the absence of coronary artery disease. This is exaggerated when exposed to stress like exercise. These dysfunctions coupled with dysfunction in peripheral vasculature in CMCM translate into profound compromise in overall exercise reserve.

2.2 A central role for mitochondrial dysfunction in CMCM

2.2.1 Normal role of mitochondria

Myocardial contractile function is energy (ATP) dependent. Mitochondria are the major site of substrate oxidation and ATP production in cardiomyocytes. In addition, mitochondria also contribute to intracellular ROS generation. It is by oxidative phosphorylation in the mitochondrial system through which the oxidation of energy substrates in a cell is coupled to the activity of ATP synthase in the mitochondrial inner membrane. The activity of ATP synthase is powered by the electrochemical gradient existing across the mitochondrial inner membrane. The ATP produced drives energy demanding reactions not only in the mitochondrion but also in the cytoplasm.

2.2.2 Abnormal mitochondrial morphology and function

Lines of evidence have shown that mitochondrial dysfunction contributes to the development of insulin resistance and metabolic syndrome. The causes of mitochondrial dysfunction are complex, but over-nutrition and sedentary life style are among the best known causes of mitochondrial dysfunction (Kim et al., 2008). The cardio-metabolic conditions such as insulin resistance, diabetes, hypertension, dyslipidemia and sub-clinical hypothyroidism are characterized by altered mitochondrial function. Visceral obesity and related cardio-metabolic disorders are linked to defective mitochondrial biogenesis and oxidative metabolism with decreased ATP production. The hypertrophy-related changes in myocardium are likely related to mitochondrial structural and functional alterations that leads to altered mitochondrial efficiency for substrate oxidation and ATP production. Studies have revealed distinct patterns in mitochondrial structural and functional alterations in pathological and physiological cardiac hypertrophy. Among many signaling pathways that conspire to impair mitochondrial function include, decreased expression or activity of transcriptional regulators that govern mitochondrial biogenesis and oxidative capacity (i.e. PGC-1α, ERRα, and PPAR-α) and decreased transcription of mitochondrial DNA. Increased G-protein-coupled receptor signaling activates Class1B PI3Kγ that leads to constitutive activation of Akt, which may repress mitochondrial function. Activation of HIF-1α leads to a PPAR-α mediated increase in FA uptake and lipogenesis that may promote lipotoxicity, which could further impair mitochondrial function. Reduced cardiolipin content and remodeling of the mitochondrial proteome also contribute to mitochondrial dysfunction. Mitochondrial dysfunction promotes oxidative stress that leads to a vicious cycle of progressive mitochondrial damage.

At functional level, activities of mitochondrial complex I and III reduce at the stage of compensated cardiac hypertrophy, but this is accompanied by reduced mitochondrial ROS and oxidative damage that only becomes evident after the transition to heart failure. Hypertrophied hearts do not lose mitochondrial membrane potential in the context of ischemia and re-perfusion injury. However, the increase in mitochondrial membrane potential correlates with an increased risk of arrhythmias. By the time compensated hypertrophy progresses to pathological LV hypertrophy, altered mitochondrial morphology and function are evident. Pathological hypertrophic cardiomyopathy displays swollen cardiac mitochondria with disrupted cristae and substantial mitochondrial DNA depletion.

Mitochondrial membrane permeabilization is a rate limiting step of apoptosis and is mediated by the mitochondrial permeability transition pore (mtPTP). mtPTP is a nonspecific pore, permeable to all molecules of less than 1.5 kDa and is formed by the voltage-dependent anion channel (VDAC), members of the pro- and anti-apoptotic Bax/Bcl2 protein family, cyclophilin D and adenine nucleotide translocase (ANT). The ANT mediates nucleotide transfer from mitochondria to cytosol. The ATP synthesized in the mitochondria is exchanged for cytosolic adenosine diphosphate (ADP) by ANT to provide a continuous supply of ADP to mitochondria. ATP/ADP exchange by ANT is essential for the maintenance of ATP synthase activity.

On the other hand, in states of impaired function of ATP/ADP exchange, ANT plays a major role in generating ROS and inducing cell apoptosis (Kim et al., 2010). Thus, impaired ANT activity could contribute to deficient energy availability in pathological cardiac hypertrophy. Reduced level of cardiac ANT has been reported in some, but not all models of pressure overload cardiac hypertrophy. Additional proteins that were proposed to be part of the mtPTP complex are hexokinase, creatine kinase, and peripheral benzodiazepine receptor. mtPTP opening causes swelling of the mitochondrial matrix and rupture of outer membrane.

Cardiolipin, an important component and one of the most abundant phospholipid of the inner mitochondrial membrane, is essential for the optimal function of numerous enzymes that are involved in mitochondrial energy metabolism, where it regulates the activity of the mitochondrial electron transport chain, ATP synthesis and mitochondrial bioenergetics (Abel & Doenst, 2011). Abundance of linoleic acid and close proximity to the site of ROS production, i.e. the inner mitochondrial membrane make cardiolipin particularly more susceptible to damage by oxidative stress. Cardiolipin is identified as the only phospholipid in mitochondria that undergoes early oxidation during apoptosis (Kagan et al., 2005). Cardiolipin peroxidation by ROS thus affects its binding with cytochrome c and affects the activity of complex I, III, and IV of the mitochondrial respiratory chain (Paradies et al., 2004). Mitochondrial cardiolipin content is reduced in heart failure and ischemia/reperfusion and correlates with reduced electron transport chain activities. Patients with obesity and insulin resistance have poorer outcomes after myocardial infarction compared with lean subjects. These changes are associated with reduced myocardial cardiolipin content (Sparagna et al., 2007). Thus, reduced myocardial cardiolipin content contributes to the reduced mitochondrial efficiency in diabetes and metabolic syndrome and may exacerbate the progression of CMCM.

3. Diagnosis

Cardiac dysfunction caused by a constellation of metabolic abnormality may have variety of presentations. On one hand it includes myocardial dysfunction and coronary artery disease and on the other hand it may be arrhythmias and sudden death. When a patient presents with features of heart failure like, exercise intolerance, fatigue, and dyspnea with exertion as prominent symptoms in background of metabolic abnormalities like impaired glucose metabolism, dyslipidemia and hypertension with or without subclinical hypothyroidism then CMCM should be considered.

Clinical assessment of patients of heart failure with metabolic disorder should start with a thorough history followed by evaluation of pulmonary function to rule out non cardiac causes of dyspnoea. This should be followed by evaluation of functional limitations and status of the structural defect in the heart. Thereafter, causes of heart failure and extent of compromise in hemodynamic (perfusion and volume) status should be assessed. Because progression of heart failure is relatively rapid in metabolically challenged patients, it is very important to identify defects early in asymptomatic patients in order to prevent progression to symptomatic disease.

Laboratory evaluation of patients should start with complete blood count, urinalysis, serum electrolytes, blood urea nitrogen, serum creatinine, fasting blood glucose (glycohemoglobin), lipid profile and liver function tests. Thyroid dysfunctions may be subclinical with normal serum free T4 (fT4), free T3 (fT3) levels but deranged serum thyroid stimulating hormone (TSH) levels. Use of biomarkers for diagnosis of heart failure includes a number of neuroendocrine hormones, including norepinephrine, angiotensin II, renin, aldosterone, vasopressin and most recently BNP. Association of abnormal levels of these biomarkers with abnormal myocardial function and the unfavorable prognostic significance are increasingly being recognized and used. Patients with history of diabetes and elderly patients who are at high risk of developing myocardial dysfunction have a high prevalence of elevated plasma BNP levels. Thus, these high risk populations with elevated plasma levels of BNP or NT-proBNP can be identified for detailed evaluation of cardiac functions by echocardiography and/or cardiopulmonary exercise testing (CPET).

Insulin resistance can be an important etiologic factor in the development of heart failure with metabolic disorder as adaptive responses of myocardium to different stress are compromised in presence of insulin resistance. Insulin resistance has strong correlation with development of hypertension, left ventricular hypertrophy and left ventricular dysfunction and subsequent development of heart failure. There is also increased prevalence of myocardial ischemia in patients with insulin resistance and heart failure itself causes insulin resistance (Wilson, 2001; Nikolaidis et al., 2004). Evidence of insulin resistance should be evaluated by measuring fasting insulin levels.

Assessment of myocardial wall thickness, LV size and pericardium by comprehensive two-dimensional Echocardiography along with Doppler imaging are useful diagnostic tests in the evaluation of patients of heart failure. The most common abnormality associated with insulin resistance and diabetes mellitus is abnormality in diastolic function which is independent of ischemic heart disease (Fang et al., 2004; Schannwell et al., 2002). Evaluation of ventricular filling pattern by color Doppler imaging evaluating diastolic dysfunction becomes important for diagnosing such symptomatic patients who have preserved ejection fraction. A comprehensive echocardiographic examination helps in these distinctions when more than one abnormality affects the cardiac functions.

Most of the above mentioned methods of evaluation examine patients at rest, thus have limitations. Physical limitations during exercise, like shortness of breath and fatigue are caused by dynamic dysfunctions in myocardium occurring under stress and may not manifest at rest. Thus, markers of diminished cardiac reserve often go undetected by echocardiography. Stress echocardiography can detect ventricular dysfunction including wall motion abnormalities (hypokinesia, akinesia, dyskinesia or diastolic dysfunction) when exposed to stress either by dobutamin or exercise. This can pick up early cases with compromsied ventricular functions, however, peripheral components of heart failure may still not be factored in it.

CPET is a well-established method of evaluating cardiopulmonary functions in heart failure. This is highly reproducible measurement and helps in differentiation of cause of symptoms associated with heart failure. Using CPET for evaluation of limitation in cardiac functions in the patients with heart failure associated with metabolic disorder will not only evaluate dynamic response of heart to physiological stress but also peripheral component of hemodynamics which often coexists. Symptoms such as fatigue and disproportionate dyspnoea may be explained by inadequate and inappropriate vascular responsiveness (capillary recruitment) to demand generated by exercising skeletal muscles (Joshi et al., 2010). Maximal aerobic capacity (peak VO_2), Ve/VCO_2 and oxygen uptake efficiency slope (OUES) parameters obtained from CPET aids in early diagnosis of subtle pathology and helps in following the progression of the disease. These have important prognostic value also.

Impedance cardiography can be used non-invasively to measure hemodynamic parameters to diagnose covert cases of CMCM. Experimental studies in diabetic patients measuring stroke volume and cardiac output by impedance cardiography at the time of rest and exercise suggest, compromise in cardiac reserve even in the absence of any clinical symptoms of heart failure (Joshi et al., 2010). Compromise in cardiac reserve was contributed to, by an inappropriate increase in stroke volume due to diastolic compromise exaggerated by increase in heart rate. There was decrease in stroke volume and it had to be compensated for, by further increase in heart rate to maintain cardiac output. This "inflexion point", the heart rate at which the stroke volume starts decreasing, occurred at a relatively low heart rate. Recent evidence that limiting heart rate increase has favorable outcome in heart failure independent of beta blockade suggests ways of managing this dysfunction (Swedberg et al., 2010). There is speculation as to what should be the target heart rate to be achieved with such therapy. Perhaps studies such as done by Joshi et al., may provide the answer.

4. Treatment

Routine management of heart failure depending upon the status of decompensation, should be integral part of any case of CMCM. Along with this, therapy directed to pathophysiology like insulin resistance, hypothyroid state, lipid abnormality and therapies modulating the metabolic properties of myocytes should be considered.

4.1 Improving insulin resistance

Therapies which reduce insulin resistance improves outcome. There are evidence to support that therapies directed to treat heart failure also reduce insulin resistance even in non-heart failure population. Similarly, exercise improves both heart failure outcome and insulin sensitivity in non-ischemic heart failure (Kemppainen et al., 2003). Angiotensin converting enzyme inhibitor and angiotensin receptor blockers also improve insulin sensitivity in addition to their effect on heart failure (Yusuf et al., 2000; Pfeffer et al., 2003).

Drug therapy improving insulin resistance in CMCM can be at multiple levels. Different approaches consisting of lowering circulating FFA levels, facilitating glucose uptake and metabolism have been identified. These can be both anti-diabetic medication and metabolic modulator.

Drugs improving insulin sensitivity like metformin and thiazolidinediones are expected to improve outcome in cardiomyopathy associated with insulin resistance. Metformin can also improve calcium handling in myocytes (Ren et al., 1999), however, potential of causing lactic acidosis limits its utility in heart failure, especially in the context of renal dysfunction. Insulin or insulin-secretagogues could be another option as they directly promote glucose metabolism and decrease circulating FFAs but they have also failed in different animal models (Ren et al., 1996). Insulin therapy is expected to reduce catecholamine-induced myocardial damage in the heart however like with thizolidinediones, there is danger of fluid retention and hypoglycemia that may be detrimental. Several studies attempting to demonstrate the beneficial effects of tight glycemic control with insulin and secretagogues have failed to show any superiority and in fact have resulted in higher cardiovascular events.

Under the circumstances of insulin resistance, the body's compensatory mechanisms (hyperinsulinemia, up-regulation of the RAAS, catecholamines, vasopressin) are maladaptive and can further worsen the cardiomyopathy. Many counter-regulatory hormones like epinephrine, norepinephrine, glucagon, cortisol, growth hormone are upregulated and increases insulin resistance and alter glucose disposition (Nikolaidis et al., 2004). They also contribute to the pathogenesis of cardiomyopathy. Adrenergic blockade with carvedilol, long acting metoprolol and nebivolol improves myocardial efficiency by reducing consumption of FFA by myocardium and increasing preference to glucose as fuel (Nikolaidis et al., 2006) because chronic stimulation of beta-receptor seen in cardiac decompensation is known to inhibit insulin-mediated glucose uptake and insulin receptor activation (Morisco et al., 2005). These patients are expected to achieve dramatic responses to angiotensin converting enzyme inhibition and beta-adrenergic blocking therapy, often with recovery of LVEF to normal or near-normal levels.

Limiting increase in heart rate independent of beta blockade has been shown to be of benefit in heart failure; ivabradine therapy in patients with systolic dysfunction and resting sinus rhythm of more than 70 bpm despite beta blockers or in beta blocker intolerant patients (Swedberg et al., 2010).

4.2 Metabolic modulators

Metabolic modulators target molecular metabolism within the myocardium and decrease consumption of FFA while increasing metabolism of glucose. Currently these drugs are used as antianginals as they increase energy efficiency in myocardium. Inhibitor of final enzyme in β-oxidation of FFA trimetazidine improves myocardial energy stores by increasing myocardial ATP/phosphocreatine levels (Aussedat et al., 1993). Trimetazidine improved LVEF and NYHA class in a study in 65 heart failure patients (Fragasso et al., 2006). Notably, benefits were more in nonischemic cardiomyopathy than the ischemic cardiomyopathy subgroup. Similarly perhexiline inhibit FFA metabolism and has demonstrated substantial improvements in LVEF, VO_2max and quality of life in a clinical trial with 56 heart failure patients (Lee et al., 2005). However, hepatotoxicity and peripheral neuropathy associated with perhexiline limits its clinical utility. Ranolazine is a third metabolic modulator which can potentially be used in CMCM to switch from FFA to glucose.

Although role of thyroid hormone therapy in treatment of heart failure is still not clear, its role in improvement of LV function, remodeling and microcirculation are being investigated. Use of l-thyroxin both in frank cases of hypothyroid and subclinical hypothyroid has shown reversal of structural abnormalities detected by echocardiography and is accompanied by clinical improvement. Gene therapies to modify thyroid hormone receptor or deiodinase expression and activity along with thyroid hormone replacement with T3 and/or T4, use of thyroid hormone analogs (e.g. diiodothyropropionic acid) will need further studies for proving its efficacy and safety in management of such cases (Gerdes & Iervasi, 2010).

4.3 Emerging therapies

4.3.1 AGE inhibitors and breakers

It is well established that AGEs, a heterogeneous group of molecules formed by the non-enzymatic reaction of reducing sugars with free amino groups of proteins, lipids and nucleic acids contribute significantly to diabetic complications, both macro- and micro-vascular.

4.3.1.1 Pharmacological intervention against AGE formation in vivo

Classically, efforts to target AGE-related complications had been approached either with intentions to inhibit the ongoing process of AGE formation or to cleave already formed AGE protein-protein crosslinks.

4.3.1.2 Pharmacological approach to inhibition of AGE crosslink formation

Accumulation of substantial evidence indicating AGEs as one of the culprits for diabetic complications, triggered active search for intervention in the process "by pharmacological approaches. Careful study of structural aspects lead researchers to target ketone group of the 1-amino-1-deoxyfructose residue in the amadori product, which was the key to subsequent AGE-forming reactions and that chemical deactivation of this ketone group would prevent AGE formation (Ulrich & Cerami, 2001).

Aminoguanidine was one such compound identified having desirable features to be studied for its ability to inhibit AGE crosslink formation. Prior to be explored for its AGE inhibition capabilities, some published reports existed for its experimental use in humans for unrelated purposes, without significant side-effects. During subsequent years, several researchers demonstrated effectiveness of aminoguanidine in inhibiting AGE formation in vivo in a wide variety of systems and tissues.

Usefulness of aminoguanidine has also been demonstrated in improving left ventricular end-diastolic (LVED) compliance in streptozotocin induced diabetic rats. Simultaneous administration of aminoguanidine with AGE-modified albumin prevented consequent glomerular hypertrophy (Bucala & Vlassara, 1995). Clinical utility with aminoguanidine was limited by its side effect potential, which was due to its inhibitory effect on diamine oxidase. This inhibition of diamineoxidase, results in an increase in histamine levels with attendant risk of vascular and respiratory complications. Aminoguanidine being a hydrazine derivative, its association with antihistone and antinuclear cytoplasmic antibody results in a clinical situation similar to lupus.

Few other less talked inhibitors of AGE formation have been reported, however none of them have reached advanced trials in humans. Pyridoxamine, a derivative of vitamin B6 has been suggested to prevent the degradation of protein-amadori intermediates to protein-AGE products. It is shown to reduce hyperlipidemia and prevents AGE formation in rats (Wu et al., 2011; Degenhardt et al., 2002; Stitt et al., 2002). Some preliminary clinical trials evaluating effect in diabetic nephropathy with this agent have been performed (Williams et al., 2007).

OPB-9195, a thiazolidine derivative has shown to be inhibitor of advanced glycation and to produce some benefits in attenuating progression of nephropathy in spontaneous diabetic rats (Nakamura et al., 1997). There is no current clinical experience with this compound nor is there any evidence for planned clinical trials.

LR-90, yet another compound capable of inhibiting AGE formation is being studied for its usefulness pre-clinically. Evidence are available for evaluating this compound in diabetic nephropathy and retinopathy (Figarola et al., 2008; Bhatwadekar et al., 2008). The compound has also shown to possess some anti-inflammatory properties (Figarola et al., 2007) with the potential for additional protective effects against diabetic vascular complications. However, future developmental strategy for this compound is not yet fully disclosed.

4.3.1.3 Pharmacological approach to cleave preformed AGE cross-linkages

Although attractive, approach to prevent AGE formation suffers from limitation of being unable to break preformed AGE crosslinkages. Thus, AGE breaker compounds are more desirable, as they open possibility for restoration of AGE damaged tissue to their original functionality, without relying on the body's much-slower, removal and repair mechanisms. Two such molecules, a thiazolium compound alagebrium (ALT-711) and pyridinium derivative TRC4186 are being evaluated for the treatment of heart failure in patients who are metabolically challenged.

Algebrium: Upon administration to various animal models of diabetes, it has resulted in an improvement in large-vessel elasticity, decrease in stiffness and peripheral resistance

(Wolffenbuttel et al., 1998; Candido et al., 2003), an attenuation in several functional and structural manifestations of diabetes related nephropathy (Peppa et al., 2006). Clinical studies with alagebrium in patients having uncontrolled systolic hypertension, of whom only an insignificant number were diabetic, found that the data did not indicate a treatment-related benefit (Zieman et al., 2007). Pulse wave velocity and arterial pressures, indicators of conduit vessel stiffness, were unchanged; however, brachial flow mediated dilatation, an indicator of endothelial function, was improved. In the DIAMOND study in elderly and PEDESTAL in adults with diastolic heart failure, alagebrium significantly decreased left ventricular mass, improved left ventricular diastolic filling and improved effort tolerance assessed by the 6-minute walk test. However, the trials did not meet the primary endpoint of improvement in ejection fraction. Here again, diabetes or impaired control of glycemia was not a precondition for inclusion of patients. Subsequently, further development of this compound is terminated.

TRC4186: TRC4186/TRC4149 is shown to act via multiple mechanisms, which include breaking of pre-formed AGE cross-links, reducing accumulation of carbohydrate as well as lipid derived AGEs and a potent free radical scavenging activity. Treatment of diabetic spontaneously hypertensive (SHR) rats, with TRC4149 resulted in a reduced AGE burden as evident by reduced immunochemical staining for AGE and significant reduction in VCAM expression in aorta. Ultimately, the combined actions translate into better preservation of endothelial function as well as an improved cardiac function (Pathak et al., 2008). Evaluation of TRC4186 in a more complex animal model of metabolic syndrome, ob-ZSF1 rats, demonstrated its capability to attenuate overall disease progression. The compound successfully prevented rise in blood pressure following salt loading and preserved ventricular functions. Although the exact mechanism of AGE breaking is not very clear, reduction in AGE load and all ensuing downstream events, including attenuation of the associated inflammatory response, likely contributed to the improvement observed on treatment with TRC4186. These outcomes are substantially supported by suitable histopathological and immunohistochemical findings (Joshi et al., 2009).

AGE breakers are likely to be beneficial in diabetic heart failure patients in whom there is usually a significant component of diastolic dysfunction and vascular unresponsiveness, when assessed for meaningful clinical endpoints such as physical attributes of Minnesota Living with Heart Failure Questionnaire and OUES, that are able to assess not only myocardial reserve but also vascular (nutritive perfusion) reserve. Other measures such as NT pro-BNP would be useful to assess diastolic dysfunction and fluid retention that could be exaggerated in patients with compromised renal function, a common co-morbidity in these patients. TRC4186, currently under investigation for use in diabetic patients has successfully completed phase 1 clinical trial and results of its phase 2 clinical trial Prospective Evaluation of AGE Breaker in Heart Failure (PEACH-F) are awaited.

Researchers have also focus on the possibility of preventing AGE-RAGE interaction thereby preventing subsequent deleterious downstream events contributing to AGEs related pathophysiology. Conceptually this has been attained by infusing soluble RAGE (sRAGE), and by RAGE antibodies. Though it is clear that blocking AGE receptors using antibodies would prevent AGE-RAGE interaction; it remains yet to be elucidated as to whether sRAGE acts as an antagonist inhibiting RAGE dependent signaling pathways, or scavenge AGEs and AGE precursor from circulation (Zieman & Kass, 2004). There are presently no small molecule inhibitors of RAGE, and this approach has yet to be tested in clinical studies.

Finally, intracellular signalling pathways upregulated by AGEs can be inhibited by AGE signal transduction inhibitors (e.g. PK-C inhibitors incadronate disodium, cerivastatin, and curcumin) (Peyroux & Sternberg, 2006).

4.3.2 Emerging therapy targeting mitochondrial energetics

Visceral obesity and related cardiometabolic disorders are linked to defective mitochondrial biogenesis and oxidative metabolism with a decreased ATP production. The defective mitochondrial function, a common pathophysiologic feature of these cardiometabolic disorders is a key etiopathological factor exacerbating the CMCM.

The effectiveness of beta-adrenergic blockers and angiotensin-converting enzyme inhibitors to improve ventricular function in patients with heart failure, may be, due in part to the action of these agents in decreasing energy demand. Other compounds that may also have beneficial effects in hypertrophied hearts include vanadyl sulfate, which improves tolerance of ischemia by stimulating membrane glucose transport, and propionyl-L-carnitine, which prevents myocardial mechanical alterations associated with pressure overload. There is evidence that administration of propionyl-L-carnitine increases both glucose and palmitate oxidation in hypertrophied hearts and improves the efficiency of translating ATP production into cardiac work.

On this basis, a restoration of metabolic demand by restoring mitochondrial energy efficiency may have potential as a new therapeutic treatment of the hypertensive heart and heart failure (Fujii et al., 2004). Although as yet no agent exists that promote mitochondrial biogenesis, PGC-1 alpha has generated interest. Sirt1 activators have also shown potential to increase mitochondrial biogenesis. The nitric oxide-cGMP–dependent pathway may also control mitochondrial biogenesis and may ameliorate energy deficiency in heart failure. Indeed, phosphodiesterase 5 inhibitors such as sildenafil that increase cGMP have, in preliminary studies, improved LV function and exercise capacity in heart failure.

The implications for thyroid hormones on the efficiency of energy expenditure and the handling of ROS are important. One of the thyroid hormone analog, DIPTA has been tested for heart failure in early clinical trials; however agents with greater therapeutic margin are yet desirable. Thus, there is still much scope for research into the energetic effects of thyroid hormones. The preclinical evidence of TRC150094 has shown potential to improve mitochondrial substrate oxidation capacity and mitochondrial efficiency as well as improve various cardiometabolic risks with acceptable safety (Cioffi et al., 2010; Zambad et al., 2011). However this molecule is yet to be proven in a clinical setting. The discovery of such newer agents improving mitochondrial energetics will help to explore the role of these agents in the treatment of CMCM. It would be interesting to follow the progress of some investigational drugs such as TRC150094 which are in early clinical development.

5. Conclusion and key learning

- Diabetes, hypertension, dyslipidemia and thyroid dysfunction often occur concomitantly in metabolically challenged individuals who are overweight. When present together, their effect on myocardium as well as on the vasculature contribute significantly to the clinical manifestations of patients diagnosed with heart failure not predominantly due to epicardial Coronary Artery Disease (cardio-metabolic cardiomyopathy).

- Impairment in mitochondrial energetics resulting in inflexibility in fuel utilization has a significant role in development and progression of CMCM.
- Currently recommended diagnostic methods such as Echocardiography and tissue Doppler imaging are carried out at rest and may result in underestimation of heart failure in the absence of a suitable provocative diagnostic method capable of assessing the ability of the heart to augment cardiac output (cardiac reserve) on exertional demand.
- Dynamic assessment of cardiac response during exercise with assessment of peripheral flow, distribution and nutritive perfusion such as CPET may provide an objective and sensitive measure of cardiac and microvascular correlates of the composite with better correlation to clinical manifestation and possibly also help in more accurately assessing the onset and progress of cardiovascular malfunction.
- Some of the newer emerging non-conventional diagnostic methods and therapies may offer a solution for the management of CMCM.

6. References

Abel, E. D. & Doenst, T. (2011). Mitochondrial adaptations to physiological vs. pathological cardiac hypertrophy. *Cardiovascular Research,* Vol.90, No.2, pp. 234-242, ISSN 1755-3245.

Ashrafian, H.; Frenneaux, M. P. & Opie, L. H. (2007). Metabolic mechanisms in heart failure. *Circulation,* Vol. 16, No.4, pp. 434-448, ISSN 0009-7322.

Aussedat, J.; Ray, A.; Kay, L.; Verdys, M.; Harpey, C. & Rossi, A. (1993). Improvement of long-term preservation of isolated arrested rat heart: beneficial effect of the antiischemic agent trimetazidine. *Journal of Cardiovascular Pharmacology,* Vol.21, No.1, pp. 128-135, ISSN 1533-4023.

Bhatwadekar, A.; Glenn, J. V.; Figarola, J. L.; Scott, S.; Gardiner, T. A.; Rahbar, S. & Stitt, A. W. (2008). A new advanced glycation inhibitor, LR-90, prevents experimental diabetic retinopathy in rats. *British Journal of Ophthalmology,* Vol.92, No.4, pp. 545-547, ISSN 1468-2079.

Borradaile, N. M.; Han, X.; Harp, J. D.; Gale, S. E.; Ory, D. S. & Schaffer, J. E. (2006). Disruption of endoplasmic reticulum structure and integrity in lipotoxic cell death. *Journal of Lipid Research,* Vol.47, No.12, pp. 2726-2737, ISSN 1539-7262.

Bucala, R. & Vlassara, H. (1995). Advanced glycosylation end products in diabetic renal and vascular disease. *American Journal of Kidney Disease,* Vol.26, No.6, pp. 875-888, ISSN 0272-6386.

Candido, R.; Forbes, J. M.; Thomas, M. C.; Thallas, V.; Dean, R. G.; Burns, W. C.; Tikellis, C.; Ritchie, R. H.; Twigg, S. M.; Cooper, M. E. & Burrell, L. M. (2003). A breaker of advanced glycation end products attenuates diabetes-induced myocardial structural changes. *Circulation Research,* Vol.92, No.7, pp. 785-792, ISSN 1524-4571.

Carley, A. N. & Severson, D. L. (2008). What are the biochemical mechanisms responsible for enhanced fatty acid utilization by perfused hearts from type 2 diabetic db/db mice? *Cardiovascular Drugs and Therapy,* Vol.22, No.2, pp. 83-89, ISSN 1573-7241.

Carley, A. N. & Severson, D. L. (2005). Fatty acid metabolism is enhanced in type 2 diabetic hearts. *Biochimica et Biophysica Acta,* Vol.1734, No.2, pp.112-126, ISSN 0006-3002.

Cioffi, F.; Zambad, S. P.; Chhipa, L.; Senese, R.; Busiello, R. A.; Tuli, D.; Munshi, S.; Moreno, M.; Lombardi, A.; Gupta, R. C.; Chauthaiwale, V.; Dutt, C.; de Lange, P.; Silvestri, E.; Lanni, A. & Goglia, F. (2010). TRC150094, a novel functional analog of iodothyronines, reduces adiposity by increasing energy expenditure and fatty acid oxidation in rats receiving a high-fat diet. *The FASEB Journal*, Vol.24, No.9, pp. 3451-3461, ISSN 1530- 6860.

Clarke, P. M.; Glasziou, P.; Patel, A.; Chalmers, J.; Woodward, M.; Harrap, S. B. & Salomon, J. A. (2010). Event rates, hospital utilization, and costs associated with major complications of diabetes: a multicountry comparative analysis. *PLoS Med*, Vol.7, No.2, pp. e1000236, ISSN 1549-1676.

Degenhardt, T. P.; Alderson, N. L.; Arrington, D. D.; Beattie, R. J.; Basgen, J. M.; Steffes, M. W.; Thorpe, S. R. & Baynes, J. W. (2002). Pyridoxamine inhibits early renal disease and dyslipidemia in the streptozotocin-diabetic rat. *Kidney International*, Vol.61, No.3, pp. 939-950, ISSN 1523-1755.

Dillmann, W. (2010). Cardiac hypertrophy and thyroid hormone signaling. *Heart Failure Reviews*, Vol.15, No.2, pp. 125-132, ISSN 1573-7322.

Dickstein, K.; Cohen-Solal, A.; Filippatos, G.; McMurray, J. J.; Ponikowski, P.; Poole-Wilson, P. A.; Stromberg, A.; van Veldhuisen, D. J.; Atar, D.; Hoes, A. W.; Keren, A.; Mebazaa, A.; Nieminen, M.; Priori, S. G.; Swedberg, K.; Vahanian, A.; Camm, J.; De, C. R.; Dean, V.; Dickstein, K.; Filippatos, G.; Funck-Brentano, C.; Hellemans, I.; Kristensen, S. D.; McGregor, K.; Sechtem, U.; Silber, S.; Tendera, M.; Widimsky, P. & Zamorano, J. L. (2008). ESC Guidelines for the diagnosis and treatment of acute and chronic heart failure 2008: the Task Force for the Diagnosis and Treatment of Acute and Chronic Heart Failure 2008 of the European Society of Cardiology. Developed in collaboration with the Heart Failure Association of the ESC (HFA) and endorsed by the European Society of Intensive Care Medicine (ESICM). *European Heart Journal*, Vol.29, No.19, pp. 2388-2442, ISSN 1522-9645.

Elliott, P.; Andersson, B.; Arbustini, E.; Bilinska, Z.; Cecchi, F.; Charron, P.; Dubourg, O.; Kuhl, U.; Maisch, B.; McKenna, W. J.; Monserrat, L.; Pankuweit, S.; Rapezzi, C.; Seferovic, P.; Tavazzi, L. & Keren, A. (2008). Classification of the cardiomyopathies: a position statement from the European Society Of Cardiology Working Group on Myocardial and Pericardial Diseases. *European Heart Journal*, Vol.29, No.2, pp. 270-276, ISSN 1522-9645.

Fang, Z. Y.; Prins, J. B. & Marwick, T. H. (2004). Diabetic cardiomyopathy: evidence, mechanisms, and therapeutic implications. *Endocrine Reviews*, Vol.25, No.4, pp. 543-567, ISSN 0163-769X.

Figarola, J. L.; Shanmugam, N.; Natarajan, R. & Rahbar, S. (2007). Anti-inflammatory effects of the advanced glycation end product inhibitor LR-90 in human monocytes. *Diabetes*, Vol.56, No.3, pp. 647-655, ISSN 1939-327X.

Figarola, J. L.; Loera, S.; Weng, Y.; Shanmugam, N.; Natarajan, R. & Rahbar, S. (2008). LR-90 prevents dyslipidaemia and diabetic nephropathy in the Zucker diabetic fatty rat. *Diabetologia*, Vol.51, No.5, pp. 882-891, ISSN 1432-0428.

Fragasso, G.; Palloshi, A.; Puccetti, P.; Silipigni, C.; Rossodivita, A.; Pala, M.; Calori, G.; Alfieri, O. & Margonato, A. (2006). A randomized clinical trial of trimetazidine, a partial free fatty acid oxidation inhibitor, in patients with heart failure. *Journal of American College of Cardiology*, Vol.48, No.5, pp. 992-998, ISSN 0735-1097.

Fujii, N.; Nozawa, T.; Igawa, A.; Kato, B.; Igarashi, N.; Nonomura, M.; Asanoi, H.; Tazawa, S.; Inoue, M. & Inoue, H. (2004). Saturated glucose uptake capacity and impaired fatty acid oxidation in hypertensive hearts before development of heart failure. *American Journal of Physiology Heart and Circulatory Physiology,* Vol.287, No.2, pp. H760-H766, ISSN 1522-1539.

Garvey, W. T.; Hardin, D.; Juhaszova, M. & Dominguez, J. H. (1993). Effects of diabetes on myocardial glucose transport system in rats: implications for diabetic cardiomyopathy. *American Journal of Physiology Heart and Circulatory Physiology,* Vol.264, No.3, pp. H837-H844, ISSN 1522-1539.

Gerdes, A. M. & Iervasi, G. (2010). Thyroid replacement therapy and heart failure. *Circulation,* Vol.122, No.4, pp. 385-393, ISSN 0009-7322.

Goldin, A.; Beckman, J. A.; Schmidt, A. M. & Creager, M. A. (2006). Advanced glycation end products: sparking the development of diabetic vascular injury. *Circulation,* Vol.114, No.6, pp. 597-605, ISSN 0009-7322.

He, Z.; Way, K. J.; Arikawa, E.; Chou, E.; Opland, D. M.; Clermont, A.; Isshiki, K.; Ma, R. C.; Scott, J. A.; Schoen, F. J.; Feener, E. P. & King, G. L. (2005). Differential regulation of angiotensin II-induced expression of connective tissue growth factor by protein kinase C isoforms in the myocardium. *The Journal of Biology and Chemistry,* Vol.280, No.16, pp. 15719-15726, ISSN 1083-351X.

Herrero, P.; Peterson, L. R.; McGill, J. B.; Matthew, S.; Lesniak, D.; Dence, C. & Gropler, R. J. (2006). Increased myocardial fatty acid metabolism in patients with type 1 diabetes mellitus. *Journal of American College of Cardiology,* Vol.47, No.3, pp. 598-604, ISSN 0735-1097.

Jessup, M.; Abraham, W. T.; Casey, D. E.; Feldman, A. M.; Francis, G. S.; Ganiats, T. G.; Konstam, M. A.; Mancini, D. M.; Rahko, P. S.; Silver, M. A.; Stevenson, L. W. & Yancy, C. W. (2009). 2009 focused update: ACCF/AHA Guidelines for the Diagnosis and Management of Heart Failure in Adults: a report of the American College of Cardiology Foundation/American Heart Association Task Force on Practice Guidelines: developed in collaboration with the International Society for Heart and Lung Transplantation. *Circulation,* Vol.119, No.14, pp. 1977-2016, ISSN 0009-7322.

Joshi, D.; Gupta, R.; Dubey, A.; Shiwalkar, A.; Pathak, P.; Gupta, R. C.; Chauthaiwale, V. & Dutt, C. (2009). TRC4186, a novel AGE-breaker, improves diabetic cardiomyopathy and nephropathy in Ob-ZSF1 model of type 2 diabetes. *Journal of Cardiovascular Pharmacology,* Vol.54, No.1, pp. 72-81, ISSN 1533-4023.

Joshi, D.; Shiwalkar, A.; Cross, M. R.; Sharma, S. K.; Vachhani, A. & Dutt, C. (2010). Continuous, non-invasive measurement of the haemodynamic response to submaximal exercise in patients with diabetes mellitus: evidence of impaired cardiac reserve and peripheral vascular response. *Heart,* Vol.96, No.1, pp. 36-41, ISSN 1468-201X.

Kagan, V. E.; Tyurin, V. A.; Jiang, J.; Tyurina, Y. Y.; Ritov, V. B.; Amoscato, A. A.; Osipov, A. N.; Belikova, N. A.; Kapralov, A. A.; Kini, V.; Vlasova, I. I.; Zhao, Q.; Zou, M.; Di, P.; Svistunenko, D. A.; Kurnikov, I. V. & Borisenko, G. G. (2005). Cytochrome c acts as a cardiolipin oxygenase required for release of proapoptotic factors. *Nature Chemical Biology,* Vol.1, No.4, pp. 223-232, ISSN 1552-4450.

Kemppainen, J.; Tsuchida, H.; Stolen, K.; Karlsson, H.; Bjornholm, M.; Heinonen, O. J.; Nuutila, P.; Krook, A.; Knuuti, J. & Zierath, J. R. (2003). Insulin signalling and resistance in patients with chronic heart failure. *The Journal of Physiology,* Vol.550, No.1, pp. 305-315, ISSN 1469-7793.

Kim, J. A.; Wei, Y. & Sowers, J. R. (2008). Role of mitochondrial dysfunction in insulin resistance. *Circulation Research,* Vol.102, No.4, pp. 401-414, ISSN 1524-4571.

Kim, E. H.; Koh, E. H.; Park, J. Y. & Lee, K. U. (2010). Adenine nucleotide translocator as a regulator of mitochondrial function: implication in the pathogenesis of metabolic syndrome. *Korean Diabetes Journal,* Vol.34, No.3, pp. 146-153, ISSN 2093-2650.

Kinugawa, K.; Minobe, W. A.; Wood, W. M.; Ridgway, E. C.; Baxter, J. D.; Ribeiro, R. C.; Tawadrous, M. F.; Lowes, B. A.; Long, C. S. & Bristow, M. R. (2001). Signaling pathways responsible for fetal gene induction in the failing human heart: evidence for altered thyroid hormone receptor gene expression. *Circulation,* Vol.103, No.8, pp. 1089-1094, ISSN 0009-7322.

Ku, P. M.; Chen, L. J.; Liang, J. R.; Cheng, K. C.; Li, Y. X. & Cheng, J. T. (2011). Molecular role of GATA binding protein 4 (GATA-4) in hyperglycemia-induced reduction of cardiac contractility. *Cardiovascular Diabetology,* Vol.10, No.1, pp. 57, ISSN 1475 - 2840.

Lee, L.; Campbell, R.; Scheuermann-Freestone, M.; Taylor, R.; Gunaruwan, P.; Williams, L.; Ashrafian, H.; Horowitz, J.; Fraser, A. G.; Clarke, K. & Frenneaux, M. (2005). Metabolic modulation with perhexiline in chronic heart failure: a randomized, controlled trial of short-term use of a novel treatment. *Circulation,* Vol.112, No.21, pp. 3280-3288, ISSN 0009-7322.

Miyata, T.; Saito, A.; kurokawa, K. & van Ypersele de S.C. (2001). Advanced glycation and lipoxidation end products: reactive carbonyl compounds-related uraemic toxicity. *Nephrology Dialysis Transplantation,* Vol.16, No.4, pp. 8-11, ISSN 1460-2385.

Morisco, C.; Condorelli, G.; Trimarco, V.; Bellis, A.; Marrone, C.; Condorelli, G.; Sadoshima, J. & Trimarco, B. (2005). Akt mediates the cross-talk between beta-adrenergic and insulin receptors in neonatal cardiomyocytes. *Circulation Research,* Vol.96, No.2, pp. 180-188, ISSN 1524-4571.

Nakamura, S.; Makita, Z.; Ishikawa, S.; Yasumura, K.; Fujii, W.; Yanagisawa, K.; Kawata, T. & Koike, T. (1997). Progression of nephropathy in spontaneous diabetic rats is prevented by OPB-9195, a novel inhibitor of advanced glycation. *Diabetes,* Vol.46, No.5, pp. 895-899, ISSN 1939-327X.

Nikolaidis, L. A.; Sturzu, A.; Stolarski, C.; Elahi, D. Shen, Y. T. & Shannon, R. P. (2004). The development of myocardial insulin resistance in conscious dogs with advanced dilated cardiomyopathy. *Cardiovascular Research,* Vol.61, No.2, pp. 297-306, ISSN 1755-3245.

Nikolaidis, L. A.; Poornima, I.; Parikh, P.; Magovern, M.; Shen, Y. T. & Shannon, R. P. (2006). The effects of combined versus selective adrenergic blockade on left ventricular and systemic hemodynamics, myocardial substrate preference, and regional perfusion in conscious dogs with dilated cardiomyopathy. *Journal of American College of Cardiology,* Vol.47, No.9, pp. 1871-1881, ISSN 0735-1097.

Ozasa, N.; Furukawa, Y.; Morimoto, T.; Tadamura, E.; Kita, T. & Kimura, T. (2008). Relation among left ventricular mass, insulin resistance, and hemodynamic parameters in type 2 diabetes. *Hypertension Research,* Vol.31, No.3, pp. 425-432, ISSN 0916-9636.

Paradies, G.; Petrosillo, G.; Pistolese, M.; Di, V. N.; Federici, A. & Ruggiero, F. M. (2004). Decrease in mitochondrial complex I activity in ischemic/reperfused rat heart: involvement of reactive oxygen species and cardiolipin. *Circulation Research,* Vol.94, No.1, pp. 53-59, ISSN 1524-4571.

Pathak, P.; Gupta, R.; Chaudhari, A.; Shiwalkar, A.; Dubey, A.; Mandhare, A. B.; Gupta, R. C.; Joshi, D. & Chauthaiwale, V. (2008). TRC4149 a novel advanced glycation end product breaker improves hemodynamic status in diabetic spontaneously hypertensive rats. *European Journal of Medical Research,* Vol.13, No.8, pp. 388-398, ISSN 0949-2321.

Paulus, W. J. European Study Group on Diastolic Heart Failure. (1998). How to diagnose diastolic heart failure. *European Heart Journal,* Vol.19, No.7, pp. 990-1003, ISSN 1468-201X.

Peppa, M.; Brem, H.; Cai, W.; Zhang, J. G.; Basgen, J.; Li, Z.; Vlassara, H. & Uribarri, J. (2006). Prevention and reversal of diabetic nephropathy in db/db mice treated with alagebrium (ALT-711). *American Journal of Nephrology,* Vol.26, No.5, pp. 430-436, ISSN 1421-9670.

Pereira, L.; Matthes, J.; Schuster, I.; Valdivia, H. H.; Herzig, S.; Richard, S. & Gomez, A. M. (2006). Mechanisms of [Ca2+]i transient decrease in cardiomyopathy of db/db type 2 diabetic mice. *Diabetes,* Vol.55, No.3, pp. 608-615, ISSN 1939-327X.

Peyroux, J. & Sternberg, M. (2006). Advanced glycation endproducts (AGEs): Pharmacological inhibition in diabetes. *Pathol Biol (Paris),* Vol.54, No.7, pp. 405-419, ISSN 0369-8114.

Pfeffer, M. A.; Swedberg, K.; Granger, C. B.; Held, P.; McMurray, J. J.; Michelson, E. L.; Olofsson, B.; Ostergren, J.; Yusuf, S. & Pocock, S. (2003). Effects of candesartan on mortality and morbidity in patients with chronic heart failure: the CHARM-Overall programme. *Lancet,* Vol.362, No.9386, pp. 759-766, ISSN 0140-6736.

Ren, J.; Dominguez, L. J.; Sowers, J. R. & Davidoff, A. J. (1996). Troglitazone attenuates high-glucose-induced abnormalities in relaxation and intracellular calcium in rat ventricular myocytes. *Diabetes,* Vol.45, No.12, pp. 1822-1825, ISSN 1939-327X.

Ren, J.; Dominguez, L. J.; Sowers, J. R. & Davidoff, A. J. (1999). Metformin but not glyburide prevents high glucose-induced abnormalities in relaxation and intracellular Ca2+ transients in adult rat ventricular myocytes. *Diabetes,* Vol.48, No.10, pp. 2059-2065, ISSN 1939-327X.

Sarzani, R.; Salvi, F.; ssi-Fulgheri, P. & Rappelli, A. (2008). Renin-angiotensin system, natriuretic peptides, obesity, metabolic syndrome, and hypertension: an integrated view in humans. *Journal of Hypertension,* Vol.26, No.5, pp. 831-843, ISSN1473-5598.

Schannwell, C. M.; Schneppenheim, M.; Perings, S.; Plehn, G. & Strauer, B. E. (2002). Left ventricular diastolic dysfunction as an early manifestation of diabetic cardiomyopathy. *Cardiology,* Vol.98, No.1-2, pp. 33-39.

Shanmugam, N.; Figarola, J. L.; Li, Y.; Swiderski, P. M.; Rahbar, S. & Natarajan, R. (2008). Proinflammatory effects of advanced lipoxidation end products in monocytes. *Diabetes,* Vol.57, No.4, pp. 879-888, ISSN1939-327X.

Solomon, S. D.; Appelbaum, E.; Manning, W. J.; Verma, A.; Berglund, T.; Lukashevich, V.; Cherif, P. C.; Smith, B. A. & Dahlof, B. (2009). Effect of the direct Renin inhibitor aliskiren, the Angiotensin receptor blocker losartan, or both on left ventricular mass in patients with hypertension and left ventricular hypertrophy. *Circulation,* Vol.119, No.4, pp. 530-537, ISSN 0009-7322.

Sopel, M. J.; Rosin, N. L.; Lee, T. D. & Legare, J. F. (2011). Myocardial fibrosis in response to Angiotensin II is preceded by the recruitment of mesenchymal progenitor cells. *Laboratory Investigation,* Vol.91, No.4, pp. 565-578, ISSN 0023-6837.

Sparagna, G. C.; Chicco, A. J.; Murphy, R. C.; Bristow, M. R.; Johnson, C. A.; Rees, M. L.; Maxey, M. L.; McCune, S. A. & Moore, R. L. (2007). Loss of cardiac tetralinoleoyl cardiolipin in human and experimental heart failure. *Journal of Lipid Research,* Vol.48, No.7, pp. 1559-1570, ISSN 1539-7262.

Stitt, A.; Gardiner, T. A.; Alderson, N. L.; Canning, P.; Frizzell, N.; Duffy, N.; Boyle, C.; Januszewski, A. S.; Chachich, M.; Baynes, J. W. & Thorpe, S. R. (2002). The AGE inhibitor pyridoxamine inhibits development of retinopathy in experimental diabetes. *Diabetes,* Vol.51, No.9, pp. 2826-2832, ISSN 1939-327X.

Struthers, A. D. & Unger, T. (2011). Physiology of aldosterone and pharmacology of aldosterone blockers. *European Heart Journal Suppl,* Vol.13 (suppl B), B27-B30 ISSN 1554-2815.

Swedberg, K.; Komajda, M.; Bohm, M.; Borer, J. S.; Ford, I.; Dubost-Brama, A.; Lerebours, G. & Tavazzi, L. (2010). Ivabradine and outcomes in chronic heart failure (SHIFT): a randomised placebo-controlled study. *Lancet,* Vol.376, No.9744, pp. 875-885, ISSN ISSN 0140-6736.

Ulrich, P. & Cerami, A. (2001). Protein glycation, diabetes, and aging. *Recent Progress in Hormone Research,* Vol.56, pp. 1-21, ISSN 0079-9963.

Van, H. L.; Hamdani, N.; Handoko, M. L.; Falcao-Pires, I.; Musters, R. J.; Kupreishvili, K.; Ijsselmuiden, A. J.; Schalkwijk, C. G.; Bronzwaer, J. G.; Diamant, M.; Borbely, A.; van, d., V; Stienen, G. J.; Laarman, G. J.; Niessen, H. W. & Paulus, W. J. (2008). Diastolic stiffness of the failing diabetic heart: importance of fibrosis, advanced glycation end products, and myocyte resting tension. *Circulation,* Vol.117, No.1, pp.43-51, ISSN ISSN 0009-7322.

Vetter, R.; Rehfeld, U.; Reissfelder, C.; Weiss, W.; Wagner, K. D.; Gunther, J.; Hammes, A.; Tschope, C.; Dillmann, W. & Paul, M. (2002). Transgenic overexpression of the sarcoplasmic reticulum Ca2+ATPase improves reticular Ca2+ handling in normal and diabetic rat hearts. *The FASEB Journal,* Vol.16, No.12, pp. 1657-1659, ISSN 1530-6860.

Williams, M. E.; Bolton, W. K.; Khalifah, R. G.; Degenhardt, T. P.; Schotzinger, R. J. & McGill, J. B. (2007). Effects of pyridoxamine in combined phase 2 studies of patients with type 1 and type 2 diabetes and overt nephropathy. *American Journal of Nephrology,* Vol.27, No.6, pp. 605-614, ISSN 1421-9670.

Wolffenbuttel, B. H.; Boulanger, C. M.; Crijns, F. R.; Huijberts, M. S.; Poitevin, P.; Swennen, G. N.; Vasan, S.; Egan, J. J.; Ulrich, P.; Cerami, A. & Levy, B. I. (1998). Breakers of advanced glycation end products restore large artery properties in experimental diabetes. *Proceedings of the National Academy of Sciences U. S. A.,* Vol.95, No.8, pp. 4630-4634, ISSN 0027-8424.

Wilson, P. W. (2001). Diabetes mellitus and coronary heart disease. *Endocrinology Metabolism Clinics of North America,* Vol.30, No.4, pp. 857-881, ISSN 0889-8529.

Wu, E. T.; Liang, J. T.; Wu, M. S. & Chang, K. C. (2011). Pyridoxamine prevents age-related aortic stiffening and vascular resistance in association with reduced collagen glycation. *Experimental Gerontology*, Vol.46, No.6, pp. 482-488, ISSN 1873-6815.

Yusuf, S.; Sleight, P.; Pogue, J.; Bosch, J.; Davies, R. & Dagenais, G. (2000). Effects of an angiotensin-converting-enzyme inhibitor, ramipril, on cardiovascular events in high-risk patients. The Heart Outcomes Prevention Evaluation Study Investigators. *New England Journal of Medicine*, Vol.342, No.3, pp. 145-153. ISSN 1533-4406.

Zambad, S. P.; Munshi, S.; Dubey, A.; Gupta, R.; Busiello, R. A.; Lanni, A.; Goglia, F.; Gupta, R. C.; Chauthaiwale, V. & Dutt, C. (2011). TRC150094 attenuates progression of nontraditional cardiovascular risk factors associated with obesity and type 2 diabetes in obese ZSF1 rats. *Diabetes, Metabolic Syndrome and Obesity: Targets and Therapy*, Vol. 6, No. 4, pp. 5-16, ISSN 1178-7007.

Zieman, S. & Kass, D. (2004). Advanced glycation end product cross-linking: pathophysiologic role and therapeutic target in cardiovascular disease. *Congestive Heart Failure*, Vol.10, No.3, pp. 144-149, ISSN 1751-7133.

Zieman, S. J.; Melenovsky, V.; Clattenburg, L.; Corretti, M. C.; Capriotti, A.; Gerstenblith, G. & Kass, D. A. (2007). Advanced glycation endproduct crosslink breaker (alagebrium) improves endothelial function in patients with isolated systolic hypertension. *Journal of Hypertension*, Vol.25, No.3, pp. 577-583, ISSN 1473-5598.

5

Insulin Resistance and Cardiomyopathy

Jiung-Pang Huang and Li-Man Hung
Department and Graduate Institute of Biomedical Sciences and Healthy Aging Research Center, College of Medicine, Chang Gung University, Tao-Yuan
Taiwan

1. Introduction

During the past two decades, a striking increase in the number of people with metabolic syndrome has taken place worldwide. With the increased risk worldwide of not only type 2 diabetes mellitus (T2DM), but also of cardiovascular disease from the metabolic syndrome, there is an urgent need for strategies to prevent the emerging global epidemic (1-4). Insulin-mediated glucose metabolism varies widely in healthy human beings, and the more insulin resistant an individual, the more insulin they must secrete in order to prevent the development of T2DM. However, the combination of insulin resistance and compensatory hyperinsulinemia increases the likelihood that an individual will be hypertensive, and have a dyslipidemia characterized by a high plasma triglyceride (TG) and low high-density lipoprotein cholesterol (HDL-C) concentration. Given the rapid increase in the number of clinical syndromes and abnormalities associated with insulin resistance/hyperinsulinemia, it is reasonable to suggest, that the cluster of these changes related to the defect in insulin action be included within the term, insulin resistant syndrome.

Under physiological conditions, insulin in the heart is for the regulation of the substrate employed in the contraction/ relaxation cycle and cell growth (5-9). Decreased insulin sensitivity reduces cardiac performance leading to left ventricular hypertrophy, diastolic dysfunction, and heart failure (10-12). Several mechanisms are known to contribute to the myocardial dysfunction including, reduced energy production due to decreased mitochondrial respiration and pyruvate dehydrogenase activity, oxidative stress, defective cardiac contractility, and intracellular Ca^{2+} regulatory proteins such as myosin, titin, sarcoendoplasmic reticulum Ca^{2+}-ATPase (SERCA), phospholamban, and Na^{+}-Ca^{2+} exchanger (13, 14). The high incidence of cardiac problems in patients with metabolic syndrome warrants a more stringent clinical management. Although a wide variety of pharmacological targets and agents have been discovered, the clinical management of cardiovascular risk associated with metabolic syndrome is still dismal.

2. Diabetic cardiomyopathy

It has been reported that diabetic patients suffer from heart failure with normal coronary arteries and with no other obvious aetiology for heart failure (3, 4). This phenomenon has led to the use of the term "diabetic cardiomyopathy" (DCM). The term now includes diabetic individuals with diastolic dysfunction, the prevalence of which may be as high as

60% in well-controlled T2DM individuals (12, 15). Thereby, subclinical left ventricular dysfunction may be a very common feature in diabetes, in addition to the increased prevalence of coronary heart disease (16-21). In experimental rodent models, myocardial contractile dysfunction independent of coronary artery disease has also been demonstrated in db/db, ob/ob, and Zucker rodent models, supporting the existence of an obesity-related cardiomyopathy and a diabetic cardiomyopathy (3, 22). In addition, mice with a selective cardiomyocyte only deletion of the insulin receptor (CIRKO mice) have reduced insulin-stimulated glucose uptake and also have a modest decrease in contractile function, thereby implicating insulin resistance as a contributing factor in the development of contractile dysfunction in the metabolic syndrome (23, 24).

3. Metabolic disturbances and cardiomyopathy

It is well recognized that insulin regulates the critical steps in intermediary metabolism of many tissues (including skeletal muscle, adipose tissue, and liver) and consequently maintains metabolic homeostasis within the body. However, many other tissues including the heart also express insulin receptors and their important functions may be regulated by insulin. Insulin resistance is an important risk factor for the development of hypertension, atherosclerotic heart disease, left ventricular hypertrophy and dysfunction, and heart failure. It reflects a disturbance of insulin-mediated glucose metabolism and can potentially worsen metabolic efficiency of both skeletal and cardiac muscle. Recently, the relationship between insulin resistance and cardiac contractile dysfunction has been investigated by generating a new insulin resistant animal rat model on a high cholesterol-fructose (HCF) diet. The HCF diet-induced insulin resistance not only occurred in metabolic-response tissues but also in the heart as well. These results indicate cardiac insulin resistance-associated metabolic alterations may consequently lead to the development of cardiomyopathy and contractile dysfunction (25).

Diabetes causes metabolic dysregulation and contains numerous risk factors which are associated with cardiomyopathy and heart failure. Extensive cellular and molecular studies have elucidated putative process of metabolic disturbances in the pathogenesis of cardiac dysfunction in diabetes (Table.1) (26). The metabolic disturbances in the development of cardiomyopathy are listed below.

3.1 Increased triglycerides (TG) and nonesterified fatty acids (NEFAs)

Hyperlipidemia is one of the features of obesity induced T2DM. When circulating NEFAs are greater than the oxidative capacity of the heart, NEFAs are stored as intramyocardial triglycerides. Both NEFAs and TG contribute to cardiac lipotoxicity and worsened heart failure (27-32). High levels of circulating NEFAs promote insulin resistance by impairment of insulin-Akt activation and compensatory hyperinsulinemia (27, 33-36). NEFAs also induce the activation of atypical protein kinase C (PKC)θ, which is a serine/threonine kinase that phosphorylates and subsequently activates IκB kinase. Then IκB kinase phosphorylates insulin receptor substrate-1 (IRS-1) serine residues which inhibit the ability of IRS-1 to bind to SH2 domains of the p85 regulatory subunit of phosphatidylinositol 3-kinase (PI3K), and consequently impair insulin signal transduction (36). NEFAs not only trigger the development of cardiac insulin resistance but also lead to the development of myocardial contractile dysfunction. NEFAs can directly alter myocardial contractility by increasing NEFA flux into the myocardium. A recent study suggests that increasing the entry of fatty acyl coenzyme A (CoA) into the cardiomyocytes may modulate the K_{ATP} channel opening during the contractile state of the myocardium (37). Activation of K_{ATP} channel contributes to shortening of the action potential and decreases trans-sarcolemmal calcium flux and subsequent myocardial contractility (37).

TRIGGERS	MEDIATORS	EFFECTORS	TARGETS
NEFA	↑ Acyl CoA	↑ K^{+}_{ATP} CHANNEL	↓ ACTIVATOR Ca^{++}
	↑ ATYPICAL PKC ↑ PTEN	↓ Akt-1 ACTIVATION	INSULIN RESISTANCE
	↑ TNF α	↑ CERAMIDE	MYOCYTE APOPTOSIS
HYPERGLYCEMIA	↑ ROS → ↑ PARP ↓ ↓ GAPDH	↑ PKC	CALCIUM HOMEOSTASIS
		↑ HEXOAMINE	CONTRACTILE PROTEINS
		↑ POLYOL FLUX	
		↑ AGE	MATRIX PROTEINS
HYPERINSULINEMIA INSULIN RESISTANCE	PI3K/Akt-1	↓ GSK-3 β ↑ mTOR	MYOCYTE HYPERTROPHY
	↑ MAP KINASE	↑ Ras/ ↑ Rho	↑ PROTEIN SYNTHESIS

Table 1. The relationship between diabetic metabolic disturbances (triggers) and the mediators, effectors, and intracellular targets that lead to a diabetic cardiomyopathic phenotype. (Modified from Poornima IG, Parikh P, Shannon RP. Diabetic cardiomyopathy: the search for a unifying hypothesis. *Circ Res*. 2006; 98: 596-605.)

3.2 Hyperglycemia

Hyperglycemia leads to increasing glucose oxidation. Brownlee and colleagues have elucidated that hyperglycemia generates reactive oxygen species (ROS) and consequently mediates tissue injury (38, 39). In fact, mitochondria generate high levels of ROS which lead to damage of DNA and inhibit the activity of glyceraldehyde phosphate dehydrogenase (GAPDH) (39, 40). On the other hand, hyperglycemia also shifts the glucose glycolytic pathway into alternative pathways that are considered mediators of hyperglycemia induced cellular injury (26). The damage resulting from hyperglycemia includes elevation of advanced glycation end products (AGEs), hexosamine and polyol pathway, activation of beta 2 isoform PKC and alteration of myocardial structure and function (41-47). In addition, it has been suggested that hyperglycemia is linked to altering the expression and function of both the ryanodine receptor (RyR) and sarco/endoplasmic reticulum Ca^{2+}-ATPase (SERCA), and this alteration may contribute to impair myocardial systolic and diastolic function (26).

3.3 Insulin resistance and hyperinsulinemia

Insulin resistance is prevalent in chronic heart failure patients with idiopathic dilated cardiomyopathy (12, 48). Furthermore, insulin resistance is a primary etiology factor in the development of nonischemic heart failure (HF) (49). The cardiac insulin action and how insulin resistance leads to the development of cardiomyopathy are discussed in detail below.

4. The cardiac action of insulin

The heart is an energy-consuming organ that requires a constant supply of fuel and oxygen in order to maintain its intracellular ATP level, which is essential for the uninterrupted myocardial contraction/relaxation cycle. Oxidation of fatty acids supplies approximately 70% of the heart's energy needs, while glucose and lactate may account for up to 30% of total ATP production. The energy requirements of the heart could be covered for a short period by the breakdown of intracellular stored glycogen and lipid droplets, but a longer duration would rely on the uptake of exogenous glucose and long chain fatty acid (LCFA). Circulating insulin and increased contractile activity are the two major signals responsible for acute increases in cardiac substrate uptake, enabled by inducing transporter translocation from intracellular stores to the sarcolemma (Fig.1) (5).

Under normal physiological conditions, the main role of insulin on the heart is the regulation of substrate utilization. Insulin regulates cardiac metabolism by modulating glucose and fatty acid transport, glycolysis, glycogen synthesis, lipid metabolism, protein synthesis, growth, contractility, and apoptosis in the cardiomyocytes (5). The actions of insulin are mediated by binding to specific cell surface receptors (insulin receptor, InsR). Each cardiomyocyte is expressed at levels of about 10,000 to 100,000 receptors of InsR. The InsR is a tetrameric enzyme comprising two extracellular α-subunits and two transmembrane β-subunits (5). The binding of insulin to the extracellular domain of InsR triggers the activation of intrinsic tyrosine kinase activity of the β-subunits of the receptor. This leads to an autotransphosphorylation of the receptor where one β-subunit phosphorylates the other on several tyrosine residues. Once activated and phosphorylated, InsR binds via its phosphotyrosine residues and phosphorylates a series of downstream elements, including the insulin receptor substrate (IRS) family and Shc (5, 50). This recruitment and activation lead to the activation of two main pathways, the phosphatidylinositol 3-kinase (PI3K) and the mitogen-activated protein kinase (MAPK) pathway respectively. PI3K is considered to be the main player of the metabolic action of insulin, whereas the MAPK pathway is principally involved in cell growth and differentiation in the heart (Fig.2) (50, 51).

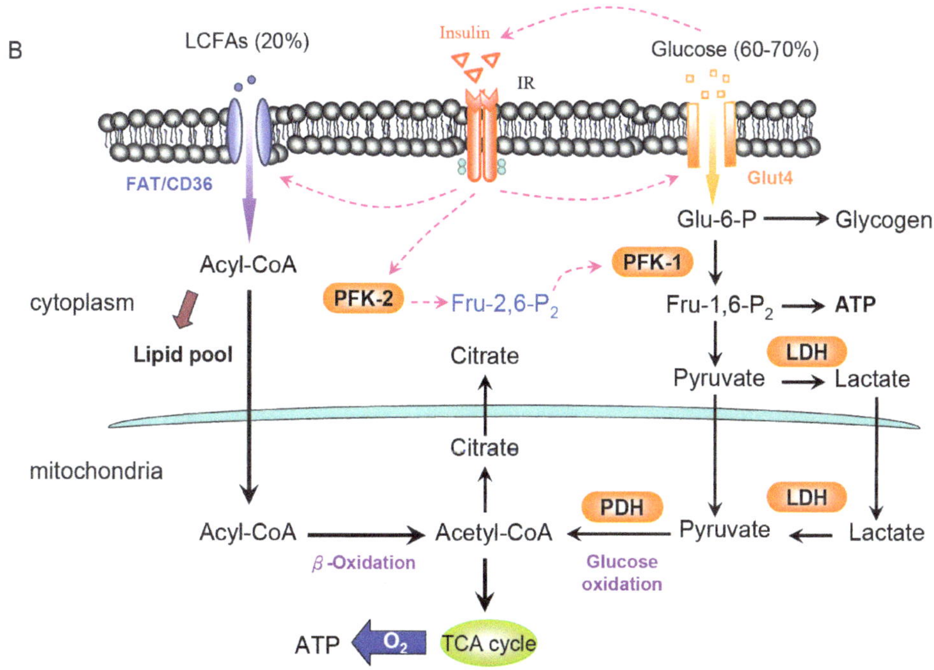

Fig. 1. Cardiac metabolism under control (A) and insulin (B) conditions. Under control conditions, ATP production comes from fatty acids and glucose oxidation. Fatty acid is the privileged substrate used by the heart, the β-oxidation inhibiting glucose oxidation via the Randle cycle. When glucose and insulin plasma levels increase, glucose becomes the main energy-providing substrate. Indeed, insulin induces Glut4 translocation and PFK-2 activation, leading to the concomitant stimulation of glucose uptake and glycolysis. (Modified from Bertrand L, Horman S, Beauloye C, Vanoverschelde JL. Insulin signalling in the heart. *Cardiovasc Res*. 2008; 79: 238-248.)

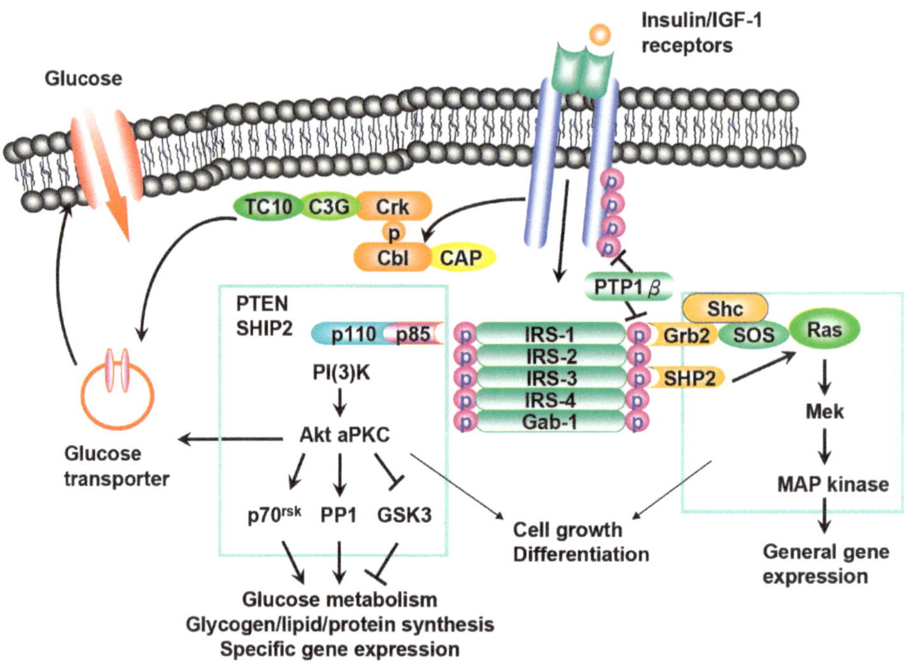

Fig. 2. Signal transduction in insulin action. The insulin receptor is a tyrosine kinase that undergoes autophosphorylation, and catalyses the phosphorylation of cellular proteins such as members of the IRS family, Shc, and Cbl. These pathways act in a concerted fashion to coordinate the regulation of vesicle trafficking, protein synthesis, enzyme activation and inactivation, and gene expression, which results in the regulation of glucose, lipid, and protein metabolism. (Modified from Saltiel AR, Kahn CR. Insulin signalling and the regulation of glucose and lipid metabolism. *Nature*. 2001; 414: 799-806.)

Insulin mediation of glucose uptake depends on the presence of glucose transporters (Gluts) at the plasma membrane. Glut1 and Glut4 are the two glucose transporters expressed in the heart; however, Glut4 is considered to be the main contributor for the insulin stimulated glucose uptake (52, 53). The role of the PI3K/PKB/Akt-signalling in the insulin-stimulated Glut4 translocation has been well established (54). Insulin not only stimulates glucose uptake, it also induces LCFA uptake in cardiomyocytes (55, 56). Insulin stimulates LCFA uptake by translocation of LCFA transporter (FAT/CD36) to the plasma membrane in the cardiomyocytes (57, 58).

Insulin also promotes protein synthesis by phosphorylation and dephosphorylation of several translational factors and ribosomal proteins through PI3K/AKT/mTOR pathway (59, 60). Activation of mTOR mainly regulates two translational factors which are 4E-binding protein-1 (4E-BP1) and the p70 ribosomal S6 protein kinase (p70S6K). Additionally, PKB/AKT also regulates GSK-3 and the forkhead transcription factor (FOXO) family, participating in the modulation of protein translation and promoting the atrogene transcriptional program (61). In addition to affecting energy metabolism, Akt activation also modulates several cellular functions which inhibit apoptosis, stimulate myocyte hypertrophy/fibrosis, and enhance nitric oxide production. Therefore, an absent insulin response can lead to less nitric oxide production, more apoptosis, and alterations in myocardial structure (62-65). Fig.3 elucidates the multiple biological functions of PKB/Akt (63).

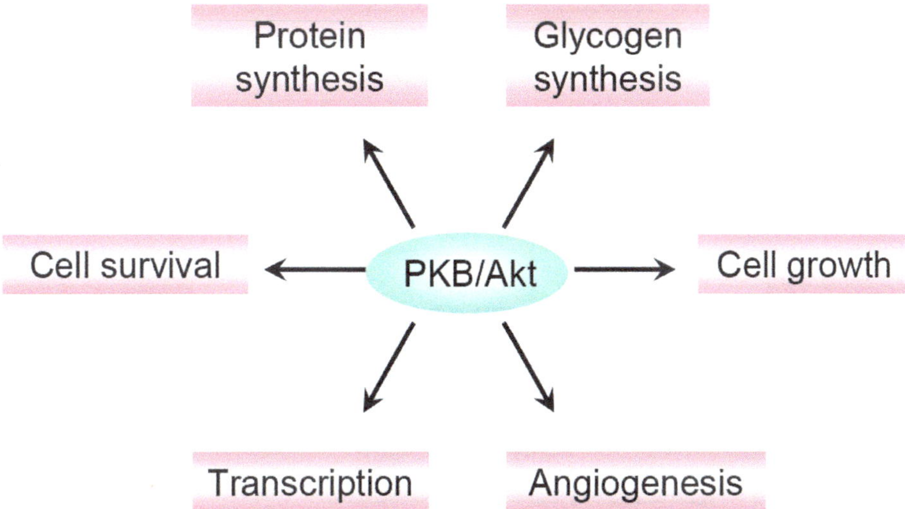

Fig. 3. Central role of protein kinase B (PKB)/Akt in multiple cellular responses. PKB/Akt control numerous of key cellular events. (Modified from Brazil DP, Hemmings BA. Ten years of protein kinase B signalling: a hard Akt to follow. *Trends Biochem Sci*. 2001; 26: 657-664.)

5. Insulin resistance induced cardiomyopathy

Insulin resistance describes an impaired biological response to insulin, and in the early stages, the plasma insulin level is increased. Although the increased insulin level may compensate for resistance to some biological actions of insulin, it may result in overexpression of actions in tissues that retain normal or slightly impaired sensitivity to insulin. In general, insulin resistance can be due to a prereceptor, receptor, or postreceptor abnormality (66). The insulin resistance induced cardiomyopathy may contain the following features.

5.1 Hypertension

Clinical studies reveal that insulin resistance and hyperinsulinemia is related to hypertension (67, 68). Mechanisms for the development of hypertension in insulin resistance and hyperinsulinemia include activation of the sympathetic nervous system, renal sodium retention, transmembrane cation transport alteration, growth-promoting effects of vascular smooth muscle cells, and vascular hyperreactivity (66, 69, 70). Fig. 4 is a schematic representation of the hypothetical relationships between obesity, insulin resistance, and hypertension (70).

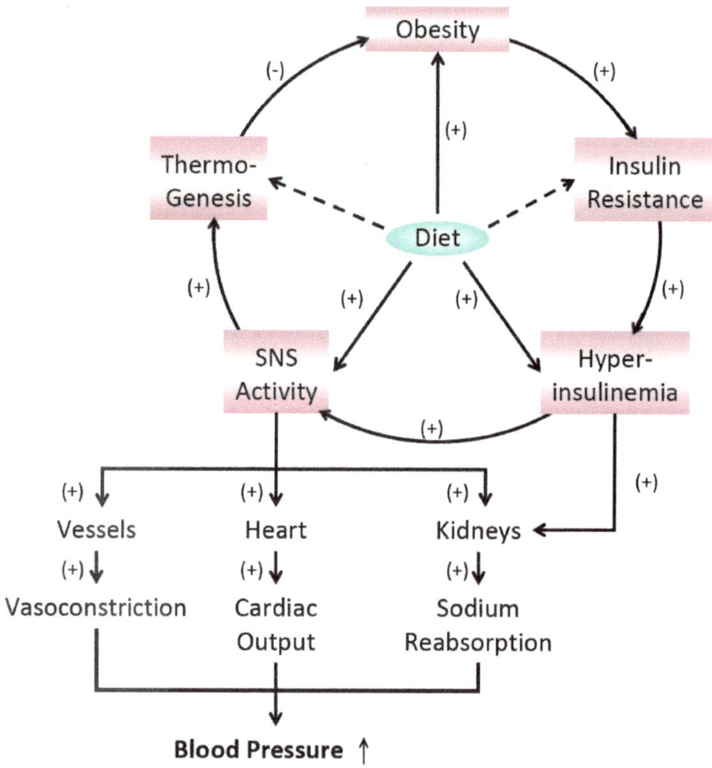

Fig. 4. Multiple role of insulin resistance to hypertension. Insulin resistance as a physiologic mechanism to restore energy balance, activate sympathetic stimulation, and leading to hypertension. The steady-state hyperinsulinemia, acting at the level of the kidney, and the consequent sympathetic stimulation of the vasculature, heart, and kidneys result in hypertension. Plus signs denote positive or stimulatory effects, the minus sign a negative or inhibitory effect, and the dotted line the direct effects of food on insulin resistance and metabolic rate. (Modified from Reaven GM, Lithell H, Landsberg L. Hypertension and associated metabolic abnormalities--the role of insulin resistance and the sympathoadrenal system. *N Engl J Med.* 1996; 334: 374-381.)

5.2 Ventricular hypertrophy

Previous studies have demonstrated that left ventricular hypertrophy and heart failure may be associated with insulin resistance (71-73). Insulin and insulin growth factor-1 (IGF-1) may exert a direct growth-promoting effect on cardiomyocytes (74, 75) and lead to cardiomyocyte hypertrophy. On the other hand, diabetes and insulin resistance are a disorder of metabolic regulation. Many acute metabolic changes alter the cellular signal transduction cascades and are believed to be involved in the adaptation of the heart to changes in its environment. PI3K, PKC and Ca^{2+}, all play a role in cardiac adaptation to regulate metabolism in the heart (76). Adrenergic activation induced hypertension may also stimulate pressure overload hypertrophy as an adaptation process (77).

5.3 Dilated cardiomyopathy and heart failure

Many studies have confirmed a strong correlation between nonischemic cardiomyopathy and diabetes, with a dramatically increased prevalence of diabetes in the dilated cardiomyopathy population (78). Additionally, abnormal glucose tolerance and insulin resistance in patients with idiopathic dilated cardiomyopathy (IDCM) has been described (49, 79). It is almost clear that insulin resistance itself is not enough to trigger dilated cardiomyopathy as the majority of patients with insulin resistance do not develop dilated cardiomyopathy. Insulin resistance is more likely to create an abnormal environment, rather than causing another stressor (e.g., pressure/volume overload, metabolic inbalance, energy defect or decreased perfusion). Insulin resistance makes the heart unable to maintain homeostasis of its energy and function, which may favor the development of cardiomyopathy and heart failure (45, 80, 81). Fig. 5 shows the relationships/mechanism between insulin resistance and heart failure (49).

5.4 Cardiac mitochondria abnormalities and ROS elevation

ROS is the one-electron reduction of O_2 to superoxide by nicotinamide adenine dinucleotide phosphate (NADPH) oxidase, which contributes to ROS generation, especially in chronic pathological states (82, 83). Mitochondria provide another significant source of cardiomyocyte ROS, particularly under acute stress. Insulin resistance impaired mitochondrial biogenesis and oxidative phosphorylation, is associated with myocardial dysfunction (84). Insulin resistance-induced hyperglycemia also directly enhances ROS generation and protein damage which leads to mitochondrial apoptosis and degradation (84). In addition, activation of the renin angiotensin aldosterone system (RAAS) is associated with increasing oxidative stress (85). The oxidative stress can impair glucose transport/utilization as well as mitochondrial ATP generation and intracellular Ca^{2+} regulatory proteins. Abnormalities in Ca^{2+} signaling/flux and myofilament functions, contribute to the cardiomyopathy changes and defective cardiac contractile function (86-87). In the 1980s, Przyklenk K et al. demonstrated that superoxide dismutase (SOD) plus catalase improve myocardial contractile function in the canine model (88). A recent study also points out that cardiac overexpression of catalase rescues insulin resistance induced myocardial contractile dysfunction (89).

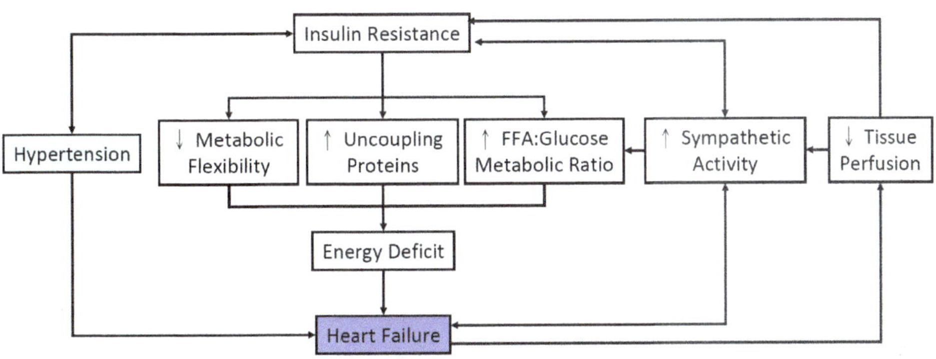

Fig. 5. Relationships/mechanism between insulin resistance to heart failure. (Modified from Witteles RM, Fowler MB. Insulin-resistant cardiomyopathy clinical evidence, mechanisms, and treatment options. *J Am Coll Cardiol*. 2008; 51: 93-102.)

6. Animal models for diabetic or insulin resistant cardiomyopathy

The impairment of glucose uptake, glycolysis, and pyruvate oxidation has been observed in both, types 1 and type 2 diabetes. In addition, attenuation of insulin function augments lipolysis and increases FFA release from adipose tissue. These abnormalities play a crucial role in the development of cardiomyopathy. Recently, several diabetic and insulin resistant animal models which include chemical (STZ-diabetes), genetic defect (*ob/ob* and *db/db* mice and Zucker diabetic fatty rats), and western diets (high fat, high fructose, high cholesterol, and high choleserol with fructose diets) diabetic induced animals, have been used to elucidate the pathophysiological processes of insulin resistance related cardiomyopathy.

6.1 Type 1 diabetes model

Streptozotocin (STZ) is a chemical generating the production of ROS which damages the pancreas with loss of function and reduced insulin production, by triggering DNA fragmentation (90, 91). The STZ-diabetic animal model can be employed for assessing the mechanisms of insulin dependent non-obese diabetes and screening potential therapies for the treatment of this condition. The characteristics of STZ-diabetes-induced cardiomyopathy include the alteration of contractile protein synthesis, abnormality of diastolic pressure-volume relationships, impairment of cardiac contractility, and incomplete relaxation of the myocardium (92, 93-97). The STZ-induced diabetics have metabolic disturbances especially, an increased plasma free fatty acid concentration (98-100). Insulin treatment reverses STZ-diabetes-induced cardiomyopathy suggesting that insulin deficiency is the major reason leading to the development of diabetic cardiomyopathy but not due to a primary cardiotoxic effect of STZ (92, 101). Resveratrol (RSV), a natural antioxidant derived from grapes, has been suggested to improve cardiac contractile function in STZ-diabetic rats (102). Moreover, the angiotensin II blocker losartan, restores cardiomyocyte functional properties in STZ-diabetic rats (103).

6.2 *Ob/ob* and *db/db* mice model

Obesity is closely associated with insulin resistance and serves as a major risk factor for the development of T2DM. Leptin or leptin receptor gene deficiency mice (*ob/ob* and *db/db* mice) are commonly used animal models for the study of T2DM. The *ob/ob* and *db/db* mice exhibit an increase of hepatic lipogenesis and gluconeogenesis resulting in increased insulin secretion by the pancreas due to the hyperglycemia and hyperlipidemia, which begins a vicious cycle of insulin resistance. Recently, contractile dysfunction independent of coronary artery disease has also been demonstrated in db/db and ob/ob mice, supporting the existence of an obesity-related cardiomyopathy and a diabetic cardiomyopathy (104-108). These genetically defective mice show a decrease in glucose oxidation rates and an increase of FFA oxidation and myocardial oxygen consumption (MVO_2), resulting in impaired cardiac efficiency (106, 108). Moreover, *ob/ob* hearts show a decrease in mitochondrial oxidative capacity, an increase of fatty acid-induced mitochondrial uncoupling, and deleterious effects on global cellular Ca^{2+} homeostasis (109, 110). As observed in STZ-diabetic rats, *db/db* mice also have excessive ROS generation, which causes cardiomyocyte damage and augmentation of apoptosis (110, 111).

6.3 Zucker diabetic fatty rat (ZDF rat)

The Zucker rat (leptin receptor gene deficient) was bred to be a genetic model for research in obesity and hypertension, and T2DM. Obese Zucker rats exhibit hyperlipidemia, hypercholesterolemia, and insulin resistance. The cardiac contractile functions and carbohydrate oxidation rates are reduced and fatty acid utilization is increased in the Zucker rat heart (28, 112-115). In contrast, several studies indicate that Zucker rats display insulin resistance without overt signs of diabetes (hyperglycemia and hyperlipidemia). These rats also show a normoglycemia phenomenon and absence of significant cardiac contractile dysfunction (116,117). Taken together, the genetic defect (leptin or leptin receptor)-induced cardiomyopathy may include several characteristics which contribute to impair myocardial contractility in diabetes mellitus. These are: (a) disturbance of substrate metabolism, (b) impairment of calcium homeostasis, (c) increased oxidative stress, (d) upregulation of the renin-angiotensin system, and (e) impairment of mitochondrial biogenesis and function (3).

6.4 Diet induced insulin resistance and cardiomyopathy

Based on previous reviews, it is widely accepted that disturbance of substrate metabolism is a key factor in the induction of insulin resistance and cardiomyopathy. Both genetic and environmental factors contribute to the development of metabolic abnormalities. Several experimental studies have demonstrated that the macronutrient composition of a diet is an important environmental determinant of the quality of insulin action (118, 119). High-fat and high-fructose intakes have been shown to contribute to conditions such as hyperlipidemia, glucose intolerance, hypertension, and atherosclerosis (120, 121). In addition, brief feeding of an excessive atherogenic diet (chow with 45% kcal from fat and 2% cholesterol) produces striking features of metabolic syndrome and coronary artery disease (122). High sugar intake is linked to an increased risk of heart disease. Simple sugars are the primary source of high triglycerides and very low-density lipoproteins (LDL), which are independent risk factors for atherosclerosis. Sugar lowers high-density lipoprotein (HDL) cholesterol and raises LDL cholesterol along with blood pressure. In addition, it has been suggested that fructose induced hyperuricemia results in endothelial dysfunction and insulin resistance, and might be a causal mechanism of the metabolic syndrome (123).

6.4.1 High fat diet (HFD)

With long term high fat intake, the response to a chronic high plasma concentration of long-chain fatty acids is that the heart is forced to increase the uptake of fatty acid. This switch in metabolic substrate uptake is accompanied by an increased presence of the fatty acid transporter FAT / CD36 at the cardiomyocyte sarcolemma. This shifts oxidation towards FA rather than glucose oxidation, and results in the development of cardiac insulin resistance and ultimately diabetic cardiomyopathy (124). It is unquestionable that chronic feeding with a high fat diet causes insulin resistance. The implication is that it decreases insulin-stimulated Akt phosphorylation, whereas cardiac basal Akt phosphorylation is elevated (124). HFD also causes cardiac lipotoxicity which may contribute to the development of diabetic cardiomyopathy (125). Additionally, hypertrophic growth and structural alterations in the context of disease is in the end maladaptive, because it will progress to, contractile dysfunction, decompensation and ultimately heart failure.

6.4.2 High fructose diet

High-fructose intake is shown to contribute to conditions such as hyperlipidemia, glucose intolerance, hypertension, and atherosclerosis (126). The preference of fructose in the lipogenesis pathway contributes to induce hyperlipidemia, in particular, a marked increase of postprandial triglyceride (TG) concentration (Fig.6) (127-129). Fructose intake is associated with an increasing incidence of insulin resistance and insulin-resistant related hypertension and cardiomyopathy (130, 131). High fructose induced insulin resistance may manifest as alterations in insulin activated PI3K/Akt pathway leading to reduced, Glut4 translocation, glucose uptake, and cardiomyocyte growth and survival. Upregulation of lipid metabolism in fructose-fed rats increases ROS production and damages the cardiomyocyte. In addition, ROS-induced dephosphorylation of Akt at Serine473 residue has been reported to participate in the insulin resistance (132).

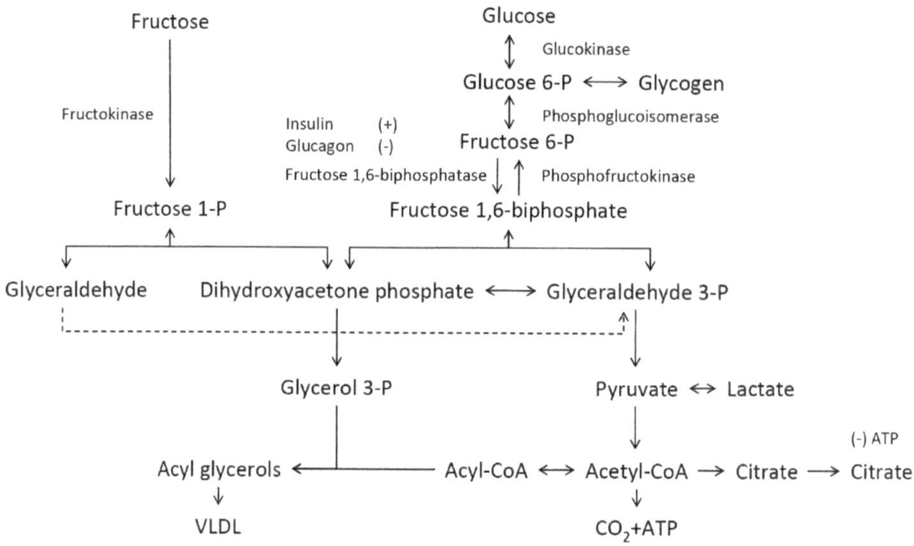

Fig. 6. Specific utilization of fructose and the glucose utilization in the liver. Hepatic fructose metabolism begins the phosphorylation by fructokinase. Fructose carbon enters the glycolytic pathway at the triose phosphate level. Thus, fructose bypasses the major control point by which glucose carbon enters glycolysis (phosphofructokinase), where glucose metabolism is limited by feedback inhibition by citrate and ATP. This allows fructose to serve as an unregulated source of both glycerol-3-phosphate and acetyl-CoA for hepatic lipogenesis. (Modified from Elliott SS, Keim NL, Stern JS, Teff K, Havel PJ. Fructose, weight gain, and the insulin resistance syndrome. *Am J Clin Nutr*. 2002; 76: 911-922.)

6.4.3 High cholesterol and fructose diet (HCF)

Brief feeding of an excessively atherogenic diet (chow with 45% kcal from fat and 2% cholesterol) produces striking features of metabolic syndrome and coronary artery disease (122). Numerous studies show that high cholesterol induces chronic inflammation. It is reported that the addition of a small amount of cholesterol to a western-type diet is associated with chronic systemic inflammation, as evidenced by an increase in atherosclerosis and circulating inflammatory protein levels (133, 134). Specifically, a study proposes the concept that, dietary cholesterol worsens adipose tissue macrophages independent of weight gain (133). This observation is consistent with the notion that adipose tissue inflammation and dysregulation of adipokines secretion contribute to the development of systemic insulin resistance (135). Our laboratory study reveals that a high cholesterol-fructose (HCF) diet also induces insulin resistance not only in metabolic-responsive tissues (i.e. liver and muscle) but also in the heart as well (25). Insulin-stimulated cardiac glucose uptake was significantly reduced after 15 weeks of HCF feeding, and cardiac insulin resistance was associated with blunted Akt-mediated insulin signaling along with GLUT4 translocation. The basal FATP1 (fatty acid transporter 1) levels were increased in HCF rat hearts. The cardiac performance of the HCF rats showed a marked reduction (25). Our results indicate that high-cholesterol food and sugar-sweetened beverages that lead to maladaptive metabolic processes may interfere with the action of insulin and increase susceptibility for the development of cardiomyopathy (25).

7. Potential therapies in insulin resistant related cardiomyopathy

Insulin resistance is an important risk factor for the development of hypertension, atherosclerotic heart disease, left ventricular hypertrophy and dysfunction, and heart failure (136-138). It reflects a disturbance of glucose metabolism and can potentially worsen the metabolic efficiency of both skeletal and cardiac muscle. The exact mechanisms of cardiac insulin resistance leading to and progression of, left ventricular contractile dysfunction are not fully elucidated. Currently, the most promising potential medical therapies for insulin resistant cardiomyopathy can be divided into 2 broad categories which are, metabolic modulators and diabetic medications (Table.2)(49).

Medication	Mechanism	Other/Side-effects
Metabolic modulators		
Trimetazidine	↓ FFA metabolism	Not approved In U.S.
Perhexiline	↓ FFA metabolism	Not approved In U.S.,liver/neuro-toxicity
Ranolazine	↑ Glu metabolism	Might not be primary mechanism, ↑ QT interval
L-carnitine	↑ FFA/Glu metabolism	
Diabetic medications		
Insulin	↑ Ins	Hypoglycemia
Sulfonylureas	↑ Ins	Hypoglycemia
Metformin	↑ Ins sensitivity	Lactic acidosis (rare)
TZDs (glitazones)	↑ Ins sensitivity	Fluid retention/edema
GLP-1	↑ Ins/ ↑ Ins sensitivity	Very short half-life (1-2 min)
Exenatide	↑ Ins/ ↑ Ins sensitivity	Nausea/weight loss, subcutaneous injection
DPP-IV inhibitor	↑ Ins/ ↑ Ins sensitivity	

Table 2. Potential treatments for insulin resistant cardiomyopathy. (Modified from Witteles RM, Fowler MB. Insulin-resistant cardiomyopathy clinical evidence, mechanisms, and treatment options. *J Am Coll Cardiol*. 2008; 51: 93-102.)

1. Metabolic modulators which increase glucose metabolism, decrease FFA metabolism, and potentially enhance myocardial contractile efficiency are e.g. Trimetazidine, Perhexiline, Ranolazine, and L-carnitine.
2. Diabetic medications enhancing insulin sensitivity (TZDs) might theoretically be the most attractive therapies to improve insulin resistant related cardiomyopathy. These agents work on the activation of PPARγ, a transcription factor that promotes insulin sensitivity and decreases circulating FFA, and increases myocardial glucose uptake (139).

Moreover, several newly developed classes of antidiabetic medications have been discovered recently. Glucagon-like peptide 1(GLP1) treatment, results in promotion of post prandial insulin secretion and improvement of insulin sensitivity (140). GLP1 infusion improves left ventricular function, hemodynamic status, and cardiac efficiency (141). In addition, angiotensin converting enzyme inhibitors (ACEI), angiotensin II receptor blockers and statins all affect glucose metabolism (142-144); although combined therapy involving a diuretic agent and a calcium-channel blocker is required (145). Interestingly, a recent study shows that RSV and insulin combination treatment has preventive effects on diabetes-associated cardiovascular dysfunction. However, when a diabetic individual has suffered an acute heart attack the synergistic actions of combination treatment were nullified and the advantage of RSV was antagonized by insulin. This study provides valuable advice for using insulin and RSV in patients with diabetes and those diabetic individuals with ischemic heart disease (102).

8. Summary and conclusion

Insulin plays an important physiological role in coupling metabolic and cardiac homeostasis under healthy conditions. Loss of normal insulin action (insulin resistance) on the heart makes the heart unable to maintain homeostasis of its energy and function, which may favor the development of cardiomyopathy and heart failure. It is almost clear that insulin resistance itself is not enough to trigger dilated cardiomyopathy as the majority of patients with insulin resistance do not develop dilated cardiomyopathy. Insulin resistance is more likely to create an abnormal environment, rather than causing another stressor.

9. References

[1] Aronson D, Rayfield EJ, Chesebro JH. Mechanisms determining course and outcome of diabetic patients who have had acute myocardial infarction. *Ann Intern Med.* 1997; 126: 296-306.

[2] Gu K, Cowie CC, Harris MI. Diabetes and decline in heart disease mortality in US adults. *JAMA.* 1999; 281:1291-1297.

[3] Boudina S, Abel ED. Diabetic cardiomyopathy revisited. *Circulation.* 2007;115: 3213–3223.

[4] Rubler S, Dlugash J, Yuceoglu YZ, Kumral T, Branwood AW, Grishman A. New type of cardiomyopathy associated with diabetic glomerulosclerosis. *Am J Cardiol.* 1972; 30: 595- 602.

[5] Bertrand L, Horman S, Beauloye C, Vanoverschelde JL. Insulin signalling in the heart. *Cardiovasc Res.* 2008; 79: 238-248.

[6] Gary D. Lopaschuk, Clifford D.L. Folmes and William C. Stanley. *Circulation Research.* 2007; 101: 335-347.

[7] Heineke J, Molkentin JD. Regulation of cardiac hypertrophy by intracellular signalling pathways. *Nat Rev Mol Cell Biol.* 2006; 7: 589–600.

[8] Wang Y. Mitogen-activated protein kinases in heart development and diseases. *Circulation.* 2007; 116: 1413-1423.

[9] Proud CG. Ras, PI3-kinase and mTOR signaling in cardiac hypertrophy. *Cardiovasc Res.* 2004; 63: 403-413.

[10] Hintz KK, Aberle NS, Ren J. Insulin resistance induces hyperleptinemia, cardiac contractile dysfunction but not cardiac leptin resistance in ventricular myocytes. *International Journal of Obesity.*2003; 27: 1196–1203.

[11] Mureddu GF, Greco R, Rosato GF, Cella A, Vaccaro O, Contaldo F, de Simone G. Relation of insulin resistance to left ventricular hypertrophy and diastolic dysfunction in obesity. *Int J Obes Relat Metab Disord.* 1998; 22: 363-368.

[12] Swan JW, Anker SD, Walton C, Godsland IF, Clark AL, Leyva F, Stevenson JC, Coats AJ. Insulin resistance in chronic heart failure: relation to severity and etiology of heart failure. *J Am Coll Cardiol.* 1997; 30: 527-532.

[13] Hayat SA, Patel B, Khattar RS, Malik RA. Diabetic cardiomyopathy: mechanisms, diagnosis, and treatment. *Clin Sci.* 2004; 107: 539–557.

[14] Voulgari C, Papadogiannis D, Tentolouris N. Diabetic cardiomyopathy: from the pathophysiology of the cardiac myocytes to current diagnosis and management strategies. *Vasc Health Risk Manag.* 2010; 6: 883-903.

[15] Poirier P, Bogaty P, Garneau C, Marois L, Dumesnil JG. Diastolic dysfunction in normotensive men with well-controlled type 2 diabetes: importance of maneuvers in echocardiographic screening for preclinical diabetic cardiomyopathy. *Diabetes Care.* 2001; 24: 5-10.

[16] Grundy SM, Benjamin IJ, Burke GL, Chait A, Eckel RH, Howard BV, Mitch W, Smith SC, Sowers JR: Diabetes and cardiovascular disease: A statement for healthcare professionals from the American Heart Association.. *Circulation.* 1999; 100: 1134–1146.

[17] Chatham JC, Forder JR, McNeill JH: *The Heart in Diabetes.* Norwell, MA: Kluwer Academic Publishers, 1996.

[18] Lagadic-Gossmann D, Buckler KJ, Le Prigent K, Feuvray D. Altered Ca2+ handling in ventricular myocytes isolated from diabetic rats. *Am J Physiol.* 1996; 270(5 Pt 2):H1529-H1537.

[19] Ren J, Davidoff AJ. Diabetes rapidly induces contractile dysfunctions in isolated ventricular myocytes. *Am J Physiol.* 1997; 272(1 Pt 2): H148-H158.

[20] Margonato A, Gerundini P, Vicedomini G, Gilardi MC, Pozza G, Fazio F. Abnormal cardiovascular response to exercise in young asymptomatic diabetic patients with retinopathy. *Am Heart J.* 1986; 112: 554-560.

[21] Mirsky I. Assessment of diastolic function: suggested methods and future considerations. *Circulation.* 1984; 69: 836-841.

[22] Pelleymounter MA, Cullen MJ, Baker MB, Hecht R, Winters D, Boone T, Collins F. Effects of the obese gene product on body weight regulation in ob/ob mice. *Science*. 1995; 28; 269: 540-543.
[23] Hu P, Zhang D, Swenson L, Chakrabarti G, Abel ED, Litwin SE. Minimally invasive aortic banding in mice: effects of altered cardiomyocyte insulin signaling during pressure overload. *Am J Physiol Heart Circ Physiol*. 2003; 285: H1261-1269.
[24] McQueen AP, Zhang D, Hu P, Swenson L, Yang Y, Zaha VG, Hoffman JL, Yun UJ, Chakrabarti G, Wang Z, Albertine KH, Abel ED, Litwin SE. Contractile dysfunction in hypertrophied hearts with deficient insulin receptor signaling: possible role of reduced capillary density. *J Mol Cell Cardiol*. 2005; 39: 882-892.
[25] Deng JY, Huang JP, Lu LS, Hung LM. Impairment of cardiac insulin signaling and myocardial contractile performance in high-cholesterol/fructose-fed rats. *Am J Physiol Heart Circ Physiol*. 2007; 293: H978-H987.
[26] Poornima IG, Parikh P, Shannon RP. Diabetic cardiomyopathy: the search for a unifying hypothesis. *Circ Res*. 2006; 98: 596-605.
[27] An D, Rodrigues B. Role of changes in cardiac metabolism in development of diabetic cardiomyopathy. *Am J Physiol Heart Circ Physiol*. 2006; 291: H1489-H1506.
[28] Chiu HC, Kovacs A, Ford DA, Hsu FF, Garcia R, Herrero P, Saffitz JE, Schaffer JE. A novel mouse model of lipotoxic cardiomyopathy. *J Clin Invest*. 2001; 107: 813-822.
[29] Christoffersen C, Bollano E, Lindegaard ML, Bartels ED, Goetze JP, Andersen CB, Nielsen LB. Cardiac lipid accumulation associated with diastolic dysfunction in obese mice. *Endocrinology*. 2003; 144: 3483-3490.
[30] Pillutla P, Hwang YC, Augustus A, Yokoyama M, Yagyu H, Johnston TP, Kaneko M, Ramasamy R, Goldberg IJ. Perfusion of hearts with triglyceride-rich particles reproduces the metabolic abnormalities in lipotoxic cardiomyopathy. *Am J Physiol Endocrinol Metab*. 2005; 288: E1229-H1235.
[31] Yagyu H, Chen G, Yokoyama M, Hirata K, Augustus A, Kako Y, Seo T, Hu Y, Lutz EP, Merkel M, Bensadoun A, Homma S, Goldberg IJ. Lipoprotein lipase (LpL) on the surface of cardiomyocytes increases lipid uptake and produces a cardiomyopathy. *J Clin Invest*. 2003; 111: 419-426.
[32] Zhou YT, Grayburn P, Karim A, Shimabukuro M, Higa M, Baetens D, Orci L, Unger RH. Lipotoxic heart disease in obese rats: implications for human obesity. *Proc Natl Acad Sci U S A*. 2000; 97: 1784-1789.
[33] Shah A, Shannon RP. Insulin resistance in dilated cardiomyopathy. *Rev Cardiovasc Med*. 2003; 4 Suppl 6: S50-S57.
[34] Shulman GI. Cellular mechanisms of insulin resistance. *J Clin Invest*. 2000; 106: 171-176.
[35] Birnbaum MJ. Turning down insulin signaling. *J Clin Invest*. 2001; 108: 655-659.
[36] Kim JK, Kim YJ, Fillmore JJ, Chen Y, Moore I, Lee J, Yuan M, Li ZW, Karin M, Perret P, Shoelson SE, Shulman GI. Prevention of fat-induced insulin resistance by salicylate. *J Clin Invest*. 2001; 108: 437-446.
[37] Liu GX, Hanley PJ, Ray J, Daut J. Long-chain acyl-coenzyme A esters and fatty acids directly link metabolism to K(ATP) channels in the heart. *Circ Res*. 2001; 88: 918-924.
[38] Du X, Matsumura T, Edelstein D, Rossetti L, Zsengellér Z, Szabó C, Brownlee M. Inhibition of GAPDH activity by poly(ADP-ribose) polymerase activates three

major pathways of hyperglycemic damage in endothelial cells. *J Clin Invest.* 2003 112: 1049-1057.

[39] Nishikawa T, Edelstein D, Du XL, Yamagishi S, Matsumura T, Kaneda Y, Yorek MA, Beebe D, Oates PJ, Hammes HP, Giardino I, Brownlee M. Normalizing mitochondrial superoxide production blocks three pathways of hyperglycaemic damage. *Nature.* 2000; 404: 787-790.

[40] Du XL, Edelstein D, Rossetti L, Fantus IG, Goldberg H, Ziyadeh F, Wu J, Brownlee M. Hyperglycemia-induced mitochondrial superoxide overproduction activates the hexosamine pathway and induces plasminogen activator inhibitor-1 expression by increasing Sp1 glycosylation. *Proc Natl Acad Sci U S A.* 2000; 97: 12222-12226.

[41] Bidasee KR, Nallani K, Yu Y, Cocklin RR, Zhang Y, Wang M, Dincer UD, Besch HR Jr. Chronic diabetes increases advanced glycation end products on cardiac ryanodine receptors/calcium-release channels. *Diabetes.* 2003; 52: 1825-1836.

[42] Candido R, Forbes JM, Thomas MC, Thallas V, Dean RG, Burns WC, Tikellis C, Ritchie RH, Twigg SM, Cooper ME, Burrell LM. A breaker of advanced glycation end products attenuates diabetes-induced myocardial structural changes. *Circ Res.* 2003; 92: 785-792.

[43] Herrmann KL, McCulloch AD, Omens JH. Glycated collagen cross-linking alters cardiac mechanics in volume-overload hypertrophy. *Am J Physiol Heart Circ Physiol.* 2003; 284: H1277-H1284.

[44] Clark RJ, McDonough PM, Swanson E, Trost SU, Suzuki M, Fukuda M, Dillmann WH. Diabetes and the accompanying hyperglycemia impairs cardiomyocyte calcium cycling through increased nuclear O-GlcNAcylation. *J Biol Chem.* 2003; 278: 44230-44237.

[45] Galvez AS, Ulloa JA, Chiong M, Criollo A, Eisner V, Barros LF, Lavandero S. Aldose reductase induced by hyperosmotic stress mediates cardiomyocyte apoptosis: differential effects of sorbitol and mannitol. *J Biol Chem.* 2003; 278: 38484-38494.

[46] Koya D, King GL. Protein kinase C activation and the development of diabetic complications. *Diabetes.* 1998; 47: 859-866.

[47] Wakasaki H, Koya D, Schoen FJ, Jirousek MR, Ways DK, Hoit BD, Walsh RA, King GL. Targeted overexpression of protein kinase C beta2 isoform in myocardium causes cardiomyopathy. *Proc Natl Acad Sci U S A.* 1997; 94: 9320-9325.

[48] Paolisso G, De Riu S, Marrazzo G, Verza M, Varricchio M, D'Onofrio F. Insulin resistance and hyperinsulinemia in patients with chronic congestive heart failure. *Metabolism.* 1991; 40: 972-977.

[49] Witteles RM, Fowler MB. Insulin-resistant cardiomyopathy clinical evidence, mechanisms, and treatment options. *J Am Coll Cardiol.* 2008; 51: 93-102.

[50] Saltiel AR, Kahn CR. Insulin signalling and the regulation of glucose and lipid metabolism. *Nature.* 2001; 414: 799-806.

[51] Deprez J, Bertrand L, Alessi DR, Krause U, Hue L, Rider MH. Partial purification and characterization of a wortmannin-sensitive and insulin-stimulated protein kinase that activates heart 6-phosphofructo-2-kinase. *Biochem J.* 2000; 347 Pt 1:305-312.

[52] Zorzano A, Sevilla L, Camps M, Becker C, Meyer J, Kammermeier H, Muñoz P, Gumà A, Testar X, Palacín M, Blasi J, Fischer Y. Regulation of glucose transport, and

glucose transporters expression and trafficking in the heart: studies in cardiac myocytes. *Am J Cardiol.* 1997; 80: 65A-76A.

[53] Abel ED. Glucose transport in the heart. *Front Biosci.* 2004; 9: 201-215.

[54] Watson RT, Pessin JE. Bridging the GAP between insulin signaling and GLUT4 translocation. *Trends Biochem Sci.* 2006; 4: 215-222.

[55] Coort SL, Bonen A, van der Vusse GJ, Glatz JF, Luiken JJ. Cardiac substrate uptake and metabolism in obesity and type-2 diabetes: role of sarcolemmal substrate transporters. *Mol Cell Biochem.* 2007; 299(1-2): 5-18.

[56] Glatz JF, Bonen A, Ouwens DM, Luiken JJ. Regulation of sarcolemmal transport of substrates in the healthy and diseased heart. *Cardiovasc Drugs Ther.* 2006; 20: 471-476.

[57] Luiken JJ, Koonen DP, Willems J, Zorzano A, Becker C, Fischer Y, Tandon NN, Van Der Vusse GJ, Bonen A, Glatz JF. Insulin stimulates long-chain fatty acid utilization by rat cardiac myocytes through cellular redistribution of FAT/CD36. *Diabetes.* 2002; 51: 3113-3119.

[58] Dyck DJ, Steinberg G, Bonen A. Insulin increases FA uptake and esterification but reduces lipid utilization in isolated contracting muscle. *Am J Physiol Endocrinol Metab.* 2001; 281: E600-E607.

[59] Hedhli N, Pelat M, Depre C. Protein turnover in cardiac cell growth and survival. *Cardiovasc Res.* 2005; 68: 186-196.

[60] Proud CG. Signalling to translation: how signal transduction pathways control the protein synthetic machinery. *Biochem J.* 2007; 403: 217-234.

[61] Sandri M, Sandri C, Gilbert A, Skurk C, Calabria E, Picard A, Walsh K, Schiaffino S, Lecker SH, Goldberg AL. Foxo transcription factors induce the atrophy-related ubiquitin ligase atrogin-1 and cause skeletal muscle atrophy. *Cell.* 2004; 117: 399-412.

[62] Asbun J, Villarreal FJ. The pathogenesis of myocardial fibrosis in the setting of diabetic cardiomyopathy. *J Am Coll Cardiol.* 2006; 47: 693-700

[63] Brazil DP, Hemmings BA. Ten years of protein kinase B signalling: a hard Akt to follow. *Trends Biochem Sci.* 2001; 26: 657-664.

[64] Lawlor MA, Alessi DR. PKB/Akt: a key mediator of cell proliferation, survival and insulin responses? *J Cell Sci.* 2001; 114(Pt 16): 2903-2910.

[65] Stühlinger MC, Abbasi F, Chu JW, Lamendola C, McLaughlin TL, Cooke JP, Reaven GM, Tsao PS. Relationship between insulin resistance and an endogenous nitric oxide synthase inhibitor. *JAMA.* 2002; 287: 1420-1426.

[66] Hunter SJ, Garvey WT. Insulin action and insulin resistance: diseases involving defects in insulin receptors, signal transduction, and the glucose transport effector system. *Am J Med.* 1998; 105: 331-345.

[67] Ferrannini E, Buzzigoli G, Bonadonna R, Giorico MA, Oleggini M, Graziadei L, Pedrinelli R, Brandi L, Bevilacqua S. Insulin resistance in essential hypertension. *N Engl J Med.* 1987; 317: 350-357.

[68] Shen DC, Shieh SM, Fuh MM, Wu DA, Chen YD, Reaven GM. Resistance to insulin-stimulated-glucose uptake in patients with hypertension. *J Clin Endocrinol Metab.* 1988; 66: 580-583.

[69] Sowers JR, Sowers PS, Peuler JD. Role of insulin resistance and hyperinsulinemia in development of hypertension and atherosclerosis. *J Lab Clin Med*. 1994; 123: 647-652.

[70] Reaven GM, Lithell H, Landsberg L. Hypertension and associated metabolic abnormalities--the role of insulin resistance and the sympathoadrenal system. *N Engl J Med*. 1996; 334: 374-381.

[71] Ingelsson E, Sundström J, Arnlöv J, Zethelius B, Lind L. Insulin resistance and risk of congestive heart failure. *JAMA*. 2005; 294: 334-341.

[72] Ho KK, Pinsky JL, Kannel WB, Levy D. The epidemiology of heart failure: the Framingham Study. *J Am Coll Cardiol*. 1993; 22(4 Suppl A): 6A-13A.

[73] Verdecchia P, Reboldi G, Schillaci G, Borgioni C, Ciucci A, Telera MP, Santeusanio F, Porcellati C, Brunetti P. Circulating insulin and insulin growth factor-1 are independent determinants of left ventricular mass and geometry in essential hypertension. *Circulation*. 1999; 100: 1802-1827.

[74] Hill DJ, Milner RD. Insulin as a growth factor. *Pediatr Res*. 1985; 19: 879-886.

[75] Ito H, Hiroe M, Hirata Y, Tsujino M, Adachi S, Shichiri M, Koike A, Nogami A, Marumo F. Insulin-like growth factor-I induces hypertrophy with enhanced expression of muscle specific genes in cultured rat cardiomyocytes. *Circulation*. 1993; 87: 1715-1721.

[76] Doenst T, Taegtmeyer H. alpha-adrenergic stimulation mediates glucose uptake through phosphatidylinositol 3-kinase in rat heart. *Circ Res*. 1999; 84: 467-474.

[77] Kariya K, Karns LR, Simpson PC. An enhancer core element mediates stimulation of the rat beta-myosin heavy chain promoter by an alpha 1-adrenergic agonist and activated beta-protein kinase C in hypertrophy of cardiac myocytes. *J Biol Chem*. 1994; 269: 3775-3782.

[78] Bertoni AG, Tsai A, Kasper EK, Brancati FL. Diabetes and idiopathic cardiomyopathy: a nationwide case-control study. *Diabetes Care*. 2003; 26: 2791-2795.

[79] Witteles RM, Tang WH, Jamali AH, Chu JW, Reaven GM, Fowler MB. Insulin resistance in idiopathic dilated cardiomyopathy: a possible etiologic link. *J Am Coll Cardiol*. 2004; 44: 78-81.

[80] Nikolaidis LA, Sturzu A, Stolarski C, Elahi D, Shen YT, Shannon RP. The development of myocardial insulin resistance in conscious dogs with advanced dilated cardiomyopathy. *Cardiovasc Res*. 2004; 61: 297-306.

[81] Dávila-Román VG, Vedala G, Herrero P, de las Fuentes L, Rogers JG, Kelly DP, Gropler RJ. Altered myocardial fatty acid and glucose metabolism in idiopathic dilated cardiomyopathy. *J Am Coll Cardiol*. 2002; 40: 271-277.

[82] Selemidis S, Sobey CG, Wingler K, Schmidt HH, Drummond GR. NADPH oxidases in the vasculature: molecular features, roles in disease and pharmacological inhibition. *Pharmacol Ther*. 2008; 120: 254-291.

[83] Lambeth JD. NOX enzymes and the biology of reactive oxygen. *Nat Rev Immunol*. 2004; 4: 181-189.

[84] Ren J, Pulakat L, Whaley-Connell A, Sowers JR. Mitochondrial biogenesis in the metabolic syndrome and cardiovascular disease. *J Mol Med* (Berl). 2010; 88: 993-1001.

[85] Cooper SA, Whaley-Connell A, Habibi J, Wei Y, Lastra G, Manrique C, Stas S, Sowers JR. Renin-angiotensin-aldosterone system and oxidative stress in cardiovascular insulin resistance. *Am J Physiol Heart Circ Physiol*. 2007; 293: H2009-H2023.

[86] Choi KM, Zhong Y, Hoit BD, Grupp IL, Hahn H, Dilly KW, Guatimosim S, Lederer WJ, Matlib MA. Defective intracellular Ca(2+) signaling contributes to cardiomyopathy in Type 1 diabetic rats. *Am J Physiol Heart Circ Physiol*. 2002; 283: H1398-H1408.

[87] Dong F, Li Q, Sreejayan N, Nunn JM, Ren J. Metallothionein prevents high-fat diet induced cardiac contractile dysfunction: role of peroxisome proliferator activated receptor gamma coactivator 1alpha and mitochondrial biogenesis. *Diabetes*. 2007; 56: 2201-2212.

[88] Przyklenk K, Kloner RA. Superoxide dismutase plus catalase improve contractile function in the canine model of the "stunned myocardium". *Circ Res*. 1986; 58: 148-156.

[89] Dong F, Fang CX, Yang X, Zhang X, Lopez FL, Ren J. Cardiac overexpression of catalase rescues cardiac contractile dysfunction induced by insulin resistance: Role of oxidative stress, protein carbonyl formation and insulin sensitivity. *Diabetologia*. 2006; 49: 1421-1433.

[90] Kakkar R, Mantha SV, Radhi J, Prasad K, Kalra J. Increased oxidative stress in rat liver and pancreas during progression of streptozotocin-induced diabetes. *Clin Sci* (Lond). 1998; 94: 623-632.

[91] Szkudelski T. The mechanism of alloxan and streptozotocin action in B cells of the rat pancreas. *Physiol Res*. 2001; 50: 537-546.

[92] Huang JP, Huang SS, Deng JY, Hung LM. Impairment of insulin-stimulated Akt/GLUT4 signaling is associated with cardiac contractile dysfunction and aggravates I/R injury in STZ-diabetic rats. *J Biomed Sci*. 2009; 16:77.

[93] Fein FS, Kornstein LB, Strobeck JE, Capasso JM, Sonnenblick EH. Altered myocardial mechanics in diabetic rats. *Circ Res*. 1980; 47: 922-933.

[94] Regan TJ, Lyons MM, Ahmed SS, et al. Evidence for cardiomyopathy in familial diabetes mellitus. *J Clin Invest*. 1977; 60: 885–899.

[95] Regan TJ, Ettinger PO, Khan MU, et al. Altered myocardial function and metabolism in chronic diabetes mellitus without ischemia in dogs. *Circ Res*. 1974; 35: 222–237.

[96] Garber DW, Neely JR. Decreased myocardial function and myosin ATPase in hearts from diabetic rats. *Am J Physiol*. 1983; 244: H586– H591.

[97] How OJ, Aasum E, Severson DL, Chan WY, Essop MF, Larsen TS. Increased myocardial oxygen consumption reduces cardiac efficiency in diabetic mice. *Diabetes*. 2006; 55: 466-473.

[98] Penpargkul S, Schaible T, Yipintsoi T, Scheuer J. The effect of diabetes on performance and metabolism of rat hearts. *Circ Res*. 1980; 47: 911-921.

[99] Ogihara M, Tokumitsu Y, Ui M. Metabolic alterations in normal and streptozotocin-diabetic rats in vivo: influence of prolonged starvation. *Jpn J Pharmacol*. 1984; 34: 307-311.

[100] Malone JI, Cuthbertson DD, Malone MA, Schocken DD. Cardio-protective effects of carnitine in streptozotocin-induced diabetic rats. *Cardiovasc Diabetol.* 2006; 19; 5: 2.

[101] Schaible TF, Malhotra A, Bauman WA, Scheuer J. Left ventricular function after chronic insulin treatment in diabetic and normal rats. *J Mol Cell Cardiol.* 1983; 15: 445-458.

[102] Huang JP, Huang SS, Deng JY, Chang CC, Day YJ, Hung LM. Insulin and resveratrol act synergistically, preventing cardiac dysfunction in diabetes, but the advantage of resveratrol in diabetics with acute heart attack is antagonized by insulin. *Free Radic Biol Med.* 2010; 49: 1710-1721.

[103] Raimondi L, De Paoli P, Mannucci E, Lonardo G, Sartiani L, Banchelli G, Pirisino R, Mugelli A, Cerbai E. Restoration of cardiomyocyte functional properties by angiotensin II receptor blockade in diabetic rats. *Diabetes.* 2004; 53: 1927-1933.

[104] Wolf G. Insulin resistance associated with leptin deficiency in mice: a possible model for noninsulin-dependent diabetes mellitus. *Nutr Rev.* 2001; 59: 177-179.

[105] Buchanan J, Mazumder PK, Hu P, Chakrabarti G, Roberts MW, Yun UJ, Cooksey RC, Litwin SE, Abel ED. Reduced cardiac efficiency and altered substrate metabolism precedes the onset of hyperglycemia and contractile dysfunction in two mouse models of insulin resistance and obesity. *Endocrinology.* 2005; 146: 5341-5349.

[106] Belke DD, Larsen TS, Gibbs EM, Severson DL. Altered metabolism causes cardiac dysfunction in perfused hearts from diabetic (db/db) mice. *Am J Physiol Endocrinol Metab.* 2000; 279: E1104-E1113.

[107] Mazumder PK, O'Neill BT, Roberts MW, Buchanan J, Yun UJ, Cooksey RC, Boudina S, Abel ED. Impaired cardiac efficiency and increased fatty acid oxidation in insulin-resistant ob/ob mouse hearts. *Diabetes.* 2004; 53: 2366-2374.

[108] Boudina S, Sena S, O'Neill BT, Tathireddy P, Young ME, Abel ED. Reduced mitochondrial oxidative capacity and increased mitochondrial uncoupling impair myocardial energetics in obesity. *Circulation.* 2005; 112: 2686-2695.

[109] Fauconnier J, Andersson DC, Zhang SJ, Lanner JT, Wibom R, Katz A, Bruton JD, Westerblad H. Effects of palmitate on Ca($^{2+}$) handling in adult control and ob/ob cardiomyocytes: impact of mitochondrial reactive oxygen species. *Diabetes.* 2007; 56: 1136-1142.

[110] Barouch LA, Gao D, Chen L, Miller KL, Xu W, Phan AC, Kittleson MM, Minhas KM, Berkowitz DE, Wei C, Hare JM. Cardiac myocyte apoptosis is associated with increased DNA damage and decreased survival in murine models of obesity. *Circ Res.* 2006; 98: 119-124.

[111] Cai L, Li W, Wang G, Guo L, Jiang Y, Kang YJ. Hyperglycemia-induced apoptosis in mouse myocardium: mitochondrial cytochrome C-mediated caspase-3 activation pathway. *Diabetes.* 2002; 51: 1938-1948.

[112] Young ME, Guthrie PH, Razeghi P, Leighton B, Abbasi S, Patil S, Youker KA, Taegtmeyer H. Impaired long-chain fatty acid oxidation and contractile dysfunction in the obese Zucker rat heart. *Diabetes.* 2002; 51: 2587-2595.

[113] Chatham JC, Seymour AM. Cardiac carbohydrate metabolism in Zucker diabetic fatty rats. *Cardiovasc Res*. 2002; 55: 104-112.

[114] Wang P, Lloyd SG, Zeng H, Bonen A, Chatham JC. Impact of altered substrate utilization on cardiac function in isolated hearts from Zucker diabetic fatty rats. *Am J Physiol Heart Circ Physiol*. 2005; 288: H2102-H2110.

[115] Rösen P, Herberg L, Reinauer H. Different types of postinsulin receptor defects contribute to insulin resistance in hearts of obese Zucker rats. *Endocrinology*. 1986; 119: 1285-1291.

[116] Coort SL, Hasselbaink DM, Koonen DP, Willems J, Coumans WA, Chabowski A, van der Vusse GJ, Bonen A, Glatz JF, Luiken JJ. Enhanced sarcolemmal FAT/CD36 content and triacylglycerol storage in cardiac myocytes from obese zucker rats. *Diabetes*. 2004; 53: 1655-1663.

[117] Carley AN, Severson DL. Fatty acid metabolism is enhanced in type 2 diabetic hearts. *Biochim Biophys Acta*. 2005; 1734: 112-126.

[118] Axen KV, Dikeakos A, Sclafani A. High dietary fat promotes syndrome X in nonobese rats. *J Nutr*. 2003; 133: 2244-2249.

[119] Bessesen DH. The role of carbohydrates in insulin resistance. *J Nutr*. 2001; 131: 2782S-2786S.

[120] Mann JI. Diet and risk of coronary heart disease and type 2 diabetes. *Lancet*. 2002; 360: 783-789.

[121] Storlien LH, Kraegen EW, Jenkins AB, Chisholm DJ. Effects of sucrose vs starch diets on in vivo insulin action, thermogenesis, and obesity in rats. *Am J Clin Nutr*. 1988; 47: 420-427.

[122] Dyson MC, Alloosh M, Vuchetich JP, Mokelke EA, Sturek M. Components of metabolic syndrome and coronary artery disease in female Ossabaw swine fed excess atherogenic diet. *Comp Med*. 2006; 56: 35-45.

[123] Nakagawa T, Tuttle KR, Short RA, Johnson RJ. Hypothesis: fructose-induced hyperuricemia as a causal mechanism for the epidemic of the metabolic syndrome. *Nat Clin Pract Nephrol*. 2005; 1: 80-86.

[124] Ouwens DM, Diamant M, Fodor M, Habets DD, Pelsers MM, El Hasnaoui M, Dang ZC, van den Brom CE, Vlasblom R, Rietdijk A, Boer C, Coort SL, Glatz JF, Luiken JJ. Cardiac contractile dysfunction in insulin-resistant rats fed a high-fat diet is associated with elevated CD36-mediated fatty acid uptake and esterification. *Diabetologia*. 2007; 50: 1938-1948.

[125] Schaffer JE. Lipotoxicity: when tissues overeat. *Curr Opin Lipidol*. 2003; 14: 281-287.

[126] Kuczmarski RJ, Flegal KM, Campbell SM, Johnson CL. Increasing prevalence of overweight among US adults. The National Health and Nutrition Examination Surveys, 1960 to 1991. *JAMA*. 1994; 272: 205-211.

[127] Bantle JP, Raatz SK, Thomas W, Georgopoulos A. Effects of dietary fructose on plasma lipids in healthy subjects. *Am J Clin Nutr*. 2000; 72: 1128-1134.

[128] Teff KL, Elliott SS, Tschöp M, Kieffer TJ, Rader D, Heiman M, Townsend RR, Keim NL, D'Alessio D, Havel PJ. Dietary fructose reduces circulating insulin and leptin, attenuates postprandial suppression of ghrelin, and increases triglycerides in women. *J Clin Endocrinol Metab*. 2004; 89: 2963-2972.

[129] Elliott SS, Keim NL, Stern JS, Teff K, Havel PJ. Fructose, weight gain, and the insulin resistance syndrome. *Am J Clin Nutr*. 2002; 76: 911-922.

[130] Hwang IS, Ho H, Hoffman BB, Reaven GM. Fructose-induced insulin resistance and hypertension in rats. *Hypertension*. 1987; 10: 512-516.

[131] Mellor KM, Bell JR, Young MJ, Ritchie RH, Delbridge LM. Myocardial autophagy activation and suppressed survival signaling is associated with insulin resistance in fructose-fed mice. *J Mol Cell Cardiol*. 2011; 50: 1035-1043.

[132] Cao J, Xu D, Wang D, Wu R, Zhang L, Zhu H, He Q, Yang B. ROS-driven Akt dephosphorylation at Ser-473 is involved in 4-HPR-mediated apoptosis in NB4 cells. *Free Radic Biol Med*. 2009; 47: 536-547.

[133] Subramanian S, Han CY, Chiba T, McMillen TS, Wang SA, Haw A 3rd, Kirk EA, O'Brien KD, Chait A. Dietary cholesterol worsens adipose tissue macrophage accumulation and atherosclerosis in obese LDL receptor-deficient mice. *Arterioscler Thromb Vasc Biol*. 2008; 28: 685-691.

[134] Lewis KE, Kirk EA, McDonald TO, Wang S, Wight TN, O'Brien KD, Chait A. Increase in serum amyloid a evoked by dietary cholesterol is associated with increased atherosclerosis in mice. *Circulation*. 2004; 110: 540-545.

[135] Berg AH, Scherer PE. Adipose tissue, inflammation, and cardiovascular disease. *Circ Res*. 2005; 96: 939-949.

[136] Ferrannini E, Iozzo P. Is insulin resistance atherogenic? A review of the evidence. *Atheroscler Suppl*. 2006; 7: 5-10.

[137] Govindarajan G, Whaley-Connell A, Mugo M, Stump C, Sowers JR. The cardiometabolic syndrome as a cardiovascular risk factor. *Am J Med Sci*. 2005; 330: 311-318.

[138] Paternostro G, Pagano D, Gnecchi-Ruscone T, Bonser RS, Camici PG. Insulin resistance in patients with cardiac hypertrophy. *Cardiovasc Res*. 1999; 42: 246-253.

[139] Hällsten K, Virtanen KA, Lönnqvist F, Janatuinen T, Turiceanu M, Rönnemaa T, Viikari J, Lehtimäki T, Knuuti J, Nuutila P. Enhancement of insulin-stimulated myocardial glucose uptake in patients with Type 2 diabetes treated with rosiglitazone. *Diabet Med*. 2004; 21: 1280-1287.

[140] Salehi M, D'Alessio DA. New therapies for type 2 diabetes based on glucagon-like peptide 1. *Cleve Clin J Med*. 2006; 73: 382-389.

[141] Nikolaidis LA, Elahi D, Hentosz T, Doverspike A, Huerbin R, Zourelias L, Stolarski C, Shen YT, Shannon RP. Recombinant glucagon-like peptide-1 increases myocardial glucose uptake and improves left ventricular performance in conscious dogs with pacing-induced dilated cardiomyopathy. *Circulation*. 2004; 110: 955-961.

[142] Freeman DJ, Norrie J, Sattar N, Neely RD, Cobbe SM, Ford I, Isles C, Lorimer AR, Macfarlane PW, McKillop JH, Packard CJ, Shepherd J, Gaw A. Pravastatin and the development of diabetes mellitus: evidence for a protective treatment effect in the West of Scotland Coronary Prevention Study. *Circulation*. 2001; 103: 357-362.

[143] Pfeffer MA, Swedberg K, Granger CB, Held P, McMurray JJ, Michelson EL, Olofsson B, Ostergren J, Yusuf S, Pocock S; CHARM Investigators and Committees. Effects of candesartan on mortality and morbidity in patients with chronic heart failure: the CHARM-Overall programme. *Lancet*. 2003; 362: 759-766.

[144] Yusuf S, Sleight P, Pogue J, Bosch J, Davies R, Dagenais G. Effects of an angiotensin-converting-enzyme inhibitor, ramipril, on cardiovascular events in high-risk patients. The Heart Outcomes Prevention Evaluation Study Investigators. *N Engl J Med*. 2000; 342: 145-153.

[145] Williams B, Poulter NR, Brown MJ, Davis M, McInnes GT, Potter JF, Sever PS, McG Thom S; British Hypertension Society. Guidelines for management of hypertension: report of the fourth working party of the British Hypertension Society, 2004-BHS IV. *J Hum Hypertens*. 2004; 18: 139-185.

6

Thyrotoxic Cardiomyopathy

Alina Yu. Babenko, Alekber A. Bairamov,
Elena N. Grineva and Eugenia O. Ulupova
Almazov Federal Heart, Blood and Endocrinology Centre, St. Petersburg, Russia

1. Introduction

1.1 Thyrotoxicosis and thyrotoxic cardiomyopathy – Current state

Thyrotoxicosis is a common syndrome, and according to the Wickham Survey its prevalence is 2% among women and 0.2% in men in the areas with normal iodine consumption. Over the 20-year follow-up the incidence of thyrotoxicosis was 0.8:1000 in women and 0.6:1000 in men (Bird et al,1977).

Subclinical thyrotoxicosis (ST) is defined by low or undetectable serum thyrotropin stimulating hormone (TSH) and normal free thyroxin (FT4) and free triiodthyronin (FT3) concentrations (Biondi & Cooper, 2008). Although thyroid hormones are defined as being within normal range in patients with ST, they are often at the upper limit of the reference range, and thus sufficiently increased to suppress TSH and potentially produce abnormal tissue effects.

The prevalence of subclinical thyrotoxicosis varies from 0.6 to 16% % (Biondi et al., 2002; Wang & Crapo, 1997; Samuels, 1998) depending on such risk factors as age (it is twice higher in elderly people), iodine deficiency (5-times higher in the areas of iodine deficiency), and decreased TSH level. All authors agree that ST is more common compared to overt thyrotoxicosis.

There are exogenous (iatrogenic) and endogenous causes of thyrotoxicosis. Exogenous thyrotoxicosis usually is subclinical and mainly is caused by suppressive therapy with L-thyroxin leading to the decrease of TSH below normal values. It is commonly present in postoperative patients with differentiated thyroid cancer (papillary and follicular) as the mean of cancer recurrence prevention. This group of patients gets prolonged (2 years and longer) high-dose L-thyroxin therapy, and is considered in studies regarding side-effects of suppressive treatment. At the same time patients with benign thyroid nodules get short courses (6-12 months) of suppressive therapy, leading to a less decrease of TSH (above 0,1 mIU/l). According to the majority of data 1/2-2/3 of ST cases are exogenous (Figge et al., 1994; Canaris et al., 2002; Hoogendoorn et al., 2004).

Endogenous thyrotoxicosis can be also divided into immune (Graves' disease, "Hashitox") and non-immune (toxic (pretoxic) thyroid adenoma and toxic multinodular goiter) (Ross, 1996; Marqusee et al., 1998; Al-Abadi, 2001). Graves' disease is the most common cause of overt thyrotoxicosis.

Thyrotoxic cardiomyopathy (TCMP) is a threatening complication of thyrotoxicosis increasing risk of disability and mortality. Until recently myocardial alterations observed in thyrotoxicosis were considered favorable regarding prognosis because of the high reversibility if euthyroid state is quickly achieved. However, long-term follow-up studies demonstrated that the involution of the changes is not always complete. Some irreversible histological alterations of myocardium are found in patients who had thyrotoxicosis in past: necrosis of the hypertrophied myocytes and fibrosis development (Ortmann et al., 1999). Myocardial fibrosis has been also detected by radioimmunoimaging with antimyosin antibodies in patients with TCMP complicated by heart failure (HF) (Martí et al., 1997).

There is a current evidence that even successfully treated thyrotoxicosis is associated with the worse prognosis. Thus, cardiovascular (hypertension, valvular diseases, heart failure, and to a lesser extent coronary artery disease) mortality is 1.2 higher in these patients, and cerebrovascular mortality is 1.4 higher than in general population (Osman et al., 2002). Persistent cardiovascular alterations are considered an evident cause of the increased mortality in thyrotoxicosis (Metso et al., 2007; Sheu et al., 2010). Health effects of subclinical thyrotoxicosis are not fully recognized, and some questions are still unsolved. However, quite large amount of publications of the last two decades verify deleterious effects of thyrotoxicosis, and uppermost, on cardiovascular system (Biondi et al., 2002). Moreover, there is evidence of the increased mortality in subclinical thyrotoxicosis (Sgarbi, 2010). Thus, in British study among patients over 60 years of age mortality (5 year follow-up) in subjects with TSH below normal values was about twice that of euthyroid subjects (Parle et al., 2001). Cardiovascular diseases were the most common cause of lethal events. Therefore, cardiovascular complications of thyrotoxicosis are of great medical importance.

2. Definition – Epidemiology of thyrotoxic cardiomyopathy and its clinical variants

Thyrotoxic cardiomyopathy defines a myocardial damage caused by the toxic effects of abundant thyroid hormones (TH) (Report of the 1995 WHO/ISFC) that result in altered energy production by myocytes (oxidative phosphorylation, glycolysis), intracellular metabolism (protein synthesis) and myofibril contractile function (Klein, 1990).

The main manifestations of thyrotoxic cardiomyopathy (TCMP) are left ventricular hypertrophy (LVH) (Ching et al., 1996, Dorr et al., 2005), heart rhythm disturbances (usually, atrial fibrillation (AF)) (Dunn et al., 1986; Frost et al., 2004), dilation of the heart chambers and heart failure (HF) (Dougherty & Craige, 1973; Siu et al., 2007), pulmonary hypertension (PH) (Chu et al., 2002; Rubin & Badesch, 2006), and diastolic dysfunction. Epidemiology data on TCMP are currently lacking. This is due to the lack of diagnostic criteria and to the late introduction of the term "thyrotoxic cardiomyopathy" in clinical and research practice that occurred only after implementation of WHO classification of cardiomyopathies (Report of the 1995 WHO/ISFC).

Meanwhile et al. (1959) found that 4 out of 9 postmortem examinations detected no other cause for severe congestive HF but thyrotoxicosis, and that 64 out of 150 patients (43%) with thyrotoxicosis had cardiovascular complications in the absence of any known pre-existing heart disease.

The available evidence provides only data on the incidence of TCMP manifestations, including the most severe ones - AF and HF.

The incidence of heart rhythm disturbances in thyrotoxicosis varies in a wide range. Sinus tachycardia is the most common occurring in 42%-73% [Burggraaf J et al 2001, Cacciatori V, et al. 1996]. Tachycardia at rest and during sleep is a typical symptom in thyrotoxicosis.

Heart rate at rest is known to be one of the most important reserve parameters and a predictor of fatal cardiovascular complications. Elevated resting heart rate is associated with higher mortality. Risk of death from all causes is three-times higher in subjects with resting heart rate of 90-99 versus 60 beats per minute. Predictive value of heart rate is higher in hypertensive people and those with coronary artery disease. High resting heart rate might cause worsening of hypertension, increases risk of acute cardiovascular events, coronary artery disease, fatal ventricular arrhythmias as the most common causes of a sudden death, blood pressure elevation and heart failure development. Sinus bradycardia is rather rare in thyrotoxicosis.

Atrial fibrillation takes second place among heart rhythm disturbances occurring in 9%-23% of thyrotoxic patients compared to 0.4%-1.0% in general population (Petersen & Hansen, 1988; Presti & Hart, 1989; Parle et al., 1991; Frost et al., 2004). This is the most common cardiovascular complication of thyrotoxicosis), and is associated with high morbidity and mortality related to the thromboembolism (Staffurt et al., 1977). The complication rate varies widely and will be discussed later. Thus, Sandler and Wilson (1959) and Petersen and Hansen (1988) found 14% and 14.9% occurrence of atrial fibrillation, respectively, in the population of subjects without concomitant heart disease. In a study of women with different cardiac pathology atrial fibrillation was diagnosed in 67% of subjects with thyrotoxicosis (Ladenson, 1993).

Subclinical thyrotoxicosis is associated with the increased risk of atrial fibrillation (Auer et al., 2001). In the Framingham study at 20-year follow-up the incidence of AF was 25% in patients with low TSH that is 3 times as high as in euthyroid patients (7%) (Sawin et al., 1994). The prevalence of AF seems to be comparable in overt and subclinical thyrotoxicosis. According to Auer J. et al. (2001) it was 13.8% in patients with overt thyrotoxicosis, 12.7 % in subclinical thyrotoxicosis, and 2.3 % in euthyroid subjects (Auer et al., 2001). Extrasystole (5%-7%), paroxysmal tachycardia (0.2%-3.3%) and atrial flutter (approximately 1.4%) rarely occur in thyrotoxicosis. 24-hour ECG monitoring studies demonstrated that atrial heart rhythm disturbances are typical for thyrotoxicosis while ventricular ones usually occur only in severe cases and in subjects with concomitant cardiovascular diseases (table1).

Arrhythmias	Frequency (%)
Sinus tachycardia	42-73
Atrial fibrillation	9-23
Extrasystole	5-7
Atrial flutter	1,2-2,3
Paroxysmal tachycardia	0,2-3,3
AV-block	2,7-5
Sick sinus syndrome can develop in elderly people	

Table 1. Arrhythmias in thyrotoxicosis

The evidence on **left ventricular hypertrophy** (LVH) prevalence is not enough. On the one hand, some authors found the increase in left ventricular myocardium mass in both overt (Nixon et al., 1979; Auer et al., 2001; Dorr et al., 2005; Marcisz et al., 2006) and subclinical (Ching et al., 1996; Biondi, 1999, 2000; Auer, 2001) thyrotoxicosis. On the other hand, there are not enough studies considering LVH occurrence in thyrotoxicosis and factors contributing its development, geometry type (eccentric or concentric), and reversibility.

According to the epidemiology study (1510 patients over 45 years of age) by M. Dörr et al. (2005) LVH was diagnosed in 57,1% of patients with thyrotoxicosis, compared to 10.5% in euthyroid individuals. Therefore, thyrotoxicosis was considered an independent predictor of LVH (odds ratio, 13.65; 95% confidence interval, 2.83–65.75; $p < 0.01$). We have analyzed the occurrence of LVH and factors contributing its development and reversibility among in-patients with thyrotoxicosis. The LVH occurrence was 22.7% that is lower compared to the mentioned data. We included patients under 55 years of age without concomitant cardiovascular pathology, and this could be a possible reason for the lower prevalence (Babenko et al., 2011).

The increase of left ventricular myocardial mass index (LVMMI) was demonstrated in all studies regarding subclinical thyrotoxicosis (Ching et al., 1996; Auer, 2001), however, the values did not meet diagnostic criteria for left ventricular hypertrophy (Biondi, 1999, 2000).

Only women with overt thyrotoxicosis, unlike those with subclinical thyrotoxicosis, had high values of LVMMI (meeting LVH criteria) associated with the decrease of end-diastolic left ventricular volume and development of concentric LVH (CLVH), as reported by Donatelli M et al. (2003) on the other hand, the majority of studies demonstrate increase of both LVMMI and end-diastolic left ventricular volume and development of eccentric LVH (ELVH) (Levina, 1989; Marcisz et al., 2006; Babenko et al., 2007, 2008, 2011).

Concentric remodeling of left ventricle occurs in ST (Biondi et al., 2002; Donatelli et al., 2003), while eccentric remodeling is more common in overt thyrotoxicosis.

Prevalence of heart failure also widely varies - from 12% to 68% (Forfar et al., 1982; Hrnciar, 2002; Roffi et al., 2003); up to 90% of patients with thyrotoxicosis and HF develop AF (Siu et al., 2007).

Dilated TCMP as a threatening complication of thyrotoxicosis should be mentioned (Goland et al., 1999). Siu C-W. et al. (2007) reported 1% occurrence of **dilated thyrotoxic cardiomyopathy** in patients with thyrotoxicosis, and one thirds of cases is irreversible. Thyrotoxicosis accounts for 1% of the reasons of dilated TCMP (Lutton et al., 2001).

Association between thyrotoxicosis and pulmonary hypertension (PH) has been described as early as in the beginning of 1980s (Mier et al., 1989) and the linking mechanisms are discussed till nowadays (Yanai-Landau et al., 1995; Barst & Loyd, 1998; Menzel et al., 2000; Armigliato et al., 2006). Graves' (autoimmune) disease accounts for the most cases of PH: 47-65% of patients with diffuse goiter have PH (Mercé et al., 2005, Armigliato et al., 2006; Yung et al., 2006), such a high prevalence can be explained by both severe form of thyrotoxicosis and autoimmune effects (Yanai-Landau et al., 1995; Chu et al., 2002). The occurrence of PH in subclinical thyrotoxicosis is almost unknown. According to our data, the prevalence of PH was 29% in ST, and 39.6% in overt thyrotoxicosis.

The prevalence of mitral valve prolapse is 18-41% in thyrotoxicosis compared to 6-20% in general population (Brauman et al., 1985, Kahaly, 1986, Evangelopoulou et al., 1999).

3. The pathogenesis of thyrotoxic cardiomyopathy and its manifestations

3.1 Cardiovascular effects of thyroid hormones

Thyroid hormones (TH) affect cardiovascular system through three main intracellular processes in cardiomyocytes: energy production (oxidative phosphorylation, glycolysis), protein synthesis and cardiomyofibril contractility (Dillmann, 1990; Klein et al., 2000, 2001).

Alteration of energy production. Myocardial oxygen consumption increases in thyrotoxicosis. The number of mitochondria and their functional activity grows leading to the enhancement of adenosine triphosphate (ATP) production. However, in severe thyrotoxicosis, despite the increased oxygen consumption, the efficiency of its utilization decreases significantly. This follows altered oxidative phosphorylation resulted from the abnormal oxidative enzyme activity (decrease of myocardial ATP and creatine phosphate levels results in glycolysis activation) (Golber & Kandror, 1972).

Direct and indirect effects on myocardial of abundant TH **result in alteration of cardiomyofibril contractility**. **Direct effects** involve transcription of some genes regulating function of cardiomyiocytes, vascular smooth muscle cells (SMC) and other structural units (Dillmann, 1990; Klein et al., 2000, 2001)(Fig.1). Triiodothyronine (T3) is a biologically active thyroid hormone that enters cardiomyocytes through specific transporters located in the cellular membrane, and binds thyroid hormone receptor (THR) in the nucleus (Dillmann,1990; Everts et al., 1996). Nowadays two types of THR are known: homodimer (THR/THR) and heterodimer - 9-cis retinoic acid receptor (THR/RXR). Active forms of these receptors affect gene expression through binding specific DNA response elements, so called thyroid hormone-sensitive elements (TRE), located in the promoter region of T3-sensitive genes (Brent, 1994; Everts et al., 1996; Fazio et al., 2004). Gene transcription is augmented in the regions encoding alpha-myosine heavy chains (MNC-a), Ca^{2+}-ATPase of sarcoplasmatic reticulum of the cardiomyocytes, Ca^{2+}-K^{+}-ATPase Ca^{2+}- -uretic, beta1-adrenergic receptors, troponine I and Ca^{+}-uretic peptide. Three types of myosine isoforms are distinguished: V1 consisting of the MNC-alpha/alpha chains, V2 - consisting of MNC-alpha/beta chains, and V3 - consisting of MNC-beta/beta chains. High levels of TH affect myosine isoform expression and lead to the enhanced synthesis of V1 isoform and decrease of V3 isoform. ATPase being more active in MNC-alpha/alpha myosine chains compared to MNC-beta/beta chains, the velocity of myofibril contractions increases (Klein & Ojamaa, 2000, 2001) (Fig.1).

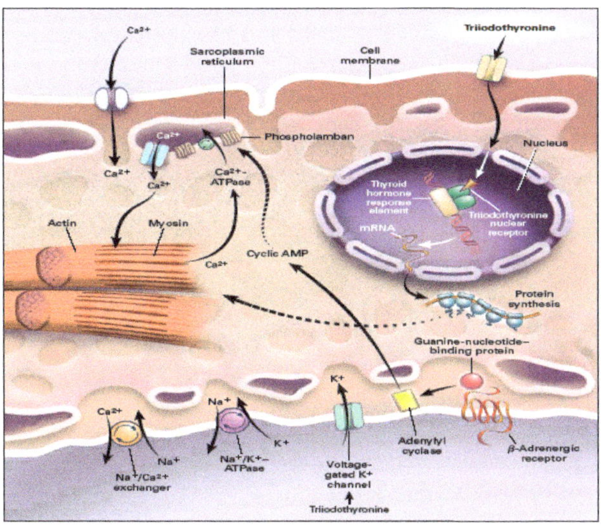

Fig. 1. Genom and nongenom effects of triiodthyronine in cardiomyocytes (from Klein& Ojamaa, 2000)

Indirect myocardial effect of abundant thyroid hormones include Ca^{2+} release from the intracellular depots and their subsequent reuptake by sarcoplasmic reticulum. The latter results from the enhanced Ca^{2+} ATPase (SERCA) expression and phospholamban suppression that are involved in the regulation of calcium intramyocyte concentration during cardiac cycle (systole and diastole). This leads to the increase of peak strain of cardiomyofibrils and shortening of the ventricular systole. Abundant thyroid hormone have been shown to induce expression of ryanodine receptors facilitating calcium (Ca2+) release from sarcoplasmic reticulum, thus amplifying contraction and myocardial hypertrophy. Moreover, high levels of TH cause intracellular calcium mobilization directly affecting L-type of Ca2+-channels (Dillmann , 1990, Kiss et al., 1994; Klein & Ojamaa, 2000, 2001)(Fig.1).

Therefore, high levels of TH contribute to the increased myocardial contractility through enhanced transcription of the genes encoding heavy chains of myocine beta-isoform and calcium-dependent ATPase, induced protein synthesis and augmented calcium and glucose myocardial consumption. In addition, thyroid hormones cause 50-70% reduction of the **systemic vascular resistance** (SVR) through direct and indirect (increase of tissue thermogenesis and lactate hyperproduction) effects on vascular smooth muscle cells leading to the decrease of diastolic blood pressure (DBP) and the increase of end-diastolic left ventricular volume. In particular, TH are known to induce nitric oxide production causing vasodilatation through direct effects on vascular smooth muscle cells (Ishikawa et al., 1989; Klein & Ojamaa, 2000, 2001; Vargas et al., 2006). Moreover, high levels of TH lead to the increase of circulating blood volume and venous return through the following mechanisms: aldosterone-renin system activation, enhancement of erythropoietin synthesis and renal sodium reabsorption (Jiménez et al., 1982; Marchant et al., 1993; Klein & Ojamaa, 2000, 2001; Vargas et al., 2006). Renal juxteglomerular complex is activated when DBP is reduced (Büssemaker et al., 2003). In addition, T3 directly stimulates rennin substrate synthesis by liver (Ganong WF. 1982). The reduction of BP and SVR induces production of rennin and aldosterone resulting in the increase of circulating blood volume and end-diastolic volume that finally amplifies workload on heart (Klein & Ojamaa, 2000, 2001; Vargas et al., 2006) (fig.2).

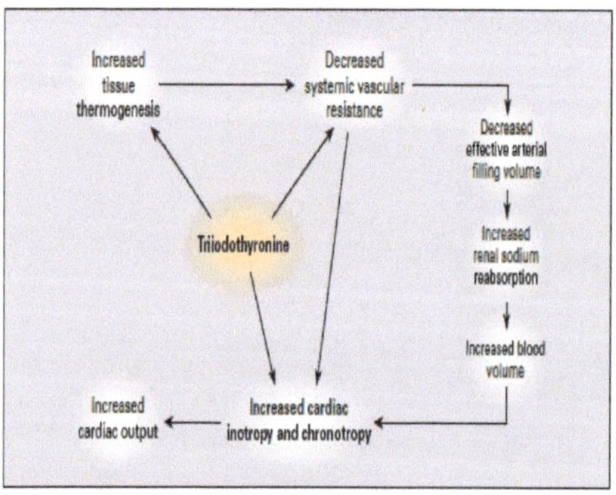

- The diagram shows the way in which triiodothyronine increases cardiac output by affecting tissue oxygen consumption (thermogenesis),
- vascular resistance, blood volume, cardiac contractility, and heart rate

(from Klein I. and Ojamaa K. 2001)

Fig. 2. Effects of Thyroid Hormone on Cardiovascular Hemodynamics

Tachycardia is a typical feature of thyrotoxicosis (Nordyke, 1988; Cacciatori, 1996; Biondi, 2000). It is caused by the faster diastolic depolarization associated with the shortening of action potential of the sinoatrial node (Osman et al., 2002). In general, the TH effects on pacemaker and conductive cardiac system include acceleration of systolic and diastolic depolarization and shortening of action potential, as well as of refractory period of atrial and atrioventricular myocytes. The latter can result in the increase of AF occurrence in thyrotoxicosis. Other mechanisms include augmentation of the pressure in left atrium, ischemia and left atrial premature ectopic heart beats (Bielecka-Dabrowa et al., 2009).

Thyroid hormones regulate some myocardial genes encoding synthesis of ion channels (K^+/Na^+-ATPase, Ca^+/Na^+- exchanger and potential-depending potassium channels) in cell membrane. These extranuclear effects involve the transport of aminoacids, glucose and calcium through cell membrane. Therefore, T3 can alter the activity of various ion channels (including sodium, potassium and calcium channels) located in cell membrane. (Bielecka-Dabrowa et al., 2009). In particular, phospholipid and Ca-dependent proteinkinase, cAMP-dependent proteinkinase, and Ca2+-calmodulin complex as the components of signal transmission system are involved in the T3 non-genomic cell effects. Thus, non-genomic actions of thyroid hormones include regulation of intracellular ion levels and their intracellular distribution. Changing transmembrane ion transport TH affect electrophysiologic features of cardiomyocytes (Kim & Smith, 1984). T3-induced expression of L-type calcium channels leads to the following: less calcium ions enter cardiomyocytes through L-type channels, and action potential gets shorter (Freedberg et al., 1970).

The occurrence of atrial rhythm disturbances (atrial fibrillation, atrial premature heart beats) is higher at thyrotoxicosis, while the rate of ventricular arrhythmias is comparable with the one in general population (Osman et al., 2002). Atrial and ventricular myocardial sensitivity to thyroid hormones is different that can be the cause of the variation in atrial and ventricular arrhythmia prevalence. High atrial sensitivity to arrhythmogenic thyroid effects is due to the high β-adrenoreceptor density at the surface of atrial cardiomyocytes and to the different autonomic innervation of atria and ventricles (Polikar et al., 1993; Lombardi et al., 1994). Golf et al. (1985) found that β-adrenoreceptor density in right atria of human heart samplings is more than twice as high as in left ventricle. Higher β-adrenoreceptor density in thyrotoxicosis is associated with the greater catecholamine myocardial sensitivity. Androgens up-regulate expression of the β-adrenoreceptor genes leading to their density increase. This can explain higher susceptibility to heart rhythm disturbances in men compared to one of women.

Expression of potential-dependent K+-channels in atria is 30% as high as in ventricles (Ojamaa et al., 1999). Expression of genes encoding both β-adrenoreceptor and potential-dependent K+-channels depends on thyroid hormones that induce heart rhythm disturbances. Experimental mice studies demonstrated that duration of atrial action potential is shorter, and atrial delayed rectifier potassium current (ultra rapid - Ikur and slow - Iss) mediating repolarization is greater in thyrotoxicosis. RNA messenger level and expression of genes of K+-channels (Kv1.5 и Kv2.1) were shown to be higher in both atria that also leads to the greater density of delayed rectifier potassium channels (Ikur и Iss) in hyperthyroidism. Thyroid effects on action potential and delayed rectifier potassium current are more expressed in right atrium compared to left one resulting in low interatrial difference of action potential duration (Bielecka-Dabrowa et al., 2009).

Shortening of atrial action potential in thyrotoxicosis is associated with the shorter duration of effective refractory period facilitating re-entry foci developing. On the other hand, normal interatrial difference of action potential is of great importance for synchronous atrial contraction (regarding right-sided location of the sinus node). Spontaneous ectopic activity, particularly in left atrium, can increase leading to atrial heart rhythm disturbances (atrial fibrillation) when the interatrial action potential difference is reduced (Bielecka-Dabrowa, 2009).
Pulmonary veins are known to initiate paroxysmal atrial fibrillation that can be due to the increased spontaneous activity of that region. Shorter action potential of the cardiomyocytes located in pulmonary veins associated with the shortening of refractory period and facilitating re-entry onset was shown in experimental thyrotoxicosis models (Chen, 2002). Incubation with thyroid hormones increased spontaneous activity in pulmonary vein cardiomyocytes similar to its effect on sinoatrial node cells. Trigger activity is supposed to underlie spontaneous activity of pulmonary veins (Bielecka-Dabrowa et al., 2009).

3.2 Pathogenesis of clinical manifestations of thyrotoxic cardiomyopathy

Tachycardia in thyrotoxicosis develops due to the faster diastolic depolarization associated with the shortening of action potential of the sinoatrial node cells [Osman F et al. 2002]. Sinus bradycardia can develop in case of congenital disorders or sick sinus syndrome. The latter, as well as abnormal heart rhythm can result from the decreased reserves of the mediator acetylcholine.
Mechanisms of arrhythmogenesis are discussed in the former chapter. Pathogenesis of heart rhythm disorders is not clear, and the following pathogenetic factors are being discussed: toxic effects of thyroid hormones, increased sympathetic activity, reduced intracellular potassium level (Table 2).

Effects of thyroid hormones	Pathogenesis of influence of thyroid hormones
Toxic influence on myocardium (amplification cardiomyofibril contractility and hypertrophy right atrium and left ventricule of heart)	Alteration oxidative phosphorylation. Increase synthesis of protein, action of enzymes, uptake of O_2 Alteration power processes and changes of K+/Na+-pump - increase velocity of diastolic depolarization
Increase sensitivity of SNS	Increase of number of β1-adrenoreceptors
Decrease of intracellular pool of potassium	Hyperfunction of heart and increase of action of simpatoadrenal influence
Change of vascular reactivity	Hyperrelaxations vascular myocites

Table 2. Pathogenesis of arrhythmias in thyrotoxicosis

Cardiac hyperfunction and increased adrenergic stimulation contribute the loss of intracellular potassium ions leading to heart rhythm disorders. Atrial dystrophic alterations associated with the structural myocardial heterogeneity are a confounding factor for atrial fibrillation. Exposure to any additional factor increasing myocardial heterogeneity can result in the complete myocardial uncoupling inducing heart rhythm disturbances. Atrial dilation, increased excitability of atria associated with the myocardial heterogeneity mediating functional conductive disorders underlie re-entry arrhythmias. Re-entry associated with the frequent focal activity are supposed to be the main mechanism of atrial fibrillation and flutter in thyrotoxicosis.

Increased cardiac output and reduced system vascular resistance (SVR) in thyrotoxicosis commonly lead to the amplification of pulse amplitude. Hemodynamics is altered in thyrotoxicosis as it has been mentioned above. The changes include elevation of heart rate, stroke and minute volumes, acceleration of blood flow, decrease of systemic vascular resistance (Fig.3), and resulting changes of blood pressure - systolic blood pressure is moderately increased, while diastolic blood pressure is within normal values or decreased. Thus pulse pressure goes up. The recent studies have demonstrated arterial stiffening and low SVR in thyrotoxicosis (Palmieri et al., 2004). Therefore, high levels of thyroid hormones cause systolic blood pressure (BP) elevation leading to **isolated systolic hypertension** in elderly patients with decreased arterial elasticity due to the atherosclerotic vascular lesion. The prevalence of isolated systolic hypertension is significantly higher in patients with thyrotoxicosis compared to euthyroid subjects (Marcisz et al., 2001). ST can resulting in an increase in nighttime systolic and mean blood pressure (Botella-Carretero et al, 2004). It appears to be one of the factors for LVH development in thyrotoxicosis.

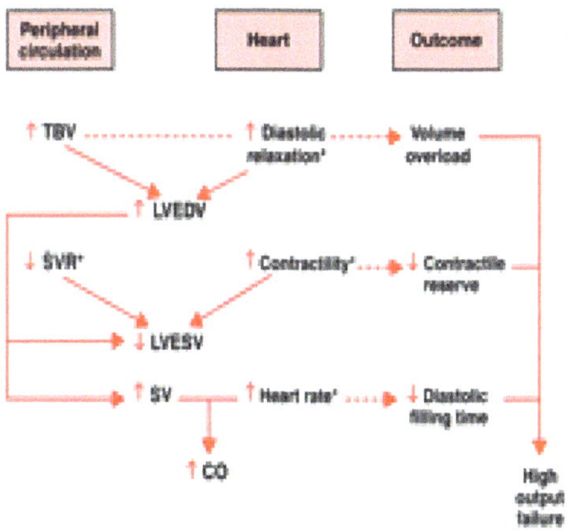

TBV- total blood volume;
LVEDV - left ventricular end diastolic volume; LVESV - left ventricular end systolic volume;
SV - stroke volume;
SVR - systemic vascular resistance;
CO - cardiac output;
↑ increase; ↓ decrease.
Solid arrows indicate direct effects, and dashed arrows potential outcomes.
*Features for which T3 is directly responsible. (from A Toft, N Boon 2000)

Fig. 3. Effects of hyperthyroidism on the cardiovascular system and the possible outcomesEccentric type of LVH, as a result of low SVR and volume overload on the heart, is a typical feature of thyrotoxicosis. However, there are data showing both normal LV geometry (Levina, 1989; Babenko, 2008), and LVH (eccentric type (Levina, 1989; Marcisz et al., 2006; Babenko et al., 2008, 2011) as well as concentric one (Donatelli et al., 2003) in patients with thyrotoxicosis. It depends on the degree of cardiovascular damage influenced by the variety of factors that will be discussed later.

Reduced **functional cardiac reserve** and physical load tolerance are also common in thyrotoxicosis because tachycardia at rest prevents from the increase of heart rate and effusion fraction and from the SVR lowering at physical load.

Pulmonary hypertension (PH) (mean pulmonary pressure more than 25 mmHg at rest and more than 30 mmHg at load) is frequently reported at overt thyrotoxicosis. Pulmonary hypertension is often associated with valvular insufficiency (of tricuspid and mitral valves) due to the papillary muscles dysfunction (Whitner et al., 2005; Mercé et al., 2005). Patients with Graves' disease are more likely to have myxomatous degeneration and prolapse of mitral valve as a consequence of endocardium involvement compared to subjects with toxic multinodular goiter (Kahaly, 1987).

There are two possible mechanisms of valve involvement in Graves' disease. First mechanism includes induction of glycosaminoglycan synthesis in endocardium (similar to one in retrobulbar space in ophthalmopathy) leading to the valve cusp thickening (Kahaly, 1987). The second one implies the reduced tone of papillary muscles and their consequent overstretching resulting in prolapse of mitral valve cusps in left atrium during ventricular systole (Brauman et al., 1985).

Pulmonary hypertension develops due to Kitaev reflex - spasm of pulmonary arterioles leading to the increase of pulmonary resistance (Okura & Takatsu, 1994). Thyroid hormones seem to affect pulmonary vessels in a rather different way compared to other vessels as they cause SVR reduction and circulating blood volume elevation. Blood pressure decreases in resistive vessels due to the vasodilatation effect of TH, and increases in pulmonary vessels. This is possibly mediated by endothelial dysfunction (Okura & Takatsu, 1994), and by the accelerated metabolism of pulmonary vasodilatation substances, such as acetylcholine, observed in patients with severe thyrotoxicosis (Okura & Takatsu, 1994; Nakchbandi et al., 1999). In addition, autonomic imbalance, in particular, sympathetic hyperactivity and lower vagal tone (Burggraaf et al., 2001), caused by hyperthyroidism facilitates further pulmonary vasoconstriction and PH development. Autoimmune mechanism might be an additional factor for PH development (Yanai-Landau et al., 1995; Barst & Loyd, 1998; James et al., 2002).

The diagnosis of heart failure in thyrotoxic patients is complex, because classic symptoms of heart failure including tachycardia and dyspnea, occur at the onset of hyperthyroidism due to both toxic effects of thyroid hormones on sinoatrial node and respiratory centre and intercostal muscles weakness. Heart failure (HF) develops in thyrotoxicosis because of the isotonic contraction (volume overload) of left ventricle and mixed overload (both volume and resistance overload) of right ventricle, thus right ventricular HF is more common for hyperthyroid state. Concomitant tricuspid valve insufficiency and regurgitation can worsen the situation (Whitner et al., 2005). Mitral valve prolapse is a common disorder in thyrotoxicosis, but it is rarely symptomatic.

Heart failure (HF) associated with thyrotoxicosis is more common in elderly rather than in young patients, and the mechanisms are better studied in aged group. Elderly subjects usually have co-existing cardiovascular diseases (coronary artery disease, valvular heart disease, arterial hypertension) leading to the functional and structural cardiac alterations, thus, myocardium contractility is easily impaired in case of increased myocardial load caused by hyperthyroidism. Elderly patients with heart rhythm disturbances, such as atrial fibrillation (AF), have the highest risk of HF development, because AF is usually associated with the increased heart rate followed by functional impairment of cardiomyocytes. Younger patients without cardiovascular pathology more often develop "high output heart failure" (Okura & Takatsu, 1994). This type of HF is characterized by the myocardial hypercontractility. HF with low output and heart chambers dilation (dilated thyrotoxic cardiomyopathy) can develop in young patients in case of the long-lasting severe thyrotoxicosis (Manger et al., 1988; Soh & Croxson, 2008). However, long duration of hyperthyroidism is not always evident, so the mechanisms are not fully understood.

Autoimmune mechanisms were considered possible (Kahaly, 1987; Koshiyama et al., 1996), but the hypothesis was denied afterwards (Fatourechi & Edwards, 2000). Two hypotheses are discussed nowadays. According to the first one two diseases are supposed to coexist in one individual - Graves' disease and idiopathic dilated cardiomyopathy (IDC). It is supported by their common pathogenesis - genetic predisposition determined by the HLA haplotypes (Limas & Limas, 1989; Olson et al., 1992) and common association of IDC and autoimmune thyroid diseases (Marković et al., 2005). According to the second hypothesis long-lasting myocardial hypertrophy can transform into dilation, and heart chamber dilation can develop in untreated prolonged overt and even subclinical thyrotoxicosis (Soh & Croxson, 2008).

Therefore, there are two main mechanisms of heart failure development in thyrotoxicosis: 1) tachycardia-induced HF with left ventricular dysfunction (left ventricular HF) is most common in patients with AF; 2) right ventricular HF resulted from volume overload of right ventricle due to the increased circulating blood volume and venous return is characterized by right ventricular dilation, enlargement of the tricuspid valve ring and tricuspid insufficiency and is frequently associated with pulmonary hypertension (Okura & Takatsu, 1994; Xenopoulos et al., 1996; Whitner et al., 2005).

Three stages of thyrotoxic cardiomyopathy are defined: hyperkinetic (with preserved left ventricular function, but at physical load left ventricular effusion fraction does not increase), normokinetic (a compensatory stage with a reversible myocardial hypertrophy and preserved cardiac output), and hypokinetic stage (decompensation stage with low cardiac output and stroke volume, either reversible or irreversible heart chamber hypertrophy and dilation).

High occurrence of thromboembolic events (higher than in general population) is typical for thyrotoxicosis, and even in absence of AF. Endothelial dysfunction is a possible explanation for high rate of thromboembolism: altered vasodilation response to acetylcholine exposure (Faber et al., 2001, Napoli et al., 2001), as well as elevated level of humoral substances Von Willebrand factor (Cucuianu et al., 1987; Squizzato et al., 2007), plasminogen activator, endothelin (Baumgartner-Parzer et al., 1997) confirm thrombogenesis activation in thyrotoxicosis (Homoncik et al., 2007). ST has been recently shown to have a prothrombogenic effects (Horne et al., 2004; Erem, 2006). Increased activity of Von Willebrand factor (Coban et al., 2006) and elevated fibrinogen level (Dörr et al., 2001) were demonstrated at ST.

4. Clinical manifestations and diagnostic tests of thyrotoxic cardiomyopathy

The most common symptoms of thyrotoxic cardiomyopathy are palpitations, chest pain (cardialgia), dyspnea, irregular heart beats. Tachycardia and heart rhythm disturbances, systolic hypertension, orthostatic hypotension, heart enlargement, systolic murmur maximal over mitral valve and bubbling rales in case of HF are the most common findings at physical examination. Tachycardia at rest and during sleep and significant increase of heart rate at minimal physical exertion are typical for thyrotoxicosis. Tachycardia is position-independent and resistant to therapy by cardiac glycosides. Usually there is a direct relation between tachycardia intensity and the severity of diffuse goiter. Heart rate increases up to 120-140 beats per minute, and up to 160 beats per minute and more on movement, at physical and emotional exertion. Patients complain of pulsation in the neck, head and abdomen. Atrial fibrillation can develop in both clinical thyrotoxicosis and subclinical and latent forms. Thus, as a potential cause thyrotoxicosis should be excluded in all patients with persistent atrial fibrillation resistant to antiarrhythmic drugs. Thyroid dysfunction is the cause of 46% of arrhythmias of this type. Paroxysmal atrial fibrillation at the onset of thyrotoxicosis usually turns into permanent form with the progression of the disease. There is a particular form of thyrotoxicosis characterized by paroxysmal atrial fibrillation with normal sinus rhythm or bradycardia without any other symptoms of thyrotoxicosis. The level of thyroid hormones is crucial to make the diagnosis in such cases. Physical examination reveals tachycardia and ascending apex beat. The cardiac borders are expanded to the left, the heart sounds are intensive, first heart sound is loud, and systolic murmur can be heard. Systolic blood pressure is increased, while diastolic blood pressure is within normal values or decreased (resulting in high pulse pressure, or pulse amplitude). Water retention is usual, and edema can be found even in patients with preserved ejection fraction. If the symptoms are persistent after successful treatment of thyrotoxicosis coexistent cardiovascular pathology should be excluded. In otherwise healthy individuals palpitations are associated with female sex and age older than 50 years, dyspnea is linked to female sex and increased level of T4>30 pmol/l. After euthyroid state restoration dyspnea can persist in smoking subjects (Osman et al., 2007).

Heart failure is associated with the pleural effusions, and right ventricular heart failure is more prevalent in diffuse goiter (Levina, 1989). Patients with dilated thyroid cardiomyopathy reveals cardiomegaly and pulmonary congestion (Soh & Croxson, *2008)* and all spectre clinical sins of heart failure.

Diagnosis. ECG changes include high, sharp P and T waves, atrial fibrillation, and extrasystole. ST segment depression and T wave inversion might be also present without angina pectoris, and are due to metabolic changes. ECG changes are reversible if the thyroid hormone levels are normalized.

Dilation of both ventricles and conus pulmonalis expansion are typical radiological signs in severe thyrotoxicosis. Conus pulmonalis expansion and right ventricle enlargement form mitral configuration of the heart. However, there is no left atrium enlargement at oblique view unlike the changes in mitral stenosis.

Pulmonary edema is another radiological sign in thyrotoxicosis. Echocardiography finds left ventricular hypertrophy including posterior wall and interventricular septum thickening, increase of end-diastolic volume and of left ventricular myocardial mass. Mitral valve prolapse is a common finding in thyrotoxicosis. The dilation of all heart chambers and decreased systolic function of left ventricle can be found in dilated thyrotoxic cardiomyopathy.

Perfusion scintigraphy of the heart with thallium chloride 201 demonstrates diffuse or small-focal decrease of cardiomyocyte metabolic activity. This diagnostic method enables assessment of the intact cardiomyocytes, and is helpful to exclude myocardial damage at early stages of the disease.

Stress-echocardiography is useful for assessment of functional myocardial reserve.

Increased levels of thyroid hormones and TSH suppression are crucial parameters to confirm the underlying cause (thyrotoxicosis) of the clinical findings.

5. The impact of various factors in clinical manifestations of thyrotoxic cardiomyopathy

5.1 Left atrial dilation and atrial fibrillation

Right atrial hypertrophy associated with dilation and verified by ECG was found in 30.5% of patients with thyrotoxicosis, left atrial hypertrophy - in 13.7%, and the hypertrophy of both atria was found in 11.8% patients.

Atrial fibrillation occurrence in thyrotoxicosis widely varies depending on the studied population. Age, sex, severity and intensity of hyperthyroidism, and concomitant cardiovascular diseases affect the incidence of atrial fibrillation.

Age-dependence is well-known: the risk of AF development increases as patients get older. Thus, at 10-year follow-up the incidence of atrial fibrillation was 25% in patients over 65 years of age with thyrotoxicosis, even its subclinical form, and this is threefold risk of patients with normal TSH (7%). The prevalence of AF was 21% in total cohort patients with clinical thyrotoxicosis (Iwasaki T et al, 1989), and 31% in subjects over 40 years old, while there was no single case of AF in individuals younger than 40 years. In another study 25% of thyrotoxic subjects over 60 years old had AF compared to 5% in younger group (Agner et al., 1984). Regression analysis performed by Nakazawa H. (2000) demonstrated a clear age-dependence of AF prevalence increasing stepwise till the maximal values in patients older than 70 years.

Male sex is another risk factor for AF (Staffurt et al., 1977). Toft A. & Boon N (2000) reported up to 50% prevalence of AF in males aged 60 years with hyperthyroidism.

The impact of the **duration of thyrotoxicosis** is less investigated. AF is quite rare (less than 2%) at onset of overt thyrotoxicosis (Nakazawa et al., 2000) and in patients under 40 years old without concomitant cardiovascular diseases Toft A. & Boon N (2000). The following factors are considered the most significant for AF development in young subjects without concomitant cardiovascular pathology: thyrotoxicosis duration (p=0,0005, OR=72 (6,6-794)), male sex (OR=10,4 (3,0-36,0), p=0,0003), and heart rate (OR=1,07 (1,03-1,11) p=0,0001) (Babenko et al., 2011). These factors are also important in case of coexistent heart pathology. Having examined 40 628 patients with thyrotoxicosis Frost (2004), showed that the highest risk of AF is associated with male sex, coronary artery disease and congestive HF. J. Mercé et al. (2005) found higher occurrence of AF in thyrotoxic patients with symptomatic insufficiency of either mitral or tricuspid valves (40% vs. 14%, P=0,02 in mitral regurgitation, and 86% vs. 3%,P=0,01 in tricuspid regurgitation).

Data on the effect of thyrotoxicosis intensity (overt or subclinical) are controversial. Auer et al.(2001) reported similar relative risk of AF in both subclinical and overt thyrotoxicosis (12,7 % and 13,8%, respectively). According to other data, AF occurrence in ST was 7% compared to 16% in clinical thyrotoxicosis (Babenko et al., 2011). There is an association between atrial fibrillation occurrence and type of predominantly elevated thyroid hormone (T3 or T4). Thus, atrial fibrillation occurs in 36% patients if T3 is elevated, in 13% - if T4 is increased, and in 21% - if the levels of both thyroid hormones are high. Therefore, the highest occurrence of atrial fibrillation was observed in the thyrotoxicosis due to isolated T3 excess. However, the difference could be explained by the different duration of the disease: isolated T3 thyrotoxicosis develops in nodal thyroid autonomy that is characterized by the long-term asymptomatic period and slow increase of thyroid hormone level at first leading to subclinical thyrotoxicosis, and then to T3 thyrotoxicosis. Conversion to sinus rhythm was reported only in 19% of patients with atrial fibrillation and at subclinical thyrotoxicosis. Risk factors for atrial fibrillation are listed in table 3.

Standard ECG could be used to identify high-risk patients at subclinical thyrotoxicosis: those with a short P-R interval who are predisposed to reentrant atrioventricular nodal tachycardia (Biondi B et al, 1998) and those with higher maximum P wave duration and P wave dispersion who are predisposed to AF (Aras D et al, 2005). In predisposed patients (those with two functionally distinct AV nodal conduction patterns), l-thyroxine (l-T4) suppressive therapy may increase the occurrence of reentrant-atrioventricular nodal tachycardia because of the enhanced atrial excitability, which increases the number of atrial premature beats, and the shortening of the refractory period of the conducting tissue (Biondi B et al, 1998). Moreover, by measuring P maximum and P wave dispersion values, one could theoretically identify the patients with ST that are at high risk of AF (Aras D et al, 2005). Holter ECG could be performed before starting l-T4 treatment in doses that suppress TSH to potentially identify patients who may be less tolerant to l-T4 treatment.

Age
Male sex
Duration of hyperthyroidism
Heart rate
Concomitant cardiovascular diseases

Table 3. Risk factors for atrial fibrillation development.

5.2 Left ventricular hypertrophy

LVMMI is influenced by T3 level, systolic BP level and body mass index in patients with thyrotoxicosis (Marcisz et al., 2006). Eccentric left ventricular remodeling is predominant, and treatment and restoration of euthyroid state is not associated with LVMI normalization (9-month follow-up).

Sex also affects the occurrence of left ventricular hypertrophy (LVH) in thyrotoxic patients: the incidence of LVH is higher in men than in women (21,3% vs. 30,6%, respectively, OR=3,6; CI (1,8; 7,4); p=0,05). Eccentric type of LVH was present in 18,2%, and concentric one - in 4,3%, concentric remodeling occurred in 7,4% of patients (Babenko et al., 2011).

LVH rate increases in older population, however, the age-dependence is different in men and women. Correlation between LVMI and age is significant in general population (r=0,22, p=0,0007), and in females (r=0,27, p=0,0002), compared to non-significant association in males (r=0,10, p=0,58). More precise analysis showed that these parameters are related nonlinearly, and variability of LVMI increases in older subjects. Non-linear regression analysis defined an age threshold of 44 years: LVMI does not change up to this limit, and increases rapidly in older subjects for more than 10 g/m^2. It is even more evident in females: mean LVMI is 90±20 g/m^2 in women younger 44 years, and 105±25 g/m^2 - in older ones. The prevalence of left ventricular hypertrophy increases significantly from 11 up to 36% (OR=4,4; CI (2,1; 9,1), p=0,0002). Similar LVMI increase is observed in males - from 117±27 to 124±36 g/m^2, but changes of LVMI values and LVH prevalence are not significant because of the high LVMI variability (and smaller group) (p=0,63) (Babenko et al., 2011).

Atrial fibrillation is another factor associated with both LVH presence and severity (LVMI value) (Babenko et al., 2011).

The factors affecting left ventricular hypertrophy in subclinical thyrotoxicosis are not completely established. Shapiro L.C. et al. (1997) did not find LVH development in long-lasting ST (9,2±5,4 years) and very low TSH - 0,001 mIU/l in subjects with endogenous ST (mean age 45±10 years (27-63)). Biondi B. et al. (2000) reported significant increase of LVMI (162±24 g/m^2) in an age-matching group (43±9 years (27-69)) with endogenous ST but with higher TSH values (0,15 mIU/l) and shorter duration of subclinical thyrotoxicosis (6 months), however, it should be mentioned that 80% of the group were women. The same authors (Biondi et al., 1999) also demonstrated positive correlation between LVMI and duration and dozing of L-thyroxin treatment in patients with endogenous ST. There is

evidence of different underlying mechanisms of LVH development in clinical and subclinical thyrotoxicosis (Donatelli et al., 2003), although the degree of LVH is comparable. LVH was shown to develop even in ST with normal heart rate, blood pressure and systolic left ventricular function that indicates the direct trophic effect of TH.
LVMI is higher in patients with subclinical thyrotoxicosis of variable etiology (iatrogenic, autoimmune hyperthyroidism caused by subclinical Graves' disease and nonimmune hyperthyroidism at pretoxic thyroid adenoma) compared to age- and sex-matching control group (p<0,005). LVH prevalence is 39% (43 patients, 45,5% in males and 38,4% in females) in ST. There was no difference in etiology and duration of ST. Male sex is a risk factor for LVH in ST as well as in clinical hyperthyroidism (Babenko et al., 2011).
Age and systolic blood pressure are two other risk factors for left ventricular hypertrophy (Babenko et al., 2007). Therefore, risk factors for left ventricular hypertrophy and atrial fibrillation development are different (Table 4)

Age
Male sex
Duration of thyrotoxicosis
Systolic blood pressure
Concomitant cardiovascular diseases

Table 4. Risk factors for left ventricular hypertrophy

5.3 Pulmonary hypertension

J. Mercé et al. (2005) analyzed data on pulmonary hypertension and its risk factors. Pulmonary hypertension (PH) occurs in 41% of thyrotoxic patients. Patients with thyrotoxicosis and symptomatic mitral or tricuspid insufficiency have higher pulmonary pressure: 53,8 vs. 34,9 mmHg, P=0,0001 in mitral insufficiency, 43,9 vs. 35,12 mmHg, P =0,07 in tricuspid insufficiency. There is no relationship between PH and following factors: age, sex, the cause of hyperthyroidism, cardiovascular or other symptoms, heart rate and type of heart rhythm disturbance, the level of thyroperoxidase antibodies, TSH, and TH. Pulmonary hypertension persisted in 16% of subjects after euthyroid state restoration. We found 39% prevalence of PH in thyrotoxicosis, and pulmonary pressure lowered till normal values in 61.5% of patients after persistent euthyroidism was achieved. The increase of pulmonary pressure was associated with free thyroxine level before treatment (r=0,5, p=0,0001), age (r=0,25, p=0,002) and endothelial vasodilatation function (the lower the response in reactive hyperemia test, the higher pulmonary pressure, r=-0,37, p=0,002). Right ventricular diameter positively correlated with pulmonary pressure (r=0,36, p=0,0001), and was considered a predictor of PH as there was 100% elevation of pulmonary pressure in patients with initial right ventricular dilation and normal pulmonary pressure.
According to our data pulmonary hypertension occurs in 29.6% of patients with subclinical thyrotoxicosis. The occurrence was highest (37,5%) in subjects with endogenous nonimmune ST (autonomic thyroid nodules). Free T3 and the degree of TSH suppression had the greatest impact. Thus, there was a positive correlation between pulmonary pressure and free T3 level (r=0,56, p<0,001), and negative - with TSH (r=-0,34, p<0,005). Higher level of T3 appears to be the reason of the greater elevation of pulmonary pressure in nonimmune endogenous ST (Babenko et al., 2008).

5.4 Heart failure

Risk factors of heart failure (HF) development in thyrotoxicosis are not well understood. As reported by Siu C-W et al. (2007), 5.8 % thyrotoxic patients developed heart failure, and AF was an independent predictor of HF (OR 37,4, (CI 9,72- 144,0, p <0,001)). 47% had left ventricular dysfunction (EF < 50%) that was more severe in patients with the lowest serum TSH level. Male sex was related with heart failure development (OR 26,6 (CI 2,6-272,5), p = 0,006). Left ventricular dysfunction and heart chamber dilation were present in one third of patients with restored euthyroidism. Patients with preserved output (ejection fraction 55% vs. 30 %, p <0.001) and lower functional class of heart failure (NYHA) demonstrate better outcome (reverse changes) (1.2 (0.1) vs. 2.5 (0.2), p <0.001).

The following main predictors of HF development in thyrotoxicosis (Babenko et al., 2011) are defined by multifactorial analysis: systolic blood pressure and free T3 level before treatment, dilation of left ventricle and to a lesser extent of other heart chambers.

To sum up, duration of hyperthyroidism, sex (male) and age are the main predictors of development of thyrotoxic cardiomyopathy and its clinical manifestations (left atrial dilation, atrial fibrillation, LVH, HF).

6. Predictive and therapeutic approach to thyrotoxic cardiomyopathy based on its risk stratification

Therapeutic approach should consider the factors affecting developing of thyrotoxic cardiomyopathy (TCMP) because persistent cardiac alterations have negative impact on cardiovascular prognosis.

European guidelines on management of toxic diffuse goiter offer the following strategy: conservative treatment by antithyroid drugs should be administered for 18 months with the following withdrawal in case of remission achieved, otherwise non-medication (irreversible) treatment is strongly recommended.

Persistent euthyroid state achievement is of great importance in management of thyrotoxic cardiomyopathy symptoms, while greater duration and older age are associated with worse cardiovascular prognosis. In our study (Babenko et al., 2011) median duration of hyperthyroidism was 10 (6; 16) months in women without left ventricular hypertrophy (LVH) and 10 (6; 15) in men, while it was up to 20 (9; 40) months in women with LVH (p=0,006) and up to 19 (12; 30) in men with left ventricular hypertrophy (p=0,09). Therefore, left ventricular hypertrophy risk is low in thyrotoxicosis lasting for less than 10 months, but it is significantly higher in more prolonged disease. In addition, left ventricular hypertrophy risk was higher in women over 44 years old, but it was age-dependent in men. Age and sex differences should be considered in clinical practice, and early non-medication treatment (after 8-10 months of antithyroid therapy) should be recommended in all male subjects and in women older 44 years. On the other hand, left ventricular hypertrophy in a newly diagnosed thyrotoxicosis is the sign of the long-lasting pathology, and its total duration is longer than mentioned periods. These subjects should undergo irreversible treatment earlier. Systolic hypertension worsens cardiovascular prognosis and it must be effective curation.

The choice of non-medication therapy- surgery or radioiodine intervention - is not easy in patients with thyrotoxic cardiomyopathy. Surgical treatment is associated with the high peri- and intraoperative risk, and radioiodine therapy is linked to the worse prognosis. The latter is due to the radioactive thyreoiditis development leading to the "leakage" thyrotoxicosis, causing atrial fibrillation recurrence, vasospasm and cardiovascular events (myocardial infarction, stroke, pulmonary thromboembolism). I131 treatment is associated with the high early mortality at 1-2 months after intervention that coincides with the time of radioactive thyreoiditis onset.

Because increasing cardiovascular risk is present in older ST patients, treatment of endogenous ST (antithyroid drugs or radioiodine) is recommended to these patients. Restoration of euthyreoidism improves cardiovascular parameters (reduction in heart rate and the number of atrial and ventricular premature beats, LVMI and cardiac output) (Biondi and Cooper, 2008).

At older patients it is necessary to avoid whenever possible exogenous ST. Recent guidelines do not recommend suppressive therapy with l-T4 (to suppress serum TSH to below 0.1 mIU/liter) of benign thyroid nodules. Long-term suppressive therapy with serum TSH concentrations below 0.1 mIU/liter is recommended for DTC patients with persistent disease and a high risk of recurrence. Beta-blockade might be considered in high-risk thyroid cancer patients with adrenergic hyperresponsiveness to l-T4 (Biondi et al, 2005).

Symptomatic therapy of thyrotoxic cardiomyopathy should consider underlying pathogenetic mechanisms. Regarding high β-adrenoreceptor density, tachycardia due to increased adrenergic activity and volume heart load, β-blockers and diuretics should be administered. Diuretics are of great importance in patients with congestion symptoms (edema, dyspnea). Beta-blockers do not influence the release of thyroid hormones and are used to decrease sympathetic hyperactivity, thus leading to the reduction of cardiac load and myocardial oxygen demand. The choice of β-blocker is a highly debated question till nowadays. On the one hand, antithyroid activity of non-selective β-blockers (e.g. propranolol) is well-known . There is evidence that beta-blockers (propranolol) affect metabolism of thyroid hormones by inhibition of deiodinase type 2 in different tissues including cardiomyocytes and contributing transformation of T4 to inactive T3 – reversible hormone (Fig 4).

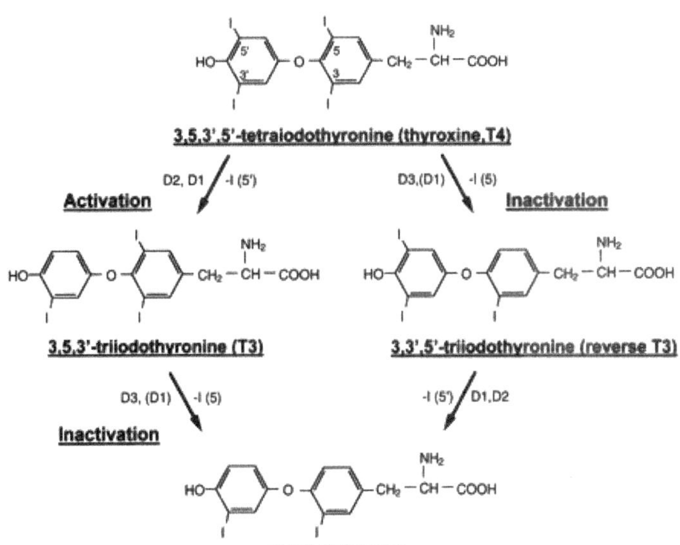

Fig. 4. Structures and interrelationships between the principal iodothyronines activated or inactivated by the selenodeiodinases (from A. Bianco, 2002)

Deiodinases are the selenoenzymes regulating thyroxine (T4) transformation into triiodothyronine (T3) (Bianco et al. 2002, Kohrle, 1999). Type 1 deiodinase (D1) is present in liver, kidneys and thyroid gland (Bianco et al. 2002, Peeters et al. 2003) and is supposed to play the key role in active circulating hormone T3 production (Kohrle, 1999). Type 2 deiodinase (D2) enables T3 production in the following tissues: central nervous system, pituitary gland, brown adipose tissue, myocardium, somatic muscles, osteocytes; and it is less expressed in liver and kidneys (Bianco et al. 2002, Kohrle, 1999, Peeters et al 2006). Thus, D2 plays the key role in local tissue T3 production, however D2 activity in somatic muscles makes a major contribution to serological markers output (Peeters et al, 2006, Maia, 2005) . Therefore, free T3 concentration in tissues depends on both T4 synthesis in thyroid gland and, correspondingly, circulating T4 concentration, and deiodinase activity in tissues. D1 contribution varies from 15-39% in the most of studies to 80% (Bianco et al. 2002, Pilo, 1990) (fig.5). T3 tissue concentration less depends on plasma thyroid hormone levels as D2 activity can contribute to a larger T3 tissue output. As a result, T3 concentration differs a lot in various organs and tissues. For example, T3 saturation usually is about 50% in liver and kidneys while it amounts to 95% in central nervous system (Bianco A et al. 2002). According to scientific data, type 2 deiodinase activity rises many times in some tissues in patients with Graves' disease. Thus, high D2 activity was revealed in thyroid tissue extracted from patient with Graves' disease at surgery (Salvatore et al, 1996). There are data showing that thyrotoxicosis clinical manifestations do not always correlate with circulating thyroid hormone concentration. B.Biondi et al. (2000) using questionnaire (with special symptoms scale) revealed manifested thyrotoxic symptoms in some patients with subclinical thyrotoxicosis. Cardiovascular examination of these patients (Echocardiography (EchoCG), bicycle ergometry, electrocardiography, etc.) also revealed severe pathologic changes (high atrial arrhythmia prevalence, left ventricular hypertrophy, diastolic dysfunction).

Heart lesions similar to ones described in thyrotoxicosis patients were revealed in experiments involving mice with induced high D2 gene expression activity in cardiomyocytes (Pachucki et al, 2001).

Based on these data it was supposed that the severity of many pathologic changes including cardiovascular abnormalities in patients with Graves' disease can be associated with both circulating hormone level and deiodinase-dependent T3 tissue production. In particularly, energy consumption in skeletal muscles was shown to correlate with free thyroxin (FT4) and TSH circulating levels, but not with free triiodothyronine level (FT3) (Canani et al, 2005). Type 2 deiodinase is assumed to play the key role in T3 tissue concentration changes, at least, in the tissues (such as myocardium, vessel wall) with high D2 gene expression.

Latter studies showed clinical impact of certain polymorphisms of deiodinase genes. One of these is found in humans and includes D2 polymorphisms characterized by threonine (Thr) changed for alanine (Ala) in codone 92 (D2 Thr92Ala).

Ala/Ala homozygous patients demonstrate lower D2 tissue activity compared to Ala/Thr heterozygous and Thr/Thr homozygous patients. Therefore, this polymorphism can decrease T3 effects in tissues with high D2 gene expression (Bianco et al. 2002, Kohrle, 1999). Therefore, this polymorphism is suggested to influence clinical manifestations and the severity of heart damage in patients with thyrotoxicosis.

Our study shows that Thr92Ala D2 polymorphism can impact clinical course of Graves' disease and heart damage (Grineva et al, 2009).

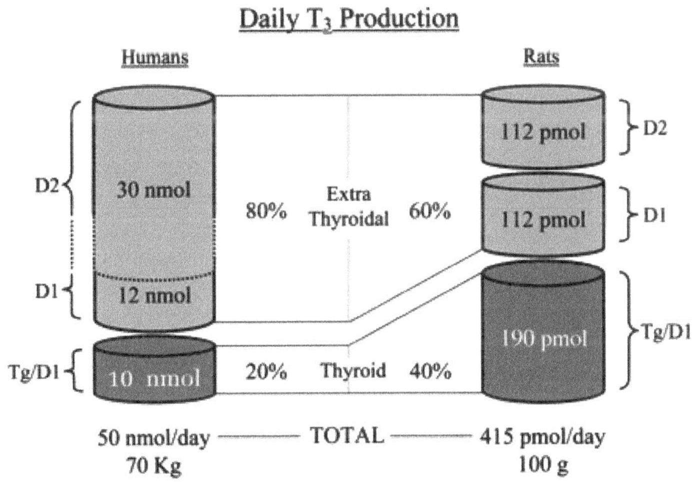

Fig. 5. Pathways of T_3 production in humans and rats. The dotted lines in the cylinder representing human extrathyroidal production reflect the uncertainty about the exact contributions of D1 and D2 to this pool. Values given are based on the studies cited in the text. Values for rats are normalized to 100 g body weight (from A. Bianco, 2002)

T3 level and T3/T4 index before treatment are considered as predictors of Graves' disease remission. We show significant differences between these parameters depending on Thr92Ala D2 polymorphism occurrence prove its role as a predictor of Graves' disease prognosis. It is confirmed by considerable difference in disease duration in groups of patients with various genotype. Thr92Ala D2 polymorphism seems to be protective as disease duration and relapse prevalence were considerably lower in Ala/Ala homozygous patients. This leads to inhibition of T3 effects in tissues with high D2 expression, such as: heart, thyroid and pituitary gland. Our data prove that Thr92Ala D2 polymorphism can impact clinical manifestations of Graves' disease including thyroid volume gain and heart rate. Ala/Ala homozygous patients reveal lower heart rate than heterozygous and Thr/Thr homozygous ones. All these clinical features (lower hormone level and heart rate, less thyrotoxicosis duration) contribute to less severe thyrotoxic cardiomyopathy in Ala/Ala homozygous patients.

Ala/Ala genotype of D2 polymorphism is also protective lowering total LVH risk and negative prognostic types of remodeling (concentric hypertrophy and dilatation of chambers), in particular. Therefore, medications leading to the decrease of deiodinase 2 activity could result in the reduced clinical manifestations of TCMP, however, no evidence is still available (Grineva et al, 2009).

However, only high doses of propranolol (more than 160 mg daily) can significantly decrease T3 plasma level (for approximately 30%), and it can result in severe reduction of blood pressure in the majority of patients (normotensive ones) as far as only some of them develop systolic hypertension.

On the other hand, β1-adrenoreceptor density is the first to be increased in thyrotoxicosis. Selective β1-blockers are supposed to be more effective. However, the advantage of any certain β-blocker in TCMP management is not evident, thus, the choice is based on the other advantages, e.g. dosage: once- or twice-daily drugs are preferred. It should be stated that elderly subjects as well as patients with low output HF and low blood pressure level are at high risk of hypotension (in particular, postural hypotension) development when treated by beta-blockers. (15)Low doses of cardioselective beta-blockers - betaxolol, atenolol, metoprolol - are preferable in this group of patients and in subjects who have relative contraindications (eg. bronchial obstruction) to beta-blockers. Beta-blockers are usually administered while euthyroid state is achieved, and then the doses are gradually diminished and withdrawn, in some cases if necessary low doses are maintained for a long time. The latter includes sustained tachycardia resistant to antithyroid therapy, heart rhythm disturbances such as extrasystole and atrial fibrillation; heart failure due to the forceful cardiac contractions. Beta-blockers are also used before the effects of antithyroid drugs or radioiodine are apparent, as well as in thyrotoxic storm and as a part of preoperative care.

Combination therapy by beta-blockers and antithyroid drugs has certain cardiovascular benefits compared to monotherapy. However, individual beta-blocker susceptibility should be assessed. Decrease of heart rate and absence of side effects are the main signs of the correct dosing. Significant positive clinical effect is usually apparent after 5-7 days of therapy by beta-blocker, including reduction of sympathetic hyperactivity and related symptoms, decrease of heart rate (in sinus rhythm as well as in atrial fibrillation), extrasystoles are less frequent or disappear, in some cases atrial fibrillation converts to sinus rhythm.

In patients with exogenous ST, the administration of a beta-blocking drug reduced the increased heart rate and left ventricular mass (Fazio et al, 1995). Therefore, beta-adrenergic blocking drugs should reduce the cardiovascular risk, and thus they might be considered for patients requiring long-term TSH suppressive therapy, especially symptomatic patients with high-risk thyroid cancer in which more aggressive TSH suppression may be required (Biondi and Cooper, 2008).

Cardiac glycosides usually are not indicated in thyrotoxicosis even in patients with severe HF. They lead to systole enhancement, diastole prolongation, being vagotropic they slow down cardiac conductivity, in particular atrioventricular conduction. Thyrotoxicosis is characterized by hyperkinetic hemodynamics, delayed atrioventricular conduction, and cardiac glycosides are even dangerous as digitalis intoxication easily develops. Thyrotoxic patients are usually resistant to antiarrhythmic drugs, and amiodarone (containing one third of iodine) can induce severe therapy-resistant thyrotoxicosis, including thyrotoxic crisis.

Efficacy of AF treatment depends on several factors. Younger age (under 50 years), absence of HF symptoms or other coexistent cardiovascular pathology, short duration (<4 month) and paroxysmal AF, normal systolic blood pressure and fast hypothyroidism achievement by antithyroid medication are the main predictors of sinus rhythm restoration that is observed in about one third of patients. **Spontaneous conversion to sinus rhythm** usually occurs at 3-month persistent euthyroid state. Otherwise standard guideline-based management of atrial fibrillation should be applied. The indirect relation between probability of successful cardioversion and duration of atrial fibrillation from any cause should be considered before the procedure (either pharmacologic or electrical cardioversion). Warfarin should be prescribed in patients with persistent AF, or aspirin should be considered in case of contraindications to anticoagulation therapy.

7. Conclusion – Up-to-date prevention of thyrotoxic cardiomyopathy and future prospects

LVH used to be considered reversible in TCMP patients as it was mentioned above. In basic animal research thyroxine induced LVH was found to be completely reversible when euthyroidism was achieved. Nixon et al. (1979) and Ching et al.(1996) demonstrated LVMI reduction after euthyroidism restoration in patients with thyrotoxicosis. However, it was not proven in more prolonged studies when thyroid function was normalized by thymasol therapy (Merillon et al.1989, Makaruk et al., 1998), According to Marcisz et al (2006) cardiac function and output, as well as systolic blood pressure were altered even after euthyroid state was restored, compared to healthy control group. It could result from TH-induced expression of the genes of contractile proteins and β-adrenoreceptors. Reversible changes might not be complete and would take longer time.

Beta-adrenergic effects have been investigated for years. Some authors confirmed beta-blocker benefits for LVH prevention in animal models, while others did not. A number of articles have been recently published regarding the impact of rennin-angiotensin system on LVH development and potential role of angiotensin converting enzyme inhibitors (ACEi) in LVH prevention and treatment in thyrotoxicosis. However, all available data are provided by experimental studies. As far as LVH is a common indication for ACEi we studied their effects in humans with TCMP. We found non-complete, but more pronounced reverse changes of LVH and left atrial dilation in patients treated by ACEi (Babenko et al. 2006).

Therefore, recent studies demonstrated high risk of irreversible LVH and left atrial dilation in AF in prolonged thyrotoxicosis and/or in elderly patients. The risk is high even after euthyroidism restoration by antithyroid medication. Beta-blockers and ACEi contribute to a better reversibility of the alterations, but complete recovery is not observed. Therefore, non-reversible (non-medication) treatment seems to be beneficial in a high-risk patients (males, women over the age of 44 years, systolic hypertension) regarding TCMP prevention.

Delayed diagnosis of thyrotoxicosis is of great medical importance as TCMP may manifest at first examination. These patients should be considered for non-medication treatment immediately after euthyroidism is restored.

8. References

Agner T. et al. (1984). A reevaluation of atrial fibrillation in thyrotoxicosis. *Dan Med Bull* 1984, 31:157-159.

Al-Abadi A. (2001). Subclinical thyrotoxicosis. *Postgrad Med J* . 2001;77:29

Aras D, et al (2005) Simple electrocardiographic markers for the prediction of paroxysmal atrial fibrillation in hyperthyroidism. Int J Cardiol 99:59–64

Armigliato M. et al. (2006). Hyperthyroidism as a cause of pulmonary arterial hypertension: a prospective study. *Angiology*. 2006 Oct-Nov;57(5):600-6.

Auer J. et al. (2001) Subclinical hyperthyroidism as a risk factor for atrial fibrillation. *Am Heart J* 2001, 142:838-842

Babenko A. et al. 2006. «Effect of ingibitors converting enzime on echocardiography parametrs at a thyrotoxicosis» poster of 31 annual meting ETA, Italy, Napoly, 2-6.09.

Babenko A. (2006). «Influence of subclinical thyrotoxicosis of varius genesis on cardiovascular system». *«Scientific notes of S-Petersburg Medical Uneversity named after Pavlov »* 2006, V.13, №4, p.65-69.

Babenko A. (2007) «Remodeling of cardiovascular system at thyreotoxicosis, its influense on vital prognosis» «Arterial hypertension» 2007 V.13, № 1 p.14-21.

Babenko A. (2008) «Character of geometry at clinical and subclinical thyrotoxicosis» «Vestnik of S-Petersburg Uneversity» s. 11 «Medicine», Vol. 4, dec. 2008 г., p.40-46.

Babenko A. et al. (2011). Analisis of contribution of various factors in development and type of remodeling left ventricule at thyreotoxicosis. *Bulleten of Almazov Federal Heart, Blood and Endocrinology Centre*. - 2011. - N 2 (в печати)

Barst RJ & Loyd JE. (1998). Genetics and immunogenetic aspects of primary pulmonary hypertension *Chest.* 1998;114;231-236.

Baumgartner-Parzer S.M. et al. (1997). Increase by triiodothyronine of endothelin-1, fibronectin and von Willebrand factor in cultured endothelial cells . *J. Endocrinol.* 1997. Vol. 154, No. 2. P. 231-239.

Bianco A et al (2002). Biochemistry, Cellular and Molecular Biology, and Physiological Roles of the Iodothyronine Selenodeiodinases. *Endocrine Reviews* 2002; 23(1): 38-89.

Bielecka-Dabrowa A et al. (2009) The mechanisms of atrial fibrillation in hyperthyroidism Review. *Thyroid Research* V.2

Biondi B, et al (1998) Clinical case seminar: reentrant atrioventricular nodal tachycardia induced by levothyroxine. *J Clin Endocrinol Metab* 83:2643–2645

Biondi B. et al. (1999). Effects of chronic subclinical hyperthyroidism from levothyroxine on cardiac morphology and function. *Cardiologia*. - 1999. Vol. 44. P. 443-449.

Biondi B. et al. (2000). Endogenous subclinical hyperthyroidism affects quality of life and cardiac morphology and function in young and middle-aged patients. *J Clin Endocrinol Metab.* 2000; 85: 4701–4705.

Biondi B. et al. (2002). Effects of Subclinical Thyroid Dysfunction on the Heart. *Ann Intern Med*, Dec. 3, 2002; 137(11): 904–914

Biondi B. et al. (2002). Effects of thyroid hormone on cardiac function: the relative importance of heart rate, loading conditions, and myocardial contractility in the regulation of cardiac performance in human hyperthyroidism. *J Clin Endocrinol Metab.* 2002; 87: 968–974.

Biondi B, Filetti S, Schlumberger M 2005 Thyroid hormone therapy and thyroid cancer: a reassessment. *Nat Clin Pract EndocrinolMetab* 1:32–40 363.

Biondi B. & Cooper D. (2008). The clinical significance of subclinical thyroid dysfunction. *Endocr Rev* 2008;29:76-131.

Bird T et al. The spectrum of thyroid disease in a community: the Whickham survey. 1977. www.feedback@ist-world.org.

Botella-Carretero JI et al. (2004) Chronic thyrotropin-suppressive therapy with levothyroxine and shortterm overt hypothyroidism after thyroxine withdrawal are associated with undesirable cardiovascular effects in patients with differentiated thyroid carcinoma. *Endocr Relat Cancer* 11:345–356

Brauman A. et al. (1985). Mitral valve prolapse in hyperthyroidism of two different origins. *Br Heart J.* 1985. Vol. 53. - P.374-377.

Brent G (1994). The molecular basis of thyroid hormone action. *N Engl J Med* 1994, 331:847-853

Burggraaf J. et al. (2001) Sympathovagal imbalance in hyperthyroidism. *Am J Physiol Endocrinol Metab.* 2001. 281: P190-195.

Büssemaker E. et al. (2003). Hyperthyroidism enhances endothelium-dependent relaxation in the rat renal artery. *Cardiovascular Research.* 2003. Vol.59. P.181–188.

Cacciatori V. et al. (1996). Power spectral analysis of heart rate in hyperthyroidism. *J Clin Endocrinol Metab.* 1996; 81: 2828–2835.

Canaris G et al. (2000). The Colorado thyroid disease prevalence study. *Arch Intern Med.* 2000;160:526-34.

Canani LH, et al (2005) The Type 2 Deiodinase A-G (Thr92Ala) Polymorphism Is Associated with Decreased Enzyme Velocity and Increased Insulin Resistance in Patients with Type 2 Diabetes Mellitus. . *J Clin Endocrinol Metab.* 2005; 90(6): 3472-3478.

Cappola A. et al. (2006). Thyroid Status, Cardiovascular Risk, and Mortality in Older Adults. *JAMA.* 2006. Vol. 295. P.1033-1041

Chen Y et al. (2002). Effects of thyroid hormone on the arrhythmogenic activity of pulmonary vein cardiomyocytes. *J Am Coll Cardiol* 2002, 39:366-372

Ching G. et al. (1996). Cardiac hypertrophy as a result of long-term thyroxine therapy and thyrotoxicosis. *Heart.* 1996.Vol.75. P. 363-368.

Chu J. et al. (2002). FCCP High Prevalence of Autoimmune Thyroid Disease in Pulmonary Arterial Hypertension. *Chest.* 2002;122:1668-1673

Coban E. et al. (2006) Endothelial dysfunction in subjects with subclinical hyperthyroidism. *J Endocrinol Invest* 29:197–200

Cucuianu M. et al. (1987). High levels of plasma von Willebrand factor in hyperthyroidism. *Rev Roum Med* 25:205–210

Dillmann W. (1990). Biochemical basis of thyroid hormone action in the heart. *Am J Med.* 1990. 88:626–630

Donatelli M. et al. (2003). Cardiac changes in subclinical and overt hyperthyroid women: retrospective study. *Int J Cardiol.* 2003. Vol. 90. P.:159-164.

Dorr M. et al. (2001). Low serum thyrotropin is associated with high plasma fibrinogen. *Thyroid.* 2001. Vol. 11. P. 153-160.

Dorr M. et al. (2005). The association of thyroid function with cardiac mass and left ventricular hypertrophy. *J Clin Endocrinol Metab.* 2005; 90: 673–677.

Dougherty M & Craige E. (1973). Apathetic hyperthyroidism presenting as tricuspid regurgitation. *Chest* 1973;63:767–72.

Dunn M. et al. (1989). Antithrombotic therapy in atrial fibrillation. *Chest.* 1989;95(2 Suppl):118S-127S.

Erem C (2006) Blood coagulation, fibrinolytic activity and lipid profile in subclinical thyroid disease: subclinical hyperthyroidism increases plasma factor X activity. *Clin Endocrinol (Oxf)* 64:323–329

Evangelopoulou M. et al. (1999). Mitral valve prolapse in autoimmune thyroid disease: an index of systemic autoimmunity? *Thyroid.* 1999. Vol. 9. P. 973-977

Everts M et al. (1996). Uptake of thyroid hormone in neonatal rat cardiac myocytes. *Endocrinology* 1996, 137:4235-4242

Faber J et al. (2001). Haemodynamic changes following treatment of subclinical and overt hyperthyroidism. *Eur J Endocrinol* 2001;145:391–6

Fazio S. et al. 2004. Effects of Thyroid Hormone on the Cardiovascular System. *Recent Progr Horm Res* 2004, 59:31-50

Figge J et al. (1994). The clinical evaluation of patients with subclinical hyperthyroidism and free triiodothyronine (free T_3) toxicosis. *Am J Med* 1994;96:229-234

Forfar J. et al. (1982). Abnormal left ventricular function in hyperthyroidism: evidence for a possible reversible cardiomyopathy. *N Engl J Med.* 1982. Vol. 307. P.1165-1175.

Freedberg A et al. (1970). The effect of altered thyroid state on atrial intracellular potentials. *J Physiol* 1970, 207:357-369

Frost L. et al. (2004). Hyperthyroidism and risk of atrial fibrillation or flutter: a population-based study. *Arch.Intern.Med.* 2004. Vol.164. P.1675–1678.

Ganong W (1982). Thyroid hormones and renin secretion. *Life Science.* 1982. Vol.30. P.577-584.

Gerdes A et al. (1985). Failure of propranolol to prevent chronic hyperthyroid induced cardiac hypertrophy and multifocal cellular necrosis in the rat. *Can J Cardiol.* 1985 Sep-Oct;1(5):340-5.

Goland S. et al. (1999) Dilated cardiomyopathy in thyrotoxicosis. *Heart* 1999;81:444-445.

Golber L & Kandror V 1972. *Thyreotoxic Heart.* Moscow, Russia.

Golf S et al. (1985). Beta-adrenoceptor density and relative number of beta-adrenoceptor subtypes in biopsies from human right atrial, left ventricular, and right ventricular myocard. *Cardiovasc Res* 19:636–641.

Grineva E. (2009) Type 2 deiodinase Thr92Ala polymorphism impact on clinical course and myocardial remodeling in patients with Graves' disease. *Cell Cycle.* Vol.8. Is.16 P.2565-2570.

Hoogendoorn E et al. (2004). Subclinical hyperthyroidism: to treat or not to treat? *Postgraduate Medical Journal* 2004;80:394-398

Homoncik M. et al. (2007) Altered platelet plug formation in hyperthyroidism and hypothyroidism. *J. Clin. Endocrinol.Metab.* 2007. Vol. 92, No. 8. P. 3006-3012.

Horne M et al. (2004). Is thyroid hormone suppression therapy prothrombotic? *J Clin Endocrinol Metab 2004* 89 4469–4473

Hrnciar J. (2002). Cor thyreotoxicum. Part I - new findings about its etiopathogenesis and diagnosis. Overview of the problem based on 35 years' experience. *Vntr Lek.* 2002. Vol. 48(1). P. 38-43.

Ikram H. (1977). Haemodynamic effects of beta-adrenergic blockade in hyperthyroid patients with and without heart failure. *BMJ 1977*;i:1505-7.

Ishikawa T. et al. (1989). Thyroid hormones directly interact with vascular smooth muscle strips. *Molecular Pharmaceutics.* 1989. Vol.35. P.760–765.

Iwasaki T. et al. (1989) Echocardiographic studies on the relationship between atrial fibrillation and atrial enlargement in patients with hyperthyroidism of Graves' disease. *Cardiology.* 1989. Vol.76. N 1. P.10-17.

Jiménez E. et al. (1982). Effects of hyper-and hypothyroidism on the basal levels of angiotensin I and kinetic parameters of renin angiotensin system in male rats. *Revista Española de Fisiologia.* 1982. Vol.38. P.149–154.

Kahaly G. (1987). Graves' disease and mitral valve prolapse. *JAMA.* 1987. Vol.257.-P. 22-28.

Kim D & Smith T (1984). Effect of thyroid hormone on sodium pump sites, sodium content, and contractile response to cardiac glycosides in cultured chick ventricular cells. *J Clin Invest* 1984, 74:1481-1488

Kiss E et al. (1994). Thyroid hormone induced alterations in phospholamban protein expression. Regulatory effects on sarcoplasmic reticulum calcium transport and myocardial relaxation. *Circ Res* 75:245–251.

Klein I. (1988). Thyroxine-induced cardiac hypertrophy: time course of development and inhibition by propranolol. *Endocrinology*. 1988. № 123. P.203–210.

Klein I. (1990). Thyroid hormone and the cardiovascular system. *Am. J. of Medicine*. 1990. № 88. P.631–637.

Klein I & Levey GS. (2000). The cardiovascular system in thyrotoxicosis. In: Braverman LE, Utiger RD, eds. *The thyroid*, 8th ed. Philadelphia: Lippincott-Raven, 2000;596-604.

Klein I. & Ojamaa K. (2001). Thyroid hormone and cardiovascular system. *N Engl J Med*, 2001Vol. 344, No. 7 February 15, p.501-509.

Kobori H et al. (1999). Local renin-angiotensin system contributes to hyperthyroidism-induced cardiac hypertrophy. *J. Endocrinol*. 1999. V.160, I. 1, 43-47.

Kohrle J. Local activation and inactivation of thyroid hormones: the deiodinase family. Mol Cell Endocrinol. 1999 May 25; 151(1-2):103-19.

Ladenson P. (1993). Thyrotoxicosis and the heart: something old and something new[Editorial]. *J Clin Endocrinol Metab*. 1993. Vol. 77. P. 332-333.

Levina L. (1989). *Heart at endocrine diseases*. Leningrad, Russia.

Lombardi G. et al. (1994). *Heart and Thyroid*. Wien. - P.86-91.

Lutton S. et al. (2001) *Cardiomyopathy and myocardial failure*.

Maia A et al (2005) Type 2 iodothyronine deiodinase is the major source of plasma T3 in euthyroid humans. *J.Clin. Invest*. 2005; 115: 2524–2533

Makaruk B et al. (1998). Changes of echocardiographic indices of the left cardiac ventricle systolic function during thyrostatic therapy. *Polish J Endocrinol*, 1998; 49: 307-12.

Manger J et al. (1988). Congestive heart failure and sudden death in a young woman with thyrotoxicosis. *West J Med* 1988; 149:86-91

Marchant C.et al. (1993). Renin-angiotensin system in thyroid dysfunction in rats. *J.of Cardiovascular Pharmacology*. – 1993. – Vol.22. – P.449–455.

Marcisz C et al.(2001). Influence of short-time application of a low sodium diet on blood pressure in patients with hyperthyroidism or hypothyroidism during therapy. *Am J Hypertens*. 2001; 14: 995–1002

Marcisz C. et al. (2006). Left ventricular mass in patients with hyperthyroidism. *Med Sci Monit*. 2006. 12(11) P.481-486.

Marqusee E et al. (1998). Subclinical thyrotoxicosis. Endocrinol Metab Clin North Am. 1998;27:37-49

Martí V et al. (1997). Myocardial damage does not occur in untreated hyperthyroidism unless associated with congestive heart failure. *Am Heart J*. 1997 Dec;134(6):1133-7

Menzel T et al. (2000). Pathophysiology of impaired right and left ventricular function in chronic embolic pulmonary hypertension: changes after pulmonary thromboendarterectomy. *Chest* 118: 897–903, 2000.

Mercé J. et al. (2005). Cardiovascular abnormalities in hyperthyroidism: A prospective Doppler echocardiographic study. *Am. J.Medicine* (2005) 118, 126-131.

Merillon J et al. (1981). Left ventricular function and hyperthyroidism. *Br Heart J*, 1981; 46: 137-43.

Metso, S. et al. (2007) Increased Cardiovascular and Cancer Mortality after Radioiodine Treatment for Hyperthyroidism *J Clin Endocrinol Metab* 2007;92:2190-2196

Mier A et al (1989) Reversible respiratory muscle weakness in hyperthyroidism. *Am Rev Respir Dis* 139,529-533

Nakazawa H et al. (2000). Is there a place for the late cardioversion of atrial fibrillation? A long-term follow-up study of patients with post-thyrotoxic atrial fibrillation. *Eur Heart J.* 2000; 21: 327–333.

Nakchbandi I et al. (1999) Pulmonary Hypertension Caused by Graves' Thyrotoxicosis* Normal Pulmonary Hemodynamics Restored by ^{131}I Treatment *Chest.* 1999;116:1483-1485.

Napoli R et al. (2001) Impact of Hyperthyroidism and Its Correction on Vascular Reactivity in Humans. *Circulation.* 2001;104:3076

Nordyke R et al. (1988) Graves' disease: influence of age on clinical findings. *Arch Intern Med.* 1988; 148: 626–631.

Nixon J et al. (1979). Alterations in left ventricular mass and performance in patients treated effectively for hyrotoxicosis. A comparative echocardiographic study. *Am J Med.* 1979 Aug;67(2):268-76 .

Ojamaa K et al. (1999) Regulation of rat cardiac Kv1.5 gene expression by thyroid hormone is rapid and chamber specific. *Endocrinology.* 1999.140:3170–3176.

Okura H & Takatsu Y. (1994) High-Output Heart Failure as a Cause of Pulmonary Hypertension. *Intern. Med.* Vol. 33, No. 6 June 1994

Ortmann C et al. (1999) Inflammation of the cardiac conduction system in a case of hyperthyroidism. *Int J. Legal. Med.* 1999. № 112. - P.271–274.

Osman F. et al. (2000) Cardiac rhythm abnormalities in thyrotoxicosis—the explanation for excess vascular mortality *J.Endocrinology.* - 2000. - Vol.164. -P.321.

Osman F. et al. (2002). Cardiac Dysrhythmias and Thyroid Dysfunction - The Hidden Menace? *J Clin Endocrinol Metab.* 2002 Vol. 87, No. 3 963-967.

Osman F. et al. (2007) Cardiovascular Manifestations of Hyperthyroidism Before and After Antithyroid Therapy. *J Am Coll Cardiol,* 2007; 49:71-81

Pachucki J, et al (2001) Type 2 Iodothyronine Deiodinase Transgene Expression in the Mouse Heart Causes Cardiac-Specific Thyrotoxicosis. *Endocrinology.* 2001; 142(1): 13-20.

Palmieri E et al. (2004) Myocardial contractility and total arterial stiffness in patients with overt hyperthyroidism: acute effects of beta1-adrenergic blockade. *Eur J Endocrinol.* 2004; 150: 757–762.

Paran Y et al. (2006) Pulmonary hypertension and predominant right heart failure in thyrotoxicosis. *Resuscitation.* 2006; 69: 339–341.

Parle J. et al.(2001). A single low serum thyrotrophin (TSH) concentration predicts increased all-cause and cardiovascular mortality in older persons in the community: a 10-year cohort study. *Lancet.* 2001. Vol.358. P.861–865.

Parle J. et al. (1991). Prevalence and follow-up of abnormal thyrotrophin (TSH) concentrations in the elderly in the United Kingdom. *Clin Endocrinol* (Oxf). 1991. № 34. P.77-83.

Peeters R et al (2003). Polymorphisms in Thyroid Hormone Pathway Genes Are Associated with Plasma TSH and Iodothyronine Levels in Healthy Subjects? *J Clin Endocrinol Metab.* 2003; 88(6): 2880-2888.

Peeters R et al. (2006). Genetic variation in thyroid hormone pathway genes; polymorphisms in the TSH receptor and the iodothyronine deiodinases. *Eur. J. Endocrinol.* 2006; 155(5): 655-662.

Petersen P. & Hansen J.M. (1988) Stroke in thyrotoxicosis with atrial fibrillation. *Stroke.* 1988. Vol.19. P.15–18.

Pilo A et al. (1990) Thyroidal and peripheral production of 3,5,3'-triiodothyronine in humans by multicompartmental analysis. Am J Physiol 1990; 258:715–726

Polikar R. et al. The thyroid and the heart. *Circulation.* 1993.Vol. 87. P.1435-1441.

Presti C. & Hart R. Thyrotoxicosis, atrial fibrillation, and embolism, revisited. *Am.Heart J.* 1989. Vol.117. P.976-977.

Report of the 1995 World Health Organization/International Society and Federation of Cardiology Task Force on the Definition and Classification of Cardiomyopathies. *Circulation.* 1996. Vol. 93. P. 841-842

Roffi M. et al. (2003) Thyrotoxicosis and the cardiovascular system: Subtle but serious effects. *Cleveland Clinic Journal Of Medicine.* 2003. Vol. 70.P. 57-63.

Ross D (1996) Subclinical thyrotoxicosis. In: Braverman LE, Utiger RD, eds. Werner and Ingbar's *The Thyroid*: A Fundamental and Clinical Text. 7th ed. Philadelphia: Lippincott Williams & Wilkins; 1996:1016-20.

Rubin L. & Badesch D. (2006) Thyrotoxicosis as a Risk Factor for Pulmonary Arterial Hypertension. *Ann Intern Med,* February 7, 2006; 144(3): 222 - 223.

Salvatore D, et al (1996). Type 2 iodothyronine deiodinase is highly expressed in human thyroid. *J Clin Invest* 1996; 98:962–968.

Samuels M (1998) Subclinical thyroid disease in the elderly. *Thyroid.*1998;8:803-13

Sandier G. & Wilson G. (1959)The nature and prognosis of heart disease in thyrotoxicosis: a review of 150 patients treated with I^{131}. *QJM* 1959. Vol. 28. P. 347-352.

Sawin C. T. et al.(1994) Low serum thyrotropin concentrations as a risk factor for atrial fibrillation in older persons. *N Engl J Med.* 1994. Vol. 331.-P. 1249-1254.

Scivoletto R. et al. (1986) Thyroid hormones and vascular reactivity: role of the endothelial cell. *Eur. J. Pharm.* 1986. Vol.129. P.271–278.

Shapiro L et al. (1997) Minimal cardiac effects in asymptomatic athyreotic patients chronically treated with thyrotropin-suppressive doses of l-thyroxine. *J Clin Endocrinol Metab.* 1997;82:2592-5.

Sgarbi J et al (2010) Subclinical thyroid dysfunctions are independent risk factors for mortality in a 7.5-year follow-up: the Japanese-Brazilian thyroid study.*Eur J Endocrinol* 2010;162:569-77.

Siu C-W. et al. (2007) Incidence, clinical characteristics and outcome of congestive heart failure as the initial presentation in patients with primary hyperthyroidism. *Heart* 2007;93:483-487.

Soh M & Croxson M. (2008) Fatal thyrotoxic cardiomyopathy in a young man. *BMJ.* 2008; 337: a531

Squizzato A. et al. (2007) Thyroid Dysfunction and Effects on Coagulation and Fibrinolysis: A Systematic Review. *J Clin Endocrinol Metab.*2007. Vol. 92, No. 7 2415-2420

Staffurt J et al. (1977) Arterial embolism in thyrotoxicosis with atrial fibrillation. *Br Med J* 1977, 2:688-690

Toft A & Boon N (2000) Thyroid disease and the heart. *Heart* 2000;84:455-460

Yanai-Landau H et al (1995) Autoimmune aspects of primary pulmonary hypertension. *Pathobiology.* 1995;63(2):71-5.

Yung C. et al. (2006) Hemodynamic Changes in Hyperthyroidism-Related Pulmonary Hypertension: A Prospective Echocardiographic Study. *J Clin Endocrinol Metab.* 2006 Vol. 92, No. 5 1736-1742

Vargas F et al. (2006) Vascular and renal function in experimental thyroid disorders. *Eur. J. Endocrinol.,* 2006, Vol 154, I 2, 197-212.

Wang C & Crapo L (1997)The epidemiology of thyroid disease and implications for screening. [PMID: 9074859] *Endocrinol Metab Clin North Am.* 1997;26:189-218

Whitner T. et al. (2005) Hyperthyroidism. Presenting as Isolated Tricuspid Regurgitation and Right Heart Failure. *Tex Heart Inst J.* 2005; 32(2): 244–245.

Woeber K (1992) Thyrotoxicosis and the heart. *N Engl J Med* 1992;327:94-98.

Xenopoulos NP et al.(1996) Severe right heart failure in a patient with Graves' disease. *Clin Cardiol* 1996;19:903–5.

7

Taurine Depletion-Related Cardiomyopathy in Animals

Takashi Ito and Junichi Azuma
Hyogo University of Health Sciences
Japan

1. Introduction

Taurine is a nontoxic β-amino acid and a normal constituent of the human diet found in animal food sources, especially fishes and shell fishes. It is found in very high concentration in cardiac tissue, and represents approximately 60% of free amino acid pool in the mammalian heart. Mammalian cardiac taurine contents vary among the spices. Cats are known to be the species most susceptible to taurine deficiency due to poor synthetic capacity. On the other hand, rats have high amount of taurine in the heart, liver and skeletal muscle. Therefore, it may be the natural providence that cats chase rats.

While biosynthesis of taurine in heart is limited, the major determinant of myocardial taurine is uptake from plasma. The concentration in myocardium is approximately 100 times higher than that in plasma, indicating active transport process from the plasma. The biochemical aspects of its transport mechanism including changes in taurine content resulting from modification of uptake into and leakage from myocardial cells by physiological (β-adrenergic stimulation), pharmacological (guanidinoethyl sulfonate or β-alanine) and pathophysiological (congestive heart failure, ischemia, hypoxia or cardiomyopathy) interventions have been quite well documented. However, these physiological and pathophysiological roles in heart remain uncertain.

Taurine is known to possess a variety of biological actions including calcium handling, osmoregulation, anti-oxidation, bile acid conjugation and so on. In heart, some physiological or pharmacological effects have been reported, as shown in Table 1. Meanwhile, it has been discovered in 1980s that taurine deficient diet causes dilated

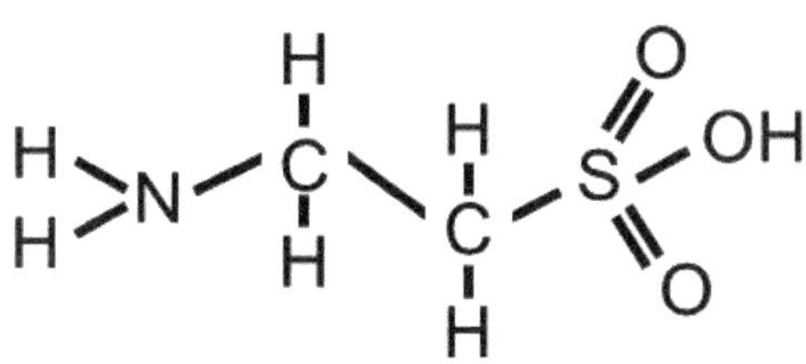

Fig. 1. Taurine (2-aminoethanesulfonic acid)

1.	Positive inotropy at low calcium concentrations
2.	Negative inotropy at high calcium concentrations
3.	Potentiation of digitalis inotropy
4.	Antagonism of negative inotropy
5.	Retardation of lesion development in calcium overload myopathy
6.	Protection against drug-induced cardiotoxicity
7.	Protection against calcium paradox- and oxygen paradox- induced myocardial injury
8.	Antiarrythmia
9.	Modulation of cardiac calcium current
10.	Antiapoptotic effect

Table 1. Action of taurine on the heart

cardiomyopathy (DCM) implicated with taurine depletion in house cats. Thereafter, taurine depletion-related cardiomyopathy has been reported in foxes and dogs. It has been reported that amount of taurine intake is widely varied among individuals in human and correlates to mortality rate caused by ischemia heart diseases in epidemiologic studies (Yamori et al., 2001, 2009), indicating taurine depletion may also occur in human. Hence, taurine depletion-induced DCM should be focused as one of the etiology of cardiomyopathy in human. In this chapter, we introduce taurine depletion-related cardiomyopathy in animals. Moreover, mechanisms underlying the pathogenesis of taurine depletion-related cardiomyopathy have been investigated, while the mechanisms remain uncertain. Studies by using β-alanine and guanidinoethane sulfonate (GES) which are the inhibitors of taurine influx into cells through taurine transporter are very useful to evaluate the molecular mechanism. Further, the genetically engineered mice knocking out taurine transporter have been recently developed. These mice also exhibited the cardiomyopathy with cardiac atrophy. We also describe recent evidences and possible mechanisms which should associate with the taurine depletion-related cardiomyopathy.

Furthermore, a lot of studies support the beneficial effect of taurine on cardiomyopathy and heart failure in animal model as well as in human. In the latter half of this chapter, we describe the pharmacological effects of taurine supplementation against heart diseases.

2. Taurine depletion-related cardiomyopathy

2.1 Cats

Taurine depletion-related DCM was firstly identified in domestic cats in 1980s. Pion et al. reported that low taurine concentration in plasma is a major causal factor of DCM in pet cats (Pion et al., 1987). They analyzed the pet cats having a diagnosis of heart failure in hospital, and found that 22 of 23 cats with echocardiographic evidence of DCM had low concentration of plasma taurine. Moreover, treatment of taurine (0.5 g administered twice daily) improved cats echocardiographically in 2-week period after treatment. At the end all cats were clinically and echocardiographically normal and were no longer receiving medication of their heart failure. In further study, the authors prospectively evaluated the long term benefits of administering taurine to cats with moderate to severe DCM (Pion et al., 1992). They compared the survival times of this prospectively evaluated population to the other population which were diagnosed as DCM before the discovery of the role of taurine deficiency in the cause of cardiomyopathy. As a result, all cats that survived more than 30 days remained clinically stable despite withdrawal of all medications except taurine. The clinical response and 1-year survival rate of 58% in the taurine treatment group represents a marked improvement compared with a 1-year survival rate of 13% in the retrospectively evaluated population.

Further, Novotny et al. examined the intrinsic contraction-relaxation properties of left ventricle using perfused hearts isolated from cats maintained by taurine-deficient diet with or without taurine supplementation (Novotny et al., 1991). They demonstrated that coronary-perfused hearts from the taurine deficient cats did not achieve isovolumic systolic pressure and ±dP/dt max values of the magnitude generated by heart from taurine-treated cats. They also identified that the pressure-volume relation curve resulted from isovolumic heart preparations of taurine-deficient cats were shifted downward and to the right of control curves, indicating inotropic depression and increased chamber compliance or distensibility. Therefore, these data illustrate the myocardial contractile dysfunction and LV chamber dilatation in hearts from taurine-deficient cats.

Subsequent control study with cats also showed the evidence that dietary taurine deficiency induces myocardial failure (Novotny et al., 1994). Novotny et al. evaluated left ventricular function using M-mode echocardiography in cats maintained on a taurine deficient diet for 6-15 months. At 4 months from the onset of the study, plasma taurine concentration of cats fed taurine-deficient diet is 12 nmol/mL, while baseline value is 227 nmol/mL. They demonstrated that 74% of taurine-deficient cats experienced greater than 25% reductions in fraction shortening values and 91% had a greater than 25% increase in LV end-systolic short axis diameter values in response to taurine deficient diet. The average reduction of fraction shortening was 37%. Moreover, the study with colony-source cats revealed that the greatest rate of change occurred during the first four months in taurine-deficient cats. The authors concluded that while DCM was observed in some cats, decreased systolic pump function and increased LV end-systolic short axis diameter were more consistent findings.

Pion reported in 2004 that in their repeated studies, approximately 25% of all (n>100) cats depleted of taurine for more than 2 years developed overt myocardial failure (Pion, 2004). He mentioned that the other factors required for taurine developed overt myocardial failure are unknown, and that nutritional taurine deficiency combined with other causes of myocardial stress, such as congenital or acquired left ventricle overload, toxic, ischemic, nutritional, endocrine or metabolic problems, may lead to synergistic complicating effects. Furthermore, he noted that taurine deficiency in cats may be a direct result of inadequate amounts of taurine in the diet, such commercial pet food, in most cases and is thus preventable.

2.2 Foxes

Foxes are also known to have low taurine synthesis capacity. Moise et al. reported the relationship between taurine deficiency and DCM in foxes (Moise et al., 1991). They found that plasma taurine concentration in foxes from farms with a history of death caused by DCM was less than that in foxes without family history of cardiac death. Furthermore, they demonstrated that the activity of hepatic cysteinesulfinic acid decarboxylase which is a rate-limiting enzyme in taurine synthesis from cysteine was less in foxes with DCM, suggesting that inadequate cysteinesulfinic acid decarboxylase activity may contribute to susceptibility to dietary taurine deficiency. Also, the therapy with taurine supplementation for 2 months in foxes with DCM reduced cardiac size, resolved pulmonary edema and improved systolic function, indicating DCM was reversed.

2.3 Dogs

Taurine is not an essential amino acid in dogs. Normal dogs fed diets with little or no taurine maintain plasma and whole blood taurine concentration similar to those found in normal cats. The activity of cysteinesulfinic acid decarboxylase is high in dog compared to the cat. Therefore, until recently, it was thought that taurine deficiency was not a clinical issue to consider when managing canine patients (Pion, 2004).

Soon after the identification of taurine deficiency myocardial failure in cats, Pion who firstly identified taurine depletion-related DCM in cats,, as mentioned above, began administering taurine to dogs with DCM (Kramer et al., 1995; Pion, 2004). Then he and his colleagues found that plasma taurine concentration was low in 17% of dogs with DCM studied, although there were no significant differences in the average of plasma taurine concentrations between dogs with DCM and the control dogs. They also identified that a certain breeds, such as American Cocker Spaniel and Golden Retriever, with DCM had low plasma taurine concentrations, while it was not decreased in the breeds that are more commonly afflicted with DCM. Recently, DCM associated with low taurine concentration has been reported in American Cocker Spaniel, Golden Retriever, Dalmatian, boxer, Newfoundland, Portuguese water dog, English setter, Alaskan malamute and Scottish terrier (Freeman et al., 1996; Kittleson et al., 1997; Pion et al., 1998; Fascetti et al., 2003; Alroy et al., 2005; Belanger et al., 2005). Additionally, Ko et al. reported that taurine biosynthesis rate was lower in large dogs than small dogs (Ko et al., 2007), which may be associated with the greater incidence of taurine deficiency-related cardiomyopathy in large dogs than in small dogs.

2.4 Rodents

In contrast to foxes and cats, the size of the intracellular taurine pool of most animal species remains fairly constant even with significant reductions in dietary taurine content. Despite resistance to depletion, tissue taurine levels can be decreased by treatment of these animals with a taurine transport inhibitors, such β-alanine or GES, which interfere with taurine uptake by the tissues. However, Mozaffari et al. reported that GES treatment for 3 weeks resulted in the decrease in cardiac taurine content from 77 to 34 micromoles/g dry wet weight, while it did not affect myocardial contraction as assessed by perfusion technique (Mozaffari et al., 1986). Thus, although taurine depletion model induced by β-alanine and GES is a good model to analyze the physiological role of taurine deficiency, as described below, treatment of these animals with a taurine transport inhibitor does not generally cause sufficient taurine deficiency to promote the development of severe, overt pathology.

2.5 Taurine transporter knockout mice

Therefore, a more effective means of producing taurine deficiency in rodents is the formation of taurine transporter- (TauT-) null animals. Recently, transgenic mice lacking TauT gene have been generated by us and the other group. A variety of disorders have been reported in various tissues, such as eye, kidney, heart, muscle and so on, accompanied with drastic taurine deficiency in TauTKO mice (Heller-Stilb et al., 2002; Warskulat et al., 2007).

We demonstrated that taurine influx was eliminated in the cells isolated from TauTKO mice, indicating loss of taurine transport activity in TauTKO mice (Ito et al., 2008). Tissue taurine level is severely decreased in several tissues. Especially, cardiac taurine could not be detected in TauTKO mice, and skeletal muscle taurine level is decreased by 96% in TauTKO mice compared with wild-type mice. Then, we determined the cardiac phenotype of TauTKO mice. TauTKO mice exhibited a decrease in heart weight concomitant with a lower body weight than their control littermates. According to histological analyses, it was found that the ventricular wall was thinning and the ventricle lumen was dilated in the TauTKO heart compared to their wild-type littermates (Fig. 2). Moreover, the size of cardiomyocyte was markedly decreased in the TauTKO heart, indicating cardiac atrophy in TauTKO mice. Based on echocardiographic analysis, ejection fraction was diminished in the old TauTKO mice, indicating that cardiac function was eventually compromised in the TauTKO mice. Moreover, detailed functional analysis on Langendorff perfused heart also demonstrated the age-dependent cardiac dysfunction, such as a decrease in peak positive dp/dt and an increase in negative dp/dt as well as decreased ejection fraction in TauTKO mice (unpublished data). It is well established that the expression of fetal genes, including atrial natriuretic peptide (ANP), brain natriuretic peptide (BNP) and β-myosin heavy chain (β-MHC), is reactivated in heart failure (Rajabi et al., 2007). These cardiac failure markers were significantly elevated in TauTKO mice. Consistent with the cardiac function, the inductions of these genes were more significant in the old TauTKO mice. Thus, these data indicate that knockout of the TauT gene leads to an age-dependent DCM. Furthermore, in contrast to the orderly myofibrillar architecture present in wild-type cardiac muscle, electron microscopy revealed pronounced myofibrillar fragmentation, disruption of the outer mitochondrial membrane and cellular vacuolization in TauTKO hearts.

On the other hand, in another TauTKO model reported by Warskulat et al., TauTKO mice exhibited a largely normal phenotype under both control and stimulated conditions, as assessed by magnetic resonance imaging, echocardiography, and isolated heart studies (Warskulat et al., 2004). Only vasodilation was enhanced in isolated perfused TauTKO hearts during dobutamine stimulation. A possible reason for the inconsistent results between two TauTKO models is the difference of genetic background, since difference of inbred strains affects the cardiovascular phenotypes and susceptibilities against pathological stressors in mice (Barrick et al., 2007; Deschepper et al., 2004). Meanwhile, Warskulat et al. also reported that biomarker genes for heart failure, including ANP, BNP and a cardiac ankyrin repeat protein (CARP), are upregulated in TauTKO hearts, which is consistent with our TauTKO model (Warskulat et al., 2006). Furthermore, they also demonstrated that the TauTKO hearts showed a switch from α-actin 1 (skeletal muscle type, α- SKA) to α-actin 2 (smooth muscle type, α-SKA) expression. α-SMA is generally expressed in developing muscle cells, and α-SKA and α-cardiac actin (α-CAA) become upregulated and replace α-SMA during final steps of myogenesis (Tondeleir et al., 2009; Woodcock-Mitchell et al., 1988). Thus, it may be due to a reactivation of fetal gene program which is observed in pathologically hypertrophied or failing heart. Indeed, induction of smooth muscle actin has been reported in heart of DCM patients and in hypertrophied or failing heart in experimental animals. Therefore, they concluded that these hearts may be more susceptible to failure under further exogenous stresses.

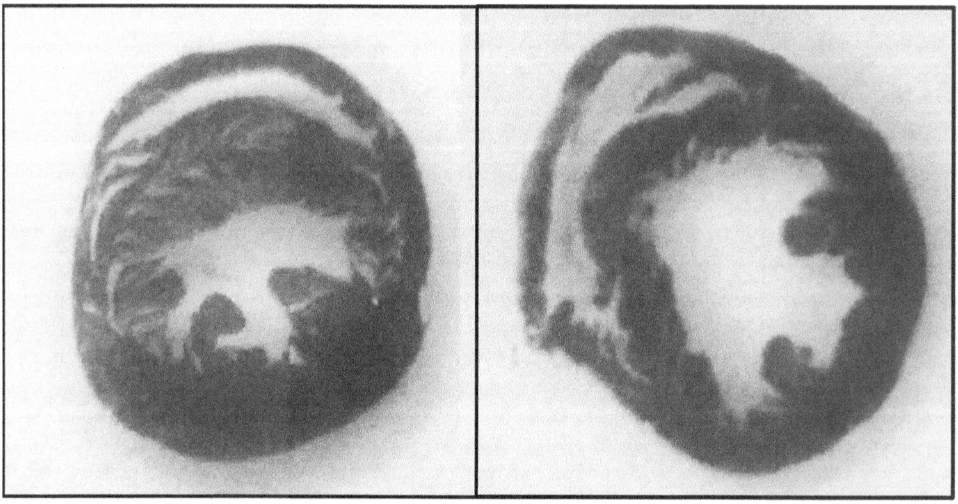

Fig. 2. Histological analysis of heart sections from WT and TauTKO mice. Heart sections were stained by hematoxylin-eosin staining method. Left: WT, Right: TauTKO. Thinning of the ventricular walls and septum and dilatation of the ventricular lumen are observed in the heart section of TauTKO mice. Ito et al. (2008)

3. Possible mechanisms for taurine depletion-related cardiomyopathy

3.1 Carbohydrate metabolism

Although the molecular mechanisms underlying the taurine depletion-related cardiomyopathy remain unclear, some potential mechanisms have been suggested.

Mozaffari et al. demonstrated that taurine depletion altered myocardial carbohydrate metabolism (Mozaffari et al., 1986). They identified that the major effect of GES treatment was stimulation in the rate of glycolysis and lactate production in rats. Furthermore, they found the activation of phosphofructokinase and a decrease in citrate in GES-treated hearts, which may relate to the activation of glycolysis. The authors concluded that taurine-depleted hearts exhibit abnormal energy metabolism and these changes may take on added importance in the stressed myocardium.

Furthermore, we reported that drug-induced taurine depletion of rat heart led to high energy phosphate metabolism due to the accumulation of free CoA, free carnitine and long-chain acylcarnitine, but a small decrease in long-chain fatty acyl-CoA (Harada et al., 1990).

Lomberdini reported the role of taurine depletion on the phosphorylation of specific protein in cardiac tissue. They demonstrated that 6-week treatment of GES in tap water increased in the phosphorylation of about 44kDa protein present in the mitochondrial fraction of the rat heart (Lombardini, 1996). Later, he identified that the 44kDa protein was pyruvate dehydrogenase which is responsible for transforming pyruvate into acetyl-CoA (Lombardini, 1998). This data suggest the role of taurine depletion in the carbohydrate metabolism through the regulation of pyruvate dehydrogenase activity. The reduction of this enzyme activity gives an explanation for the activation of lactate production in taurine-depleted hearts of GES-treated rats.

3.2 Electrophysiology and excitation-contraction coupling

Lake et al. reported the effect of GES-induced taurine depletion on electrophysiology (Lake et al., 1987). They identified an increase in the duration of ventricular action potentials in GES-treated rats and it accounted for the prolongation of QT interval by using electrocardiograms, suggesting the increased susceptibility against arrhythmias. Further, they have explored the idea that taurine deficiency may enhance vulnerability to arrhythmias in GES-treated rats operated with left coronary artery occlusion (Lake, 1992). As a result, they observed that taurine depleted animals had more and longer episodes of ventricular tachycardia and fibrillation, indicating that taurine deficient animals appear to be more susceptible to ischemia-induced arrhythmia.

Lake et al. also investigated the influence of taurine depletion to excitation-contraction coupling. They first identified that papillary muscle isolated from GES-treated rats generated tensions two third of control (Lake, 1990, 1992). Importantly, they observed small deficits in sensitivity to calcium and calcium recirculation through sarcoplasmic reticulum, but the magnitude of these change did not appear adequate to account for >40% loss in maximal calcium-activated force generation. Furthermore, Eley et al. reported that ventricular trabeculas from GES-treated rats exhibited the reductions in isometric twitch force, and demonstrated that substantial deficit in force development in taurine-depleted trabeculas was consistent with a reduced population of force generators and decreases in sarcomere proteins, but not intracellular calcium handling (Eley et al., 1994). Thus, they concluded that the inability of taurine depleted myocardium to generate the force is related to a loss of contractile proteins, which may be related to etiology of taurine depletion-related cardiomyopathy.

3.3 Osmoregulation

One of the most important biological actions of taurine is osmoregulation. In TauTKO models, compensatory induction of other organic osmolytes and osmotic stress related genes have been reported. Warskulat et al. found increases in the cytosolic concentration of various organic osmolytes, such as glutamine, alanine, glycine and glycerophosphorylcholine. Moreover, mRNA level of the system An amino acid transport protein was higher in the heart of TauTKO than of WT mice, concomitant with the increase in amino acids (Warskulat et al., 2004). Consistently, we also found increases in several genes responsive to osmotic stress, such as heat shock protein (Hsp70), amino acid transporters (Slc38a2, Slc38a4) and S100 calcium binding protein (S100A4), in TauTKO hearts (Ito et al., 2008), indicating the activation of some signal pathways responsible for regulating intracellular Osmotic balance. Thus, these data suggest that taurine depletion impairs the cellular osmotic balance, which, in turn, may activate the compensatory mechanism against osmotic stress.

Although the role of myocardial osmotic imbalance in etiology of cardiomyopathy is unknown, several possibilities are expected. First, it may be associated with ion movement in cardiac cells. When a cell is subjected to hyperosmotic stress, organic osmolytes, such as taurine, are accumulated, which minimizes the movement of water and the resulting decrease in cell volume. By contrast, hypoosmotic stress, which increases cell volume, leads to a loss of taurine and a decrease in intracellular osmolality. Although the regulatory volume change is usually transient, in the case of the cardiomyocyte of the TauTKO mouse there is a chronic decrease in cell volume. It is assumable that taurine depletion leads the accumulation of intracellular electrolytes and results in the impairment of the cell volume regulation in cardiac muscles. It may be also associated with prolongation of the QT interval observed in GES-treated rats, as mentioned above. The role of osmoregulation in ion movement has been reviewed by Schaffer et al. (Schaffer et al., 2000).

Second, organic osmolytes have been reported to play as chemical chaperones in mammalian cells, while osmotic stress and the disturbance of ion balance also impair the membrane and protein stability (Howard et al., 2003; Yancey, 2005). Based on our electron microscopic analyses, a number of organelle collapses, such as myofibril and mitochondrial breakdowns were found in TauTKO hearts. Similarly, a decrease in contractile proteins has been observed in the heart of GES-treated rats. We assume that these findings are likely associated with the loss of macromolecular stability due to osmotic imbalance which is resulted from taurine depletion.

3.4 The role of taurine in Renin-angiotensin-aldosterone system

Renin-angiotensin-aldosterone system (RAAS) plays a crucial role in the development of heart failure through the cardiac remodelling, as well as an increase in body fluid and impairment of vascular function. We previously demonstrated that taurine treatment suppressed angiotensin II-induced hypertrophic responses, including an increase in surface cell area and an induction in hypertrophic marker genes, in the cultured cardiac myocyte (Azuma et al., 2000). Moreover, while angiotensin II induced apoptosis in the cultured cardiac myocyte, Schaffer et al. have demonstrated that taurine depletion by exposure to β-alanine enhanced the angiotensin-II induced apoptosis (Schaffer et al., 2003). They also demonstrated that this effect of taurine depletion was mediated by enhanced increases in Bax and c-Jun N-terminal kinase, which are proapoptotic proteins. These beneficial actions of taurine against angiotensin II may relate to taurine depletion-related cardiomyopathy. Furthermore, taurine might prevent angiotensin II-induced oxidative stress through the inhibition of NADPH oxidase. Grishko et al. has demonstrated that angiotensin II-induced cell death is associated with the ROS production through the activation of NADPH oxidase in the cultured cardiac myocyte (Grishko et al., 2003). Recently, Li et al. have reported that treatment with taurine prevented the cardiac myocyte from the apoptosis induced by phenylephrine (Li et al., 2009). They also found that taurine treatment suppressed the oxidative stress induced by phenylephrine through the inhibition of NADPH oxidase activation. Thus, it is assumable that inhibition of NADPH oxidase may be a critical pathway of the antiapoptotic effect of taurine against angiotensin II-induced cell apoptosis.

Further studies may provide key elements on the molecular mechanism of taurine depletion-related cardiomyopathy.

4. Pharmacological effects of taurine on cardiomyopathy and heart failure

4.1 Animal models

The useful effect of taurine against cardiomyopathy was firstly reported by McBroom and Welty in cardiomyopathic hamster BIO 14.6 (McBroom & Welty, 1977). They demonstrated that taurine treatment for 4 weeks decreased calcium overload in cardiomyopathic hamsters. Subsequently, Azari et al. examined the effect of taurine in controlling calcium overload and necrotic lesion severity in advanced stages of cardiomyopathy (Azari et al.,

1980). They demonstrated that oral taurine given for 1 month was effective in decreasing in cardiac calcium concentration and subsequent severity of lesion in myopathic hamsters. Thereafter, we and others reported that taurine has protective activity against myocardial damage in experimental models caused by massive doses of isoproterenol or doxorubicin and by calcium paradox phenomenon. We demonstrated that oral administration of taurine in chick treated with toxic dose of isoproterenol suppressed the increased lipoperoxide and the decreased phospholipid (Ohta et al., 1988), suggesting that the beneficial effect of taurine may be due to inhibition of lipid peroxidation and calcium accumulation and due to protection against the deterioration of membrane phospholipids.

Furthermore, we reported the effect of taurine on doxorubicin-induced cardiotoxicity in mice (Hamaguchi et al., 1988). Taurine administration attenuated doxorubicin-induced biochemical alterations, such as the depletion of creatine phosphokinase, glutamic oxaloacetic transaminase and lactate dehydrogenase activities, in the myocardium. Moreover, taurine significantly improved the survival rate of the mice treated with doxorubicin.

Additionally, to confirm the effect of taurine against heart failure, we tested whether daily oral treatment with taurine had any effect upon the survival rate and hemodynamics in animal model for Chronic heart failure (CHF) induced artificially by aortic regurgitation (Azuma et al., 1985b; Takihara et al., 1986). Cumulative mortality rate at 8 weeks following aortic regurgitation was 10% in taurine treated rabbits compared with 53% in non-treated rabbits. On the hemodynamic study, the mean value of max dP/dt was significantly decreased in rabbit with aortic regurgitation without taurine. Taurine produced a marked increase in max dP/dt compared to non-treated animals, indicating that taurine improved the contractility in heart failure. Therefore, we concluded that taurine prevents the rapid decline of CHF and consequently prolongs the life expectancy.

4.2 Clinical studies

In 1974, Huxtable and Bresseler have reported that the left ventricular taurine content in patients who died of CHF was twice that in patients who died of other causes and had no cardiac pathology (Huxtable and Bressler, 1974). Subsequently, increased myocardial taurine content has been also reported in experimental animals with heart failure. It is still unclear whether the increase in myocardial taurine is causal factor in heart failure or whether this is secondary to factor related to the disease process, such as compensatory mechanism. Based on the concept of replacement therapy for deficiency symptom, such as hormone or vitamin, administration of taurine to patients with heart failure was not accepted around that time in Japan. However, since many evidence has been accumulated to show that taurine exerts various beneficial actions, including positive inotropic activity, and is useful to animals with cardiomyopathy, as described above, we dared to test the effect of taurine in patients with CHF. In 1982-1992, we have reported some clinical studies in which we evaluated the usefulness of taurine administration in the treatment of CHF.

Firstly, we have observed that the administration of taurine to the patient suffering from CHF alleviated their physical signs and symptoms (Azuma et al., 1982; Azuma et al., 1983). In open pilot study, the clinical efficacy of oral taurine administration was studied in 24 patients with CHF (New York Heart Association (NYHA) functional class; II-IV) as a result from various heart diseases, including congenital heart failure, acquired valvular disease, cardiomyopathy, ischemic heart diseases and hypertension heart diseases. The severity of heart failure was scored based on the clinical signs (diastolic gallop rhythm, pulsus alternans, positive hepatojugular reflex, pulmonary crackles, neck vein distension, hilar congestion on chest x-lay film, cardiomegaly on chest x-lay film, pleural effusion, peripheral edema, ascites, decreased urinary output, tachycardia and weight gain) and symptoms (orthopnea, paroxysmal nocturnal dyspnea, dyspnea on exertion, fatigue, anorexia, nausea, vomiting, and palpitation) and on roentgenographic data. The benefit for taurine treatment in patients was estimated by the difference between their pretreatment and post-treatment scores. In 19 of 24 patients taurine administration for 4 weeks improved the severity of CHF. Moreover, 13 of 15 patients who were designated as NYHA class III or IV before receiving taurine were designated as NYHA class II after they completed the study.

Subsequently, we conducted another clinical study to elucidate whether oral administration of taurine to conventional management could improve the systolic time intervals in 14 patients with CHF by a placebo-controlled, double blind, crossover method (Azuma et al., 1985a; Azuma et al., 1985b). As well as prior clinical study, the effect of taurine was observed in improvement of the NYHA class, pulmonary crackles and chest-film abnormality, and was superior to placebo. Importantly, pre-ejection period index was reduced after 4 weeks of treatment with taurine, indicating the improvement of left ventricular function. Thus, these studies have confirmed the clinical usefulness of taurine in CHF.

Furthermore, in an attempt to further clarify the effect of taurine on CHF and to define its clinical position as the therapeutic agent for heart failure, we conducted a double-blind comparative study using coenzyme Q10 as a control agent (Azuma et al., 1989; Azuma et al., 1992). In this study a total of 158 patients from 26 hospitals were randomized, and finally 138 patients were divided three treatment groups; daily dose of taurine 3g, taurine 6g and coenzyme Q10 30mg. Taurine were given orally daily for 8 weeks and the patients continued to receive their prescribed conventional drugs. Improvements of NYHA functional classes were observed both of 3 groups. Moreover, significant improvements compared with baseline were noted in the severity of the objective signs, including hepatomegaly and edema in 3 groups. However, no significant differences were observed in the changes of NYHA class and objective signs. We also tested the effect of taurine on the left ventricular performance using echocardiography, and significant improvements were also noted in the parameters of cardiac output in the taurine 3g group; systolic volume, cardiac output, ejection fraction (EF) and mean velocity of circumferential fiber shortening (mVcf) in the taurine 6g group, whereas coenzyme Q10 possessed no such pharmacological activity. Thus, this study confirms that the therapeutic effects of taurine compare favorably to CoQ10. Moreover, only 3.8% of patients treated with 6g of taurine experienced minor problems, including slight anorexia and soft feces, indicating the safety of taurine.

These studies illustrated that taurine is an effective agent for the treatment of heart failure without any adverse effects. Nowadays, powder of taurine is clinically used for patients with CHF in Japan.

Since RAAS plays a central role in the pathology of CHF and taurine antagonizes against angiotensin II-induced cell damage in vitro studies, as described above, a systemic clinical study is necessary to evaluate the benefit of taurine against RAAS in future.

5. Conclusion

In this chapter, we reviewed 1) the taurine depletion-related cardiomyopathy in cats, foxes, dogs, and genetically engineered mice lacking taurine transporter and 2) the pharmacological benefit of taurine in patients and experimental animal models with heart failure. In these animals, it is apparent that taurine deficient diet causes taurine depletion in plasma and heart, which in turn leads to cardiomyopathy. Urinary taurine concentration in human, which can represent the amount of taurine intake, varies by more than 10 times among individuals; therefore, taurine depletion may also occur in human. Although taurine depletion-related cardiomyopathy has not been reported so far, taurine deficiency should be considered as a potential pathogenesis of heart failure and/or cardiomyopathy. Meanwhile, whereas myocardial taurine content is increased in failing heart, taurine administration is "paradoxically" useful to patients with heart failure. Since an increment of myocardial taurine may be due to the activation of active transport of taurine, taurine supplementation might be necessary for some patients with failing heart as compensatory mechanism to maintain the cardiac function. To verify the unsolved problems, the physiological role of taurine in heart must be fully clarified.

It should be noted that the increasing rate of plasma taurine concentration after taurine administration varies widely among individuals (Brons et al., 2004). Additionally, there may be some genetic polymorphisms of taurine transporter which affects the taurine transport activity in human genome. Now it is well known that polymorphisms influence disease risk, drug efficacy and side-effect. Therefore, we suppose that the genetic polymorphisms of taurine transporter or the other molecules involved in the kinetics of taurine may contribute to the variation of plasma and tissue taurine concentrations. Thus, it will be plausible to find out the genetic polymorphisms which determine the variation of tissue taurine content and the rate of rise in plasma taurine after taurine administration, which will help us elucidate the role of taurine deficiency in the etiology of human cardiomyopathy.

6. Acknowledgment

This review work is partially supported by a research grant from Taisho Pharmaceutical Co. Ltd. (Japan).

7. References

Alroy, J.;Rush, J.E.&Sarkar, S. (2005). Infantile dilated cardiomyopathy in Portuguese water dogs: correlation of the autosomal recessive trait with low plasma taurine at infancy. *Amino Acids*, Vol.28, No.1,pp. 51-56, ISSN 0939-4451

Azari, J.;Brumbaugh, P.&Huxtable, R. (1980). Prophylaxis by taurine in the hearts of cardiomyopathic hamsters. *Journal of Molecular and Cellular Cardiology*, Vol.12, No.12,pp. 1353-1366, ISSN 0022-2828

Azuma, J.;Hasegawa, H.;Sawamura, A.;Awata, N.;Harada, H.;Ogura, K.&Kishimoto, S. (1982). Taurine for treatment of congestive heart failure. *International Journal of Cardiology*, Vol.2, No.2,pp. 303-304, ISSN 0167-5273

Azuma, J.;Hasegawa, H.;Sawamura, A.;Awata, N.;Ogura, K.;Harada, H.;Yamamura, Y.&Kishimoto, S. (1983). Therapy of congestive heart failure with orally administered taurine. *Clinical Therapeutics*, Vol.5, No.4,pp. 398-408, ISSN 0149-2918

Azuma, J.;Katsume, H.;Kagisgima, T.;Furukawa, K.;Awata, N.;Ishiyama, T.;Yamagami, T.;Ishikawa, H.;Iwata, H.;Kishimoto, S.&Yamamura, Y. (1989). Clinical evaluation of taurine in congestive heart failure - a double-blind comparative study using CoQ10 as a control drug. In *Taurine and The Heart*, H. Iwata; J.B. Lombardini&T. Segawa, eds. pp. 75-97,ISBN 0-89838-396-X,Boston, Kluwer academic publishers.

Azuma, J.;Sawamura, A.&Awata, N. (1992). Usefulness of taurine in chronic congestive heart failure and its prospective application. *Japanese Circulation Journal,* Vol.56, No.1,pp. 95-99, ISSN 0047-1828.

Azuma, J.;Sawamura, A.;Awata, N.;Ohta, H.;Hamaguchi, T.;Harada, H.;Takihara, K.;Hasegawa, H.;Yamagami, T.;Ishiyama, T.&et al. (1985a). Therapeutic effect of taurine in congestive heart failure: a double-blind crossover trial. *Clinical Cardiology,* Vol.8, No.5,pp. 276-282, ISSN 0160-9289

Azuma, J.;Takihara, K.;Awata, N.;Sawamura, A.;Ohta, H.;Hamaguchi, T.;Tanaka, Y.;Fukuda, K.&Kishimoto, S. (1985b). Taurine and failing heart: experimental and clinical aspects. *Progress in Clinical and Biological Research,* Vol.179,pp. 195-213, ISSN 0361-7742

Azuma, M.;Takahashi, K.;Fukuda, T.;Ohyabu, Y.;Yamamoto, I.;Kim, S.;Iwao, H.;Schaffer, S.W.&Azuma, J. (2000). Taurine attenuates hypertrophy induced by angiotensin II in cultured neonatal rat cardiac myocytes. *European Journal of Pharmacology,* Vol.403, No.3,pp. 181-188, ISSN 0014-2999

Barrick, C.J.;Rojas, M.;Schoonhoven, R.;Smyth, S.S.&Threadgill, D.W. (2007). Cardiac response to pressure overload in 129S1/SvImJ and C57BL/6J mice: temporal- and background-dependent development of concentric left ventricular hypertrophy. *American journal of physiology Heart and circulatory physiology,* Vol.292, No.5,pp. H2119-2130, ISSN 0363-6135

Belanger, M.C.;Ouellet, M.;Queney, G.&Moreau, M. (2005). Taurine-deficient dilated cardiomyopathy in a family of golden retrievers. *Journal of the American Animal Hospital Association,* Vol.41, No.5,pp. 284-291, ISSN 1547-3317

Brons, C.;Spohr, C.;Storgaard, H.;Dyerberg, J.&Vaag, A. (2004). Effect of taurine treatment on insulin secretion and action, and on serum lipid levels in overweight men with a genetic predisposition for type II diabetes mellitus. *European Journal of Clinical Nutrition,* Vol.58, No.9,pp. 1239-1247, ISSN 0954-3007

Deschepper, C.F.;Olson, J.L.;Otis, M.&Gallo-Payet, N. (2004). Characterization of blood pressure and morphological traits in cardiovascular-related organs in 13 different inbred mouse strains. *Journal of Applied Physiology,* Vol.97, No.1,pp. 369-376, ISSN 8750-7587

Eley, D.W.;Lake, N.&ter Keurs, H.E. (1994). Taurine depletion and excitation-contraction coupling in rat myocardium. *Circulation Research,* Vol.74, No.6,pp. 1210-1219, ISSN 0009-7330

Fascetti, A.J.;Reed, J.R.;Rogers, Q.R.&Backus, R.C. (2003). Taurine deficiency in dogs with dilated cardiomyopathy: 12 cases (1997-2001). *Journal of the American Veterinary Medical Association,* Vol.223, No.8,pp. 1137-1141, ISSN 0003-1488

Freeman, L.M.;Michel, K.E.;Brown, D.J.;Kaplan, P.M.;Stamoulis, M.E.;Rosenthal, S.L.;Keene, B.W.&Rush, J.E. (1996). Idiopathic dilated cardiomyopathy in Dalmatians: nine cases (1990-1995). *Journal of the American Veterinary Medical Association,* Vol.209, No.9,pp. 1592-1596, ISSN 0003-1488

Grishko, V.;Pastukh, V.;Solodushko, V.;Gillespie, M.;Azuma, J.&Schaffer, S. (2003). Apoptotic cascade initiated by angiotensin II in neonatal cardiomyocytes: role of DNA damage. *American Journal of Physiology Heart and circulatory physiology,* Vol.285, No.6,pp. H2364-2372, ISSN 0363-6135

Hamaguchi, T.;Azuma, J.;Awata, N.;Ohta, H.;Takihara, K.;Harada, H.;Kishimoto, S.&Sperelakis, N. (1988). Reduction of doxorubicin-induced cardiotoxicity in mice by taurine. *Research Communications in Chemical Pathology and Pharmacology,* Vol.59, No.1,pp. 21-30, ISSN 0034-5164

Harada, H.;Cusack, B.J.;Olson, R.D.;Stroo, W.;Azuma, J.;Hamaguchi, T.&Schaffer, S.W. (1990). Taurine deficiency and doxorubicin: interaction with the cardiac sarcolemmal calcium pump. *Biochemical pharmacology,* Vol.39, No.4,pp. 745-751, ISSN 0006-2952

Heller-Stilb, B.;van Roeyen, C.;Rascher, K.;Hartwig, H.G.;Huth, A.;Seeliger, M.W.;Warskulat, U.&Haussinger, D. (2002). Disruption of the taurine transporter gene (taut) leads to retinal degeneration in mice. *The FASEB journal,* Vol.16, No.2,pp. 231-233, ISSN 1530-6860

Howard, M.;Fischer, H.;Roux, J.;Santos, B.C.;Gullans, S.R.;Yancey, P.H.&Welch, W.J. (2003). Mammalian osmolytes and S-nitrosoglutathione promote Delta F508 cystic fibrosis transmembrane conductance regulator (CFTR) protein maturation and function. *The Journal of Biological Chemistry,* Vol.278, No.37,pp. 35159-35167, ISSN 0021-9258

Huxtable, R.&Bressler, R. (1974). Taurine concentrations in congestive heart failure. *Science,* Vol.184, No.142,pp. 1187-1188, ISSN 0036-8075

Ito, T.;Kimura, Y.;Uozumi, Y.;Takai, M.;Muraoka, S.;Matsuda, T.;Ueki, K.;Yoshiyama, M.;Ikawa, M.;Okabe, M.;Schaffer, S.W.;Fujio, Y.&Azuma, J. (2008). Taurine depletion caused by knocking out the taurine transporter gene leads to cardiomyopathy with cardiac atrophy. *Journal of Molecular and Cellular Cardiology,* Vol.44, No.5,pp. 927-937, ISSN 1095-8584

Kittleson, M.D.;Keene, B.;Pion, P.D.&Loyer, C.G. (1997). Results of the multicenter spaniel trial (MUST): taurine- and carnitine-responsive dilated cardiomyopathy in American cocker spaniels with decreased plasma taurine concentration. *Journal of veterinary internal medicine / American College of Veterinary Internal Medicine,* Vol.11, No.4,pp. 204-211, ISSN 0891-6640

Ko, K.S.;Backus, R.C.;Berg, J.R.;Lame, M.W.&Rogers, Q.R. (2007). Differences in taurine synthesis rate among dogs relate to differences in their maintenance energy requirement. *The Journal of nutrition,* Vol.137, No.5,pp. 1171-1175, ISSN 0022-3166

Kramer, G.A.;Kittleson, M.D.;Fox, P.R.;Lewis, J.&Pion, P.D. (1995). Plasma taurine concentrations in normal dogs and in dogs with heart disease. *Journal of Veterinary Internal Medicine / American College of Veterinary Internal Medicine,* Vol.9, No.4,pp. 253-258, ISSN 0891-6640

Lake, N. (1990). Effects of taurine depletion on excitable tissues: recent studies. *Progress in Clinical and Biological Research,* Vol.351,pp. 407-414, ISSN 0361-7742

Lake, N. (1992). Effects of taurine deficiency on arrhythmogenesis and excitation-contraction coupling in cardiac tissue. *Advances in Experimental Medicine and Biology,* Vol.315,pp. 173-179, ISSN 0065-2598

Lake, N.;de Roode, M.&Nattel, S. (1987). Effects of taurine depletion on rat cardiac electrophysiology: in vivo and in vitro studies. *Life Sciences,* Vol.40, No.10,pp. 997-1005, ISSN 0024-3205

Li, Y.;Arnold, J.M.;Pampillo, M.;Babwah, A.V.&Peng, T. (2009). Taurine prevents cardiomyocyte death by inhibiting NADPH oxidase-mediated calpain activation. *Free Radical Biology & Medicine,* Vol.46, No.1,pp. 51-61, ISSN 1873-4596

Lombardini, J.B. (1996). Taurine depletion in the intact animal stimulates in vitro phosphorylation of an approximately 44-kDa protein present in the mitochondrial fraction of the rat heart. *Journal of Molecular and Cellular Cardiology,* Vol.28, No.9,pp. 1957-1961, ISSN 0022-2828

Lombardini, J.B. (1998). Increased phosphorylation of specific rat cardiac and retinal proteins in taurine-depleted animals: isolation and identification of the phosphoproteins. *Advances in experimental medicine and biology,* Vol.442,pp. 441-447, ISSN 0065-2598

McBroom, M.J.&Welty, J.D. (1977). Effects of taurine on heart calcium in the cardiomyopathic hamster. *Journal of Molecular and Cellular Cardiology,* Vol.9, No.10,pp. 853-858, ISSN 0022-2828

Moise, N.S.;Pacioretty, L.M.;Kallfelz, F.A.;Stipanuk, M.H.;King, J.M.&Gilmour, R.F. (1991). Dietary Taurine Deficiency and Dilated Cardiomyopathy in the Fox. *American heart journal,* Vol.121, No.2,pp. 541-547, ISSN 0002-8703.

Mozaffari, M.S.;Tan, B.H.;Lucia, M.A.&Schaffer, S.W. (1986). Effect of drug-induced taurine depletion on cardiac contractility and metabolism. *Biochemicarmacology,* Vol.35, No.6,pp. 985-989, ISSN 0006-2952

Novotny, M.J.;Hogan, P.M.&Flannigan, G. (1994). Echocardiographic Evidence for Myocardial Failure Induced by Taurine Deficiency in Domestic Cats. *Canadian Journal of Veterinary Research-Revue Canadienne De Recherche Veterinaire,* Vol.58, No.1,pp. 6-12, ISSN 0830-9000.

Novotny, M.J.;Hogan, P.M.;Paley, D.M.&Adams, H.R. (1991). Systolic and Diastolic Dysfunction of the Left-Ventricle Induced by Dietary Taurine Deficiency in Cats. *American Journal of Physiology,* Vol.261, No.1,pp. H121-H127, ISSN 0002-9513.

Ohta, H.;Azuma, J.;Awata, N.;Hamaguchi, T.;Tanaka, Y.;Sawamura, A.;Kishimoto, S.&Sperelakis, N. (1988). Mechanism of the protective action of taurine against isoprenaline induced myocardial damage. *Cardiovascular research,* Vol.22, No.6,pp. 407-413, ISSN 0008-6363

Pion, P.D. (2004). Traditional and nontraditional effective and noneffective therapies for cardiac disease in dogs and cats. *Veterinary Clinics of North America-Small Animal Practice,* Vol.34, No.1,pp. 187-+, ISSN 0195-5616.

Pion, P.D.;Kittleson, M.D.;Rogers, Q.R.&Morris, J.G. (1987). Myocardial Failure in Cats Associated with Low Plasma Taurine - a Reversible Cardiomyopathy. *Science,* Vol.237, No.4816,pp. 764-768, ISSN 0036-8075.

Pion, P.D.;Kittleson, M.D.;Thomas, W.P.;Delellis, L.A.&Rogers, Q.R. (1992). Response of Cats with Dilated Cardiomyopathy to Taurine Supplementation. *Journal of the American Veterinary Medical Association,* Vol.201, No.2,pp. 275-284, ISSN 0003-1488.

Pion, P.D.;Sanderson, S.L.&Kittelson, M.D. (1998). The effectiveness of taurine and levocarnitine in dogs with heart disease. *The Veterinary clinics of North America Small animal practice,* Vol.28, No.6,pp. 1495-1514, ix, ISSN 0195-5616

Rajabi, M.;Kassiotis, C.;Razeghi, P.&Taegtmeyer, H. (2007). Return to the fetal gene program protects the stressed heart: a strong hypothesis. *Heart Failure Reviews,* Vol.12, No.3-4,pp. 331-343, ISSN 1382-4147

Schaffer, S.;Solodushko, V.;Pastukh, V.;Ricci, C.&Azuma, J. (2003). Possible cause of taurine-deficient cardiomyopathy: potentiation of angiotensin II action. *Journal of cardiovascular pharmacology,* Vol.41, No.5,pp. 751-759, ISSN 0160-2446

Schaffer, S.;Takahashi, K.&Azuma, J. (2000). Role of osmoregulation in the actions of taurine. *Amino Acids,* Vol.19, No.3-4,pp. 527-546, ISSN 0939-4451

Takihara, K.;Azuma, J.;Awata, N.;Ohta, H.;Hamaguchi, T.;Sawamura, A.;Tanaka, Y.;Kishimoto, S.&Sperelakis, N. (1986). Beneficial effect of taurine in rabbits with chronic congestive heart failure. *American Heart Journal,* Vol.112, No.6,pp. 1278-1284, ISSN 0002-8703

Tondeleir, D.;Vandamme, D.;Vandekerckhove, J.;Ampe, C.&Lambrechts, A. (2009). Actin isoform expression patterns during mammalian development and in pathology: insights from mouse models. *Cell motility and the cytoskeleton,* Vol.66, No.10,pp. 798-815, ISSN 1097-0169

Warskulat, U.;Andree, B.;Lusebrink, J.;Kohrer, K.&Haussinger, D. (2006). Switch from actin $\alpha1$ to $\alpha2$ expression and upregulation of biomarkers for pressure overload and cardiac hypertrophy in taurine-deficient mouse heart. *Biological chemistry,* Vol.387, No.10-11,pp. 1449-1454, ISSN 1431-6730

Warskulat, U.;Flogel, U.;Jacoby, C.;Hartwig, H.G.;Thewissen, M.;Merx, M.W.;Molojavyi, A.;Heller-Stilb, B.;Schrader, J.&Haussinger, D. (2004). Taurine transporter knockout depletes muscle taurine levels and results in severe skeletal muscle impairment but leaves cardiac function uncompromised. *The FASEB journal,* Vol.18, No.3,pp. 577-579, ISSN 1530-6860

Warskulat, U.;Heller-Stilb, B.;Oermann, E.;Zilles, K.;Haas, H.;Lang, F.&Haussinger, D. (2007). Phenotype of the taurine transporter knockout mouse. *Methods in enzymology,* Vol.428,pp. 439-458, ISSN 0076-6879

Woodcock-Mitchell, J.;Mitchell, J.J.;Low, R.B.;Kieny, M.;Sengel, P.;Rubbia, L.;Skalli, O.;Jackson, B.&Gabbiani, G. (1988). A-smooth muscle actin is transiently expressed in embryonic rat cardiac and skeletal muscles. *Differentiation; research in biological diversity,* Vol.39, No.3,pp. 161-166, ISSN 0301-4681

Yamori, Y.;Liu, L.;Ikeda, K.;Miura, A.;Mizushima, S.;Miki, T.&Nara, Y. (2001). Distribution of twenty-four hour urinary taurine excretion and association with ischemic heart disease mortality in 24 populations of 16 countries: results from the WHO-CARDIAC study. *Hypertension research,* Vol.24, No.4,pp. 453-457, ISSSN 0916-9636

Yamori, Y.;Liu, L.;Mori, M.;Sagara, M.;Murakami, S.;Nara, Y.&Mizushima, S. (2009). Taurine as the nutritional factor for the longevity of the Japanese revealed by a world-wide epidemiological survey. *Advances in experimental medicine and biology,* Vol.643,pp. 13-25, ISSN 0065-2598

Yancey, P.H. (2005). Organic osmolytes as compatible, metabolic and counteracting cytoprotectants in high osmolarity and other stresses. *The Journal of experimental biology,* Vol.208, No.Pt 15,pp. 2819-2830, ISSN 0022-0949

8

Drug-Induced Cardiomyopathies

Jan Klimas
Department of Pharmacology and Toxicology, Faculty of Pharmacy,
Comenius University in Bratislava,
Slovak Republic

1. Introduction

Heart failure represents one of most important causes of death in Western countries. Its high mortality originates in part from severe complications like cardiac contractile dysfunction and/or sudden cardiac death caused by ventricular arrhythmias (Shin et al. 2007). Unfortunately, significant portion of heart failure stems from use (and misuse) of several drugs and medications. Indeed, the cardiac muscle is widely known as a target of injury for many drugs and many other chemical compounds. Following their cardiotoxic action, these could be divided into two relevant categories: i) drugs and cardiotoxic substances leading to heart failure in terms of abrupt contractile performance, and ii) drugs affecting ion channels or pumps and, in most cases, leading to prolongation of cardiac repolarisation (and QT interval) and to increased risk of severe cardiac arrhythmias (such as *Torsades de Pointes*) and premature death. In some cases, it is very difficult to divide them in those categories as they have both of actions. Additionally, drug-induced cardiomyopathies not only belong to the serious adverse events of drug actions but they are widely used as experimental models for studying several cardiac conditions and diseases, offering the advantage of precise control of the onset time and can often be studied in a longitudinal fashion. This chapter covers in detail certain drug groups, as for example anthracyclines or some drugs of abuse, which are clearly associated with the development of cardiomyopathy followed by heart failure. Similarly, note is made regarding experimental models of primary or secondary drug-induced cardiomyopathies, QT prolonging agents and rhythm disturbances-triggering drugs. It must be noted that some of the mentioned substances are of clinical importance, the others have their use largely limited, but some of them lost their therapeutic use because of their cardiotoxicity.

2. Drugs inducing heart failure

Some substances cause acute cardiac depression as they lower heart rate, contractility and conduction and in certain causes even cardiac arrest. These substances include barbiturates (thiopental) or halogenated hydrocarbons (halothane, metoxyflurane and enflurane), even at concentrations used in surgery. However, many of drugs are administered chronically and are cardiotoxic and may trigger the development of cardiac injury even when used appropriately. As mentioned in ESC guidelines, there are some specific drug groups and substances which are strongly related to development of heart failure. Literally, beta-blockers, calcium antagonists, antiarrhythmics, cytotoxic agents, alcohol, cocaine and some trace elements are mentioned (Dickstein et al. 2008). Several pathophysiologic mechanisms of action have been proposed how and why drugs affect the cardiac tissue. They vary depending on the inciting agent, including direct toxic effects, neurohormonal activation, altered calcium homeostasis, and oxidative stress (Figueredo 2011). Conclusively, numerous chemicals and drugs are implicated in cardiomyopathy and even many of them remain unrecognised.

Amphetamine	Ethanol
Anabolic-androgenic steroids	Idarubicin
Anthraquinone	Imatinib
Antipsychotic phenothiazine derivates	Isoproterenol
Arnica herb	Ephedrine
Arsenic	Melarsoprol
Azidothymidine	Methamphetamine
Anagrelide	Methylphenidate
Catecholamines	Minoxidil
Cytarabine	Mitomycin
Clozapine	Mitoxantrone
Cobalt	Paclitaxel
Cocaine	Pentamidine
Chloroquine	Stibogluconate
Cyclophosphamide	Sunitinib
Daunorubicin	Trastuzumab
Diazoxide	Tricyclic antidepressants
Doxorubicin	Zidovudine

Table 1. Drugs and substances implicated in cardiomyopathy (Figueredo 2011).

2.1 Anthracyclines

In the first line, anti-cancer drugs are long recognised as strong cardiotoxic substances. Predominantly, anthracyclines are the best known and the most discussed drugs which hardly affect cardiac muscle. They were discovered in the 1960s and remain one of the mainstays of modern cancer therapy. The first two members of this group - daunorubicin (also known as daunomycin and rubidomycin) and doxorubicin (also known as adriamycin), were isolated from *Streptomyces peucetius*, a species of actinobacteria (Tan et al. 1967; Arcamone et al. 1969) and are well established as highly efficacious antineoplastic agents for various hemopoietic and solid tumors (such as breast cancer, sarcoma, ovarian and bronchogenic carcinoma as well as lymphoma, and certain forms of leukemia). Newer derivates are epirubicin and idarubicin. Despite their extensive use (and despite of the fact that they are extensively studied), their precise anticancerous mechanism is not completely understood. Most probably, it is a combination of several different actions, what accounts for the high efficiency of this class of anti-cancer drugs (Gewirtz, 1999; Minotti et al. 2004). It might include inhibition of DNA replication by intercalating between the base pairs which prevents replication of rapidly growing cancer cells (Sinha et al. 1984). However, contradictory to that, some studies have shown that at clinically relevant anthracycline concentrations, intercalation is unlikely to play a major role and stressed the topoisomerase II as the key target for anthracyclines (Binaschi et al. 2001). According to this, they act by stabilizing a reaction intermediate in which DNA strands are cut and covalently linked to tyrosine residues of topoisomerase II, which blocks subsequent DNA resealing. Failure to relax the supercoiled DNA blocks DNA replication and transcription. Other important mechanisms participating in the anticancer effects should be the apoptosis of cancer cells via the p-53 dependent pathway (Ruiz-Ruiz et al. 2003) as well as modifications of cellular proteins and organelles by formation of reactive oxygen species and lipid peroxidation (Muindi et al. 1984).

The cardiotoxicity of anthracyclines, which has been recognized shortly after their introduction in clinical practice, continues to limit their therapeutic potential and to threaten the cardiac function of many patients with cancer. Its manifestation can be diverse and may range from QT interval prolongation to acutely induced cardiac arrhythmias, changes in coronary vasomotion with consecutive myocardial ischemia, myocarditis, pericarditis, severe contractile dysfunction, and potentially fatal cardiac insufficiency (Zuppinger et al. 2007). Three distinct types of anthracycline-induced cardiotoxicity have been described (Shan et al. 1996). First, acute or subacute injury can occur immediately after treatment. This rare form of cardiotoxicity may cause transient arrhythmias, infrequently a pericarditis-myocarditis syndrome, or acute failure of the left ventricle. These manifestations usually respond promptly to the cessation of anthracycline infusion and rarely preclude further continuation of anthracycline treatment. Second, anthracyclines can induce chronic cardiotoxicity resulting in cardiomyopathy. This is a more common form of damage and is clinically the most important. Finally, late-onset anthracycline cardiotoxicity causing late-onset ventricular dysfunction and arrhythmias, which manifest years to decades after anthracycline treatment has been completed, is increasingly recognized. Both, chronic or late-onset forms most frequently lead to cardiomyopathy with a bad prognosis for the affected patients. Indeed, survival of patients with anthracycline-associated heart failure is worse than that of patients with ischemic or dilated cardiomyopathy (Felker et al. 2000). Echocardiography is currently the gold standard method for diagnosis and monitoring of anthracycline-induced cardiac impairment. Abnormalities in diastolic dysfunction detected by Doppler echocardiography likely represent early cardiotoxicity that precedes the onset of apparent systolic dysfunction (Wu 2008; Carver et al. 2008). However, some data suggest that the risk of anthracycline-associated heart failure is higher than usually estimated (Swain et al. 2003).

There are several known risk factors for anthracycline-associated cardiotoxicity. The total cumulative dose has been earlier identified as to be the major risk factor (Von Hoff et al. 1979). When focused on doxorubicine in a clinical study, the estimated cumulative percentage of patients who developed congestive heart failure at a cumulative dose of 400 mg/m^2 was 3%, increasing to 7% at 550 mg/m^2 and to 18% at 700 mg/m^2. It also was shown that doxorubicin-related congestive heart failure is schedule dependent. Consequently, modern adjuvant anthracycline regimens typically contain less than the cumulative dose associated with increased risk of cardiomyopathy (Wu 2008; Carver et al. 2008). Moreover, the incidence is lower with a once-weekly schedule when compared to a once-3-weekly schedule of doxorubicin administration (Von Hoff et al. 1979). Except of dosing schedule, the age may play a critical role - childhood as well as old age seem to be of risk. Young females who were treated with high cumulative doses of anthracyclines or with regimens of high individual doses, as well as patients of both sexes who were relatively young at the time of treatment or have had long periods of follow-up since doxorubicin therapy, appear to be at the highest risk for late cardiotoxic effects (Lipshultz et al. 1995). Patients who are younger at the time of diagnosis have the greatest reductions in left ventricular mass and the most profound increases in afterload. It was suggested that this difference could be due to the inhibition of myocardial growth by anthracycline, which would be accentuated in younger children, whose left ventricular mass is smaller (Lipshultz et al. 1991). Moreover, it was evidenced that limiting the cumulative dose of doxorubicin may not suffice to prevent late cardiotoxic effects in patients treated for cancer during childhood. Similarly, patients of advanced age (over 65 years old) may be at greater risk for congestive heart failure and may benefit from the early administration of a cardioprotectant (Swain et al. 2003). Interestingly enough, female gender is associated with a higher risk of cardiotoxicity as compared to males. Other risk factors include combination cancer therapy, prior or concomitant mediastinal radiotherapy, previous cardiac disease, and hypertension (Singal and Iliskovic 1998).

2.1.1 Mechanisms of cardiotoxicity of anthracyclines

In general, the pathophysiological mechanisms leading to chemotherapy-induced cardiomyopathy are mainly associated with myocardial cell loss, either due to apoptosis or necrosis what consequently leads to mild, moderate or even severe contractile dysfunction. The same is true for anthracyclines as well, but precise identification of exact mechanisms is frequently difficult since the majority of cancer patients is not only treated with a multitude of cancer drugs but might also be exposed to potentially cardiotoxic radiation therapy.

Similarly to antineoplastic action, the main cardiotoxic mechanism of anthracyclines is extensively under debate (Wu and Hasinoff 2005; Simůnek et al. 2009). As anthracyclines and their related compounds are well characterised as substances that lead to myocardial cell loss (Bristow et al. 1978; Mackay et al. 1994), it is likely that some of their anti-cancer mechanisms are involved in cardiotoxicity as well. In other words, cardiotoxicity may be viewed as an effect of the entire class of anthracyclines, which may indicate that it is inseparable from their antitumor effect. Early works on the pathogenesis of anthracycline cardiomyopathy had focused on DNA and protein synthesis (Pigram et al. 1972; Rosenoff et al. 1975; Levey et al. 1979). Currently, at least four hypotheses explaining the cardiotoxicity of anthracyclines have been proposed (Outomuro et al. 2007). First, in the 'iron and free-radical theory' an increased oxidative stress and antioxidant deficit have been suggested to play a major role. Although the molecular basis is not still clear enough, mitochondria is accepted as the locus where progressive molecular disorder is triggered. Second, the 'metabolic hypothesis' implicates C-13 alcohol metabolites of anthracyclines as mediators. Anthracycline alcohol metabolites can affect myocardial energy metabolism, ionic gradients, and calcium movements. Third, in the 'unifying hypothesis', chronic cardiotoxicity induced by C-13 alcohol metabolite might be primed by oxidative stress generated by anthracycline redox cycling. The two main possible mechanisms of cardiac damage that have been proposed, *i.e.* an increase calcium concentration in the interior of myocardial fibers, and damage to cell and organelle membranes by doxorubicin-generated oxygen radicals that produce an increase in the rate of endogenous lipid peroxidation, can obviously be sequentially ordered: first, doxorubicin radicals are generated and secondly they would lead, through lipid peroxidation and membrane damage, to a loss of membrane-selective permeability and towards increased calcium levels in the myocardial fibers. Fourth, the 'apoptosis hypothesis' is based on findings of myocyte cell loss through apoptosis in doxorubicin cardiomyopathy. The up-regulation of proapoptic proteins (Bax, caspases and cytochrome C), with or without the down-regulation of antiapoptotic proteins (Bcl2, Akt), has been documented and mitogen-activated protein kinases have been shown to be involved in both apoptosis and cell survival. Likewise, apoptosis is related with oxidative mechanisms as increased oxidative stress has been shown to promote apoptosis and antioxidants have been shown to inhibit this process.

Notably, the currently still prevailing hypotheses based on free radical production appeared in the centre of interest, as to be a major mechanism of anthracycline-associated cardiac dysfunction, in 1970's. And, during a time, the iron-mediated formation of reactive oxygen species and promotion of myocardial oxidative stress remains by far the most frequently proposed mechanism (Simůnek et al. 2009). It was demonstrated that anti-cancer agents whose structure contained quinone moieties could function as free radicals in NADPH-dependent microsomal oxidative reaction (Handa et al. 1975). Because superoxide dismutase inhibited this enhancement, it was suggested that the reaction precedes by formation of a free radical semiquinone which presumably then acts as both a chain initiator and in the transfer of electrons from molecular oxygen to superoxide anion. It was described that anthracyclines augments electron flow from NADPH to molecular oxygen in cardiac sarcosomes (Bachur et al. 1977) and others supported this (Myers et al. 1976; Myers et al. 1977) starting a focus on oxidative stress in explanation of cardiotoxicity of these drugs. In other words, the myocyte damage has been almost exclusively attributed to a concentration-dependent increase of intracellular oxidative stress with a consecutive increase in cytosolic calcium, mitochondrial dysfunction (Tokarska-Schlattner et al. 2006), and induction of myocyte apoptosis or necrosis (Hasinoff 1998; Gille and Nohl 1997; Doroshow 1983). Moreover, it is believed that reactive oxygen species not only lead to cell death, but also directly affect excitation-contraction coupling and calcium signaling in cardiomyocytes (Zuppinger et al. 2007). In addition to reactive oxygen species, reactive nitrogen species are also referred as to be implicated in anthracycline cardiotoxicity. The influence of anthracyclines on the NO signaling pathway has been studied in several experimental models and has been extensively reviewed (Fogli et al. 2004). It is known that anthracyclines may increase the expression of the inducible NO-synthase and so massively increase the NO production. Regarding chronic cardiotoxicity, prolonged anthracycline exposure may induce a large synthesis of byproducts of the NO-synthase mediated anthracycline redox-cycling, including $ONOO^-$, which can rapidly react with manganese-superoxide dismutase, leading to an inactivation of the enzyme (Radi et al. 2002). This results to initiation a deleterious faulty mechanism that will favour further formation of $ONOO^-$ and other NO-derived reactive nitrogen species, therefore promoting cardiomyocyte damage (Fogli et al. 2004). In addition, the generation of free radical species could lead to lipid peroxidation (primarily of the cell membrane); however, such lipid peroxidation would not indicate whether free radicals were being generated intracellularly or extracellularly (Gewirtz 1999).

The question – why is the heart so much more susceptible to the oxidative stress produced by anthracyclines than other tissues – has been widely studied. As proposed, cardiac tissue has weak antioxidant activity, since it lacks catalase (Doroshow 1983) and so cardiomyocytes could be exposed to high levels of hydrogen peroxide. In addition, cardiomyocytes are rich in mitochondria, which represent up to 50% of cardiomyocyte mass and which serve as both source and target of reactive oxygen species (Simůnek et al. 2009). Moreover, an important role has been attributed to exogenous NADH dehydrogenase. Unlike cardiac mitochondria, liver mitochondria lack the NADH-related pathway of reducing equivalents from the cytosol to the respiratory chain. As a result, liver mitochondria do not generate significant amounts of anthracycline semiquinones (Nohl et al. 2003).

One of the long reported hypotheses of cardiotoxicity of anthracyclines is based on the calcium overload (Olson et al. 1974), as they disrupt cellular and mitochondrial calcium homeostasis (Solem et al. 1994). Fleckenstein's calcium theory of myocardial cell necrosis from 1970' is widely quoted in literature as a general mechanism of myocardial cell damage (Fleckenstein et al. 1974). It must be noted that intracellular calcium dysregulation is present in all types of advanced cardiomyopathy and apparently is a late stage event that represents a final common pathway for myocardial cell damage and death. Similarly to that, anthracyclines dose-dependently increase diastolic intracellular calcium in single cardiomyocytes (Mijares and López 2001). There is a variety of modes how calcium regulating mechanism can strongly disrupt the calcium handling in cardiac cells. As anthracyclines may cross the cell surface and membranes of organelles and they, and their metabolites (doxorubicinol and daunorubicinol), may alter sarcoplasmic reticulum's calcium regulation, the recent focus is shifted to this organelle (Charlier et al. 2005; Kim et al. 2005; Park et al. 2005; Ondrias et al. 1990; Dodd et al. 1993; Arai et al. 1998). Indeed, there is now increasing evidence that depression of contractility in heart failure is linked to a malfunction of sarcoplasmic reticulum calcium release (Kirchhefer et al. 2007; Kirchhof et al. 2007). Calcium release is maintained by a macromolecular protein complex that is activated by L-type calcium current. It consists of the cardiac specific ryanodine receptor 2 (calcium release channel of sarcoplasmic reticulum), calsequestrin (calcium storage protein of sarcoplasmic reticulum), FK506-binding protein FKBP12.6, triadin, and junctin (Zhang et al. 1997; Bers 2002). Aside from cytosolic calcium, ryanodine receptor activity is also regulated by luminal calcium. Its storage and release are under the control of calsequstrin (Györke et al. 2002), whereas triadin and junctin may serve as linker proteins between calsequestrin and the ryanodine receptor. The interaction between these proteins appears to be critical for the regulation of calcium release. Importantly, anthracyclines may directly affect the calcium release complex because there is a direct anthracycline binding site on cardiac specific ryanodine receptor and on cardiac calsequestrin (Saeki et al. 2002; Park et al. 2005; Charlier et al. 2005). Indeed, it was shown that anthracyclines have biphasic effect on cardiac ryanodine receptor - initially, activate the channel, whereas after a few minutes, the channel becomes irreversibly inhibited (Ondrias et al. 1990). The ability of anthracyclines to inhibit calcium release may be more important pharmacologically than their ability to stimulate calcium release, since only nanomolar to low micromolar concentrations are required to produce inhibition, whereas release requires concentrations in the micromolar range (Olson et al. 2000). In addition to calcium regulation by sarcoplasmic reticulum, anthracyclines can affect L-type calcium channels, probably via formation of reactive oxygen species (Campbell et al. 1996), as well as Na^+/Ca^{2+} exchanger activity (Goldhaber 1996).

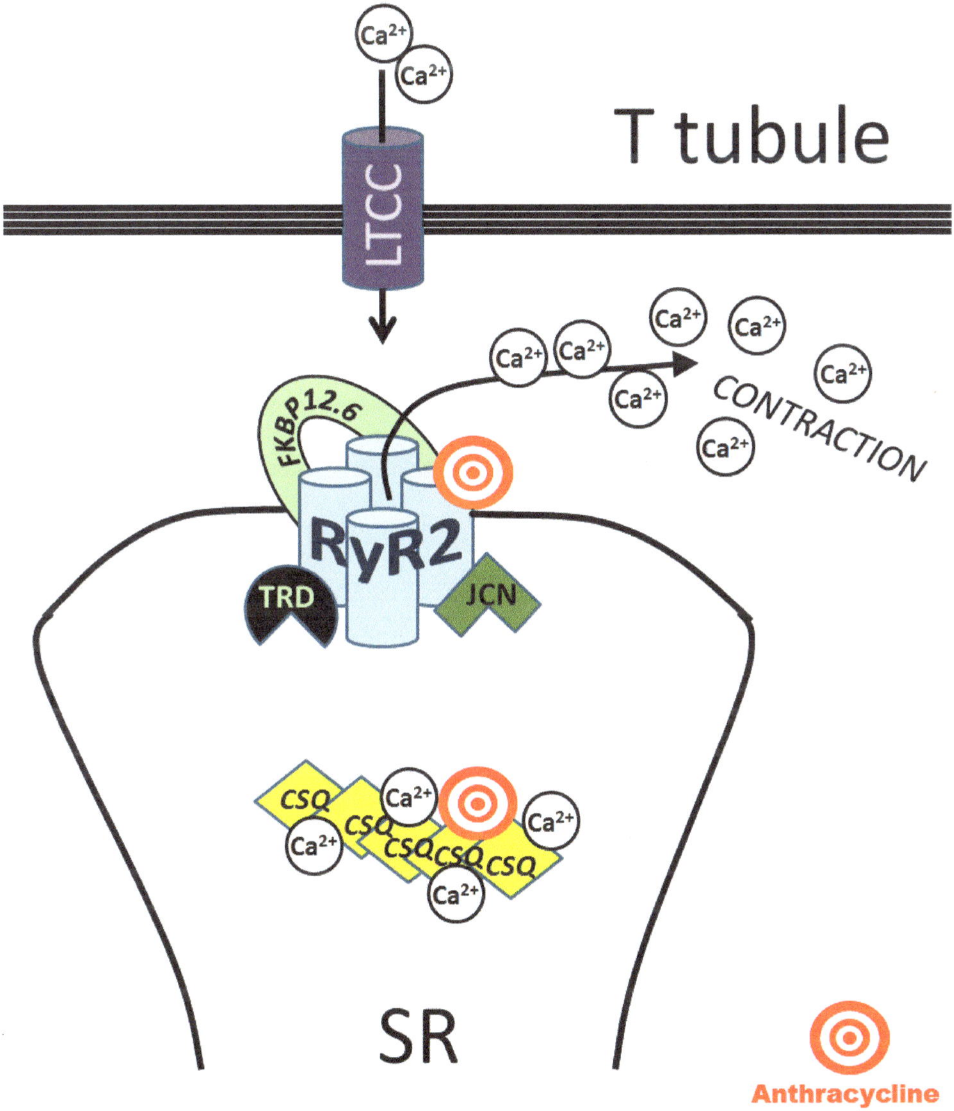

Fig. 1. Potential mechanism of anthracycline induced cardiotoxicity is based on direct binding of anthracycline on cardiac ryanodine receptor (RyR2) and/or calsequestrin (CSQ). The drug may directly modulate the calcium-induced calcium release from sarcoplasmic reticulum (SR). (Other abbreviations: LTCC - L-type Ca^{2+} channel, FKBP12.6 - FK506-binding protein 12.6, TRD - triadin, and JCN – junctin.)

Other suggested cardiotoxicity mechanisms of anthracyclines include impaired expression of various important cardiac proteins and depletion of transcription factors (Boucek et al. 1999; Aries et al. 2004), metabolism of anthracyclines into more hydrophilic and cardiotoxic substances, which subsequently accumulate in cardiomyocytes (Minotti et al. 1996), induction of mitochondrial DNA lessions (Lebrecht et al. 2005), disruption of mitochondrial bioenergetics (Tan et al. 1967), degradation of myofilamental and cytoskeletal proteins (Lim et al. 2004; Chen et al. 2006), interference with various pro-survival kinases (Peng et al. 2005) and some data suggest that the erbB2/neuregulin system might modulate anthracycline-associated cardiac toxicity, as it has been demonstrated that signaling via the erbB2 receptor can modulate doxorubicin-induced oxidative stress and myofibrillar structural damage *in vitro* (Lim t al. 2004; Sawyer et al. 2002; Pentassuglia et al. 2007). Importantly enough, all these proposed cardiotoxic pathways may contribute to cardiac cell damage, ultimately resulting in myocyte death, either by the pathway of necrosis or the pathway of apoptosis (Sawyer et al. 1999).

2.1.2 Therapy and cardioprotection against anthracycline-induced cardiotoxicity

As it is accepted that drug-induced cardiac remodelling is, similarly to other types of cardiac injury, mediated by the activation of the renin-angiotensin-aldosteron system and adrenergic system, treatment with angiotensin-converting enzyme inhibitors, angiotensin receptor blockers, aldosterone antagonists, and beta blockers are consequently used to slow the progression of disease (Mann 1999). Thus, standard treatment for systolic heart failure is indicated for treatment for both asymptomatic and symptomatic cases, with angiotensin-converting enzyme inhibitors in first line, as some trials have suggested that these drugs may reduce the incidence of left ventricular dysfunction in high risk patients after chemotherapy (Wu 2008). However, the management of such patients remains complicated.

Clinicians confront a clinical dilemma as they have to balance the efficacy of longer duration of therapy against the cardiotoxicity associated with higher cumulative doses of anthracyclines. In an effort to prevent or reduce this cardiotoxicity, numerous less cardiotoxic anthracycline analogs have been developed (epirubicin, idarubicin) such as including liposomal anthracyclines (Batist et al. 2001; Muggia and Green 1991; Muggia et al. 1997), and the cumulative and peak doses of anthracycline therapy have been diminished (Legha et al. 1982; Von Hoff et al. 1979). Another cardiotoxicity reducing strategy is based on the use of cardioprotective agents, mainly on those which might reduce oxidative stress and/or may have chelating properties. From those, dexrazoxane (also known as cardioxane) is the most investigated agent (Swain et al. 1997; Wexler et al. 1996). Moreover, it is the only approved cardioprotective agent in anthacycline chemotherapy. Interestingly, dexrazoxane prevents heart damage but there is no evidence for a difference in response rate or survival (van Dalen et al. 2011). Other agents like L-carnitine, probucol, coenzyme Q10, N-acetylcysteine, vitamin E, digoxin, enalapril, phenethylamines, deferoxamine, ethylenediaminetetraacetic acid, superoxide dismutase and monohydroxyethylrutoside are less investigated; however cardioprotective effects have been reported in numerous studies (De Leonardis et al. 1985; Elihu et al. 1998; Guthrie and Gibson 1977; Iarussi et al. 1994; Kawasaki et al. 1992; Silber et al. 2004; Singal et al. 1995; Unverferth et al. 1983; Van Acker et al. 2000). Unfortunately, none of them achieved any clinical relevance as cardioprotective agent.

2.2 Other anti-cancer agents

Several non-anthracycline based anti-cancer drugs have also been associated with significant cardiac side effects. An alkylating agent - cyclophosphamide is mainly cardiotoxic at high doses, such as those used before bone marrow or stem cell transplantation (Meinardi et al. 2000). The reported cardiotoxicity ranges from transient electrocardiographic changes and asymptomatic increases of serum levels of cardiac enzymes to more severe cardiotoxicity such as exudative pericardial effusion, ventricular hypertrophy and fatal myopericarditis and (haemorrhagic) myocardial necrosis. The onset of the latter types of cardiotoxicity is acute, with fatal consequences within 15 days. The cardiotoxic effects of cyclophosphamide probably result from direct influence on the myocardial capillaries and can probably be partly explained by damage to the endothelium with resultant increase in permeability and extravasation of plasma, red blood cells and toxic metabolites (Gottdiener et al. 1981; Fraiser et al. 1991). From the group of antimetabolites (capecitabine, cytarabine, 5-fluorouracil), the cardiotoxicity of 5-fluorouracil is the best described one. It appears to have direct toxic effects on the myocardium, although toxic effects on the coronary arteries are probably the main pathogenetic factor (Meinardi et al. 2000). Necropsy findings in humans who died from fatal myocardial infarction or cardiogenic shock after 5-fluorouracil therapy showed patchy myocardial necrosis and mononuclear inflammation unrelated to the distribution of the coronary arteries (Sasson et al. 1994). A direct interference of 5-fluorouracil with the myocardial cell metabolism leading to cellular hypoxia has been suggested from a study with an isolated perfused rat heart model (Millart et al. 1992). In addition, cases of dilated cardiomyopathy and congestive heart failure have been reported after 5-fluorouracil treatment, also suggesting a direct toxic effect on the myocardium (Schöber et al. 1993; Weidmann et al. 1995). Capecitabine may cause ischaemia and cytarabine may cause pericarditis (Wu 2008). Some risk of cardiovascular toxicity has been attributed to antimicrotubules (paclitaxel, vinca alkaloids) as well. Paclitaxel may cause hypotension or arrhythmias, both supraventricular or ventricular and atrioventricular block, and vinca alkaloids may cause ischaemia (Wu 2008).

Recently, new biological therapy opens new possibilities in the treatment of cancer. New drugs were developed with the goal to specifically inhibit selected targets and to stop cancer cell proliferation and metastasis. These targeted therapies were thought to be more effective than traditional chemotherapeutic treatments and less harmful to non-cancerous cells. However, some of the targets inhibited by these new anti-cancer drugs appear to be important also for the maintenance of cellular homeostasis of normal tissue, in particular during exposure to cytotoxic chemotherapy (Zuppinger et al. 2007). Some of the new biological anti-cancer drugs associated with myocardial contractile dysfunction are trastuzumab, imatinib, and possibly bevacizumab (Slamon et al. 2001; Tan-Chiu et al. 2005; Drímal et al. 2006; Kerkelä et al. 2006). Importantly, most of these new biological therapeutics are not cytotoxic *per se* and, therefore, need to be combined with traditional chemotherapeutics and radiation therapy. Tyrosine kinase inhibitors (sunitinib, imatinib) are small molecule agents that inhibit cellular signalling involved in tumour cell angiogenesis and proliferation. Although this targeted approach results in improved anti-tumour activity and fewer side effects, tyrosine kinases regulating non-cancer functions are also affected, leading to undesired toxic side effects, including heart failure and hypertension (Chu et al. 2007). Trastuzumab is a recombinant IgG monoclonal antibody that binds to the human epidermal growth factor receptor 2 protein and is used for treatment of breast cancer that overexpresses this growth factor. It should be noted that agents like this are still relatively new, and full understanding of long term toxicities is still evolving (Jones et al. 2007). But as expected, the combination of trastuzumab with cytotoxic agents, in particular anthracyclines, bares a significant risk of cardiotoxicity (Slamon et al. 2001; Strasser et al. 2001). Multivariate analysis for the development of cardiac dysfunction in the pivotal trastuzumab trials identified prior or concomitant anthracycline exposure, over 50 years of age, and prior cardiac disease as independent risk factors. Many of these risk factors are similar to those for doxorubicin-induced cardiac dysfunction. However, in contrast to anthracycline-induced cardiomyopathy, trastuzumab-associated cardiac dysfunction appears to be mostly reversible and non-progressive (Ewer and Lippman 2005; Ewer et al. 2005).

2.3 Stimulants

Psychomotor stimulants have a marked influence on mental function and behaviour, producing excitement and euphoria, reduced sensation of fatigue, and an increase in motor activity. Clinically, abuse of stimulants such as cocaine, ephedrine, amphetamines or methamphetamines is associated with cardiovascular action such as tachycardia, supraventricular arrhythmias, ventricular arrhythmias, impaired conduction, hypertensive crises, acute coronary syndromes, shock and cardiac arrest. A number of cellular, animal and autopsy studies, individual case reports and case series suggested that exposures of such drugs are potentially associated with structural and functional changes of myocytes, as well as clinical manifestations of cardiomyopathy and congestive heart failure (Wijetunga et al. 2003; Yeo et al. 2007). The pathogenesis is probably similar to that of catecholamine-induced cardiomyopathy, *i.e.* sympathomimetic action, as for example pathologic similarities between cocaine cardiomyopathy and those seen in pheochromocytomas suggest that chronic adrenergic stimulation may play a role in the development of cardiomyopathy. It is possible that adrenergically driven recurrent hypertensive crises ultimately result in failure of the ventricle in exactly the same way as essential hypertension, in particular when combined with inappropriate life style (Crean and Pohl 2004). Apart from that, *in vitro* experiments showed that continuous exposure to a low concentration of methamphetamine may directly facilitate the development of cellular hypertrophy (Maeno et al. 2000).

2.3.1 Amphetamines and metamphetamines

Clinically, these drugs cause central nervous system stimulation that may induce euphoria, increase alertness, intensify emotions, increase aggression, alter self-esteem, and allegedly increase sexuality. Both oral and intravenous misuses are well documented. Deaths related to intoxications from these drugs have been associated with assaults, suicides, homicides, accidents, driving impairment, and maternal-fetal and infant exposures (Albertson et al. 1999). Pharmacologically, these drugs are substrates for the neuronal uptake transporters for norepinephrine, serotonin and dopamine, and cause release of these mediators from nerve terminals in the brain. Indirectly, the hyperstimulated neurons can stimulate various other pathways. Changes in mood, excitation level, motor movement, and appetite appear to be more directly mediated by central dopaminergic alterations. Serotonin alterations may also contribute to the amphetamine-related mood changes, psychotic behavior, and aggressiveness. Cardiovascular symptoms, including chest pain, palpitations, and dyspnea, are common. The exact frequency of such events is unknown but a clinical study showed that acute coronary syndrome is common (25%) in patients hospitalized for chest pain after methamphetamine use and the frequency of other potentially life-threatening cardiac complications is not negligible. These events occur in patients with and without underlying coronary disease and may involve multiple pathophysiologic mechanisms (Turnipseed et al. 2003). When considering cardiomyopathy, the incidence of 18% has been described in subjects abusing methamphetamine (Wijetunga et al. 2003). In other clinical study, methamphetamine use was documented in 40% of young patients with cardiomyopathy and was more severe compared to other non-ischemic cardiomyopathies. This findings support the hypothesis that methamphetamine use may be a possible cause of unexplained cardiomyopathy in young patients because its widespread use (Yeo et al. 2007).

Acute and chronic cardiomyopathy from abuse is thought to be secondary to both direct cardiac toxicity and indirect amphetamine-induced hypertension, necrosis, and ischemia (Albertson et al. 1999). The 3,4-methylenedioxymethamphetamine, commonly known as ecstasy, can cause myocardial infarction, arrhythmias, and cardiomyopathy (Mizia-Stec et al. 2008; Figueredo 2011). Animal studies showed that repeated methamphetamine administration may directly induce cellular hypertrophy of cardiomyocytes, myocarditis with inflammatory infiltrates and areas of necrosis, and consequently, may cause eccentric left ventricular dilation and diastolic dysfunction, as well as contractile dysfunction in myocytes (Shenouda et al. 2009). High dose administration may lead to cardiac function disorder with disruption of microtubules and actin (Maeno et al. 2000). It was suggested that metabolites are responsible for cardiotoxicity (Shenouda et al. 2008) as 3,4-methylenedioxymethamphetamine is metabolized to catechols that can undergo redox cycling, producing reactive oxygen and nitrogen species (Bolton et al. 2000). This suggests that potential mechanisms of 3,4-methylenedioxymethamphetamine-induced cardiomyopathy are related to oxidative stress, as well as catecholaminergic stimulation. Additionally, the recreational use of 3,4-methylenedioxymethamphetamine is often characterized by a repeated pattern of frequent drug applications (binge) followed by a period of abstinence what significantly alter cardiovascular and cardiovascular reflex function and produce cardiac toxicity (Badon et al. 2002). On the other hand, experimental as well as clinical data suggest that cardiac lessions are reversible after withdrawal of methamphetamine (Islam et al. 1995; Lopez et al. 2009).

2.3.2 Cocaine

Cocaine (benzoylmethylecgonine) is an alkaloid extracted from the leaves of the *Erythroxylon coca,* a plant native to South America. It was first used as a local anesthetics in 1884 and, interestingly, was used as an ingredient in a popular cola beverage in the early 20th century (Maraj et al. 2010). Cocaine inhibits catecholamine uptake by the norepinephrine and dopamine transporters at the presynaptic adrenergic terminals, causing an accumulation of catecholamines at the postsynaptic receptor, thereby enhancing peripheral effects of sympathetic nerve activity and producing a marked psychomotor stimulant effect. Its effects resemble those of amphetamines, although it has less tendency to produce stereotyped behaviour, delusions, hallucinations and paranoia (Johanson and Fischman 1989). It also causes the release of norepinephrine and epinephrine from the adrenal medulla and thus acting as a powerful sympathomimetic agent that can cause significant central and peripheral vasoconstriction. Cocaine has multiple cardiovascular and hematologic effects that likely contribute to the development of myocardial ischemia and/or myocardial infarction. Cocaine causes increased heart rate and blood pressure in a dose-dependent fashion, as well as increased cardiac index and dP/dt. The chronotropic effects of cocaine use are intensified in the setting of alcohol use, as well as smoking. By increasing heart rate, blood pressure, and contractility, cocaine leads to increased myocardial demand. Importantly, cocaine causes coronary vasoconstriction and thrombosis and so decreases oxygen supply and induces myocardial ischemia through a variety of mechanisms (McCord et al. 2008). Acute cellular effects include changes in calcium flux that are similar to other cardiac toxins, including digoxin. Increased intracellular concentrations of calcium have been suggested as a cause of depolarisation of the cardiac membrane and, therefore, a trigger of arrhythmias.

When misused chronically, cocaine administration can reduce left ventricular function, increase end-systolic wall stress and can cause a rare form of cardiomyopathy. The exact incidence of cocaine-induced cardiomyopathy is unknown and likely underreported. The medical literature to date consists mostly of case reports describing young men with a history of cocaine abuse and reversible cardiomyopathy (Awtry and Philippides 2010). In a review of 1278 cases of dilated cardiomyopathy patients, 10 cases were related to cocaine use (Felker et al. 1999). In a study of asymptomatic apparently healthy cocaine users, left ventricular systolic dysfunction was diagnosed in 7% by radionuclide angiography performed two weeks after cocaine use (Bertolet et al. 1990). The exact mechanism by which cocaine abuse causes cardiomyopathy is not fully understood. Furthermore, the amount and duration of cocaine use necessary to develop cocaine cardiomyopathy is currently unclear. Several pharmacologic effects of cocaine appear to be directly and indirectly related to its toxic myocardial action. Importantly, cocaine has been estimated to cause the development of cardiac hypertrophy without associated increases in arterial blood pressure, heart rate, renin, aldosterone, or cortisol, indicating a direct action on cardiac tissue remodelling and leading to heart failure. Nevertheless, whether it is a consequence of cocaine cardiomyopathy or ischemic cardiomyopathy due to cocaine vascular effects remains unclear. Finally, as direct putative pathophysiologic mechanisms of cocaine-induced cardiomyopathy and myocarditis, the following has been introduced: hyperadrenergic state produces contraction band necrosis in myocardium, direct toxic effect of cocaine on myofibrils and interstitial fibrosis, and hypersensitivity reaction of myocardium to cocaine. Other mechanisms include myocardial ischemia and infarction as a consequence of increased sympathomimetic activity with increased myocardial oxygen demand, altered calcium flux across myocyte cell membrane, altered vascular endothelium integrity (reduced prostacyclin production), increased platelet thromboxane production and increased plasminogen activator inhibitor production (Maraj et al. 2010; Awtry and Philippides 2010).

Four mechanisms have been described in more detail (Awtry and Philippides 2010). All of them alters cardiac function acutely but may lead to cardiac injury in a long-term fashion. First, promotion of intracoronary thrombus formation is widely recognised. Cocaine ingestion stimulates platelet hyperaggregability and increased thromboxane production, often in the setting of coronary vasospasm. These physiologic effects promote acute intracoronary thrombus formation and myocardial ischemic events and account, in part, for the increased incidence of myocardial infarction noted in cocaine users. Acute coronary ischemia and extensive or recurrent myocardial infarction also contribute to the left ventricular dysfunction and cardiomyopathy associated with cocaine abuse. However, many cocaine abusers with severe regional or global left ventricular dysfunction do not have a clear history of obstructive coronary disease or myocardial infarction. Thus, myocardial dysfunction can result from transient ischemic insults, perhaps in the setting of vasospasm or spontaneous coronary thrombosis. Alternatively, it is likely that nonischemic mechanisms of myocyte injury may also contribute. Second, sympathomimetic effects have to be taking into account as cocaine acts as a powerful sympathomimetic agent. Stimulation of the beta-adrenergic receptors in myocardial tissue results in increased contractility and heart rate, whereas stimulation of the alpha-adrenergic receptors in coronary and peripheral arteries results in increased coronary resistance, decreased coronary blood flow, elevated blood pressure, and increased myocardial wall stress (Kloner et al. 1992). Animal studies suggest that the increased wall stress seen in acute cocaine intoxication plays an important role in the acute depression of left ventricular function. Following cocaine infusion, ejection-phase indices of left ventricular function are reduced but the effects are attributable to increased wall stress not to reduced contractility (Mehta et al. 1995). Pathologic studies showed similarities between cocaine cardiomyopathy and chronic catecholamine stimulation (Tazelaar et al. 1987). Third, increased calcium flux into myocardial cells, and fourth, enhanced oxidative stress have been suggested as co-factors (Isabelle et al. 2007). Importantly, cocaine may alter cardiac electrophysiology what results in electrocardiological abnormalities, as evidenced in numerous experimental studies. The drug prolongs the PR, QRS, QT, and QTc durations, prolongs atrioventricular nodal conduction time and maximum sinoatrial conduction time, and may trigger frequent atrial extrasystoles and atrial fibrillation and tachycardia as well as transient ventricular tachycardia (Kloner et al. 1992).

2.3.3 Ephedra (Ma Huang)

The dietary supplement ephedra, also known as *Ma Huang* and obtained from the *Ephedra sinica* plant, contains 2 alkaloids - ephedrine and its enantiomer, pseudoephedrine. In traditional Chinese medicine this plant has been used for millennia to treat disorders such as asthma, upper respiratory illnesses and seasonal allergies. In recent years ephedra has gained tremendous popularity as a diet drug because of its biochemical activity as a stimulant and a pro-thermogenic agent. The stimulant activity of ephedra suppresses appetite while the pro-thermogenic property increases the body's metabolism, all leading to improved weight loss. However, over the past decade a number of well-documented reports of ischemic stroke and adverse cardiac events such as myocardial infarction, sudden death, and cardiomyopathy linked to ephedra have lead to a FDA ban of the drug in April 2004 as a dietary supplement (Lillegard and Porterfield 2010). Pharmacologically, ephedra increases catecholamines at synaptic areas in the brain and heart and directly stimulates alpha- and beta-adrenergic receptors. Thus, it can increase heart rate, blood pressure, cardiac output, and peripheral resistance. Coronary artery spasm and pro-arrhythmic effects can account for acute events and death. Prolonged catecholamine excess with long-term ephedra use is one likely underlying mechanism for cardiomyopathy (Figueredo 2011). Importantly, ephedra is often co-abused with anabolic-androgenic steroids (Clark and Schofield 2005; Achar et al. 2010).

2.4 Anabolic-androgenic steroids

The adrenals and the testes produce various compounds that stimulate androgen receptors. Dihydrotestosterone and testosterone are the most potent, but precursors such as dehydroepiandrosterone and androstenedione also have androgenic effects. 17-carbon androgenic precursors from either the adrenals or the gonads can be converted to testosterone by 17-hydroxysteroid dehydrogenase in the testis or ovary. In target tissues where intracellular enzymes are present, the action of testosterone is mediated by metabolism. The enzyme 5alpha-reductase produces the potent androgen dihydrotestosterone in the prostate, skin, sebaceous glands and brain. Due to this tissue-specific expression of 5alpha-reductase, androgenic effects on prostate growth and male pattern baldness are largely mediated by dihydrotestosterone. Conclusively, testosterone is irreversibly converted by the enzyme 5alpha-reductase to 5alpha-dihydrotestosterone, which binds with greater affinity to the androgen receptor, or by aromatase to oestradiol, which binds to the oestrogen receptor (Kicman 2008). All steroids that are anabolic are derivatives of testosterone (Hartgens and Kuipers 2004) and are androgenic as well as anabolic, as they stimulate growth and function of male reproductive tract. Individual drugs vary in their balance of anabolic:androgen activity but none of the currently available drugs are purely anabolic. Derivatives or structural modifications of testosterone differ by its pharmacokinetics, bioavailability, or, as mentioned above, balance of androgenic to anabolic activity. The large group of anabolic-androgenic steroids include testosterone itself, all of the derivatives that are used clinically, as well as numerous plant products that at least claim to possess anabolic actions (Kuhn 2002). Importantly, the group include many agents with chemical structures derived from cholesterol that are synthesized in the liver and then metabolized to anabolic-androgenic steroids. Their structure resembles that of corticosteroids, explaining some similarities in actions in terms of renal sodium retention and hypertension (Achar et al. 2010).

2.4.1 Therapeutic use and abuse of anabolic-androgenic steroids

Predominantly, anabolic-androgenic steroids are used in the treatment of disorders of puberty, prostatic disease and hirsutism. Testosterone replacement therapy is for hypogonal men who demonstrate clinical (reduced shaving frequency, exercise endurance, libido and testicular size) and laboratory findings (reduced free or free plus albumin-bound testosterone). Testosterone replacement therapy improves physical performance, sexual function, mood and lipid profiles within four weeks in most cases. The orally active androgens methyltestosterone and fluoxymesterone are not commonly used for androgen replacement, but are commonly abused by body builders. Other orally active androgenic steroids (testolactone, oxandrolone, stanozolol, oxymetholone) and intramuscular preparations (nandrolone) have androgenic effects and are used clinically for their anabolic actions in cancer and refractory anaemia. Newly, testosterone may have therapeutic benefit and be cardioprotective in heart failure for a number of reasons. Anabolic/catabolic imbalance, which favours catabolism, is a key pathological feature of patients with severe chronic heart failure and anabolic deficiency is an important component of the imbalance (Jankowska et al. 2006). In addition, it has been shown that pharmacological augmentation of anabolic drive can result in favourable changes in the body composition, sexual function and psychological status of aging men. Moreover, testosterone is viewed as a potential natural tonic for the failing heart (Pugh et al. 2000) and testosterone therapy has been proposed as a useful add-on treatment for men with congestive heart failure as its administration increases cardiac output acutely (Pugh et al. 2003; Pugh et al. 2004; Rauchhaus et al. 2006). Indeed, there is a clinical evidence that testosterone replacement therapy regimen in men with congestive heart failure was followed by improvement in NYHA class and functional capacity (Allan and McLachlan 2004; Malkin et al. 2006).

People have been taking testosterone to restore 'vitality' since the efficacy of some hormonal component of the testes was first described by Brown-Sequard in 1889. He reported the reversal of his own aging by self-injection of a testicular extract, thereby stimulated a flurry of experimentation into the putative anti-aging effects of testicular hormones long before the identity of testosterone was confirmed. The first use to improve athletic performance occurred shortly thereafter, in 1896. A contemporary of Brown-Sequard self-administered testicular extract, then measured his finger strength (Kuhn 2002). In modern age, anabolic-androgenic steroids, which include more than 30 natural and synthetic derivatives of testosterone, were designed in 1939 to treat conditions such as eunuchoid syndromes, impotence, depression, starvation, and cryptorchidism. The first suggestion that these drugs might enhance physical performance occurred later that same year. Mass trials conducted by Nazi Germany on their own soldiers during World War II, combined with concurrent animal studies, provided compelling data to support these theories. During the 1954 Vienna world weight lifting championships, the Russian national team introduced the use of anabolic-androgenic steroids as ergogenic aids. By the 1964 Olympics, athletes from around the world were consuming the drugs. In a survey of weight lifters at the 1968 United States Olympic Training camp, 100% had taken some form of the substance. During the 1972 Olympics held in Munich, 68% of those competing in middle or short distance and field events admitted to having taken anabolic-androgenic steroids as part of their preparation for the games. Proliferation of anabolic-androgenic steroids use throughout international competition had reached such epidemic proportions that by the 1976 Olympic games they were declared banned substances (Sullivan et al. 1998). After that, anabolic-androgenic steroids continued to be used clandestinely by Olympic athletes, and its use spread quickly to high school, intercollegiate, and professional sports. According to clinical data, self-reported rates of abuse in bodybuilders and powerlifters to enhance performance range from 29% to 67% (Curry and Wagman 1999; Achar et al. 2010). Also, there is now widespread use among non-competitive bodybuilders, recreational athletes, and those who simply desire an improved physique (Dhar et al. 2005). Thus, the risk of incidence of adverse effects in general population is relatively high. In general, anabolic-androgenic steroids are abused by athletes primarily to increase lean muscle mass, enhance appearance, and improve performance. Increased cellular protein synthesis results in build-up of tissue (anabolism), especially in muscles. A variety of anabolic-androgenic steroids are often taken simultaneously (so called 'stacking'), and in doses which result in 10–100 fold increases in androgen concentrations. Administration regimens usually involve a 6–12 week cycle and are often administered in a 'pyramidal' fashion, with doses tapering from low to high to low (Payne et al. 2004). Abused substances include testosterone, its 17-beta esters, and those based on modified steroid rings (including 17-alpha derivatives).

2.4.2 Cardiac injury

Several adverse effects of steroids have been described, predominantly when taking inappropriately. In healthy men, high-dose testosterone or synthetic androgens produce small increases in muscle mass and exercise performance, while posing the risks of aggressive mood disorder, priapism, erythrocytosis, oligospermia and worsened lipid profile. Adverse hepatic effects such as blood-filled hepatic cysts (*peliosis hepatis*), hepatic adenomas and cholestatic hepatic injury have been reported primarily with oral synthetic androgens. In elderly men, androgen supplementation increases serum concentrations of prostate-specific antigen and may worsen prostate hypertrophy.

Testosterone is a potent ligand of the human androgen receptor in muscles but also directly modulates transcription, translation, and enzymatic function in numerous other tissues (Sullivan et al. 1998). Consequently, the adverse effects from use of anabolic-androgenic steroids are widespread and affect multiple organ systems, including the heart and vessels. Several actions on cardiovascular system, and predominantly on heart, have been reported. Anabolic-androgenic steroids share with endogenous steroids influences on left ventricular hypertrophic response through direct actions on the androgen receptor (Marsh et al. 1998) what is a DNA-linked ligand-activated transcription factor with homology to mineralocorticoid and progesterone steroid receptors. Androgen receptors are ubiquitously expressed, found not only in skeletal muscle cells but also in cardiac myocytes. Anabolic-androgenic steroids can cause hypertension, dyslipidemia, and impaired fasting glucose, as well as alterations in heart structure, including left ventricular hypertrophy and dilation, and impaired contraction and relaxation. Potential sequelae include hypertension, acute myocardial infarction, sudden cardiac death, abnormal cardiac repolarisation with QT interval prolongation, ventricular fibrillation triggered by exercise, atrial fibrillation, cardiac tamponade, development of dilative cardiomyopathy, and heart failure at a dose-dependent manner (Hausmann et al. 1998; Stolt et al. 1999; Du Toit et al. 2005; Karila et al. 2003; Figueredo 2011). Several case reports have linked adverse cardiac events and anabolic-androgenic steroids abuse in healthy young athletes (Stergiopoulos et al. 2008; Ahlgrim and Guglin 2009). Recently, 49 reports describing a total of 1,467 athletes has been extensively reviewed (Achar et al. 2010). In aggregate, studies evaluated lipoprotein concentrations in 643 subjects, blood pressure in 348, left ventricular dimensions in 561, and sudden death in 102. As concluded, otherwise healthy young athletes abusing anabolic-androgenic steroids may show elevated levels of low-density lipoprotein and low levels of high-density lipoprotein. Although data are conflicting, anabolic-androgenic steroids have also been linked with elevated systolic and diastolic blood pressure and with left ventricular hypertrophy that may persist after anabolic-androgenic steroid cessation. Nevertheless, mortality appears to be significantly higher in anabolic-androgenic steroids abusers than in non-abusing athletes.

The potential pathophysiological mechanisms responsible for adverse cardiac effects are incompletely understood. Four mechanisms of anabolic-androgenic steroids-induced cardiovascular toxicity have been proposed: atherogenic, thrombotic, vasospastic, and direct myocardial injury (Melchert and Welder 1995). As already mentioned, anabolic-androgenic steroids bind to androgen receptors in the heart but in arteries as well, and physiologic levels (*e.g.*, of testosterone) may have a beneficial effect on coronary arteries via endothelial release of nitric oxide and inhibition of vascular smooth muscle tone. Conversely, animal studies show that administration of high doses of anabolic-androgenic steroids may reverse this vasodilator response and lead to growth-promoting effects on cardiac tissue, as seen in hypertrophic cardiomyopathy, followed by apoptotic cell death. These effects are likely associated with increased intracellular calcium influx and calcium release from the sarcoplasmic reticulum. This increase of intracellular calcium may be directly responsible for the development of cardiac hypertrophy as well as for the activation of apoptosis (Lieberherr and Grosse 1994; Zaugg et al. 2001). Postmortem histopathological findings of young anabolic-androgenic steroid abusers include cardiac hypertrophy, what seems to be dose-dependent and reversible (Ahlgrim and Guglin 2009). In addition, several other complications have been described, such as myocardial and endocardial fibrosis, cardiac steatosis, myocardial coagulation necrosis, decreased inotropic capacity of the myocardium, and irreversibly reduced compliance of the left ventricle, and coronary atheroma (Figueredo 2011). In other studies, endomyocardial biopsy specimens have revealed increased fibrous tissue and fat droplets in the myocardium of anabolic-androgenic steroid abusers (Nieminen et al. 1996). Direct cell injury occurs by disruption of myocardial mitochondria and induction of intrafibrillar collagen dysplasia. Cell injury ensues, and scar tissue replaces dead cells, leading to fibrosis and the potential for ventricular arrhythmias. Development of hypertension also occurs, followed by left ventricular hypertrophy and structural changes to the ventricular wall. Increased ventricular septal thickness develops rapidly and is disproportionate to the expected degree of compensatory hypertrophy from resistance training. Other studies reveal increased incidence of diastolic dysfunction, greater left ventricular posterior wall thickness, and greater left ventricular end-diastolic dimensions. In this setting, sudden death may have been caused by vasospasm potentiated by diastolic dysfunction–mediated ischemia (Dhar et al. 2005). Cardiomyopathy, cardiomegaly, and biventricular dilatation induced by anabolic-androgenic steroids can occur as a result of remodelling after myocyte injury and have been noted to be reversible after discontinuation of anabolic-androgenic steroids administration (Hausmann et al. 1998). However, it is still unclear whether such detrimental effects are directly associated with the action of anabolic-androgenic steroids or they are a consequence of co-presence of developing hypertension, hyperdynamics in cardiovascular system and dysbalance in blood lipids. Moreover, athletes abusing anabolic-androgenic steroids often exhibit left ventricular hypertrophy and because the hypertrophy may relate to increased afterload from isometric exercise, the interpretation of cardiac hypertrophy in elite athletes who admit to anabolic-androgenic steroids abuse is complex. Possible associations between anabolic-androgenic steroids and left ventricular hypertrophy may be explained as secondary to hypertension or as a direct effect on the myocardium. Notably, studies in isolated human myocytes have shown that anabolic-androgenic steroids bind to androgen receptors and may directly cause hypertrophy. It was clearly demonstrated that mammalian cardiac myocytes from hearts of different species and both sexes express the androgen receptor gene (Marsh et al. 1998). Androgens are capable of mediating a hypertrophic response of cultured adult myocytes of a magnitude nearly that of the most efficacious hypertrophic stimuli identified for heart. Consequently, androgens must be considered among the neuroeffectors, paracrine factors, and hormones that act directly on the cardiac myocyte and regulate the cardiac hypertrophic response. Indeed, a clinical study suggests a distinct form of left ventricular hypertrophy, as the abuse of anabolic-androgenic steroids in weight-lifters determines some alterations of the myocardial textural parameters when analyzed by videodensitometry (Di Bello et al. 1999). In contrast to these definite findings, studies comparing echocardiographic variables between anabolic-androgenic steroids using and nonusing strength athletes have not yielded unequivocal results (Ahlgrim and Guglin 2009). Some studies have not demonstrated any structural difference with abuse (Thompson et al. 1992) or showed that the myocardial remodeling is independent from anabolic-androgenic steroid use in power athletes (Dickerman et al. 1998). Considering the high prevalence of anabolic-androgenic steroids abuse in population, the number of cases featuring associated cardiac illness reported in current literature appears rather small. Thus the type or the intensity of training might play an important role (Ahlgrim and Guglin 2009). It remains open, whether the use of anabolic-androgenic steroids is causally related to these events or is just coincidental. Some animal studies suggest that these adverse effects cardiac muscle are causal and not coincidental. In adult rat cardiomyocytes *in vitro*, anabolic-androgenic steroids induce apoptotic cell death increasing the expression of the pro-apoptotic oncogene Bax-alpha in a dose-dependent manner (Zaugg et al. 2001). When studying the cardiac cell ultrastructure, mitochondria and myofibrils show changes similar to those observed in early heart failure, *i.e.* swollen and elongated mitochondria with sparse matrix and decreased number of cristae, and myofibrils show either disintegration and widened and twisted Z-bands or a complete dissolution of the sarcomeric units (Behrendt and Boffin 1977). Long-term testosterone administration results in myocarditis characterized by interstitial oedema, round cell infiltration, and fibrosis (Imai et al. 1978). Interestingly enough, cardiac tissue was protected from testosterone cardiotoxicity by chelating agent dexrazoxan indicating that oxidative stress might be involved (Belhani et al. 2009). Additionally, it was showed that ischemia/reperfusion injury is increased when cardiac hypertrophy develops after chronically administered nandrolone (Penna et al. 2011).

Additionally, in coronary artery disease, there is a contradiction between a documented risk and the evidence that tends to suggest just the opposite. Some short-term interventional studies show that testosterone produces a modest but consistent improvement in cardiac ischemia over placebo, comparable to the effects of existing antianginal drugs as intracoronary artery infusion of testosterone causes coronary artery dilatation and not constriction as previously thought (Liu et al. 2003). Notably, reduced testosterone levels were associated with coronary artery narrowing premature atherosclerosis, increased visceral adipose tissue, hyperinsulinemia, insulin resistance, increased body mass index, reduced high density lipoprotein levels and other risk factors for myocardial infarction (Bain 2007). Similarly in experiments, administration of testosterone significantly improves recovery from global ischemia what might be associated with an attenuation of reperfusion induced intracellular calcium overload (Callies et al. 2003). In contrast to that, testosterone overdose led to increase of apoptosis of cardiac cells after ischemia/reperfusion experiments and it was suggested that testosterone has inhibitory effects on cardioprotective Heat-Shock Protein 72 expression by modulating transcription, through testosterone receptor-mediated genomic mechanisms (Kohno et al. 2007). Similarly, testosterone decreases myocardial function after ischemia/reperfusion injury what is attributed to its proinflammatory and/or proapoptotic properties (Wang et al. 2005). It was shown that testosterone decreases the activation of cardioprotective pathway of the Signal Transducer and Activator of Transduction-3 following ischemia/reperfusion injuries (Wang et al. 2009).

3. Other cardiotoxic substances

3.1 Alcohol

Similarly to stimulants, the abuse of alcohol, as a substance affecting the central nervous system, has long recognised direct toxic effects on the heart (Bing 1978). Ethanol may induce 1) direct dose-dependent myocardial damage manifested as acute effects on rhythm and left-ventricular function, and/or 2) chronic progressive left ventricular dysfunction that may remain subclinical for a long time and is known as alcoholic cardiomyopathy.

Acute harmful drinking may induce 1) changes in cardiac contractility with systolic and diastolic dysfunction, and 2) rhythm disturbances, including sudden death (Urbano-Márquez and Fernández-Solà, 2004). The acute cardiodepressive action of ethanol is well established as it reduces the force of contraction of human heart when plasma levels exceed 75 mg per 100 ml. Such an acute intoxication causes reversible myocardial dysfunction, *i.e.* it has a direct negative inotropic action with a reversible dose-dependent decrease in myocardial contractility. Most studies of isolated myocardium have sought to explain these acute and reversible changes in the force of contraction by using pharmacologic concentrations of ethanol in the 1% (by volume) range (Knochel 1983; Guarnieri and Lakatta 1990). These studies have demonstrated that ethanol has multiple effects on the myocardium, and as such could depress the force of contraction at several points in the process of electromechanical coupling, probably at the level of the myofilaments. The effect was found to be reversible by increasing the amount of calcium presented to the myofilaments or by washing out the ethanol (Guarnieri and Lakatta 1990). This cardiodepresive action of ethanol is evidenced in experimental models designed with autonomic blockade, heart denervation, or isolated cells. On the other hand, negative inotropic action of ethanol is often masked by indirect actions resulting from an enhanced release of catecholamines *in vivo*. Remarkably, the acute cardio-depressant effect of alcohol usually has fewer clinical consequences in non-alcoholic patients with normal cardiac function, but may be more relevant in patients with previous cardiac disease or in patients with alcoholic cardiomyopathy. In these patients, episodes of heart failure may be induced by acute alcohol poisoning. When considering chronotropy, the acute negative chronotropic effect with combination of augmented release of catecholamines may induce a variety of arrhythmias, known as the 'Holiday Heart' arrhythmias, with paroxysmal atrial fibrillations and ventricular premature depolarisations (Ettinger 1984). The prolongation of conduction times and a heterogeneous increase in the refractory period may be directly associated with propensity of arrhythmias. Chronic alcoholism, acute abstinence from ethanol and coexistence of electrolyte deficiencies are strong co-factors increasing the pro-arrhythmogenicity of ethanol abuse. Moreover the presence of chronic cardiomyopathy increases the risk of arrhythmias such as ventricular fibrillation or even sudden cardiac death.

Long-standing ethanol consumption may induce more important deleterious effects on the myocardium what is usually described as alcoholic cardiomyopathy manifesting as cardiac hypertrophy, disrupting contractile function and myofibrillary architecture. When comparing alcoholics with healthy controls, the alcoholics show a lower ejection fraction, a lower mean shortening fraction, a greater mean end-diastolic diameter and left ventricular enlargement. One third of the alcoholics have an ejection fraction of 55 percent or less, and when analysed using endomyocardial biopsy specimens those patients show histologically defined changes of cardiomyopathy (Urbano-Márquez et al. 1989). The chronic ventricular dysfunction develops independently of other factors such as malnutrition or vitamin deficiencies, with both systolic and diastolic dysfunction, manifested as a decrease in left-ventricular ejection fraction and disturbances in left-ventricular relaxation, respectively. These effects may first be subclinical and, later, overt clinical alcoholic dilated cardiomyopathy with left ventricular or congestive heart failure may appear. In general, one-third to one-half of alcohol consumers, in doses higher than 100 g/day for a minimum of 10 years, is affected by progressive diastolic and systolic dysfunction.

A disproportionately large majority of reported cases of alcoholic cardiomyopathy are men. In line with this, the female gender is believed to be protected from cardiovascular morbidity because of hormones (so called 'oestrogen umbrella' effect). However, this seems to be false in the case of chronic ethanol consumption. As shown in a clinical study, a third of the alcoholic women had evidence of cardiomyopathy what is comparable to men.

Despite the fact that the mean lifetime dose of alcohol in female alcoholics is only 60% that in male alcoholics, cardiomyopathy is as common in female alcoholics as in male alcoholics. Ejection fractions in women inversely correlate with the total lifetime dose of ethanol, whereas the left ventricular mass shows a direct correlation. Similarly to women, ejection fractions also correlate inversely with the total lifetime dose of ethanol in men. However, the threshold dose for the development of cardiomyopathy is considerably less in women than in men, and the decline in the ejection fraction with increasing alcohol dose is steeper. This indicates that women are more sensitive than men to the toxic effects of alcohol on cardiac muscle (Urbano-Márquez et al. 1995).

Importantly, diastolic dysfunction is the earliest sign of subclinical alcoholic cardiomyopathy. Symptoms of alcoholic cardiomyopathy are similar to other causes of low-output dilated cardiomyopathies, with shortness of breath and early fatigue during exercise, progressing to attacks of breathlessness, orthopnea, and paroxysmal nocturnal dyspnea. Negative dromotropism and lowering of the threshold level for ventricular fibrillation have been observed in chronic drinkers, leading to ventricular fibrillation and sudden death. Alcoholism also decrease the myocardial capacity at increased cardiac activity, resulting in shortness of breath due to congestion in the pulmonary vessels. Interestingly, although the development of alcoholic cardiomyopathy is independent of liver function parameters, alcoholics with cardiomyopathy have a higher incidence of liver cirrhosis. As showed in clinical study, alcoholics with diagnosed cardiomyopathy have a higher prevalence of cirrhosis than unselected alcoholics without heart disease. Similarly, actively drinking alcoholics with cirrhosis show impaired cardiac performance, whereas abstaining alcoholics with liver disease tend to manifest normal cardiac function (Estruch et al. 1995).

As already mentioned, the long-term heavy alcohol consumption (of any beverage type) is the leading cause of a nonischemic, dilated cardiomyopathy (Piano 2002). However, there appears to be a biphasic cardiovascular effect based on the chronic dose of alcohol ingested. At low to moderate doses, studies suggest that alcohol has a favourable impact on cardiovascular outcomes, *i.e.* lower incidence of myocardial infarctions and an improved survival. At chronic high-dose intake of alcohol, there is a direct relationship to elevated blood pressure. Also, prolonged exposure to alcohol increases the likelihood of developing congestive heart failure. The exact duration and intensity of alcohol consumption preceding preclinical and symptomatic heart failure is not definitively known. It is estimated that a minimum of 10 years of exposure to excessive alcohol intake leads to the onset of heart failure. However, this link to duration and amount of alcohol consumption is weak. Some heavy users of alcohol never develop a cardiomyopathy, while others who ingest only a modest amount can be at risk for developing a cardiomyopathy. Men may be more susceptible to this risk. Concurrent smoking, hypertension, and malnutrition appear highly associated with the increased risk for developing an alcoholic cardiomyopathy. The incidence of alcohol as a major contributor to cardiomyopathy has been reported to be in the range of 20%-30%, emphasizing the clinical need to recognize the risk and contribution of alcohol in heart failure patients (Lee and Regan 2002). Some studies have observed asymptomatic cardiac dysfunction in patients reporting consumption more than 90 g/day of alcohol (8-21 standard drinks) with an average duration of drinking of 15 years. The disease is characterised by ventricular dilation and systolic dysfunction, in the absence of other causative factors such as coronary disease. In preclinical stages of alcoholic cardiomyopathy, ventricular enlargement and diastolic dysfunction can be observed on echocardiography

(Piano 2002; Wu 2008). Although alcoholic cardiomyopathy may be reversible after abstention, severe cases may still progress into congestive heart failure despite a cessation of alcohol use.

The pathophysiological mechanisms underlying alcoholic cardiomyopathy are poorly understood and diverse pathogenic theories have been postulated about the mechanisms of alcohol-induced cardiac muscle damage. Except the effects of ethanol on blood lipids and systemic blood pressure, they likely involve direct myocyte injury and several direct cellular, subcellular, and molecular derangements of cardiac tissue. In past (Bing 1978), several mechanisms have been proposed such as mitochondrial effects (decreased respiratory function, loss of mitochondrial enzymes, deterioration of ultrastructure), decreased calcium uptake by sarcoplasmic reticulum, altered myocardial lipid metabolism (triglyceride accumulation, decreased fatty acid oxidation), effects by formation of acetate and acetaldehyde, non-thrombotic myocardial infarctions and nutritional defects (thiamine deficiency, protein deficiency). It was previously supposed that malnutrition (electrolyte or vitamin deficiencies) is the main pathogenic factors. However, experimental and clinical studies have clearly demonstrated that ethanol itself is a direct noxious agent to heart in a progressive, cumulative, and dose-dependent manner, and its effects are independent of nutritional, vitamin, or mineral factors. According to current knowledge, the main relevant pathogenic mechanisms of alcohol-induced damage are due to interference in carbohydrate metabolism, protein synthesis, changes in oxidative status and mitochondrial function, disruption of transduction signals, and induction of apoptosis (Urbano-Márquez and Fernández-Solà, 2004). Alcohol alters the permeability of the sarcoplasmic reticulum to calcium ions and thus reduces the efficiency by which calcium activates muscle contraction, and it reduces the synthesis of cardiac proteins in both the contractile actin-myosin complex and in mitochondria, predominantly in alcoholics with high blood pressure. Similarly, a metabolite acetaldehyde and free radicals may contribute to decreased protein synthesis as well. In addition, there is enough evidence that alcohol can induce cardiac muscle damage by increasing the expression of a certain genes, which can promote programmed cell death, resulting in muscle cell loss (Zakhari 1997). In cell cultures, the acute alcohol exposure triggers the process of apoptosis inducing the expression of the pro-apoptotic protein Bax and increased caspase-3 enzyme activity (Chen et al. 2000). However, it is also possible that other cell types or systems are activated, such as the sympathetic nervous system, renin-angiotensin system, cytokines, and natriuretic peptides which may contribute to the overall injury. Interestingly enough, the excessive use of alcohol is not the exclusive cause of development of alcoholic cardiomyopathy *per se* as not all excessive alcohol consumers develop significant myocardial damage. When taking account the high prevalence of alcohol consumption the incidence of alcoholic cardiomyopathy is relatively low in the general population (Urbano-Márquez et al., 1995). Conclusively, in addition to the toxic effect of ethanol causing apoptosis, necrosis and cell loss, other mechanisms may influence the development of cardiac functional and structural damage.

3.2 Heavy metals

Some heavy metals, as cadmium, lead and cobalt, are known to be involved in selective cardiotoxicity. They are negatively inotropic and dromotropic and may cause structural changes. As for example, cobalt has been discovered to be the cause of an endemic cardiomyopathy in heavy beer drinkers in Canada in 1966 where it was used as an additive to stabilize the froth (Alexander 1972). The cardiac muscle of autopsied patients contained a high concentration of cobalt (Sullivan et al. 1968) but to produce the cardiac disease required a combination of: 1) protein deficient diet and 2) cobalt administration (Rona and Chappel 1973). Although the amount of ingested cobalt was lower than in certain therapies, the poor general nutritional state that is typical of chronic drinkers resulted in higher susceptibility to the cardiotoxicity of cobalt. The exact mechanism for developing of cardiomyopathy is unclear but it is known that cobalt may decrease myocardial contractility by a competitive antagonism with calcium (Hashimoto et al. 1989). Amino and sulfhydryl groups of amino acids can provide protection against cobalt effects by combining with cobalt and preventing the chelation of cobalt with sulfhydryl gropus of the myocardial tissue. One lesson to be learnt from this endemic cardiomyopathy, widely known as cobalt-beer cardiomyopathy, is that effects of any given noxious agent can be compounded and exaggerated by other coexisting metabolic defects, such as protein deficiency (Rona and Chappel 1973), thiamine and zinc depletion and prior ethanolic damage to the myocardium (Alexander 1972).

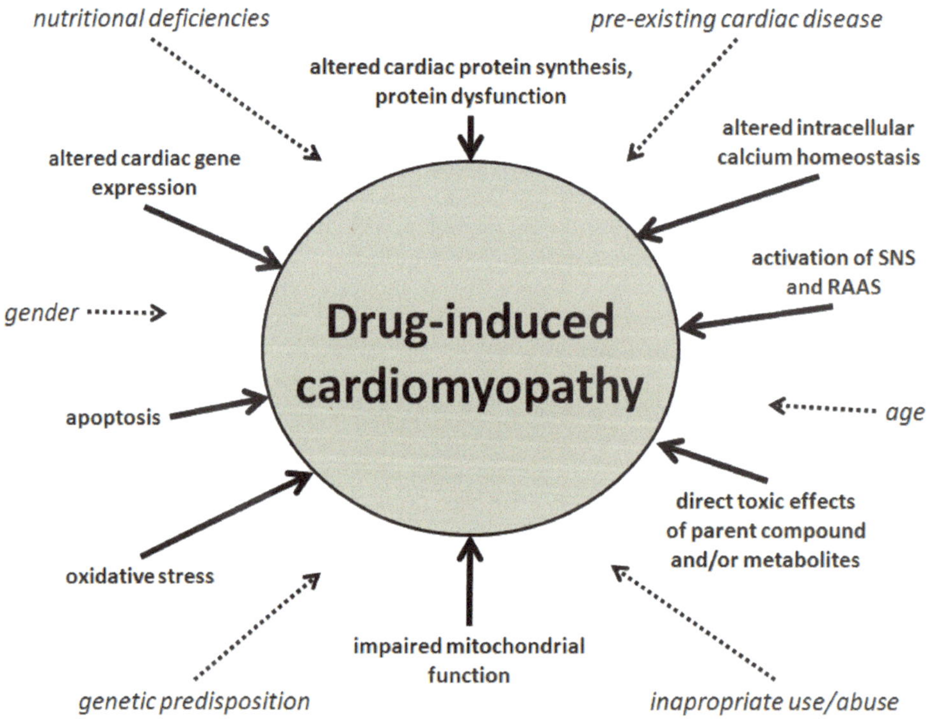

Fig. 2. Potential mechanisms (bold) and risk factors (italic) involved in drug-induced cardiomyopathies. (Abbreviations: SNS - sympathetic nervous system, RAAS - renin-angiotensin-aldosterone system.)

3.3 Experimental models of primary or secondary drug-induced cardiomyopathies

3.3.1 Catecholamines

The harmful effects of excess doses of experimentally administered catecholamines on the myocardium have been established for a long time when infarct-like lesions were produced by administration of large doses of isoproterenol (Rona et al. 1959). One of the best described models of experimental cardiomyopathies is the model of isoproterenol-induced myocardial infarction followed by cardiac hypertrophy, fibrosis and failure (Szabó et al. 1975). Similarly in clinical practice, the cardiotoxicity of catecholamines in treatment of severe asthma has been well established (Maguire et al. 1991). Moreover, catechoalmines are involved in the development of the rare 'Broken Heart Syndrome', also known as Takotsubo cardiomyopathy (Wittstein 2008). The probable mechanisms for such harmful effects of catecholamines on myocardium are not only direct effects, but also, in the case of epinephrine and isoproterenol, severe systemic hypotension with the combination producing a massive myocardial infarction. Although norepinephrine has a predominant vasopressor action, it also produces myocardial damage, which is generally of a patchy necrotic type limited to subendocardial zone occurred in patients with fatal pheochromocytoma or tetanus (Rose 1974). In past, some important mechanisms of catecholamine cardiotoxicity have been proposed: excess of calcium ions with excess excitation-contraction coupling and loss of high-energy phosphate compounds (Fleckenstein et al. 1974), increased cell membrane permeability (Rona 1985), intracellular accumulation of cyclic AMP (Lubbe et al. 1978), and increased ischemic damage (Opie et al. 1979). An important action of catecholamines is their ability to induce myocardial hypertrophy. Importantly, activation of beta-receptors induces the expression of proto-oncogenes c-fos and c-myc (Zimmer 1997). Moreover, some catecholamines induce the development of sub-endocardial fibrosis activating the proliferation of cardiac fibroblasts (Turner et al. 2003). Additionally, the role of oxidative stress (Zhang et al. 2005; Dhalla et al. 2010) and nitric oxide signalling cascade should not be neglected (Krenek et al. 2006; Krenek et al. 2009).

3.3.2 Hyperglycaemia inducing agents

Application of several drugs may lead to alterations which result in cardiac injury secondarily. One of such alteration is the long term hyperglycaemia and the development of diabetes mellitus. In experimental cardiology, two models of diabetic cardiomyopathy are widely established - streptozotocin- and alloxan-induced hyperglycaemia, diabetes and followed diabetic cardiomyopathy. Streptozotocin is a nitrosurea derivative isolated from *Streptomyces achromogenes* with broad-spectrum antibiotic and antineoplastic activity. It is a powerful alkylating agent that has been shown to interfere with glucose transport, glucokinase function and induce multiple DNA strand breaks. A single large dose of streptozotocin can produce diabetes in rodents, probably as a result of direct toxic effects characterized by a specific destruction of the pancreatic beta cells (Rees and Alcolado 2005). Streptozotocin injected rats develop severe diabetes characterized by both fasting and postprandial hyperglycemia with lack of growth in body weight and heart mass. The diabetes induced by streptozotocin can be considered as a model of both type 1 and 2 diabetes, as pancreatic islet beta cell death occurs in both types of diabetes, leading to absolute or relative insulin deficiency. Nevertheless, the model has its limits for each type. On the one hand, a single injection of streptozotocin usually does not lead to an autoimmune reaction as observed in type 1 diabetes, and on the other hand, the animals lack a significant resistance to insulin action as seen in type 2 diabetes. Nevertheless, metabolic changes typically observed in patients with diabetes, characterized by hyperglycemia and increased circulating free fatty acids, are induced. Thus, eventually the heart is exposed to the major compounds of a diabetic milieu (Dyntar et al. 2006). The developing cardiomyopathy is characterized by a decreased left ventricular performance and bradycardia under basal conditions as well as under beta-adrenergic stimulation, presence of elevated cardiac oxidative stress and changes in electrocardiograms such as the prolongation of QRS and QT interval (Howarth et al. 2005; Jankyova et al. 2009; Klimas et al. 2010). Similarly to streptozotocin, injections of alloxan induce the same blood glucose and plasma insulin responses and cause diabetes syndrome. Alloxan has two distinct pathological effects: it selectively inhibits glucose-induced insulin secretion through specific inhibition of glucokinase, the glucose sensor of the pancreatic beta cell, and it causes a state of insulin-dependent diabetes through its ability to induce reactive oxygen species formation, resulting in the selective necrosis of beta cells (Lenzen 2008). Consequently to persistent hyperglycaemia, degenerative myocardial changes are detectable in experimental settings (Mir and Darzi 2009).

3.3.3 Monocrotaline

In general, right ventricular failure is far rarer than the left ventricular failure. Experimental cardiology uses monocrotaline to induce pulmonary hypertension resulting in right ventricular hypertrophy and *cor pulmonale*. Monocrotaline is a pyrrolizidine alkaloid present in the seeds and foliage of the leguminous plant *Crotalaria spectabilis*. The administration of this alkaloid to rats produces pulmonary hypertension, hypertensive pulmonary vascular disease what results in right ventricular failure (Kay et al. 1982). The precise mechanism remains elusive but is known that to produce pulmonary insult, monocrotaline must first be activated by the liver to the putative electrophile monocrotaline pyrrole. Its stabilization by red blood cells facilitates subsequent transport to the lung where it harms the pulmonary endothelium (Lamé et al. 2000) as has been showed *in vitro* and *in vivo* as well (Boor et al. 1995).

4. Drugs inducing cardiac arrhythmias and cardiac arrest

Except of drugs inducing cellular injury or impairment resulting in depressed cardiac contractility and subsequent contractile failure, there is a number of drugs which affect ion channels and pumps and so destabilize ion homeostasis and trigger conduction defects, arrhythmias or even cardiac arrest. Importantly, these drugs do not acutely affect molecular targets but their chronic administration may affect gene expression and so change the cardiac tissue properties.

4.1 Digoxin

For more than 200 years, digoxin, a cardiotonic steroid, and its congeners have been used to treat congestive heart failure. Cardiac glycosides come from foxgloves (*Digitalis* spp.) and related plants. Nowadays, there is evidence in mammals of an endogenous digitalis-like factor closely similar to another cardiac glycoside, ouabain, and this is of potential physiological and pathological significance (Schoner 2002). Cardiotonic steroids are specific inhibitors of the the Na^+/K^+-ATP-ase of plasma membranes and this leads to an increase in the concentration of intracellular calcium via Na^+/Ca^{2+} exchanger as a secondary event. Moreover, this modulates the calcium content of the sarcoplasmic reticulum and Ca^{2+} signalling, and contributes finally to the positive inotropic effect of cardiac glycosides and an altered gene expression of proteins (Blaustein et al. 1998; Scheiner-Bobis and Schoner 2001). Because Na^+/K^+ exchange is electrogenic, inhibition of the pump by glycosides causes depolarisation, predisposing to disturbances in cardiac rhythm. Furthermore, the increased intracellular calcium causes increased after-depolarisation, leading first to bigeminy, followed eventually by ventricular tachycardia and, in certain cases, by ventricular fibrillation.

4.2 QT prolonging and Torsades de Pointes triggering drugs

The duration of QT interval measured by 12-lead electrocardiography, as a characterization of ventricular repolarisation, is one of the stable cardiac parameters widely used to describe cardiac abnormalities and safety of drugs (Klimas et al. 2008; Kmecova and Klimas 2010). The prolongation of QT interval on the surface electrocardiogram because of abnormally prolonged ventricular repolarisation is mostly referred as long QT syndrome. From a clinical perspective, it may translate into a propensity to develop syncope and sudden cardiac death. In most documented cases, death was caused by the malignant polymorphic ventricular arrhythmia called *Torsades de Pointes*. This arrhythmia is defined as a polymorphic ventricular tachycardia characterized by a 'twisting of the points' around the isoelectric line on the electrocardiogram (also formerly known as 'ballet rhythm'), and is preceded by a long QT interval (Ponte et al. 2010). Common manifestations of *Torsades de Pointes* are palpitation, symptoms of impaired cerebral circulation such as dizziness, syncope or seizures. Importantly, *Torsades de Pointes* is potentially fatal. In 20% of cases it can subsequently degenerate into ventricular fibrillation with mortality of around 10%. Predicting the development of a life-threatening arrhythmia is a hard task but, in the case of *Torsades de Pointes*, there are some useful markers. Among them, the prolongation of the QT interval is the most remarkable (Giorgi et al. 2010).

In the past few years, much attention has been focused on drugs that prolong the QT interval, potentially leading to malignant cardiac rhythm disturbances and fatal *Torsades de Pointes*. Several drugs were withdrawn from the market because they either directly caused electrocardiographic abnormality or resulted in drug-drug interactions that led to unacceptable rates of cardiotoxicity. In 1964, it was first described what would subsequently be termed drug-induced long QT syndrome with the observation that quinidine could provoke QT prolongation and arrhythmias in otherwise healthy patients (Selzer and Wray 1964). Indeed, drug administration is the most common cause of *Torsades de Pointes*. The most frequent triggers are QT-prolonging antiarrhythmics, such as quinidine, procainamide, disopyramide (class Ia) and sotalol, amiodarone, dofetilide or ibutilide (class III). With these agents, 1–8% of patients develop marked QT prolongation and *Torsades de Pointes*. On the other hand, there is a wide range of drugs developed for non-cardiovascular indications prolonging QT and inducing *Torsades de Pointes*, as well. These include high-profile drug withdrawal cases, such as terfenadine, astemizole and cisapride, as well as a variety of drugs that are in common clinical use, such as methadone, clarithromycin, erythromycin and other antibiotics, and thioridazine and other antipsychotics. An up-to-date list is maintained at the www.torsades.org website. Nevertheless, the incidence of *Torsades de Pointes* with these 'non-cardiovascular' agents is lower than with QT-prolonging antiarrhythmics (Roden 2008).

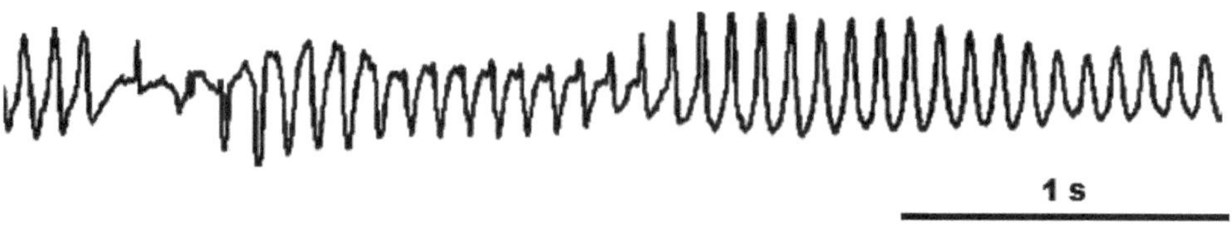

Fig. 3. The risk of *Torsades de Pointes* rises when risk factors are combined. As shown in electrocardiogram, the repeated co-administration of clarithromycin and furosemide may induce adrenergically-triggered *Torsades de Pointes* in rat (Klimas et al. 2010a).

The electrophysiological basis of QT length is the action potential of ventricular cardiomyocytes. First principles in cardiac electrophysiology dictate that an increase in QT interval must reflect an increase in action potential duration in at least some regions of the ventricle. Such increased action potential duration, in turn, must reflect an increase in inward current or a decrease in outward current (Roden 2008). Most drugs that cause *Torsades de Pointes* prolong the action potential of cardiac myocytes by blocking potassium channels (Roden 2004). Notably, the most important ionic current related to drug-induced potential of action prolongation is the delayed rectifier potassium current I_{Kr} during phase 3 of action potential. Most drugs block the I_{Kr} (Kv11.1) channel by binding to the alpha-subunits. The channel is encoded in the *human ether-a-go-go related gene* (HERG) gene. The relationship between QT prolongation and *Torsades de Pointes* has been initially supported by the fact that subjects with some forms of long QT syndrome (which have a mutation in the HERG) frequently developed *Torsades de Pointes*. Thus, extending that concept, drugs that inhibit the HERG encoded I_{Kr} channel may increase the duration of the action potential, QT interval and it might lead to *Torsades de Pointes*. In spite of this scientific evidence, the inhibition of HERG channel does not always provoke action potential and QT prolongation, mainly when the drug also blocks other ionic channels, as it happens with L-type calcium channels blockers. Moreover, some non-antiarrhythmic drugs that clearly prolong QT (as it was observed for sodium pentobarbital and ranolazine) have not been associated to *Torsades de Pointes* (Giorgi et al. 2010). However, some drugs like arsenic trioxide and pentamidine prolong the QT interval by reduced number of I_{Kr} (Kv11.1) channels on the myocardial cell membrane by causing abnormal trafficking of proteins which form the I_{Kr} (Kv11.1) channel. Importantly, only a few individuals receiving drugs that block the I_{Kr} (Kv11.1) channel develop significant QT prolongation and potentially fatal *Torsades de Pointes*. Predisposing factors include interactions with concomitantly used drugs resulting in supra-therapeutic drug levels, female gender, advanced age, bradycardia, hypokalaemia, hypomagnesaemia, ventricular hypertrophy, renal failure, central nervous system lesions, low-salt diet, congestive heart failure and nutritional disorders like prolonged starvation and anorexia nervosa. It is believed that some patients experiencing *Torsades de Pointes* may have genetic polymorphisms of genes coding for cardiac ion channels (Salvi et al. 2010).

Amiodarone	Ibutilide
Arsenic trioxide	Levomethadyl
Astemizole	Mesoridazine
Bepridil	Methadone
Chloroquine	Moxifloxacin
Chlorpromazine	Pentamidine
Cisapride	Probucol
Clarithromycin	Procainamide
Disopyramide	Quinidine
Dofetilide	Sotalol
Domperidone	Sparfloxacin
Droperidol	Terfenadine
Erythromycin	Thioridazine
Halofantrine	Vandetanib
Haloperidol	

Table 2. Drugs with a documented risk of Torsades de Pointes (Salvi et al. 2010).

5. Conclusion

The fact that drug-induced heart disease, and in particular drug-induced cardiomyopathy, does not occur more often, as would be expected from the diversity of various mechanisms, is perhaps surprising. In spite of this, cardiotoxicity remains a major problem of hundreds of pharmaceutical agents, industrial chemicals and naturally occurring products and is often a limiting factor in treatment of certain diseases. Hence, it must be taken in account in the process of clinical decision making and treatment as well as in the process of drug research and development.

6. References

Achar S, Rostamian A, Narayan SM. Cardiac and metabolic effects of anabolic-androgenic steroid abuse on lipids, blood pressure, left ventricular dimensions, and rhythm. *Am J Cardiol.* 2010;106:893-901.

Ahlgrim C, Guglin M. Anabolics and cardiomyopathy in a bodybuilder: case report and literature review. *J Card Fail.* 2009;15:496-500.

Albertson TE, Derlet RW, Van Hoozen BE. Methamphetamine and the expanding complications of amphetamines. *West J Med.* 1999;170:214-219.

Alexander CS. Cobalt-beer cardiomyopathy. A clinical and pathologic study of twenty-eight cases. *Am J Med.* 1972;53:395-417.

Allan CA, McLachlan RI. Age-related changes in testosterone and the role of replacement therapy in older men. *Clin Endocrinol (Oxf).* 2004;60:653-670.

Arai M, Tomaru K, Takizawa T, Sekiguchi K, Yokoyama T, Suzuki T, Nagai R. Sarcoplasmic reticulum genes are selectively down-regulated in cardiomyopathy produced by doxorubicin in rabbits. *J Mol Cell Cardiol.* 1998;30:243-254.

Arcamone F, Cassinelli G, Fantini G, Grein A, Orezzi P, Pol C, Spalla C. Adriamycin, 14-hydroxydaunomycin, a new antitumor antibiotic from S. peucetius var. caesius. *Biotechnol Bioeng*. 1969;11:1101-1110.

Aries A, Paradis P, Lefebvre C, Schwartz RJ, Nemer M. Essential role of GATA-4 in cell survival and drug-induced cardiotoxicity. *Proc Natl Acad Sci U S A*. 2004;101:6975-6980.

Awtry EH, Philippides GJ. Alcoholic and cocaine-associated cardiomyopathies. *Prog Cardiovasc Dis*. 2010;52:289-299.

Bachur NR, Gordon SL, Gee MV. Anthracycline antibiotic augmentation of microsomal electron transport and free radical formation. *Mol Pharmacol*. 1977;13:901-910.

Badon LA, Hicks A, Lord K, Ogden BA, Meleg-Smith S, Varner KJ. Changes in cardiovascular responsiveness and cardiotoxicity elicited during binge administration of Ecstasy. *J Pharmacol Exp Ther*. 2002;302:898-907.

Bain J. The many faces of testosterone. *Clin Interv Aging*. 2007;2:567-576

Batist G, Ramakrishnan G, Rao CS, Chandrasekharan A, Gutheil J, Guthrie T, Shah P, Khojasteh A, Nair MK, Hoelzer K, Tkaczuk K, Park YC, Lee LW. Reduced cardiotoxicity and preserved antitumor efficacy of liposome-encapsulated doxorubicin and cyclophosphamide compared with conventional doxorubicin and cyclophosphamide in a randomized, multicenter trial of metastatic breast cancer. *J Clin Oncol*. 2001;19:1444-1454.

Behrendt H, Boffin H. Myocardial cell lesions caused by an anabolic hormone. *Cell Tissue Res*. 1977;181:423-426.

Belhani D, Fanton L, Vaillant F, Descotes J, Manati W, Tabib A, Bui-Xuan B, Timour Q. Cardiac lesions induced by testosterone: protective effects of dexrazoxane and trimetazidine. *Cardiovasc Toxicol*. 2009;9:64-69.

Bers DM. Cardiac excitation-contraction coupling. *Nature*. 2002;415:198-205.

Bertolet BD, Freund G, Martin CA, Perchalski DL, Williams CM, Pepine CJ. Unrecognized left ventricular dysfunction in an apparently healthy cocaine abuse population. *Clin Cardiol*. 1990;13:323-328.

Binaschi M, Bigioni M, Cipollone A, Rossi C, Goso C, Maggi CA, Capranico G, Animati F. Anthracyclines: selected new developments. *Curr Med Chem Anticancer Agents*. 2001;1:113-130.

Bing RJ. Cardiac metabolsim: its contributions to alcoholic heart disease and myocardial failure. *Circulation*. 1978;58:965-970.

Blaustein MP, Juhaszova M, Golovina VA. The cellular mechanism of action of cardiotonic steroids: a new hypothesis. *Clin Exp Hypertens*. 1998;20:691-703.

Bolton JL, Trush MA, Penning TM, Dryhurst G, Monks TJ. Role of quinones in toxicology. *Chem Res Toxicol*. 2000;13:135-160.

Boor PJ, Gotlieb AI, Joseph EC, Kerns WD, Roth RA, Tomaszewski KE. Chemical-induced vasculature injury. Summary of the symposium presented at the 32nd annual meeting of the Society of Toxicology, New Orleans, Louisiana, March 1993. *Toxicol Appl Pharmacol*. 1995;132:177-195.

Boucek RJ Jr, Miracle A, Anderson M, Engelman R, Atkinson J, Dodd DA. Persistent effects of doxorubicin on cardiac gene expression. *J Mol Cell Cardiol*. 1999;31:1435-1446.

Bristow MR, Mason JW, Daniels JR. Monitoring of anthracycline cardiotoxicity. *Cancer Treat Rep*. 1978;62:1607-1608.

Callies F, Strömer H, Schwinger RH, Bölck B, Hu K, Frantz S, Leupold A, Beer S, Allolio B, Bonz AW. Administration of testosterone is associated with a reduced susceptibility to myocardial ischemia. *Endocrinology*. 2003;144:4478-4483.

Campbell DL, Stamler JS, Strauss HC. Redox modulation of L-type calcium channels in ferret ventricular myocytes. Dual mechanism regulation by nitric oxide and S-nitrosothiols. *J Gen Physiol*. 1996;108:277-293.

Carver JR, Ng A, Meadows AT, Vaughn DJ. Cardiovascular late effects and the ongoing care of adult cancer survivors. *Dis Manag*. 2008;11:1-6.

Charlier HA Jr, Olson RD, Thornock CM, Mercer WK, Olson DR, Broyles TS, Muhlestein DJ, Larson CL, Cusack BJ, Shadle SE. Investigations of calsequestrin as a target for anthracyclines: comparison of functional effects of daunorubicin, daunorubicinol, and trifluoperazine. *Mol Pharmacol*. 2005;67:1505-1512.

Chen DB, Wang L, Wang PH. Insulin-like growth factor I retards apoptotic signaling induced by ethanol in cardiomyocytes. *Life Sci*. 2000;67:1683-1693.

Chen Y, Daosukho C, Opii WO, Turner DM, Pierce WM, Klein JB, Vore M, Butterfield DA, St Clair DK. Redox proteomic identification of oxidized cardiac proteins in adriamycin-treated mice. *Free Radic Biol Med*. 2006;41:1470-1477.

Chu TF, Rupnick MA, Kerkela R, Dallabrida SM, Zurakowski D, Nguyen L, Woulfe K, Pravda E, Cassiola F, Desai J, George S, Morgan JA, Harris DM, Ismail NS, Chen JH, Schoen FJ, Van den Abbeele AD, Demetri GD, Force T, Chen MH. Cardiotoxicity associated with tyrosine kinase inhibitor sunitinib. *Lancet*. 2007;370:2011-2019.

Clark BM, Schofield RS. Dilated cardiomyopathy and acute liver injury associated with combined use of ephedra, gamma-hydroxybutyrate, and anabolic steroids. *Pharmacotherapy*. 2005;25:756-761.

Crean AM, Pohl JE. 'Ally McBeal heart?'-- drug induced cardiomyopathy in a young woman. *Br J Clin Pharmacol*. 2004;58:558-559.

Curry LA, Wagman DF. Qualitative description of the prevalence and use of anabolic androgenic steroids by United States powerlifters. *Percept Mot Skills*. 1999;88:224-233.

De Leonardis V, Neri B, Bacalli S, Cinelli P. Reduction of cardiac toxicity of anthracyclines by L-carnitine: preliminary overview of clinical data. *Int J Clin Pharmacol Res*. 1985;5:137-142.

Dhalla NS, Adameova A, Kaur M. Role of catecholamine oxidation in sudden cardiac death. *Fundam Clin Pharmacol*. 2010;24:539-546

Dhar R, Stout CW, Link MS, Homoud MK, Weinstock J, Estes NA 3rd. Cardiovascular toxicities of performance-enhancing substances in sports. *Mayo Clin Proc*. 2005;80:1307-1315.

Di Bello V, Giorgi D, Bianchi M, Bertini A, Caputo MT, Valenti G, Furioso O, Alessandri L, Paterni M, Giusti C. Effects of anabolic-androgenic steroids on weight-lifters' myocardium: an ultrasonic videodensitometric study. *Med Sci Sports Exerc*. 1999;31:514-521.

Dickerman RD, Schaller F, McConathy WJ. Left ventricular wall thickening does occur in elite power athletes with or without anabolic steroid Use. *Cardiology*. 1998;90:145-148.

Dickstein K, Cohen-Solal A, Filippatos G, McMurray JJ, Ponikowski P, Poole-Wilson PA, Strömberg A, van Veldhuisen DJ, Atar D, Hoes AW, Keren A, Mebazaa A, Nieminen M, Priori SG, Swedberg K; ESC Committee for Practice Guidelines (CPG). ESC guidelines for the diagnosis and treatment of acute and chronic heart failure 2008: the Task Force for the diagnosis and treatment of acute and chronic heart failure 2008 of the European Society of Cardiology. Developed in collaboration with the Heart Failure Association of the ESC (HFA) and endorsed by the European Society of Intensive Care Medicine (ESICM). *Eur J Heart Fail.* 2008;10:933-989.

Dodd DA, Atkinson JB, Olson RD, Buck S, Cusack BJ, Fleischer S, Boucek RJ Jr. Doxorubicin cardiomyopathy is associated with a decrease in calcium release channel of the sarcoplasmic reticulum in a chronic rabbit model. *J Clin Invest.* 1993;91:1697-1705.

Doroshow JH. Effect of anthracycline antibiotics on oxygen radical formation in rat heart. *Cancer Res.* 1983;43:460-472.

Drímal J, Zúrová-Nedelcevová J, Knezl V, Sotníková R, Navarová J. Cardiovascular toxicity of the first line cancer chemotherapeutic agents: doxorubicin, cyclophosphamide, streptozotocin and bevacizumab. *Neuro Endocrinol Lett.* 2006;27 Suppl 2:176-179.

Du Toit EF, Rossouw E, Van Rooyen J, Lochner A. Proposed mechanisms for the anabolic steroid-induced increase in myocardial susceptibility to ischaemia/reperfusion injury. *Cardiovasc J S Afr.* 2005;16:21-28.

Dyntar D, Sergeev P, Klisic J, Ambühl P, Schaub MC, Donath MY. High glucose alters cardiomyocyte contacts and inhibits myofibrillar formation. *J Clin Endocrinol Metab.* 2006;91:1961-1967.

Elihu N, Anandasbapathy S, Frishman WH. Chelation therapy in cardiovascular disease: ethylenediaminetetraacetic acid, deferoxamine, and dexrazoxane. *J Clin Pharmacol.* 1998;38:101-105.

Estruch R, Fernández-Solá J, Sacanella E, Paré C, Rubin E, Urbano-Márquez A. Relationship between cardiomyopathy and liver disease in chronic alcoholism. *Hepatology.* 1995;22:532-538.

Ettinger PO. Holiday heart arrhythmias. *Int J Cardiol.* 1984;5:540-542.

Ewer MS, Lippman SM. Type II chemotherapy-related cardiac dysfunction: time to recognize a new entity. *J Clin Oncol.* 2005;23:2900-2902.

Ewer MS, Vooletich MT, Durand JB, Woods ML, Davis JR, Valero V, Lenihan DJ. Reversibility of trastuzumab-related cardiotoxicity: new insights based on clinical course and response to medical treatment. *J Clin Oncol.* 2005;23:7820-7826.

Felker GM, Hu W, Hare JM, Hruban RH, Baughman KL, Kasper EK. The spectrum of dilated cardiomyopathy. The Johns Hopkins experience with 1,278 patients. *Medicine (Baltimore).* 1999;78:270-283.

Felker GM, Thompson RE, Hare JM, Hruban RH, Clemetson DE, Howard DL, Baughman KL, Kasper EK. Underlying causes and long-term survival in patients with initially unexplained cardiomyopathy. *N Engl J Med.* 2000;342:1077-1084.

Figueredo VM. Chemical cardiomyopathies: the negative effects of medications and nonprescribed drugs on the heart. *Am J Med.* 2011;124:480-488.

Fleckenstein A, Janke J, Döring HJ, Leder O. Myocardial fiber necrosis due to intracellular Ca overload-a new principle in cardiac pathophysiology. *Recent Adv Stud Cardiac Struct Metab.* 1974;4:563-580.

Fogli S, Nieri P, Breschi MC. The role of nitric oxide in anthracycline toxicity and prospects for pharmacologic prevention of cardiac damage. *FASEB J.* 2004;18:664-675.

Fraiser LH, Kanekal S, Kehrer JP. Cyclophosphamide toxicity. Characterising and avoiding the problem. *Drugs.* 1991;42:781-795.

Gewirtz DA. A critical evaluation of the mechanisms of action proposed for the antitumor effects of the anthracycline antibiotics adriamycin and daunorubicin. *Biochem Pharmacol.* 1999;57:727-741.

Gille L, Nohl H. Analyses of the molecular mechanism of adriamycin-induced cardiotoxicity. *Free Radic Biol Med.* 1997;23:775-782.

Giorgi MA, Bolaños R, Gonzalez CD, Di Girolamo G. QT interval prolongation: preclinical and clinical testing arrhythmogenesis in drugs and regulatory implications. *Curr Drug Saf.* 2010;5:54-57.

Goldhaber JI. Free radicals enhance Na+/Ca2+ exchange in ventricular myocytes. *Am J Physiol.* 1996;271(3 Pt 2):H823-H833.

Gottdiener JS, Appelbaum FR, Ferrans VJ, Deisseroth A, Ziegler J. Cardiotoxicity associated with high-dose cyclophosphamide therapy. *Arch Intern Med.* 1981;141:758-763.

Guarnieri T, Lakatta EG. Mechanism of myocardial contractile depression by clinical concentrations of ethanol. A study in ferret papillary muscles. *J Clin Invest.* 1990;85:1462-1467.

Guthrie D, Gibson AL. Doxorubicin cardiotoxicity: possible role of digoxin in its prevention. *Br Med J.* 1977;2:1447-1449.

Györke S, Györke I, Lukyanenko V, Terentyev D, Viatchenko-Karpinski S, Wiesner TF. Regulation of sarcoplasmic reticulum calcium release by luminal calcium in cardiac muscle. *Front Biosci.* 2002;7:d1454-d1463.

Handa K, Sato S. Generation of free radicals of quinone group-containing anti-cancer chemicals in NADPH-microsome system as evidenced by initiation of sulfite oxidation. *Gann.* 1975;66:43-47.

Hartgens F, Kuipers H. Effects of androgenic-anabolic steroids in athletes. *Sports Med.* 2004;34:513-554.

Hashimoto H, Yanagisawa T, Taira N. Differential antagonism of the negative inotropic effect of gentamicin by calcium ions, Bay K 8644 and isoprenaline in canine ventricular muscle: comparison with cobalt ions. *Br J Pharmacol.* 1989;96:906-912.

Hasinoff BB. Chemistry of dexrazoxane and analogues. *Semin Oncol.* 1998;25(Suppl 10):3-9.

Hausmann R, Hammer S, Betz P. Performance enhancing drugs (doping agents) and sudden death--a case report and review of the literature. *Int J Legal Med.* 1998;111:261-264.

Howarth FC, Jacobson M, Shafiullah M, Adeghate E. Long-term effects of streptozotocin-induced diabetes on the electrocardiogram, physical activity and body temperature in rats. *Exp Physiol.* 2005;90:827-835.

Iarussi D, Auricchio U, Agretto A, Murano A, Giuliano M, Casale F, Indolfi P, Iacono A. Protective effect of coenzyme Q10 on anthracyclines cardiotoxicity: control study in children with acute lymphoblastic leukemia and non-Hodgkin lymphoma. *Mol Aspects Med.* 1994;15 Suppl:s207-s212.

Imai K, Hayashi Y, Kono M. Testosterone-induced focal myocarditis in rats. I. Morphological and biochemical studies with special reference to pathogenetical mechanism and species differences. *J Toxicol Sci.* 1978;3:215-228.

Isabelle M, Vergeade A, Moritz F, Dautréaux B, Henry JP, Lallemand F, Richard V, Mulder P, Thuillez C, Monteil C. NADPH oxidase inhibition prevents cocaine-induced up-regulation of xanthine oxidoreductase and cardiac dysfunction. *J Mol Cell Cardiol.* 2007;42:326-232.

Islam MN, Kuroki H, Hongcheng B, Ogura Y, Kawaguchi N, Onishi S, Wakasugi C. Cardiac lesions and their reversibility after long term administration of methamphetamine. *Forensic Sci Int.* 1995;75:29-43.

Jankowska EA, Biel B, Majda J, Szklarska A, Lopuszanska M, Medras M, Anker SD, Banasiak W, Poole-Wilson PA, Ponikowski P. Anabolic deficiency in men with chronic heart failure: prevalence and detrimental impact on survival. *Circulation.* 2006;114:1829-1837.

Jankyova S, Kucera P, Goldenberg Z, Yaghi D, Navarova J, Kyselova Z, Stolc S, Klimas J, Racanska E, Matyas S. Pycnogenol efficiency on glycaemia, motor nerve conduction velocity and markers of oxidative stress in mild type diabetes in rats. *Phytother Res.* 2009;23:1169-1174.

Johanson CE, Fischman MW. The pharmacology of cocaine related to its abuse. *Pharmacol Rev.* 1989;41:3-52.

Jones LW, Haykowsky MJ, Swartz JJ, Douglas PS, Mackey JR. Early breast cancer therapy and cardiovascular injury. *J Am Coll Cardiol.* 2007;50:1435-1441.

Karila TA, Karjalainen JE, Mäntysaari MJ, Viitasalo MT, Seppälä TA. Anabolic androgenic steroids produce dose-dependant increase in left ventricular mass in power atheletes, and this effect is potentiated by concomitant use of growth hormone. *Int J Sports Med.* 2003;24:337-343.

Kawasaki S, Akiyama S, Kurokawa T, Kataoka M, Dohmitsu K, Kondoh K, Yamauchi M, Ito K, Watanabe T, Sugiyama S, et al. Polyoxyethylene-modified superoxide dismutase reduces side effects of adriamycin and mitomycin C. *Jpn J Cancer Res.* 1992;83:899-906.

Kay JM, Keane PM, Suyama KL, Gauthier D. Angiotensin converting enzyme activity and evolution of pulmonary vascular disease in rats with monocrotaline pulmonary hypertension. *Thorax.* 1982;37:88-96.

Kerkelä R, Grazette L, Yacobi R, Iliescu C, Patten R, Beahm C, Walters B, Shevtsov S, Pesant S, Clubb FJ, Rosenzweig A, Salomon RN, Van Etten RA, Alroy J, Durand JB, Force T. Cardiotoxicity of the cancer therapeutic agent imatinib mesylate. *Nat Med.* 2006;12:908-916.

Kicman AT. Pharmacology of anabolic steroids. *Br J Pharmacol.* 2008;154:502-521.

Kim E, Tam M, Siems WF, Kang C. Effects of drugs with muscle-related side effects and affinity for calsequestrin on the calcium regulatory function of sarcoplasmic reticulum microsomes. *Mol Pharmacol.* 2005;68:1708-1715.

Kirchhefer U, Klimas J, Baba HA, Buchwalow IB, Fabritz L, Hüls M, Matus M, Müller FU, Schmitz W, Neumann J. Triadin is a critical determinant of cellular Ca cycling and contractility in the heart. *Am J Physiol Heart Circ Physiol.* 2007;293:H3165-H3174.

Kirchhof P, Klimas J, Fabritz L, Zwiener M, Jones LR, Schäfers M, Hermann S, Boknik P, Schmitz W, Breithardt G, Kirchhefer U, Neumann J. Stress and high heart rate provoke ventricular tachycardia in mice expressing triadin. *J Mol Cell Cardiol.* 2007;42:962-971.

Klimas J, Kmecova J, Jankyova S, Yaghi D, Priesolova E, Kyselova Z, Musil P, Ochodnicky P, Krenek P, Kyselovic J, Matyas S. Pycnogenol improves left ventricular function in streptozotocin-induced diabetic cardiomyopathy in rats. *Phytother Res*. 2010;24:969-974.

Klimas J, Kmecova J, Mackovicova K, Vavrinec P, Krenek P, Kyselovic J, Ochodnicky P. Administration of clarithromycin and furosemid alters cardiac ion channel gene expression and induces beta-adrenergically evoked Torsades de Pointes in rat. *casopis*. Basic Clin Pharmacol Toxicol. 2010a;107(Suppl 1):380.

Klimas J, Stankovicova T, Kyselovic J, Bacharova L. Prolonged QT interval is associated with blood pressure rather than left ventricular mass in spontaneously hypertensive rats. *Clin Exp Hypertens*. 2008;30:475-485.

Kloner RA, Hale S, Alker K, Rezkalla S. The effects of acute and chronic cocaine use on the heart. *Circulation*. 1992;85:407-419.

Kmecova J, Klimas J. Heart rate correction of the QT duration in rats. *Eur J Pharmacol*. 2010 1;641:187-192.

Knochel JP. Cardiovascular effects of alcohol. *Ann Intern Med*. 1983;98(5 Pt 2):849-854.

Kohno H, Takahashi N, Shinohara T, Ooie T, Yufu K, Nakagawa M, Yonemochi H, Hara M, Saikawa T, Yoshimatsu H. Receptor-mediated suppression of cardiac heat-shock protein 72 expression by testosterone in male rat heart. *Endocrinology*. 2007;148:3148-3155.

Krenek P, Klimas J, Kroslakova M, Gazova A, Plandorova J, Kucerova D, Fecenkova A, Svec P, Kyselovic J. Increased expression of endothelial nitric oxide synthase and caveolin-1 in the aorta of rats with isoproterenol-induced cardiac hypertrophy. *Can J Physiol Pharmacol*. 2006;84:1245-1250.

Krenek P, Kmecova J, Kucerova D, Bajuszova Z, Musil P, Gazova A, Ochodnicky P, Klimas J, Kyselovic J. Isoproterenol-induced heart failure in the rat is associated with nitric oxide-dependent functional alterations of cardiac function. *Eur J Heart Fail*. 2009;11:140-146.

Kuhn CM. Anabolic steroids. *Recent Prog Horm Res*. 2002;57:411-434.

Lamé MW, Jones AD, Wilson DW, Dunston SK, Segall HJ. Protein targets of monocrotaline pyrrole in pulmonary artery endothelial cells. *J Biol Chem*. 2000;275:29091-29099.

Lebrecht D, Kokkori A, Ketelsen UP, Setzer B, Walker UA. Tissue-specific mtDNA lesions and radical-associated mitochondrial dysfunction in human hearts exposed to doxorubicin. *J Pathol*. 2005;207:436-444.

Lee WK, Regan TJ. Alcoholic cardiomyopathy: is it dose-dependent? *Congest Heart Fail*. 2002;8:303-306.

Legha SS, Benjamin RS, Mackay B, Ewer M, Wallace S, Valdivieso M, Rasmussen SL, Blumenschein GR, Freireich EJ. Reduction of doxorubicin cardiotoxicity by prolonged continuous intravenous infusion. *Ann Intern Med*. 1982;96:133-139.

Lenzen S. The mechanisms of alloxan- and streptozotocin-induced diabetes. *Diabetologia*. 2008;51:216-226.

Levey GS, Levey BA, Ruiz E, Lehotay DC. Selective inhibition of rat and human cardiac guanylate cyclase in vitro by doxorubicin (adriamycin): possible link to anthracycline cardiotoxicity. *J Mol Cell Cardiol*. 1979;11:591-599.

Lieberherr M, Grosse B. Adrogens increase intracellular calcium concentration and inositol 1,4,5-trisphosphate and diacylglycerol formation via a pertussis toxin-sensitive G-protein. *J Biol Chem*. 1994;269:7217-7223.

Lillegard JB, Porterfield Jr JR. Ephedra-Induced Gastric Mucosal Injury. *Case Rep Gastroenterol*. 2010;4:79-83.

Lim CC, Zuppinger C, Guo X, Kuster GM, Helmes M, Eppenberger HM, Suter TM, Liao R, Sawyer DB. Anthracyclines induce calpain-dependent titin proteolysis and necrosis in cardiomyocytes. *J Biol Chem*. 2004;279:8290-8299.

Lipshultz SE, Colan SD, Gelber RD, Perez-Atayde AR, Sallan SE, Sanders SP. Late cardiac effects of doxorubicin therapy for acute lymphoblastic leukemia in childhood. *N Engl J Med*. 1991;324:808-815.

Lipshultz SE, Lipsitz SR, Mone SM, Goorin AM, Sallan SE, Sanders SP, Orav EJ, Gelber RD, Colan SD. Female sex and drug dose as risk factors for late cardiotoxic effects of doxorubicin therapy for childhood cancer. *N Engl J Med*. 1995;332:1738-1743.

Liu PY, Death AK, Handelsman DJ. Androgens and cardiovascular disease. *Endocr Rev*. 2003;24:313-340.

Lopez JE, Yeo K, Caputo G, Buonocore M, Schaefer S. Recovery of methamphetamine associated cardiomyopathy predicted by late gadolinium enhanced cardiovascular magnetic resonance. *J Cardiovasc Magn Reson*. 2009;11:46.

Lubbe WF, Podzuweit T, Daries PS, Opie LH. The role of cyclic adenosine monophosphate in adrenergic effects on ventricular vulnerability to fibrillation in the isolated perfused rat heart. *J Clin Invest*. 1978;61:1260-1269.

Mackay B, Ewer MS, Carrasco CH, Benjamin RS. Assessment of anthracycline cardiomyopathy by endomyocardial biopsy. *Ultrastruct Pathol*. 1994;18:203-211.

Maeno Y, Iwasa M, Inoue H, Koyama H, Matoba R, Nagao M. Direct effects of methamphetamine on hypertrophy and microtubules in cultured adult rat ventricular myocytes. *Forensic Sci Int*. 2000;113:239-243.

Maguire JF, O'Rourke PP, Colan SD, Geha RS, Crone R. Cardiotoxicity during treatment of severe childhood asthma. *Pediatrics*. 1991;88:1180-1186.

Malkin CJ, Pugh PJ, West JN, van Beek EJ, Jones TH, Channer KS. Testosterone therapy in men with moderate severity heart failure: a double-blind randomized placebo controlled trial. *Eur Heart J*. 2006;27:57-64.

Mann DL. Mechanisms and models in heart failure: A combinatorial approach. *Circulation*. 1999;100:999-1008.

Maraj S, Figueredo VM, Lynn Morris D. Cocaine and the heart. *Clin Cardiol*. 2010;33:264-269.

Marsh JD, Lehmann MH, Ritchie RH, Gwathmey JK, Green GE, Schiebinger RJ. Androgen receptors mediate hypertrophy in cardiac myocytes. *Circulation*. 1998;98:256-261.

McCord J, Jneid H, Hollander JE, de Lemos JA, Cercek B, Hsue P, Gibler WB, Ohman EM, Drew B, Philippides G, Newby LK; American Heart Association Acute Cardiac Care Committee of the Council on Clinical Cardiology. Management of cocaine-associated chest pain and myocardial infarction: a scientific statement from the American Heart Association Acute Cardiac Care Committee of the Council on Clinical Cardiology. *Circulation*. 2008;117:1897-1907.

Mehta PM, Grainger TA, Lust RM, Movahed A, Terry J, Gilliland MG, Jolly SR. Effect of cocaine on left ventricular function. Relation to increased wall stress and persistence after treatment. *Circulation*. 1995;91:3002-3009.

Meinardi MT, Gietema JA, van Veldhuisen DJ, van der Graaf WT, de Vries EG, Sleijfer DT. Long-term chemotherapy-related cardiovascular morbidity. *Cancer Treat Rev.* 2000;26:429-447.

Melchert RB, Welder AA. Cardiovascular effects of androgenic-anabolic steroids. *Med Sci Sports Exerc.* 1995;27:1252-1262.

Mijares A, López JR. L-carnitine prevents increase in diastolic [CA2+] induced by doxorubicin in cardiac cells. *Eur J Pharmacol.* 2001;425:117-120.

Millart H, Brabant L, Lorenzato M, Lamiable D, Albert O, Choisy H. The effects of 5-fluorouracil on contractility and oxygen uptake of the isolated perfused rat heart. *Anticancer Res.* 1992;12:571-576.

Minotti G, Mancuso C, Frustaci A, Mordente A, Santini SA, Calafiore AM, Liberi G, Gentiloni N. Paradoxical inhibition of cardiac lipid peroxidation in cancer patients treated with doxorubicin. Pharmacologic and molecular reappraisal of anthracycline cardiotoxicity. *J Clin Invest.* 1996;98:650-661.

Minotti G, Menna P, Salvatorelli E, Cairo G, Gianni L. Anthracyclines: molecular advances and pharmacologic developments in antitumor activity and cardiotoxicity. *Pharmacol Rev.* 2004;56:185-229.

Mir SH, Darzi MM. Histopathological abnormalities of prolonged alloxan-induced diabetes mellitus in rabbits. *Int J Exp Pathol.* 2009;90:66-73.

Mizia-Stec K, Gasior Z, Wojnicz R, Haberka M, Mielczarek M, Wierzbicki A, Pstraś K, Hartleb M. Severe dilated cardiomyopathy as a consequence of Ecstasy intake. *Cardiovasc Pathol.* 2008;17:250-253.

Muggia FM, Green MD. New anthracycline antitumor antibiotics. *Crit Rev Oncol Hematol.* 1991;11:43-64.

Muggia FM, Hainsworth JD, Jeffers S, Miller P, Groshen S, Tan M, Roman L, Uziely B, Muderspach L, Garcia A, Burnett A, Greco FA, Morrow CP, Paradiso LJ, Liang LJ. Phase II study of liposomal doxorubicin in refractory ovarian cancer: antitumor activity and toxicity modification by liposomal encapsulation. *J Clin Oncol.* 1997;15:987-993.

Muindi JR, Sinha BK, Gianni L, Myers CE. Hydroxyl radical production and DNA damage induced by anthracycline-iron complex. *FEBS Lett.* 1984;172:226-230.

Myers CE, McGuire W, Young R. Adriamycin: amelioration of toxicity by alpha-tocopherol. *Cancer Treat Rep.* 1976;60:961-962.

Myers CE, McGuire WP, Liss RH, Ifrim I, Grotzinger K, Young RC. Adriamycin: the role of lipid peroxidation in cardiac toxicity and tumor response. *Science.* 1977;197:165-167.

Nieminen MS, Rämö MP, Viitasalo M, Heikkilä P, Karjalainen J, Mäntysaari M, Heikkilä J. Serious cardiovascular side effects of large doses of anabolic steroids in weight lifters. *Eur Heart J.* 1996;17:1576-1583.

Nohl H, Gille L, Kozlov A, Staniek K. Are mitochondria a spontaneous and permanent source of reactive oxygen species? *Redox Rep.* 2003;8:135-141.

Olson HM, Young DM, Prieur DJ, LeRoy AF, Reagan RL. Electrolyte and morphologic alterations of myocardium in adriamycin-treated rabbits. *Am J Pathol.* 1974;77:439-454.

Olson RD, Li X, Palade P, Shadle SE, Mushlin PS, Gambliel HA, Fill M, Boucek RJ Jr, Cusack BJ. Sarcoplasmic reticulum calcium release is stimulated and inhibited by daunorubicin and daunorubicinol. *Toxicol Appl Pharmacol.* 2000;169:168-176.

Ondrias K, Borgatta L, Kim DH, Ehrlich BE. Biphasic effects of doxorubicin on the calcium release channel from sarcoplasmic reticulum of cardiac muscle. *Circ Res.* 1990;67:1167-1174.

Opie LH, Thandroyen FT, Muller C, Bricknell OL. Adrenaline-induced "oxygen-wastage" and enzyme release from working rat heart. Effects of calcium antagonism, beta-blockade, nicotinic acid and coronary artery ligation. *J Mol Cell Cardiol.* 1979;11:1073-1094.

Outomuro D, Grana DR, Azzato F, Milei J. Adriamycin-induced myocardial toxicity: new solutions for an old problem? *Int J Cardiol.* 2007;117:6-15.

Park IY, Kim EJ, Park H, Fields K, Dunker AK, Kang C. Interaction between cardiac calsequestrin and drugs with known cardiotoxicity. *Mol Pharmacol.* 2005;67:97-104.

Payne JR, Kotwinski PJ, Montgomery HE. Cardiac effects of anabolic steroids. *Heart.* 2004;90:473-475.

Peng X, Chen B, Lim CC, Sawyer DB. The cardiotoxicology of anthracycline chemotherapeutics: translating molecular mechanism into preventative medicine. *Mol Interv.* 2005;5:163-171.

Penna C, Tullio F, Perrelli MG, Moro F, Abbadessa G, Piccione F, Carriero V, Racca S, Pagliaro P. Ischemia/reperfusion injury is increased and cardioprotection by a postconditioning protocol is lost as cardiac hypertrophy develops in nandrolone treated rats. *Basic Res Cardiol.* 2011;106:409-420.

Pentassuglia L, Timolati F, Seifriz F, Abudukadier K, Suter TM, Zuppinger C. Inhibition of ErbB2/neuregulin signaling augments paclitaxel-induced cardiotoxicity in adult ventricular myocytes. *Exp Cell Res.* 2007;313:1588-1601.

Piano MR. Alcoholic cardiomyopathy: incidence, clinical characteristics, and pathophysiology. *Chest.* 2002;121:1638-1650.

Pigram WJ, Fuller W, Hamilton LD. Stereochemistry of intercalation: interaction of daunomycin with DNA.*Nat New Biol.* 1972;235:17-19.

Ponte ML, Keller GA, Di Girolamo G. Mechanisms of drug induced QT interval prolongation. *Curr Drug Saf.* 2010;5:44-53.

Pugh PJ, English KM, Jones TH, Channer KS. Testosterone: a natural tonic for the failing heart? *QJM.* 2000;93:689-694.

Pugh PJ, Jones RD, West JN, Jones TH, Channer KS. Testosterone treatment for men with chronic heart failure. *Heart.* 2004;90:446-447.

Pugh PJ, Jones TH, Channer KS. Acute haemodynamic effects of testosterone in men with chronic heart failure. *Eur Heart J.* 2003;24:909-915.

Radi R, Cassina A, Hodara R, Quijano C, Castro L. Peroxynitrite reactions and formation in mitochondria. *Free Radic Biol Med.* 2002;33:1451-1464.

Rauchhaus M, Doehner W, Anker SD. Heart failure therapy: testosterone replacement and its implications. *Eur Heart J.* 2006;27:10-12.

Rees DA, Alcolado JC. Animal models of diabetes mellitus. *Diabet Med.* 2005;22:359-370.

Roden DM. Cellular basis of drug-induced torsades de pointes. *Br J Pharmacol.* 2008;154:1502-1507.

Roden DM. Drug-induced prolongation of the QT interval. *N Engl J Med.* 2004;350:1013-1022.

Rona G, Chappel CI, Balazs T, Gaudry R. An infarct-like myocardial lesion and other toxic manifestations produced by isoproterenol in the rat. *AMA Arch Pathol.* 1959;67:443-455.

Rona G, Chappel CI. Pathogenesis and pathology of cobalt cardiomyopathy. *Recent Adv Stud Cardiac Struct Metab.* 1973;2:407-422.

Rona G. Catecholamine cardiotoxicity. *J Mol Cell Cardiol.* 1985;17:291-306.

Rose AG. Catecholamine-induced myocardial dammage associated with phaeochromocytomas and tetanus. *S Afr Med J.* 1974;48:1285-1289.

Rosenoff SH, Brooks E, Bostick F, Young RC. Alterations in DNA synthesis in cardiac tissue induced by adriamycin in vivo-relationship to fatal toxicity. *Biochem Pharmacol.* 1975;24:1898-1901.

Ruiz-Ruiz C, Robledo G, Cano E, Redondo JM, Lopez-Rivas A. Characterization of p53-mediated up-regulation of CD95 gene expression upon genotoxic treatment in human breast tumor cells. *J Biol Chem.* 2003;278:31667-31675.

Saeki K, Obi I, Ogiku N, Shigekawa M, Imagawa T, Matsumoto T. Doxorubicin directly binds to the cardiac-type ryanodine receptor. *Life Sci.* 2002;70:2377-2389.

Salvi V, Karnad DR, Panicker GK, Kothari S. Update on the evaluation of a new drug for effects on cardiac repolarization in humans: issues in early drug development. *Br J Pharmacol.* 2010;159:34-48.

Sasson Z, Morgan CD, Wang B, Thomas G, MacKenzie B, Platts ME. 5-Fluorouracil related toxic myocarditis: case reports and pathological confirmation. *Can J Cardiol.* 1994;10:861-864.

Sawyer DB, Fukazawa R, Arstall MA, Kelly RA. Daunorubicin-induced apoptosis in rat cardiac myocytes is inhibited by dexrazoxane. *Circ Res.* 1999;84:257-265.

Sawyer DB, Zuppinger C, Miller TA, Eppenberger HM, Suter TM. Modulation of anthracycline-induced myofibrillar disarray in rat ventricular myocytes by neuregulin-1beta and anti-erbB2: potential mechanism for trastuzumab-induced cardiotoxicity. *Circulation.* 2002;105:1551-1554.

Scheiner-Bobis G, Schoner W. A fresh facet for ouabain action. *Nat Med.* 2001;7:1288-1289.

Schöber C, Papageorgiou E, Harstrick A, Bokemeyer C, Mügge A, Stahl M, Wilke H, Poliwoda H, Hiddemann W, Köhne-Wömpner CH, et al. Cardiotoxicity of 5-fluorouracil in combination with folinic acid in patients with gastrointestinal cancer. *Cancer.* 1993;72:2242-2247.

Schoner W. Endogenous cardiac glycosides, a new class of steroid hormones. *Eur J Biochem.* 2002;269:2440-2448.

Selzer A, Wray HW. Quinidine syncope paroxysmal ventricular fibrillation occuring during treatment of chronic atrial arrhythmias. *Circulation.* 1964;30:17-26.

Shan K, Lincoff AM, Young JB. Anthracycline-induced cardiotoxicity. *Ann Intern Med.* 1996;125:47-58.

Shenouda SK, Lord KC, McIlwain E, Lucchesi PA, Varner KJ. Ecstasy produces left ventricular dysfunction and oxidative stress in rats. *Cardiovasc Res.* 2008;79:662-670.

Shenouda SK, Varner KJ, Carvalho F, Lucchesi PA. Metabolites of MDMA induce oxidative stress and contractile dysfunction in adult rat left ventricular myocytes. *Cardiovasc Toxicol.* 2009;9:30-38.

Shin DD, Brandimarte F, De Luca L, Sabbah HN, Fonarow GC, Filippatos G, Komajda M, Gheorghiade M. Review of current and investigational pharmacologic agents for acute heart failure syndromes. *Am J Cardiol.* 2007;99:4A-23A.

Silber JH, Cnaan A, Clark BJ, Paridon SM, Chin AJ, Rychik J, Hogarty AN, Cohen MI, Barber G, Rutkowski M, Kimball TR, Delaat C, Steinherz LJ, Zhao H. Enalapril to prevent cardiac function decline in long-term survivors of pediatric cancer exposed to anthracyclines. *J Clin Oncol.* 2004;22:820-828.

Simůnek T, Stérba M, Popelová O, Adamcová M, Hrdina R, Gersl V. Anthracycline-induced cardiotoxicity: overview of studies examining the roles of oxidative stress and free cellular iron. *Pharmacol Rep.* 2009;61:154-171.

Singal PK, Iliskovic N. Doxorubicin-induced cardiomyopathy. *N Engl J Med.* 1998;339:900-905.

Singal PK, Siveski-Iliskovic N, Hill M, Thomas TP, Li T. Combination therapy with probucol prevents adriamycin-induced cardiomyopathy. *J Mol Cell Cardiol.* 1995;27:1055-1063.

Sinha BK, Trush MA, Kennedy KA, Mimnaugh EG. Enzymatic activation and binding of adriamycin to nuclear DNA. *Cancer Res.* 1984;44:2892-2896.

Slamon DJ, Leyland-Jones B, Shak S, Fuchs H, Paton V, Bajamonde A, Fleming T, Eiermann W, Wolter J, Pegram M, Baselga J, Norton L. Use of chemotherapy plus a monoclonal antibody against HER2 for metastatic breast cancer that overexpresses HER2. *N Engl J Med.* 2001;344:783-792.

Solem LE, Henry TR, Wallace KB. Disruption of mitochondrial calcium homeostasis following chronic doxorubicin administration. *Toxicol Appl Pharmacol.* 1994;129:214-222.

Stergiopoulos K, Brennan JJ, Mathews R, Setaro JF, Kort S. Anabolic steroids, acute myocardial infarction and polycythemia: a case report and review of the literature. *Vasc Health Risk Manag.* 2008;4:1475-1480.

Stolt A, Karila T, Viitasalo M, Mäntysaari M, Kujala UM, Karjalainen J. QT interval and QT dispersion in endurance athletes and in power athletes using large doses of anabolic steroids. *Am J Cardiol.* 1999;84:364-366.

Strasser F, Betticher DC, Suter TM. Trastuzumab and breast cancer. *N Engl J Med.* 2001;345:996.

Sullivan J, Parker M, Carson SB. Tissue cobalt content in "beer drinkers' myocardiopathy". *J Lab Clin Med.* 1968;71:893-911.

Sullivan ML, Martinez CM, Gennis P, Gallagher EJ. The cardiac toxicity of anabolic steroids. *Prog Cardiovasc Dis.* 1998;41:1-15.

Swain SM, Whaley FS, Ewer MS. Congestive heart failure in patients treated with doxorubicin: a retrospective analysis of three trials. *Cancer.* 2003;97:2869-2879.

Swain SM, Whaley FS, Gerber MC, Weisberg S, York M, Spicer D, Jones SE, Wadler S, Desai A, Vogel C, Speyer J, Mittelman A, Reddy S, Pendergrass K, Velez-Garcia E, Ewer MS, Bianchine JR, Gams RA. Cardioprotection with dexrazoxane for doxorubicin-containing therapy in advanced breast cancer. *J Clin Oncol.* 1997;15:1318-1332.

Szabó J, Csáky L, Szegi J. Experimental cardiac hypertrophy induced by isoproterenol in the rat. *Acta Physiol Acad Sci Hung.* 1975;46:281-285.

Tan C, Tasaka H, Yu KP, Murphy ML, Karnofsky DA. Daunomycin, an antitumor antibiotic, in the treatment of neoplastic disease. Clinical evaluation with special reference to childhood leukemia. *Cancer*. 1967;20:333-353.

Tan-Chiu E, Yothers G, Romond E, Geyer CE Jr, Ewer M, Keefe D, Shannon RP, Swain SM, Brown A, Fehrenbacher L, Vogel VG, Seay TE, Rastogi P, Mamounas EP, Wolmark N, Bryant J. Assessment of cardiac dysfunction in a randomized trial comparing doxorubicin and cyclophosphamide followed by paclitaxel, with or without trastuzumab as adjuvant therapy in node-positive, human epidermal growth factor receptor 2-overexpressing breast cancer: NSABP B-31.*J Clin Oncol*. 2005;23:7811-7819.

Tazelaar HD, Karch SB, Stephens BG, Billingham ME. Cocaine and the heart. *Hum Pathol*. 1987;18:195-199.

Thompson PD, Sadaniantz A, Cullinane EM, Bodziony KS, Catlin DH, Torek-Both G, Douglas PS. Left ventricular function is not impaired in weight-lifters who use anabolic steroids. *J Am Coll Cardiol*. 1992;19:278-282.

Tokarska-Schlattner M, Zaugg M, Zuppinger C, Wallimann T, Schlattner U. New insights into doxorubicin-induced cardiotoxicity: the critical role of cellular energetics. *J Mol Cell Cardiol*. 2006;41:389-405.

Turner NA, Porter KE, Smith WH, White HL, Ball SG, Balmforth AJ. Chronic beta2-adrenergic receptor stimulation increases proliferation of human cardiac fibroblasts via an autocrine mechanism. *Cardiovasc Res*. 2003;57:784-792.

Turnipseed SD, Richards JR, Kirk JD, Diercks DB, Amsterdam EA. Frequency of acute coronary syndrome in patients presenting to the emergency department with chest pain after methamphetamine use. *J Emerg Med*. 2003;24:369-373.

Unverferth DV, Jagadeesh JM, Unverferth BJ, Magorien RD, Leier CV, Balcerzak SP. Attempt to prevent doxorubicin-induced acute human myocardial morphologic damage with acetylcysteine. *J Natl Cancer Inst*. 1983;71:917-920.

Urbano-Márquez A, Estruch R, Fernández-Solá J, Nicolás JM, Paré JC, Rubin E. The greater risk of alcoholic cardiomyopathy and myopathy in women compared with men. *JAMA*. 1995;274:149-154.

Urbano-Márquez A, Estruch R, Navarro-Lopez F, Grau JM, Mont L, Rubin E. The effects of alcoholism on skeletal and cardiac muscle. *N Engl J Med*. 1989;320:409-415.

Urbano-Márquez A, Fernández-Solà J. Effects of alcohol on skeletal and cardiac muscle. *Muscle Nerve*. 2004;30:689-707.

van Acker FA, van Acker SA, Kramer K, Haenen GR, Bast A, van der Vijgh WJ. 7-monohydroxyethylrutoside protects against chronic doxorubicin-induced cardiotoxicity when administered only once per week. *Clin Cancer Res*. 2000 Apr;6(4):1337-41.

van Dalen EC, Caron HN, Dickinson HO, Kremer LC. Cardioprotective interventions for cancer patients receiving anthracyclines. *Cochrane Database Syst Rev*. 2011 Jun 15;6:CD003917.

Von Hoff DD, Layard MW, Basa P, Davis HL Jr, Von Hoff AL, Rozencweig M, Muggia FM. Risk factors for doxorubicin-induced congestive heart failure. *Ann Intern Med*. 1979;91:710-717.

Wang M, Tsai BM, Kher A, Baker LB, Wairiuko GM, Meldrum DR. Role of endogenous testosterone in myocardial proinflammatory and proapoptotic signaling after acute ischemia-reperfusion. *Am J Physiol Heart Circ Physiol.* 2005;288:H221-H226.

Wang M, Wang Y, Abarbanell A, Tan J, Weil B, Herrmann J, Meldrum DR. Both endogenous and exogenous testosterone decrease myocardial STAT3 activation and SOCS3 expression after acute ischemia and reperfusion. *Surgery.* 2009;146:138-144.

Weidmann B, Jansen W, Heider A, Niederle N. 5-Fluorouracil cardiotoxicity with left ventricular dysfunction under different dosing regimens. *Am J Cardiol.* 1995;75:194-195.

Wexler LH, Andrich MP, Venzon D, Berg SL, Weaver-McClure L, Chen CC, Dilsizian V, Avila N, Jarosinski P, Balis FM, Poplack DG, Horowitz ME. Randomized trial of the cardioprotective agent ICRF-187 in pediatric sarcoma patients treated with doxorubicin. *J Clin Oncol.* 1996;14:362-372.

Wijetunga M, Seto T, Lindsay J, Schatz I. Crystal methamphetamine-associated cardiomyopathy: tip of the iceberg? *J Toxicol Clin Toxicol.* 2003;41:981-986.

Wittstein IS. Acute stress cardiomyopathy. *Curr Heart Fail Rep.* 2008;5:61-68.

Wu AH. Cardiotoxic drugs: clinical monitoring and decision making. *Heart.* 2008;94:1503-1509.

Wu X, Hasinoff BB. The antitumor anthracyclines doxorubicin and daunorubicin do not inhibit cell growth through the formation of iron-mediated reactive oxygen species. *Anticancer Drugs.* 2005;16:93-99.

Yeo KK, Wijetunga M, Ito H, Efird JT, Tay K, Seto TB, Alimineti K, Kimata C, Schatz IJ. The association of methamphetamine use and cardiomyopathy in young patients. *Am J Med.* 2007;120:165-171.

Zakhari S. Alcohol and the cardiovascular system: molecular mechanisms for beneficial and harmful action. *Alcohol Health Res World.* 1997;21:21-29.

Zaugg M, Jamali NZ, Lucchinetti E, Xu W, Alam M, Shafiq SA, Siddiqui MA. Anabolic-androgenic steroids induce apoptotic cell death in adult rat ventricular myocytes. *J Cell Physiol.* 2001;187:90-95.

Zhang GX, Kimura S, Nishiyama A, Shokoji T, Rahman M, Yao L, Nagai Y, Fujisawa Y, Miyatake A, Abe Y. Cardiac oxidative stress in acute and chronic isoproterenol-infused rats. *Cardiovasc Res.* 2005;65:230-238.

Zhang L, Kelley J, Schmeisser G, Kobayashi YM, Jones LR. Complex formation between junctin, triadin, calsequestrin, and the ryanodine receptor. Proteins of the cardiac junctional sarcoplasmic reticulum membrane. *J Biol Chem.* 1997;272:23389-23397.

Zimmer HG. Catecholamine-induced cardiac hypertrophy: significance of proto-oncogene expression. *J Mol Med (Berl).* 1997;75:849-859.

Zuppinger C, Timolati F, Suter TM. Pathophysiology and diagnosis of cancer drug induced cardiomyopathy. *Cardiovasc Toxicol.* 2007;7:61-66.

9

Anthracycline Cardiotoxicity

Giuseppe Visani[1], Alessandro Isidori[1] and Giorgio Minotti[2]
[1]*Hematology and Stem Cell Transplant Center, Marche Nord Hospital, Via Lombroso, Pesaro,*
[2]*Center for Integrated Research and Drug Sciences, Campus Bio-Medico University, Via Alvaro del Portillo, Rome, Italy*

1. Introduction

Cancer patients who are undergoing chemotherapy have an increased risk of developing cardiovascular complications, and the risk is even greater if there is a known history of heart disease. A wide range of chemotherapy agents have been associated with cardiotoxicity. Among the serious cardiac complications related to chemotherapy, there are arrhythmias, myocardial necrosis causing a dilated cardiomyopathy and vasoocclusion or vasospasm resulting in angina or myocardial infarction.

The anthracyclines and related compounds (doxorubicin, idarubicin, epirubicin, and the anthraquinone mitoxantrone) are some of the most frequently implicated agents. Anthracyclines, including doxorubicin, are widely used in the treatment of cancer. Although topoisomerase II inhibition remains the most persuasive mechanism to explain the antitumor activity of anthracyclines, clinically relevant concentrations of anthracyclines were shown to induce apoptosis through additional mechanisms that were not bound to the topoisomerase II - p53 machinery.

However, their use is limited by cardiotoxicity and increasing survivors' susceptibility to treatment-related complications that can remarkably affect their quality of life. Surviving patients have an increased rate of heart failure, coronary artery disease, and cerebrovascular accidents compared to the general population. The specific mechanisms of anthracycline cardiotoxicity are complex and still remain unclear. Hence, determining the factors that may increase propensity to cardiotoxicity is of great importance, as is monitoring patients during and after treatment. Additionally, treatment and prevention options, such as limiting cumulative dosage, liposomal anthracyclines, and dexrazoxane, continue to be explored.

Liposomal doxorubicin has been developed with the aim of improving the therapeutics index of doxorubicin by reducing the drug's cardiotoxicity. Two liposomal formulations are currently available: non-pegylated liposomal doxorubicin (NPLD) (Myocet®, Cephalon, USA) and pegylated liposomal doxorubicin (PLD) (Caelix®/Doxil®, Schering-Plough/Orto Biothech, USA).

In this chapter, we will analyze the cardiac complications caused by the use of anthracyclines, and the potential benefit of substituting these drugs with their liposomal counterpart. Acute and chronic cardiac toxicities, together with risk factors will also be discussed. Guidelines for monitoring and drug discontinuation will be another point to be analyzed in this chapter.

2. Pharmacology

The anthracyclines represent a broad family of antibiotics that exhibit activity in numerous tumours. The first anthracyclines, doxorubicin (DOX) and daunorubicin (DNR), were isolated from Streptomyces var. Peucetius; they were shown to be composed of a tetracyclic ring system with adjacent quinone-hydroquinone moieties, a short side chain with a carbonyl group, and an aminosugar bound to the C-7 of the four-ring system. DOX and DNR only differed in the side chain terminus (-CH_2OH in DOX vs -CH_3 in DNR). Second generation anthracyclines, like epirubicin (EPI) and idarubicin (IDA), were obtained after minor chemical modifications of DOX or DNR, respectively.

When injected by standard i.v. infusion, anthracyclines show a rapid distribution phase, a high distribution volume at steady state (~15 l/kg), a slow elimination phase (successive plasma half-lives of ~ 5 minutes, ~1 hour and ~30 hours). Anthracyclines are excreted mostly through bile, which imposes special care in patients with hepatic dysfunction (Robert & Gianni, 1993). In comparison with DOX, EPI is characterized by an unique glucuronidation that accelerates its systemic body clearance and imposes administering EPI at doses 1.5 times higher than those of DOX (Innocenti F et al., 2001).

Anthracyclines have long been known to kill tumor cells by inhibiting topoisomerase II. Anthracyclines act by stabilizing a reaction intermediate in which DNA strands are cut and covalently linked to topoisomerase II, eventually impeding DNA resealing. Anthracycline intercalation into DNA plays a role in this reaction; in fact, anthracycline rings that do not intercalate into DNA probably stabilize the complex between topoisomerase II and the DNA that it has nicked (Menna et al., 2008). Anthracycline- and topoisomerase II-mediated DNA damage is followed by growth arrest in G1 and G2 and apoptosis. This is usually, but not always, relayed by p53 and the consequent induction of the WAF1/CIP1 p21 gene product, a strong inhibitor of cyclin-dependent kinases that favour cell cycle progression through the G1 to S transition (Minotti et al., 2008).

Although topoisomerase II inhibition remains the most persuasive mechanism to explain the antitumor activity of anthracyclines, clinically relevant concentrations of anthracyclines were shown to induce apoptosis through additional mechanisms that were not bound to the topoisomerase II - p53 machinery. These mechanisms include, among others, i) the activation of neutral sphingomyelinases, followed by ceramide formation and converse activation of cell death effectors (c-Jun N-terminal kinase) or down-regulation of survival pathways (Akt/protein kinase B) ii), mitochondrial dysfunction, followed by cytochrome c release and apoptosome formation iii), induction of lipid peroxidation and formation of malondialdehyde-DNA adducts, followed by the reduced activity of cyclin E- and cyclin B-associated kinase activities and growth arrest in both p53-proficient and p53-deficient cells iv), inhibition of the proteasome, followed by an accumulation of undegraded ubiquinated proteins which signal apoptosis. The mechanisms i-iii) are triggered by reactive oxygen species (ROS), that are major byproducts of anthracycline metabolism. ROS may also enable anthracyclines to damage and shorten telomeres, long sequences of base repeats that otherwise would delay cell senescence and apoptosis by preventing the degradation and ligation of the end of chromosomes; however, anthracycline-induced telomere damage and dysfunction would be relayed to apoptosis through p53 (Minotti et al, 2004).

Anthracycline treatment may be accompanied by the acquisition of a resistance phenotype through a combination of pharmacokinetic and pharmacodynamic mechanisms. On pharmacokinetic grounds, tumor resistance is caused by the reduced accumulation and/or an altered distribution of anthracyclines in tumor cells, usually mediated by overexpression of drug transporters that belong to the ATP-binding cassette family of proteins and are collectively referred to as ABC proteins (P-glycoprotein/Pgp, multidrug resistance protein 1/MRP1, breast cancer resistance protein/BCRP). On pharmacodynamic grounds, tumor resistance may be caused by such diverse mechanisms as topoisomerase II mutation or redundancy, overexpression and preferred nuclear localization of proteasome α-type subunits (leading to a anomalous degradation of topoisomerase II), genetic deletion or loss-of-function mutations of p53, overexpression of ROS-detoxifying enzymes, overexpression of Bcl-2 (leading to a diminished cytochrome c release), etc. When taken in isolation, however, none of these factors would universally predict anthracycline-resistance in a given tumor or another (Minotti et al., 2008).

3. How do anthracyclines damage the heart

The problem of anthracycline-induced cardiomyopathy and congestive heart failure (CHF) has been around for some 40 years. On ultrastructural grounds, all of the approved anthracyclines share a pattern of damage that is characterized by loss of myofibrils, dilation of the sarcoplasmic reticulum, cytoplasmic vacuolization, swelling of mitochondria, and increased number of lysosomes; however, safety threshold may differ from one anthracyclines to another. In the case of DOX, the incidence of cardiomyopathy and congestive heart failure (CHF) averages below 5% if the cumulative dose did not exceed 400-450 mg/m^2 (Swain et al., 2003) ; EPI induces CHF at doses slightly higher than equiactive to DOX (~800-900 mg/m^2). Safety limits for DNR and IDA are less firmly established because of different regimens and schedules adopted in induction or consolidation treatment of myeloproliferative disorders. With that said, cardiac events may develop at reportedly safe cumulative doses if patients presented with hypertension, arrhythmias, valvular or coronary disease, or metabolic disorders; Moreover, children and the elderly are more vulnerable than the young-adult (Minotti et al., 2010). Perhaps more importantly, we now know that subthreshold doses of anthracyclines, as commonly adopted in many oncologic settings, may cause the development of cardiotoxicity months to years after completing chemotherapy, as if "safe doses" of anthracyclines primed the heart to a subclinical damage liable to a delayed clinical manifestation (Minotti et al., 2010). Mechanisms of anthracycline cardiotoxicity should therefore be reconciled with the concept of a lifetime risk of cardiotoxicity.

Anthracycline cardiotoxicity correlates directly with drug's peak plasma concentration (Minotti et al., 2004) but correlates inversely to the levels and activity of ABC proteins that eject drugs from endothelial cells of the blood-heart barrier (Sissung et al., 2011). Once inside cardiomyocytes, much of anthracycline toxicity seems to depend on bioactivation events.

The quinone moiety of anthracyclines undergoes one-electron reduction by a number of reductases, primarily located to mitochondria; oxidation of the so-formed semiquinone with molecular oxygen regenerates the parent quinone and exposes the cell to higher than physiological levels of ROS like superoxide anion ($O_2^{\cdot -}$), hydrogen peroxide (H_2O_2), and hydroxyl radical ($\cdot OH$). Bimolecular reaction of $O_2^{\cdot -}$ with nitric oxide also generates peroxynitrite endowed with noticeable prooxidant activities. In comparison to other cell types cardiomyocytes are very rich in mitochondria, but relatively poor in ROS-detoxifying enzymes; it follows that cardiomyocytes would readily succumb to a sustained generation of ROS that eventually induced sarcomere degradation, mitochondrial dysfunction and DNA damage, disruption of cardiac-specific gene expression programs, necrotic or apoptotic death (Minotti et al., 2004). This "oxidative stress" hypothesis of cardiotoxicity gained popularity over the years and was successfully probed in transgenic mice that overexpressed antioxidant defense systems like catalase, mitochondrial manganese-dependent superoxide dismutase, metallothioneins; Interestingly, however, robust doses of antioxidants like vitamin E or N-acetylcysteine neither delayed nor mitigated cardiotoxicity induced in patients by cumulative doses of DOX (Minotti et al., 2004). The only compound consistently found to be cardioprotective in clinical settings is the iron chelator, dexrazoxane. Iron chelation would mitigate free radical reactions that otherwise caused cardiotoxicity. Another caveat in the "oxidative stress hypothesis" is the lack of a clear-and-cut relation with the lifetime risk of cardiotoxicity. Once inside cardiomyocytes anthracyclines can diffuse back toward extracellular fluids, making the intracellular drug levels decrease to below a threshold of toxic concern (Salvatorelli et al., 2009). Some investigators suggested that DOX caused an oxidative mitochondriopathy that self-maintained after DOX had been cleared from cardiomyocytes; however, self-maintaining mitochondriopathy was documented with DOX but not EPI (Lebrecht & Walker, 2007), in spite of that EPI clearly retained a potential for inducing cardiotoxicity. On balance, anthracyclines do form ROS in the relatively unprotected cardiac tissue, but compelling evidence for a cause-and-effect relationship between oxidative stress and chronic cardiomyopathy is lacking.

The lifetime risk of cardiotoxicity from anthracyclines could be better reconciled with their conversion to secondary alcohol metabolites, formed after two electron reduction of their side chain carbonyl group. Being more polar than their parent drugs, secondary alcohol metabolites are poorly cleared from cardiomyocytes and accumulate to become a long-lasting anthracycline toxic signature in the heart (Menna et al., 2008); times more potent than their parent anthracyclines at inactivating Ca^{2+}-handling proteins of the contraction-relaxation cycle or key regulators of energy metabolism and redox balance, such as cytoplasmic aconitase. Therefore, secondary alcohol metabolites may cause cardiotoxicity both during and well after the course of chemotherapy.

In clinical settings, a retrospective study of patients enrolled in the Childhood Cancer Survivor Study suggests that the V244M polymorphism of carbonyl reductase 3 associated with a higher risk to develop CHF, presumably because the methionine244 isoform of carbonyl reductase 3 shows a greater catalytic specificity toward carbonyl substrates (Blanco et al., 2008). Most recent reports suggest that gain of function CBR polymorphisms could be invoked to particularly explain CHF development in patients exposed to subthreshold cumulative doses of anthracyclines .

There are, of course, some caveats in the alcohol metabolite hypothesis of cardiotoxicity. EPI forms fewer amounts of its alcohol metabolite as compared to DOX, which is consistent with CHF developing at cumulative doses of EPI higher than equiactive to DOX (Salvatorelli et al., 2007). In contrast, DNR and IDA generate more alcohol metabolites than DOX in spite of that their cardiotoxicity was ranked similar to or less severe than that of DOX, respectively (Minotti et al., 2004). Once again, the different modalities of administration of DNR or IDA in the settings of myeloproliferative disease could be invoked to explain such discrepancy.

4. How to prevent anthracycline induced cardiotoxicity

Anthracycline cardiotoxicity coud be prevented by replacing bolus administration with slow infusions that generate lower anthracycline plasma peaks and thus mitigate a pharmacokinetic determinant of cardiotoxicity. The benefit of replacing bolus administration (5-15 min infusion) with slow infusions (24-48 h) is quite evident in adult settings but not in pediatric settings. The current thinking is that children are more vulnerable by anthracyclines; the protective benefit obtained by lowering plasma peak concentrations would therefore be offset by damage due to the longer cardiac exposure to anthracyclines (Lipshultz et al., 2002).

The notion that anthracycline-related cardiotoxicity may develop long after completing chemotherapy suggests that drugs used to treat clinically evident cardiotoxicity should be used much earlier to protect the heart against subclinical cardiotoxicity. Unfortunately, active cardiac prevention by beta-blockers, angiotensin I-converting enzyme inhibitors, or angiotensin II receptor blockers, has been explored in only few limited studies. Prophylactic commencement of angiotensin I-converting enzyme inhibitors prevented decrements of Left Ventricular Ejection Fraction (LVEF) in patients receiving high-dose chemotherapy (Cardinale et al, 2006), while prophylactic commencement of angiotensin II receptors blockers prevented transient elevations of brain natriuretic peptide in patients receiving one cycle of standard-dose chemotherapy for non-Hodgkin lymphoma (Nakamae et al., 2005). Unfortunately, prophylactic commencement of cardiovascular medications was not prospectively assessed in patients scheduled to receiving multiple cycles of standard-dose chemotherapy. The reported protective efficacy of carvedilol, mixed a1-2-b1 blocker, was observed in patients treated with anthracycline cumulative doses higher than recommended (Kalay et al., 2006) this likely amplified the protective signal of any drug that had been administered (Florenzano & Salman, 2007). Outside of these limited exploratory studies, prophylactic commencement of cardiovascular medications is uncommon or disregarded because of concerns about class-related effects such as hypotension, bradicardia, fluid retention, cough, or other discomfort.

As already mentioned, dexrazoxane was the only compound that consistently proved effective in preventing anthracycline-related cardiotoxicity. The chemical structure of dexrazoxane consists of a *bis*-ketopiperazine that diffuses in cardiomyocytes and then undergoes stepwise hydrolysis of the two piperazine rings to form one-ring open intermediates. This one-ring intermediate hydrolyses to give a diacid-diamide (code-named ADR 925) which is structurally reminiscent of EDTA and chelates iron bound to low molecular weight cellular ligands or coordinated within 3:1 anthracycline:Fe complexes (Minotti et al., 2004). When administered by intravenous push or slow infusion some 15 to 30 min before DOX at dose ratios up to 10:1 to DOX, dexrazoxane did not interfere with DOX distribution or metabolism or excretion, but reduced the incidence of cardiotoxicity. In a randomized clinical trial, women with metastatic breast cancer who received dexrazoxane prior to DOX could be treated with more cycles and higher cumulative doses of DOX (700-1,000 mg/m^2 or more) than patients in the control group. Moreover, cardiac protection was observed in patients with or without risk factors such as e.g., prior chest wall irradiation (reviewed in Minotti et al., 2004). As a matter of fact, the pharmacological properties and clinical readouts of dexrazoxane have been widely challenged. In the pharmacological field, there have been reports that dexrazoxane could protect by mechanisms other than iron chelation, like e.g., inhibition of topoisomerase II-mediated formation of DNA double-strand breaks in cardiomyocytes (Lyu et al., 2007). Accordingly, preclinical studies showed little or no cardiac protection by dexrazoxane analogues that chelated iron but failed to inhibit toposomerase II (Sterba et al. J Pharmacol Exp Ther 2006). In the clinical setting, the risk/benefit ratio of dexrazoxane was questioned in terms of hemathologic toxicities and interference with anthracycline activity. An exacerbation of anthracycline-related myelotoxicity (usually in the form of grade 3 or 4 neutropenia) is a well- known complication of the use of dexrazoxane, but other studies raised a concern that children treated with dexrazoxane were at a higher risk for second malignancies including, among others, acute myelogenous leukaemia and myelodysplastic syndrome. This latter concern was dispelled by two authoritative studies of childhood cancer survivors who had been randomized to receive anthracyclines with or without dexrazoxane as cardioprotectant (Barryet al., J Clin Oncol. 2008; Vrooman et al., Eur J Cancer. 2011). Other concerns were raised in relation to a possible interference of dexrazoxane with anthracycline activity. One single study suggested that dexrazoxane reduced response rates in women who received DOX for the treatment of advanced breast cancer (Swain et al., J Clin Oncol 1997) but many other clinical studies showed that this was not the case in either pediatric or adult settings (Swain and Vici, J Cancer Res Clin Oncol. 2004; van Dalen et al., Cochrane Database Syst Rev. 2011). In spite of the overwhelming evidence for its safety and preventative activity in a number of oncologic settings, the American Society of Clinical Oncology, Chemotherapy, and Radiotherapy Expert Panel maintained and recommended using dexrazoxane only in patients who had received more than 300 mg of DOX/m^2 and could benefit from continuing on DOX or EPI (Schuchter et al., 2002). It is our opinion that dexrazoxane should be used with less restrictions; current limitations to using it in a prophylactic manner are not supported by available evidence.

In a similar manner, oncologists should be encouraged to use liposomal formulations of DOX. These formulations approach very high peak plasma levels and longer circulating time than conventional DOX but release little or no free anthracycline in the bloodstream. Moreover, the liposomes are small enough to diffuse through the discontinuous "leaky" endothelium of tumors, but they are big enough not to diffuse through the normal microvasculature of the heart. Liposomal formulations therefore deliver high amounts of DOX in tumors but not in the heart. One liposomal DOX (Caelyx®) has polyethylene glycol embedded in the lipid layers; another formulation (Myocet®) adopts an uncoated liposome. Regardless of obvious pharmacokinetic and toxicokinetic differences between the two formulations, both proved remarkably cardiac tolerable and allowed administering high to very high cumulative doses of anthracycline. in a number of clinical settings. A recent Cochrane Intervention Review raises caution against using liposomal doxorubicin in pediatric settings or in patients diagnosed with leukaemia, but it is quite strong in concluding that liposomal formulations should be favoured in adults with a solid tumor (van Dalen et al., 2010). Despite this authoritative recommendation, clinical use of liposomal anthracycline formulations remains quite limited, primarily because of cost-related concerns. It is our opinion that liposomal doxorubicin should remain a must in certain approved settings (like e.g., ovary cancer in the case of Caelyx) and first choice in any other patients presenting with cardiovascular risk factors (as it is the case for Myocet in high risk or older patients with non Hodgkin lymphoma) (Visani & Isidori, 2011).

Preventing the risk of anthracycline-related cardiotoxicity during the lifetime means to reshape the pharmacological management of cancer survivors. Preexisting comorbidities or unfavorable lifestyle choices (hypertension, diabetes, hyperlipidemia, reduced physical activity) had long been known to increase the risk of cardiotoxicity in patients scheduled to receiving anthracyclines. The available evidence suggests that this picture should also be viewed the other way around. In comparison to siblings or age-matched subjects from the general population, previously healthy cancer survivors tend in fact to develop more comorbidities or to reduce physical activity (De Bruin et al., 2009; Jones et al., 2007). It follows that sublinical cardiotoxicity from "safe doses" of anthracyclines may progress to symptomatic events by overlapping with risk factors that matured after ending chemotherapy. This is the so-called multiple-hit hypothesis, according to which late onset cardiotoxicity originates from pharmacological and non pharmacological sequential injuries (Minotti et al, 2010). These concepts call for a new dimension of preventative cardiology, in a sense that in cancer survivors any comorbidity or unfavourable lifestyle choice should be treated earlier or more vigorously than in the general population.

5. Monitoring

There is no universally accepted guideline for monitoring patients receiving anthracyclines. Table I provides a tentative schedule that follows on suggestions by Ewer and colleagues mainly based on widely used criteria such as cumulative dose, time elapsed after chemotherapy, presence or absence of cardiovascular risk factors or preexisting cardiac disease, concerns (or symptoms) calling for unscheduled visits and cardiological inspection, dosability in any clinical center (measurements of LVEF only).

Planned Cumulative Dose (mg/m²)	**During treatment**		**After treatment**	
	No risk factors or Preexisting Cardiac Disease	One or more risk factors, Preexisting Cardiac disease	No risk factors or Preexisting Cardiac Disease	One or more risk factors, Preexisting Cardiac disease
Baseline	yes	yes		
<300	At the physician's discretion	Recommended after two-three cycles	Approx 1, 6, and 12 months after ending therapy, and then every two years unless symptoms occur	Approx 1, 6, and 12 months after ending therapy, and then every year unless symptoms occur
300-450	At the physician discretion; recommended anytime patients report on symptoms	Recommended every two cycles	Approx 1, 6, and 12 months after ending therapy, and then every year unless symptoms occur	Approx 1 month after ending therapy, and then every six months unless symptoms occur
>450	Recommended at midtherapy or earlier if symptoms occur	Recommended every two cycles or more often if symptoms occur	Approx 1 month after ending therapy, and then every six months unless symptoms occur	Approx 1 month after ending therapy, and then every six months unless symptoms occur

Table 1. General principles for monitoring LVEF in patients receiving doxorubicin. Modified after Ewer and Benjamin (2006).

Whereas the reported timetable is intrinsically correct and doable in everyday clinical practice, there are at least two disturbing points that need to be kept in mind if one wished to improve the caring of cancer patients and survivors. First, we now know that as little as 100 mg of DOX/m^2 may cause an increased risk of asymptomatic abnormalities at non-invasive cardiac tests, whereas 270 mg of DOX/m^2 introduces a measurable 4.5-fold excess risk of such abnormalities (Hudson et al, 2007). The second point is that dilative cardiomyopathy and systolic failure (reduced LVEF) have been considered for long time the only (or prevailing) clinical phenotypes of chronic cardiotoxicity from anthracyclines. Therefore, serial measurements of LVEF (whether by echocardiography or MUGA) have been adopted to measure the cardiac function of patients treated with anthracyclines. Keeping this in mind, we now know that asymptomatic diastolic dysfunction is seen in many cancer survivors with a history of prior exposure to anthracyclines. Anthracyclines, in fact, could cause diastolic elevated $[Ca^{2+}]_I$ and impaired left ventricle relaxation (stiffness) by a number of mechanisms (inhibition and/or reduced expression levels of the Ca^{2+}-ATPase that sequesters Ca^{2+} in sarcoplasmic reticulum, inhibition of the energy build-up that assists Ca^{2+} loading in mitochondria, inappropriate opening of the Ca^{2+}-gated Ca^{2+} release channel of the sarcoplasmic reticulum (ryanodine receptor 2) (Minotti et al, 2004). Long lasting diastolic dysfunction eventually increases interstitial pressure, thereby diminishing coronary conductance and causing ischemia that further aggravates Ca^{2+} overload and left ventricle wall tension (Hale et al., 2008). Reciprocal interactions between diastolic dysfunction and ischemia may remain asymptomatic for many years but eventually surface in the form of symptomatic ischemic disease and myocardial infarction. The risk of myocardial infarction in previously nonischemic Hodgkin's lymphoma survivors therefore correlated with their prior exposure to anthracyclines (Swerdlow et al., 2007). Furthermore, diastolic dysfunction and reduced coronary conductance would render the heart more vulnerable by comorbidities that diminish coronary flow or increased oxygen demand, like e.g. premature atherosclerosis or hypertension. All such concepts call for reshaping current modalities of follow up of cancer survivors. Serial measurements of LVEF should no longer be considered adequate to identify patients at risk for symptomatic cardiac events. Moreover, careful inspection of diastolic function (e.g., transmitral flow) is equally important and much needed, not to mention myocardial perfusion imaging techniques that show hypoperfusion under stress conditions. These approaches are less doable in clinical practice, leaving many patients with normal LVEF at risk for sudden or slowly developing cardiac events.

Current limitations in the monitoring of patients at risk for anthracycline related cardiotoxicity could be obviated by measuring pre- and post- infusional levels of circulating troponin (TnI), marker of toxic or ischemic cardiomyocyte necrosis. Persistent elevations of TnI were shown to anticipate LVEF decrements and other cardiac events in otherwise asymptomatic childhood cancer patients (Lipshultz et al., 1997) or in adults receiving high-dose chemotherapy (Cardinale et al., 2006). More recently, elevations of TnI were shown to anticipate LVEF decrements in women who had received sequential adjuvant chemotherapy and immunologic treatment with the anti-Erbb2 monoclonal antibody trastuzumab for the treatment of Erbb2$^+$ early breast cancer (J Clin Oncol., 2010, 28:3910-6). Unfortunately, TnI measurements are uncommon outside of limited exploratory studies; there is a lack of studies that prospectively evaluated TnI in large cohort of patients and firmly established laboratory ranges that should guide the physicians in making decisions such as adjusting the dose of anthracycline or commencing prophylactic cardiovascular medications. Similarly uncommon is the measurement of circulating natriuretic peptides, markers of left ventricular diastolic tension. On treatment elevations of natriuretic peptides were reported to anticipate chemotherapy-induced diastolic dysfunction, but such elevations were seen in patients treated with high-dose chemotherapy or in patients receiving just one cycle of standard-dose chemotherapy (Gianni et al., 2008, J. Clin. Oncol. 26; Nakamae et al., 2005). There is little information on the prognostic value of natriuretic peptides elevations during the course of cumulative standard-dose chemotherapy and at follow-up.

6. Liposomal formulations of doxorubicin

Daunorubicin (DNR) as the cell cycle non-specific anthracycline antibiotics is highly effective in treating a wide range of cancer diseases [5-7]. Its antineoplastic mechanisms are through DNA topoisomerase II inhibition, DNA intercalation, RNA synthesis inhibition, cell membranes interaction, free radicals production and induction of apoptosis [8-10]. However, the clinical use of daunorubicin is hampered by two major problems: cardiotoxicity [11] and drug resistance, as daunorubicin is a substrate for P-glycoprotein (MDR1; ABCB1) [12] and breast cancer resistance protein (BCRP;ABCG2) [13]. This limits of standard doxorubicin have moved forward the development of new liposomal formulations of the drug, which gained increasing interest in the therapy of onco-hematological malignancies and, in particular, for the treatment of breast cancer and B-cell lymphomas. In the early 1980s, liposomes were discovered to be good anthracycline carriers, reducing toxicity while retaining potent antitumor activity and therefore improving the therapeutic index of anthracyclines [14]. Liposomal formulations of doxorubicin have indeed been developed with the aim of improving the therapeutic index of doxorubicin by reducing the drug's cardiotoxicity. Nevertheless, liposomal conjugation of doxorubicin results in preferential distribution of the drug in the tumor compared with normal tissue.

Two liposomal formulations are currently available: non-pegylated liposomal doxorubicin (NPLD) (Myocet®, Cephalon, USA) and pegylated liposomal doxorubicin (PLD) (Caelix®/Doxil®, Schering-Plough/Orto Biothech, USA)

NPLD is a liposome encapsulated formulation of doxorubicin, which differs from pegylated liposomal doxorubicin, as well as from unencapsulated, conventional doxorubicin, resulting in an alteration in the pharmacokinetics and biodistribution. This results in a higher area under the curve, a smaller volume of distribution and a preferential distribution to liver, spleen, and lymphatics, when compared with conventional doxorubicin. Pre-clinical studies comparing equal doses of liposome-encapsulated doxorubicin and conventional doxorubicin showed that the use of nonpegylated liposomal doxorubicin resulted in a significantly lower cardiac and gastrointestinal toxicity, with similar anti-tumor efficacy.

The other liposomal compound, pegylated liposomal doxorubicin (PLD) (Caelix®/Doxil®, Schering-Plough/Orto Biothech, USA), is a liposomal formulation with a distinct pharmacokinetic profile characterized by an extended circulation time and a reduced volume of distribution [22]. Biodistribution animal studies indicate superior accumulation of PLD into various implanted mouse-human tumors, with an augmentation of liposomal drug tumor levels compared with free drugs [22]. The extended circulation time of pegylated liposomes and their ability to extravasate through the leaky vasculature of tumors results in the increased delivery of liposomal drug and/or radiotracers to the tumor site in patients with cancer. Pegylated liposomal doxorubicin has been approved for clinical use in a variety of cancer types due to its antitumor efficacy. However, the safety profile needs further improvement, as long as hand-foot syndrome remains a dose-limiting toxic effect of Doxil, maybe due to the considerable amount of drug being delivered to the skin owing to the drug's long circulation in the bloodstream.

7. Non-Pegylated Liposomal Doxorubicin (NPLD)

NPLD is a doxorubicin citrate complex encapsulated in a liposome, an aqueous dispersion of egg Phosphatydilcholine

and cholesterol, sterile, non-pyrogenous that traps doxorubicin by pulling it into the interior of the vesicle (TLC D-99 model) by the generation of an electropotential across the liposome membrane. This mechanism for remote loading involves the generation of a pH gradient between the inside and the extraliposomal buffer. At the end of the encapsulation process, the ratio of doxorubicin:lipid in NPLD is approximately 1:4 and the pH is in the range of 5.5–6.5. The maximum activity of doxorubicin and other anthracyclines manifests itself in the S phase of the cellular cycle.

The encapsulation of a cytostatic agent within a macromolecular vector such as a liposome reduces drastically its distribution volume, diminishing its diffusion in the organism and thus the toxicity for healthy tissues while increasing the concentration within the neoplastic tissue. In ideal conditions the drug can be transported in the circulatory system within the liposome's aqueous space and arrives to the site of the tumor in active form. Encapsulation in a liposome means the drug is protected from inactivation while in the blood stream and furthermore its diffusion through the healthy endothelium is limited, while it can diffuse through tumoral endothelium which would present discontinuities. Thus, NPLD should preferentially direct doxorubicin away from sites of potential toxicity, but leaves the tumor exposed.

7.1 Non-pegylated liposomal doxorubicin in breast cancer

NPLD was designed to reduce the cardiotoxicity of doxorubicin while preserving its antitumor efficacy. In the early 2000, the safety and efficacy of NPLD was tested in cancer patients, after the demonstration of a significantly lower cardiac and gastrointestinal toxicity, with similar anti-tumor efficacy showed by NPLD in pre-clinical studies.

The first studies were conduced in breast cancer patients. These phase III, randomized, multicenter trials were designed to test the hypothesis that NPLD, alone or in combination with other drugs, would result in significantly less cardiac toxicity than the same dose and schedule of conventional doxorubicin and other drugs, while providing comparable antitumor efficacy in first-line treatment of metastatic breast cancer.

Batist et al (Batist et al., 2001) randomized 297 patients with MBC and no prior chemotherapy for metastatic disease were randomized to receive either 60 mg/m^2 of NPLD or conventional doxorubicin (A), in combination with 600 mg/m^2 of cyclophosphamide (C), every 3 weeks until disease progression or unacceptable toxicity. Antitumor efficacy of MC versus AC was comparable: objective response rates, 43% versus 43%; median time to progression, 5.1% versus 5.5 months; median time to treatment failure, 4.6 versus 4.4 months; and median survival, 19 versus 16 months (Batist et al., 2001).

Cardiotoxicity was a primary end point parameter in all treated patients (Batist et al., 2001). Cardiac toxicity, sufficient for removal of a patient from study, was defined as a decrease in resting LVEF of ≥ 20 ejection fraction (EF) units from baseline to a final value of ≥ 50%, or a decrease of ≥ 10 EF units from baseline to a final value of less than 50%, or clinical evidence of CHF. LVEFs were assessed using serial Multigated blood-pool imaging (MUGA) scans, which have been shown to be a reliable and serially reproducible method of evaluating cardiac function in patients receiving anthracycline therapy.

To ensure accuracy and objectivity, each center was required to have its equipment and methodology used for MUGA scans reviewed and certified by a cardiologist at the Core Laboratory at Yale University before enrolling patients. During the trial, all MUGA scans were sent to the Core Laboratory at Yale, where they were read by the same cardiologist blinded to the patient's treatment (Batist et al., 2001). To minimize the risk of CHF, all scans were read in real time and results provided to the site before the next scheduled dose of anthracycline therapy. CHF was determined on the basis of a treatment-blinded review of records from patients for whom the investigator had made a diagnosis of CHF, as well as patients who had a LVEF of ≤ 30%. LVEF ≤ 30% was selected as the cutoff because these patients are at significant risk for CHF (Batist et al., 2001). The blinded review was conducted by a second cardiologist at Yale University noted for his expertise in doxorubicin-induced cardiotoxicity. All MUGA scan data were interpreted and LVEF values were estimated at a core laboratory on a blinded basis. Nine patients (6%) treated with MC developed protocol-defined cardiotoxicity compared with 33 patients (21%) treated with AC (log-rank *P* = .0001). Five cases of CHF, all in the AC arm (log-rank *P* = .02), were observed after cumulative lifetime doses ranging from 360 to 480 mg/m^2. Four of the five patients with CHF were anthracycline-naive before this study; one patient had 240 mg/m^2 of prior adjuvant doxorubicin. All other patients with cardiotoxicity had an asymptomatic decrease in LVEF of ≥ 10 EF units from baseline to a final value less than 50%. The estimated (Kaplan-Meier) median cumulative lifetime dose of doxorubicin at the first occurrence of protocol-defined cardiac toxicity was more than 2,220 mg/m^2 for the MC arm versus 480 mg/m^2 for the AC arm. The hazard ratio of 4.8 shows that patients treated with MC were 80% less likely to develop cardiotoxicity with respect to patients treated with AC.

Similarly, there was a highly significant difference in the time to onset of cardiotoxicity when measured from the start of protocol therapy. The estimated median onset of protocol-defined cardiotoxicity was more than 22 months for MC versus 10 months for AC (log-rank P = .0003). There was a gradual increase in the median change from baseline LVEF to the last posttreatment LVEF among patients treated with either regimen, but this was more pronounced in the AC-treated group (Batist et al., 2001).

In the subset of patients with recognized risk factors for cardiac toxicity, the hazard ratio was increased to 16, indicating that these patients were more than 90% less likely to develop cardiac toxicity with MC relative to AC. Four percent of MC-treated patients developed a protocol-defined cardiac event versus 22% of AC-treated patients (Batist et al., 2001). The median lifetime cumulative dose of doxorubicin at onset was 480 mg/m2 for AC versus more than 2,220 mg/m2 for MC (P = .0001) (Batist et al., 2001). Four of the five patients with CHF were in this subgroup with increased risk of cardiac toxicity (Batist et al., 2001).

In conclusion, the improved therapeutic index for NPLD predicted by the preclinical data and indicated by the phase I/II clinical trials was confirmed in this phase III, randomized, multicenter trial. Statistically significantly fewer patients treated with NPLD in combination with cyclophosphamide experienced cardiac toxicity defined by reductions in LVEF or clinical CHF (Batist et al., 2001).

Another interesting study was carried on by Harris et al (Harris et al, 2002). Two hundred twenty-four patients with MBC and no prior therapy for metastatic disease were randomized to receive either TLC D-99 (75 mg/m2) or doxorubicin (75 mg/m2) every 3 weeks, in the absence of disease progression or unacceptable toxicity. The primary efficacy endpoint was response rate. The primary safety endpoint was cardiotoxicity.

Electrocardiograms and MUGA scans were done at baseline, and after reaching a lifetime cumulative doxorubicin dose of 300, 400, 500 mg/m^2, and before each subsequent dose, at off-study, and at 3-month follow-up. All MUGA scan data were transferred electronically to a core laboratory for blinded interpretation and estimation of LVEF (Harris et al, 2002). Before the first interim analysis, endomyocardial biopsies were performed at a selected number of institutions after lifetime cumulative doxorubicin dose of 425 mg/m^2. All patients whose LVEF declined by greater than 10% to a value of greater than or equal to 50%, or by greater than 6% to a value of less than 50% were to have cardiac biopsies regardless of lifetime cumulative doses (Harris et al, 2002). All biopsies were read by a core pathologist, and the results were scored according to the Billingham scale. The purpose of biopsies was to validate the results of MUGA scans. After the first interim analysis, it was determined that MUGA scans were adequate to monitor cardiac function and cardiac biopsies were discontinued (Harris et al, 2002). All MUGA scan data were sent to an independent central laboratory for estimation and interpretation of LVEF values without knowledge of treatment arm.

Cardiac events, sufficient for removal of a patient from study, were more than twice as frequent in doxorubicin-treated patients than TLC D-99-treated patients (29% vs. 13%, log-rank P = 0.0001) (Harris et al, 2002). With the increasing lifetime cumulative dose of doxorubicin and TLC D-99, there was a gradual increase in the median change from baseline LVEF to the first post-treatment LVEF among patients treated with either agent, but this was more pronounced in the doxorubicin group (Harris et al, 2002). A Kaplan-Meier estimate of the probability of the first onset of a cardiac event as related to the lifetime cumulative dose of doxorubicin or TLC D-99 showed that risk of cardiotoxicity was much higher with doxorubicin treatment than TLC D-99 (HR = 3.56) (P = 0.0001) (Harris et al, 2002). Two patients (2%) on TLC D-99 developed clinical CHF. One patient, after 13 cycles of TLC D-99 and a cumulative dose of 1110 mg/m^2, had a decrease of 14 EF units in her LVEF to 46% and was taken off-study. Two months after the last dose she presented with shortness of breath and bilateral pleural effusions and was hospitalized for CHF. Another patient, with prior adjuvant doxorubicin dose of 290 mg/m^2 and prior chest wall irradiation, received five cycles of TLC D-99 for a total lifetime doxorubicin dose of 785 mg/m^2, and went off-study for PD. Four months after the last dose, a MUGA scan showed a LVEF of 46% (a 16-point decrease from baseline). Later, the patient received five cycles of a mitomycin plus mitoxantrone, and 11 months after the last study treatment she received a diagnosis of CHF (Harris et al, 2002). Nine patients (8%) on doxorubicin developed clinical CHF at lifetime doses of 525–765 mg/m^2. Three patients had CHF within 30 days of the last dose of study treatment, including one who died of CHF after 585 mg/m^2. All nine cases were attributed to study drug treatment (Harris et al, 2002).

Before the first interim analysis, 51 patients were treated at 8 participating institutions performing endomyocardial biopsies. Of those, 36 patients qualified for the procedure, and all 36 patients had cardiac biopsies. All biopsies were read by a core pathologist, blinded to treatment assignment, and the results were scored according to the Billingham scale. There was a significant difference between the two treatment groups favoring TLC D-99 and the number of patients who had a score of greater than or equal to 2.5 (26% vs. 71%; $P = 0.02$) (Harris et al, 2002).

Regarding efficacy, the overall response rate was 26% in both treatment groups. The median TTP was 2.9 months on TLC D-99 versus 3.1 months on doxorubicin. Median survival was 16 versus 20 months with a non significant trend in favor of doxorubicin (P = 0.09).

In another randomized study, Chan et al tried to ascertain the efficacy and tolerability of NPLD and epirubicin combined with cyclophosphamide in the first-line treatment of patients with metastatic breast cancer (Chan et al., 2004). One hundred and sixty anthracycline-naïve metastatic breast cancer patients were randomised to receive NPLD (M; 75 mg/m2) or epirubicin (E; 75 mg/m2) in combination with cyclophosphamide (C; 600 mg/m2), every 3 weeks for up to eight cycles. Cardiotoxicity was low in both treatment groups: nine patients on MC and eight on EC had asymptomatic LVEF reductions at comparable cumulative doses . For MC there were two cases at 100–299 mg/m2, four at 300–399 mg/m2 and three at 500–599 mg/m2; for EC there was one case at 200–299 mg/m2, four at 300–399 mg/m2 and three at 400–499 mg/m2. There was no clinical evidence of CHF in any patient. Overall response rates were 46% and 39% for MC and EC treatment, respectively (P=0.42). MC was superior to EC with respect to median time to treatment failure (5.7 versus 4.4 months; P=0.01) and median time to disease progression (7.7 versus 5.6 months; P=0.02). Median survival times were 18.3 and 16.0 months for MC and EC, respectively (P=0.504). Unsurprisingly, the results from this study (Chan et al., 2004) suggested that, at equimolar doses, in combination with cyclophosphamide, NPLD has modest but significant advantages over epirubicin for some efficacy end points and a non-significant trend towards improvement in others. Given the well established correlation between dose and therapeutic effect for doxorubicin, and in light of the uncertainty surrounding the optimal therapeutic dose of epirubicin, NPLD offers clinicians the opportunity to make clinical use of a drug that combines the dose/effect reliability of doxorubicin with the level of safety provided by epirubicin.

In conclusion, two studies (Batist et al., 2001; Harris et al., 2002; Chan et al, 2004) clearly demonstrated reduced cardiotoxicity of NPLD when compared to standard doxorubicin, with a superimposable antitumor efficacy of the two drugs. The third study showed a trend of higher efficacy fot NPLD with respect to epirubicin, with equal cardiotoxicity.

7.2 Non-pegylated liposomal doxorubicin in non-Hodgkin lymphoma

The first study testing the safety and efficacy of NPLD in non-Hodgkin lymphoma NHL (AIDS-related) was conducted by Alexandra Levine and coworkers in 2004 (Levine et al., 2004). The study enrolled 24 patients with newly diagnosed AIDS-related NHL (median age: 43 years). Sixty-seven percent of patients had a high or high-intermediate International Prognostic Index (IPI) scores at diagnosis. Serum LDH was high in 17 patients (71%). A total of 21 patients (88%) had extranodal disease, and 12 patients (50%) had 2 or more sites of extranodal involvement.

The primary objective of the study was to evaluate the safety and efficacy of NPLD when substituted for doxorubicin in the CHOP in patients with newly diagnosed AIDS-related non-Hodgkin's lymphoma (AIDS-NHL). NPLD at doses of 40, 50, 60, and 80 mg/m2 was given with fixed doses of cyclophosphamide (750 mg/m2), vincristine (1.4 mg/m2) and prednisone (40 mg/m2) every 21 days. The maximum tolerated dose (MTD) of NPLD was defined as the dose at which less than half of the patients on a cohort experienced a dose-limiting toxicity. No dose escalations were allowed in individual patients. The MTD of NPLD was not reached at the 80 mg/m2 dose. As a high complete response (CR) rate was seen at all dose levels, a dose of 50 mg/m2 of NPLD was chosen for the phase II portion of the trial, which was expanded to a total of 24 patients, including 10 on the initial phase I dose-escalation portion. All patients received highly active antiretroviral therapy while on chemotherapy.

The results of the study were encouraging. No dose-limiting toxicities were observed at any level, with myelosuppression being the most frequent toxicity (grade 4 neutropenia in 75% of patients, neutropenic fever in 12% and neutropenic sepsis in 8%). Overall response rate was 88%, with a CR rate of 75%, and a partial response (PR) rate of 13%. The median duration of CR was 15.6 months (range, 1.7 to 43.5 months).

Moreover, 16 out of 24 AIDS-related NHL patients were evaluated for multidrug resistance (MDR-1) expression on their hystological samples. The Authors demonstrated that this NPLD-based regimen was equally effective in both MDR-1-positive and MDR-1-negative cases. The Authors postulated that the efficacy of this regimen was eventually related to the ability of NPLD to overcome excessive drug efflux due to P-gp (MDR-1) overexpression. The MDR-1 expression did not correlate with response in this study, suggesting that NPLD might evade this resistance mechanism.

In terms of potential cardiac toxicity, left ventricular ejection fraction (LVEF) was obtained at baseline and at study termination in 19 patients. No patient developed a decline in LVEF to below normal (45%). Fourteen patients had no significant change in LVEF over time, while 5 patients (26%) experienced a 10% or greater decline, though their LVEF values still remained within normal range. None of these five patients had any signs or symptoms of cardiac dysfunction, and the values returned to baseline levels in the two patients who had follow-up cardiac studies performed, 3 months after completion of chemotherapy.

Starting from that background, the same group of the Keck School of Medicine designed in 2006 a phase I-II trial to evaluate the safety of the same regimen (NPLD, cyclophosphamide, vincristine, and prednisone every 21 days) in the treatment of newly diagnosed aggressive NHL patients (Tulpule et al., 2006).

Forty-seven patients (median age: 55 years) were enrolled in the study. The vast majority of the patients had diffuse large B-cell NHL (37/47). Liposomal doxorubicin at doses of 40 mg/m2, 50 mg/m2, 60 mg/m2, and 80 mg/m2 was given with fixed doses of cyclophosphamide (750 mg/m2), vincristine (1.4mg/m2) and prednisone (40 mg/m2). Chemotherapy cycles were repeated every 21 days.

No dose-limiting toxicities were observed at any level. Reversible grade 3/4 neutropenia was the most common toxicity (95.8%). Most non-hematologic side effects were nausea, vomiting fatigue and fever and were primarily grade 1/2 in severity. Stomatitis of mild or moderate severity was reported in 23% of patients.

Two out of 47 patients (4%) developed clinically silent cardiac toxicity, with a decline in LVEF of 20% each. None of the patients presented any symptoms of cardiotoxicity. The decline in LVEF occurred in one patient after a cumulative NPLD dose of 240mg/m2 and in the other one after a cumulative NPLD dose of 640 mg/m2. In both patients the declines returned to baseline 2 months and 6 months from discontinuation of NPLD, respectively.

Complete remissions were documented in 31 of 46 evaluable patients (67.4%) and partial remissions in 7 (15.2%), for an overall major response rate of 82.6%. Responses were attained after a median of 4 cycles of therapy. Patients with T-cell lymphomas fared poorly with this regimen, with none of them achieving a CR lasting more than 6 months.

The median duration of complete remission was 27.7 months (range, 2.4 months to 59.8 months). Reported median follow-up was 3.1 years. Median survival was not reached at the time of publication. The 2-year estimated overall suvival (OS) probability was 65% (95% CI, 50-77%), with a 3-year estimated OS probability of 59% (95%CI, 44%-73%). Nineteen patients had died at the time of publication.

Regarding the relationship between MDR-1 expression and outcome, MDR-1-related p-glycoprotein expression was assessed in lymphoma tissues from 27 patients. Eight patients (30%) was MDR-1 positive at diagnosis. No difference in CR rates were observed when comparing patients whose tumors expressed MDR-1 versus those who did not (63% in MDR-1-positive and 74% in the MDR-1-negative lymphomas, P = 0.66), indicating that NPLD might overcome MDR-1 in vivo.

Rigacci and collaborators (Rigacci et al., 2007) designed a prospective study to assess the efficacy and safety of the combination of NPLD with cyclophosphamide, vincristine, prednisone and Rituximab (R-COMP) in patients with aggressive non-Hodgkin's B-cell lymphomas and concurrent cardiac disease or pre-treated with anthracyclines.

Twenty-one patients were selected for the presence of cardiac comorbidity and/or previous treatment with anthracycline-based regimens. NPLD at a dose of 50 mg/m2 was administered in association with cyclophosphamide (750 mg/m2), vincristine (1.4mg/m2), prednisone (40 mg/m2) and rituximab (375 mg/m2) every 21 days for 4 to 6 cycles unless progression or unacceptable toxicity occurred. CR rate was 76%, whereas PR rate was 14%, with an overall response rate (ORR) of 90%. Two patients (10%) did not respond to therapy. After a median follow-up of 13 months (range 2–36 months), 2/16 CR patients relapsed, with a cumulative disease-free survival (DFS) rate of 78%.

Regarding toxicities, the Authors observed only a congestive heart failure (CHF) in one patient, among a total of 115 chemotherapy cycles administered. LVEF was evaluated after the 3rd cycle and at the end of treatment in all but one patient, who developed CHF with LVEF 20% after the first cycle of R-COMP. Between the 20 evaluable patients, median LVEF was 60% (range 38%–74%) after three cycles and 60% (range 40%–69%) at the end of the treatment. There was no significant difference between LVEF at baseline, after the 3rd cycle, and at the end of study in patients with cardiac comorbidity (52, 58 and 60%, respectively), in those without cardiac diseases (62, 61 and 60%, respectively) and in those previously treated with anthracyclines. Patients were evaluated every 6 months after the end of the study. Among the 15 patients who were followed-up for at least 12 months after the end of therapy, none of them presented any cardiac dysfunction or significant decrease of LVEF.

The Authors stated that Rituximab plus NPLD-based regimen was well tolerated and highly effective in inducing clinical responses in this group of patients at high risk for cardiac toxicity or previously treated with anthracyclines. The tolerability profile was favorable, with a low incidence of cardiac events (1/21 patients).

Visani and coworkers (Visani et al., 2008) conduced a pilot study to assess the toxicity and efficacy of the combination of NPLD with cyclophosphamide, vincristine, prednisone and

Rituximab (R-COMP) in frail and elderly patients with aggressive non-Hodgkin's B-cell lymphomas.

NPLD at a dose of 50 mg/m2 was administered in association with cyclophosphamide (750 mg/m2), vincristine (1.4mg/m2), prednisone (40 mg/m2) and rituximab (375 mg/m2) every 21 days for 4 to 6 cycles unless progression or unacceptable toxicity occurred.

Twenty frail patients (median age: 73 years), as defined by Balducci & Extermann (Balducci & Extermann,2000) with diffuse large B cell or grade IIIb follicular lymphoma, either at diagnosis (15 patients) or relapsed (5 patients), were prospectively enrolled.

Thirteen out of 20 NHL patients (65%) had a complete response (CR) and an additional 5 patients (25%) achieved a partial response (PR), with an overall response rate of 90% (ORR). Notably, the median age of the study population (73 years) was the oldest ever reported in literature of patients treated with this combinations. As a matter of fact, this population consisted of particularly elderly and frail patients with advanced disease at the time of study entry. These patients had indeed an extremely high probability of being unable to complete one of the standard anthracyclines-based regimens or to suffer from cardiotoxicity.

The treatment was relatively well-tolerated. Grade 3 or 4 neutropenia occurred in 26% of cycles and febrile neutropenia in 5%. There was no significant difference between LVEF at baseline, after the 3rd cycle, and at the end of study in 16/19 patients. Notably, 2 patients presented a CHF (NYHA 3) after 1 and 3 cycles of R-COMP, respectively and were shifted to receive an anthracycline-free regimen while in CR after R-COMP. In these 2 patients, the Authors observed a 20% decrease of the LVEF which partially recovered after medical therapy. The cumulative percentage of cardiovascular complications was 15%, higher than that reported for elderly patients treated with R-CHOP 21 or 14. However, this patient population consisted only of frail patients having a poor WHO performance status and important comorbidities.

This study demonstrated for the first time the safety and efficacy of the R-COMP 21 regimen in frail and elderly patients with aggressive NHL. Cardiotoxicity was low and a promising response rate was observed in this setting patients.

Another interesting study regarding the safety and the efficacy of the R-COMP combination was recently published (Luminari et al., 2010). Seventy-five elderly patients with diffuse large B-cell lymphoma (DLBCL) were studied. Only patients with left ventricular ejection fraction (LVEF) > or =50% were allowed. R-COMP regimen was administered every 3 weeks for three cycles, followed by additional five cycles in case of complete response (CR) or partial response.

Seventy-five patients with a median age of 72 years were registered, and 72 were evaluable for response assessment. Fifty-six percent of patients had high or high-intermediate International Prognostic Index score. Median LVEF at baseline was 61%. Thirty-eight patients had history of abnormal cardiovascular conditions. The overall response rate was 71%, with a CR rate of 57%. After a median follow-up of 33 months, the 3-year overall survival, failure-free survival, and progression-free survival rates were 72%, 39%, and 69%, respectively. Neutropenia (54%) was the most frequent grade 3-4 adverse event; 21% of patients experienced cardiac adverse events, graded as 3-4 in 4% of the cases.

8. Pegylated Liposomal Doxorubicin (PLD)

Pegylated liposomal doxorubicin (PLD) is doxorubicin confined in liposomes that have been sterically stabilized by grafting polyethylene glycol onto the surface (Stealth Liposome"). PLD has a circulation half-life of approximately 73.9 h, whereas doxorubicin has a half-life of <10 min. Prolonged circulation facilitates greater uptake of PLD liposomes by tumor tissue. PLD accumulates selectively in metastatic breast carcinoma tissue, resulting in 10-fold higher intracellular drug concentrations compared with adjacent normal tissue (Symon et al., 1999). Pegylated liposomal encapsulation also reduces plasma levels of free doxorubicin and may reduce drug delivery to normal tissue, which may reduce toxicity. Studies of PLD suggest that a dose of 45 to 50 mg/m2 every 4 weeks is well tolerated with little nausea or vomiting, mild myelosuppression, minimal alopecia, and very little cardiotoxicity.

8.1 Pegylated liposomal doxorubicin in breast cancer

The first randomized, multicenter, phase III study was designed to demonstrate that efficacy in terms of progression-free survival of pegylated liposomal doxorubicin HCl (PLD) was non-inferior to doxorubicin with significantly less cardiotoxicity in first-line treatment of women with metastatic breast cancer (MBC) (O'Brien et al., 2004). Women (n = 509) with MBC and normal cardiac function were randomized to receive either PLD 50 mg/m^2 (every 4 weeks) or doxorubicin 60 mg/m^2 (every 3 weeks). Cardiac event rates were based on reductions in left ventricular ejection fraction as a function of cumulative anthracycline dose.

In this open-label, multicenter trial, patients were randomized in a 1:1 ratio by an independent central third party according to a computer-generated randomization program. Patients received either PLD [50 mg/m2 intravenous (i.v.) infusion for up to 60 min every 4 weeks] or doxorubicin [60 mg/m2 i.v. infusion for 60 min every 3 weeks]. Patients were prospectively stratified based on three criteria to balance major prognostic risk factors between treatment groups: prior adjuvant anthracycline exposure; presence of bone metastases as only site of disease; presence of at least one cardiac risk factor (O'Brien et al., 2004). Cardiac risk factors were defined as prior mediastinal irradiation, age ≥65 years, history of heart disease (previous myocardial infarction, arrhythmia or angina, not requiring treatment) or hypertension, or diabetes requiring medical treatment.

Regarding cardiotoxicity, MUGA scans were performed to measure LVEF before onset of treatment, after 300 mg/m2 cumulative anthracycline exposure, and after every additional 100 mg/m2 of PLD and every 120 mg/m2 of doxorubicin. Compliance with the protocol on performing MUGA evaluations was high. Of the 283 patients who reached doses ≥300 mg/m2 cumulative anthracyclines, all but 20 patients (nine PLD, 11 doxorubicin) had a baseline MUGA evaluation and at least one follow-up MUGA evaluation during treatment (O'Brien et al., 2004).

Overall, 339 patients (152 PLD and 187 doxorubicin) had electronic MUGA scan data for evaluation of cardiotoxicity (baseline and at least one scan during treatment) and were included in the analysis. Patients in the PLD arm had a median cumulative anthracycline dose of 398 mg/m2 (including prior anthracycline exposure). Patients in the conventional doxorubicin arm had a median cumulative anthracycline dose of 421 mg/m2 (including prior anthracycline exposure). Fifty-eight patients (10 PLD, 48 doxorubicin) met the protocol-defined LVEF criteria for cardiotoxicity during treatment and/or follow-up. The risk of developing cardiotoxicity was significantly higher for patients receiving doxorubicin than for those receiving PLD (P <0.001, HR = 3.16 for comparison of cumulative anthracycline dose at the first, protocol-specified, cardiac event) (O'Brien et al., 2004). The increase in risk of developing cardiotoxicity on doxorubicin versus PLD was observed in all subgroups analyzed, including those at high risk for developing CHF. In the subgroup that received prior adjuvant anthracycline therapy, the risk of developing cardiotoxicity was seven-fold higher with doxorubicin than with PLD. None of the 10 PLD-treated patients who had cardiotoxicity by LVEF criteria developed clinical signs or symptoms of CHF, whereas 10 of 48 doxorubicin-treated patients who had cardiotoxicity by LVEF criteria developed signs or symptoms of CHF. Two patients in each group developed clinical CHF but did not have a corresponding decrease in LVEF. As expected with doxorubicin, the mean percentage change from baseline in LVEF was positively correlated with the increase in cumulative anthracycline dose. However, with PLD, only a 2–3% mean decrease in LVEF was observed as the cumulative anthracycline dose increased. At cumulative doses at or above 450 mg/m2, a seven-fold greater mean percentage decrease in LVEF was observed with doxorubicin versus PLD (-17.2% versus- 2.3%; mean percentage change from baseline in LVEF in doxorubicin-treated and PLD-treated patients, respectively) (O'Brien et al., 2004).

Regarding efficacy, PLD and doxorubicin were comparable with respect to PFS (6.9 versus 7.8 months, respectively) and to OS (21 and 22 months for PLD and doxorubicin, respectively. Palmar-plantar erythrodysesthesia (48% versus 2%), stomatitis (22% versus 15%) and mucositis (23% versus 13%) were more often associated with PLD than doxorubicin. In conclusion, in first-line therapy for MBC, PLD provides comparable efficacy to doxorubicin, with significantly reduced cardiotoxicity (O'Brien et al., 2004).

Another multicentric, randomized trial was published on the same year (Keller et al., 2004). This trial was designed to compare the efficacy of pegylated liposomal doxorubicin (PLD) with that of a common salvage regimen (comparator) in patients with taxane-refractory advanced breast cancer. Following failure of a first- or second-line taxane-containing regimen for metastatic disease, 301 women were randomly assigned to receive PLD (50 mg/m2 every 28 days); or comparator-vinorelbine (30 mg/m2 weekly) or mitomycin C (10 mg/m2 day 1 and every 28 days) plus vinblastine (5 mg/m2 day 1, day 14, day 28, and day 42) every 6 to 8 weeks (Keller et al., 2004). Changes in LVEF values were only assessed in patients receiving PLD. Cardiac toxicity was defined as either a decrease of ≥ 15 points from baseline or a ≥ 5-point decrease from baseline with a level below the lower limit of normal for the institution. Twenty-two patients developed LVEF changes consistent with cardiac toxicity. However, decreases in LVEF did not correlate with cumulative anthracycline dose and none of these patients developed clinical congestive heart failure. The majority (n = 14) discontinued due to progressive disease. There were four patients who discontinued treatment due to cardiac toxicity (LVEF decrease), three patients who discontinued due to noncardiac adverse events, and one patient who discontinued due to noncompliance. Progression-free survival (PFS) and overall survival (OS) were similar for PLD and comparator (Keller et al., 2004).

8.2 Pegylated liposomal doxorubicin in non-Hodgkin lymphoma

Pegylated liposomal doxorubicin has been substituted for conventional doxorubicin in the CHOP regimen in a number of trials. In phase II studies in elderly patients with diffuse large B-cell lymphoma, ORR of approximately 65% was achieved: 50% CR and 15% PR, an estimated 1-year OS of 55%, and an estimated 2-year event-free survival of 45%. Neutropenia was the only grade III-IV toxicity observed [23,24].

Cutaneous T-cell lymphoma (CTCL) is a specific niche in which PLD has proven to be very active at low doses in a similar fashion to Kaposi sarcoma [25]. A response rate of 88% (44% CR) with mean OS of 18 months was observed in a retrospective analysis of 31 patients receiving PLD at doses varying from 20-40 mg/m2 every 4 weeks. These patients had recurrent or unresponsive disease, or rapidly progressive disease [25].

Indeed, PLD has been shown to have equal efficacy and a better safety profile in the treatment of multiple myeloma, when compared with conventional doxorubicin combinations. In controlled clinical trials, PLD combined with vincristine and dexamethasone provided response rates comparable with the doxorubicin-based standard vincristine/doxorubicin/dexamethasone) therapy, but the former required less hospitalization, no central venous catheter, with a reported lower toxicity in terms of alopecia and severe leukopenia [26]. There are ongoing studies trying to establish the usefulness of newer compounds in combination with liposomal anthracyclines for the therapy of multiple myeloma.

9. Conclusions

New acquisitions, particularly in terms of pathogenetical mechanisms, have considerably changed the perception of anthracycline cardiotoxicity in patients cured after a cancer diagnosis. From a " cumulative dose" era, where caution to further treatments with anthracyclines was linked more to a mere calculation of global administered dose, we are now shifting to a more prudential approach, that considers a persistent biological damage due to anthracycline administration, and prompts us toward a better definition of measures able to control, in particular, late cardiac toxicity. One item is becoming evident: a strict cohoperation between cardiologists and oncologists/hematologists could significantly improve the life expectancy and reduce the risks of major CHF in anthracycline pretreated patients, simply not underevaluating concurrent risk factors for CHF, that must be addressed early and consistently with adequate "cardiological" therapies.

On the other hand, the pharmacological research has in some way met the challenge to reduce the toxicity of the therapy with anthracyclines, both designing new, safer, anthracycline analogues, such as liposomal compounds, and reshaping the way to use protective compounds, such as dexrazoxane, during anthracycline therapy. The possible role (and optimal way of use) of iron chelators, such as deferasirox, is still under evaluation.

Cost related issues have up to now limited the use of liposomal derivatives, except for niches of fragile patients; it should be considered, anyway, if the global,high impact on costs of cardiotoxicity in cancer survivors(in terms of disability and related treatments) could justify,expecially in the long run, the costs of an optimized treatment,with modified anthracyclines or with cardioprotectants, potentially able to reduce, in particular, the frequency of late cardiac toxicity.

10. Acknowledgments

Supported in part by AIL PESARO ONLUS.

11. References

Balducci L. & Extermann, M. (2000) Management of cancer in the older person: a practical approach. *Oncologist*, Vol 5, No3,pp 224-237.

Barry EV et al.. (2008). Absence of second malignant neoplasms in children with high risk acute lymphoblastic leukemia treated with dexrazoxane. *Journal of Clinical Oncology*,Vol 26, pp. 1106-1111

Batist, G. "et al" (2001). Reduced cardiotoxicity and preserved antitumor efficacy of liposome-encapsulated doxorubicin and cyclophosphamide compared with conventional doxorubicin and cyclophosphamide in a randomized, multicenter trial of metastatic breast cancer. *Journal of Clinical Oncology*, Vol.19, pp.1444-1454.

Blanco, J.G. "et al". (2008) Genetic polymorphisms in the carbonyl reductase 3 gene CBR3 and the NAD(P)H:quinine oxidoreductase 1 gene NQO1 in patients who developed anthracycline-related congestive heart failure after childhood cancer. *Cancer*, Vol. 112, pp. 2789–2795

Cardinale, D. "et al". (2006) Prevention of high-dose chemotherapy-induced cardiotoxicity in high-risk patients by angiotensin-converting enzyme inhibition. *Circulation*, Vol.114, pp.2474-2481.

Cowens, J.W. "et al" (1993). Initial clinical (Phase I) trial of Myocet (doxorubicin encapsulated in liposomes). *Cancer Research*, Vol.53, pp. 2796-2802.

Dean, M.; Fojo, T. & Bates, S. (2005). Tumour stem cells and drug resistance. *Nature Reviews Cancer*, Vol.5, No.4, pp.275-84.

De Bruin, M.L. "et al". (2009). Increased risk of stroke and transient ischemic attack in 5-year survivors of Hodgkin lymphoma. *Journal of the National Cancer Institute*, Vol. 101, pp 928-937.

Endicott, J.A. & Ling, V. (1989). The biochemistry of P-glycoprotein-mediated multidrug resistance. Annual Reviews of Biochemistry, Vol.58, pp.137-71.

Ewer MS and Benjamin RS (2006). Doxorubicin cardiotoxicity: clinical aspects, recognition, monitoring, treatment, and prevention, in: *Cancer and the Heart (Ewer MS and Yeh E eds)*: pp 9–32, BC Decker, Hamilton, ON, Canada. Florenzano, F. & Salman, P. (2007) Carvedilol for anthracycline cardiomyopathy prevention. *Journal of the American College of Cardiology*, Vol.49,pp. 2142-2143.

Gianni, L. " et al.". Anthracycline cardiotoxicity: from bench to bedside. *Journal of Clinical. Oncology*, Vol. 26, pp. 3777-3784.

Gabizon, A.A. (1994). Liposomal anthracyclines. *Hematology/Oncology Clinics of North America* , Vol. 8, pp. 431-50.

Hale, S.L. "et al". (2008) Late sodium current inhibition as a new cardioprotective approach. *Journal of Molecular and Cellular Cardiology*, Vol.44, pp. 954-967.

Harris, L. "et al". (2002) Liposome-encapsulated doxorubicin compared with conventional doxorubicin in a randomized multicenter trial as first-line therapy of metastatic breast carcinoma. *Cancer*, Vol.94, No.1, pp 25-36.

Hudson, M.M. "et al". (2007) Noninvasive evaluation of late anthracycline cardiac toxicity in childhood cancer survivors. *Journal of Clinical Oncology*, Vol.25. pp. 3635–3643.

Innocenti, F. "et al". (2001) Epirubicin glucuronidation is catalyzed by human UDP glucuronosyltransferase 2B7. *Drug Metab Dispos*, Vol. 29, pp 686-692.

Jones, L.W. "et al". (2007). Early breast cancer therapy and cardiovascular injury. *Journal of the American College of Cardiology*, Vol. 50, pp.1435-1441.

Kalay, N. "et al". (2006) Protective effects of carvedilol against anthracycline-induced cardiomyopathy. *Journal of the American College of Cardiology*, Vol.48, pp.2258-2264.

Lasic, D.D. (1993). Liposomes: from physics to applications, p. 575. Amsterdam: Elsevier.

Lebrecht, D. & Walker, U.A. (2007). Role of mtDNA lesions in anthracycline cardiotoxicity. *Cardiovascular Toxicology* Vol.7, pp.108-113.

Levine, A.M. "et al". (2004) Liposome-encapsulated doxorubicin in combination with standard agents (cyclophosphamide, vincristine, prednisone) in patients with newly diagnosed AIDS-related non-Hodgkin's lymphoma: results of therapy and correlates of response. *Journal of Clinical Oncology*, Vol. 22, No.13, pp.2662-2670.

Lipshultz, S.E. "et al". (2002) Doxorubicin administration by continuous infusion is not cardioprotective: the Dana-Farber 91-01 Acute Lymphoblastic Leukemia protocol. *Journal of Clinical Oncology*, Vol. 20, pp. 1677-1682.

Lipshultz, S.E. "et al". (1997). Predictive value of cardiac troponin T in pediatric patients at risk for myocardial injury. *Circulation*, Vol. 96, pp. 2641-2648

Lotfi, K.; Zackrisson, A.L. & Peterson, C. (2002) Comparison of idarubicin and daunorubicin regarding intracellular uptake, induction of apoptosis, and resistance. *Cancer Letters*, Vol. 25, No.178 (2), pp.141-9.

Luminari, S. "et al". (2010). Nonpegylated liposomal doxorubicin (MyocetTM) combination (R-COMP) chemotherapy in elderly patients with diffuse large B-cell lymphoma (DLBCL): results from the phase II EUR018 trial. *Annals of Oncology*; Vol.21, No.7, pp.1492-9.

Lyu, Y.L., "et al". (2007) Topoisomerase IIbeta mediated DNA double-strand breaks: implications in doxorubicin cardiotoxicity and prevention by dexrazoxane. Cancer Res 2007;67:8839-46; Martin E, Thougaard AV, Grauslund M, et al. Evaluation of the topoisomerase II-inactive bisdioxopiperazine ICRF-161 as a protectant against doxorubicin-induced cardiomyopathy. *Toxicology*, Vol. 255, pp.72-79.

Martino R, "et al". (2002). Cyclophosphamide, pegylated liposomal doxorubicin (Caelyx), vincristine and prednisone (CCOP) in elderly patients with diffuse large B-cell lymphoma: results from a prospective phase II study. *Haematologica*, Vol.87, pp.822-7.

Menna, P. " et al". (2008) Anthracycline Cardiotoxicity. *Topics in Current Chemistry*, Vol. 283, pp 21-44.

Minotti G, "et al". (2004). Anthracyclines: molecular advances and pharmacologic developments in antitumor activity and cardiotoxicity. Pharmacological Reviews, Vol.56, No.2, pp.185-229.

Minotti G, "et al". (2008) Anthracyclines. In: Encyclopedic Reference of Molecular Pharmacology (S. Offermanns and W. Rosenthal, eds.). Springer.

Minotti, G.; Salvatorelli, E. & Menna, P. (2010). Pharmacological Foundations of Cardio-Oncology. *Journal of Pharmacology and Experimental Therapeutics*, Vol. 334, pp. 2-8.

Muthu, M.S. & Feng, S.S. (2010). Nanopharmacology of liposomes developed for cancer therapy. *Nanomedicine*, Vol.5, No.7, pp.1017-1019.

Nakamae, H. "et al". (2005) Notable effects of angiotensin II receptor blocker, valsartan, on acute cardiotoxic changes after standard chemotherapy with cyclophosphamide, doxorubicin, vincristine, and prednisolone. *Cancer*, Vol. 104, pp. 2492-2498.

Rabbani, A.; Finn, R.M. & Ausió, J. (2005) The anthracycline antibiotics: antitumor drugs that alter chromatin structure. *Bioassays*, Vol. 27, No.1, pp.50-6.

Rifkin, R.M. "et al". (2006) Pegylated liposomal doxorubicin, vincristine, and dexamethasone provide significant reduction in toxicity compared with doxorubicin, vincristine, and dexamethasone in patients with newly diagnosed multiple myeloma: a Phase III multicenter randomized trial. *Cancer*, Vol.106, pp. 848-58.

Rigacci L., "et al". (2007). Liposome-encapsulated doxorubicin in combination with cyclophosphamide, vincristine, prednisone and rituximab in patients with lymphoma and concurrent cardiac diseases or pre-treated with anthracyclines. *Hematological Oncology*, Vol. 25, No.4, pp 198-203.

Robert, J. & Gianni, L. (1993) Pharmacokinetics and metabolism of anthracyclines. *Cancer Surv*, Vol.17, pp 219-252.

Salvatorelli, E. "et al". (2009) Doxorubicinolone formation and efflux: a salvage pathway against epirubicin accumulation in human heart. *Journal of Pharmacology and Experimental Therapeutics*, vol. 329, pp 175-184.

Salvatorelli, E. "et al". (2007). Defective taxane stimulation of epirubicinol formation in the human heart: Insight into the cardiac tolerability of epirubicin-taxane chemotherapies *Journal of Pharmacology and Experimental Therapeutics*, Vol.320, pp. 790-800.

Schuchter, L.M. "et al". (2002) American Society of Clinical Oncology Chemotherapy and Radiotherapy Expert Panel. 2002 update of recommendations for the use of chemotherapy and radiotherapy protectants: clinical practice guidelines of the American Society of Clinical Oncology. *Journal of Clinical Oncology*, Vol.20, pp.2895–2903.

Sissung, T.M. "et al". Impact of ABCB1 allelic variants on QTc interval prolongation. *Clinical Cancer Research*, Vol. 17, pp. 937-946.

Soloman, R. & Gabizon, A.A. (2008). Clinical pharmacology of liposomal anthracyclines: focus on pegylated liposomal Doxorubicin. *Clinical Lymphoma Myeloma*, Vol.8, No.1, pp. 21-32.

Symon, Z. "et al". (1999) Selective delivery of doxorubicin to patients with breast carcinoma metastases by stealth liposomes. *Cancer*, Vol. 86, pp. 72–78.

Sterba, M "et al". (2006). Cardio protective effects of a novel iron chelator, pyridoxal 2-chlorobenzoylhydrazone, in the rabbit model of daunorubicin-induced cardiotoxicity. *Journal of Pharmacology and Experimental Therapy*, Vol. 319,No. 3, pp. 1336-1347

Swain, S.M. "et al". (1997). Cardioprotection with dexrazoxane for doxorubicin-containing therapy in advanced breast cancer. *Journal of Clinical Oncology*, Vol. 15,pp. 1318-1332.

Swain, S.M. Whaley, F.S. & Ewer, M.S. (2003) Congestive heart failure in patients treated with doxorubicin: a retrospective analysis of three trials. *Cancer*, Vol.97, pp. 2869–2879.

Swain, S.M. and Vici, P. (2004). The current and future role of dexrazoxane as a cardioprotectant in anthracycline treatment: expert panel review. *Journal of Cancer Research in Clinical Oncology*, vol.130,pp.1-7

Swerdlow, A.J. "et al". (2007). Myocardial infarction mortality risk after treatment for Hodgkin disease: a collaborative British cohort study. *Journal of the National Cancer Institute*, Vol.99, pp. 206-214.

Tulpule, A. "et al". (2006). Phase I/II trial of nonpegylated liposomal doxorubicin, cyclophosphamide, vincristine, and prednisone in the treatment of newly diagnosed aggressive non-Hodgkin's lymphoma. *Clinical Lymphoma Myeloma*, Vol.7, No.1, pp. 59-64.

van Dalen, E.C. "et al". (2010). Different anthracycline derivates for reducing cardiotoxicity in cancer patients. *Cochrane Database Syst Rev*, Vol 12, CD005006.

van Dalen, E.C. "et al". (2011). Cardioprotective interventions for cancer patients receiving anthracyclines. *Cochrane Database Systematic Reviews*, Vol.6: CD003917

Visani, G. "et al". (2008). R-COMP 21 for frail elderly patients with aggressive B-cell non-Hodgkin lymphoma: a pilot study. *Leukemia & Lymphoma*, Vol.49, No.6, pp.1081-6.

Visani, G. "et al". (2005) Cyclophosphamide, pegylated liposomal doxorubicin, vincristine and prednisone (CDOP) plus rituximab is effective and well tolerated in poor performance status elderly patients with non-Hodgkin's lymphoma. *Leukemia & Lymphoma*, Vol.46, No.3, pp.477-479.

Visani, G. & Isidori, A. (2009). Nonpegylated liposomal doxorubicin in the treatment of B-cell non-Hodgkin's lymphoma: where we stand. *Expert Reviews on Anticancer Therapy*, Vol.9, No.3, pp.357-63.

Vrooman, L.M. " et al". (2011). The low incidence of secondary acute myelogenous leukaemia in children and adolescents treated with dexrazoxane for acute lymphoblastic leukaemia: a report from the Dana-Farber Cancer Institute ALL Consortium. *European Journal of Cancer*, Vol. 47, pp.1373-1379.

Weiss, R.B. (1992). The anthracyclines: will we ever find a better doxorubicin? *Semin Oncol.* 19(6):670-86.

Wollina, U. "et al". (2003) Multicenter study of pegylated liposomal doxorubicin in patients with cutaneous T-cell lymphoma. *Cancer,* Vol. 98, pp. 993-1001.

Zucchi, R. & Danesi, R. (2003) Cardiac toxicity of antineoplastic anthracyclines. *Current Medicinal Chemistry - Anti-Cancer Agents,* Vol.3, No.2, pp.151-71.

10

Cardiotonic Steroids and Cardiac Fibrosis

Sandeep Vetteth, Deepak Malhotra and Joseph I. Shapiro
University of Toledo
United States of America

1. Introduction

It is well known and has been shown that patients who have chronic renal failure tend to develop and die of cardiac causes. These patients are known to develop a cardiomyopathy that is characterized by left ventricular hypertrophy and significant diastolic dysfunction. It has also been shown that the chronic renal failure condition is characterized by significant sodium pump inhibition due to increases in the circulating levels of cardiotonic steroids (CTS) such as marinobufagenin (MBG). In this review we will try to elucidate the mechanisms involved in the pathogenesis of uremic cardiomyopathy and the role of CTS in the pathogenesis as well as the possible areas of therapeutic interventions.

2. Renal failure and cardiotonic steroids

The current treatment of patients with end stage renal failure is complicated by the tremendous cardiovascular mortality associated with it. Such patients tend to develop a cardiomyopathy characterized by marked diastolic dysfunction and left ventricular hypertrophy (LVH). These patients also have substantial increases in the circulating levels of CTS (Mohmand, Malhotra et al. 2005). Perhaps of greater importance, it has more recently been shown that patients with more modest degrees of chronic renal insufficiency have markedly worse outcomes in high cardiovascular risk settings as well as a substantial worsening of cardiovascular risk (Alsheikh-Ali, Trikalinos et al. 2011; Kreuz, Horlbeck et al. 2011)

It was proposed nearly 4 decades ago that there is accumulation of CTS in chronic renal failure that causes the inhibition of the Na/K ATPase. The patients with chronic renal failure developed some antibodies to digoxin and had false positive digoxin levels even though these patients had not been treated with digitalis (Graves 1986; Graves and Williams 1987). More recently using more definitive analytical techniques several of these CTS have been characterized. These include ouabain (Hamlyn, Blaustein et al. 1991) which is a cardenolide and marinobufagenin (MBG) and telocinobufagin (TBG) (Bagrov and Fedorova 1998; Komiyama, Dong et al. 2005) which are bufadienolides. These CTS have been considered only as drugs until recently as studies now indicate that these compounds are secreted in the body and regulated by multiple physiological stimuli such as ACTH and angiotensin II (Fedorova, Agalakova et al. 2005; Bagrov, Shapiro et al. 2009). They have also been found to play an important role in renal salt handling as well as the regulation of cardiac contractility and vascular tone (Hamlyn, Blaustein et al. 1991; Fedorova, Doris et al.

1998). Recently, many other functions of these endogenous ligands of the Na/K-ATPase have been proposed.
The mechanism of elevation of these CTS possibly includes a combination of decreased elimination and increased production, but one would anticipate an elevation as it was initially thought that the these hormones functioned as natriuretic hormones since the Na/K ATPase comprises a major sodium transporting mechanism in the kidney (de Wardener, Clarkson et al. 1971). Increases in sodium levels would be caused by decreased renal elimination due to loss of renal function. It has also been thought that the increases in the CTS effect vasoconstriction by inhibition of Na/K ATPase causing coupled activation of the Na/Ca exchanger in the vascular smooth muscles (Jaitovich and Bertorello 2010). Bricker and colleagues postulated that in order to maintain sodium homeostasis in renal failure, increases in circulating CTS were necessary, but the effects of CTS on other tissues other than the kidneys explained many of the clinical features seen in renal failure. This was termed as the trade off hypothesis for the pathogenesis of the 'uremic syndrome' (Bricker and Fine 1978) and is illustrated in figure 1. Now it is well known that the reduced pump activity has been seen in red cells, white blood cells, transporting epithelia, muscle cells, adipocytes and the cardiomyocytes (Stokes, Willcocks et al. 1986; Okamoto 1988; Takahashi, Nishimura et al. 1989; Mimura, Makino et al. 1992; Periyasamy, Chen et al. 2001).

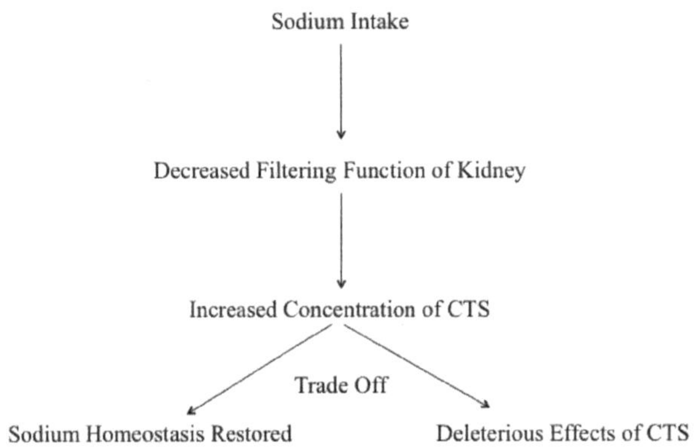

Fig. 1. Illustration of the role of cardiotonic steroids (CTS) in "trade off." With decreased filtering function, CTS concentrations increase to maintain sodium homeostasis, but these elevated hormone levels have adverse effects on different tissues.

Ouabain the prototypical CTS described in 1991 by Hamlyn and colleagues (Hamlyn, Blaustein et al. 1991) was initially thought to function as the natriuretic peptide responsible for the effects seen. However it is well known now that ouabain has high affinity to the alpha 2 and 3 isoforms of Na/K ATPase where as rat tubular cells mainly express the alpha 1 isoform which is relatively insensitive to ouabain (Sweadner 1989). However in humans the sensitivity of the different isoforms to ouabain seems to be not that significant (Croyle, Woo et al. 1997; Lingrel 2010). It is now known that ouabain probably has a more neuro-hormonal function and has been isolated from the hypothalamus and the hippocampus (Kawamura, Guo et al. 1999; Fedorova, Zhuravin et al. 2007). A new body of evidence is emerging that brain ouabain may play important role in pathogenesis of salt sensitive hypertension (Fedorova, Zhuravin et al. 2007).

More recently other CTS have been described such as MBG and TBG, which has a structure very similar to that of MBG (Bagrov, Roukoyatkina et al. 1993; Komiyama, Dong et al. 2005). They were seen to be elevated significantly in plasma of ESRD patients. The bufadienolides were first described from the skin of amphibians such as the marine toad (Bufo marinus) (Bagrov, Shapiro et al. 2009) and MBG emerged as the most important contender since it has the affinity towards the alpha 1 isoform which is the isoform present almost exclusively in the mammalian tubules. MBG at low doses also causes vasoconstriction in isolated human blood vessels (Bagrov, Roukoyatkina et al. 1995). Bagrov and colleagues have demonstrated that the levels of MBG are elevated in response to both salt loading and in the presence of experimental renal failure (Fedorova, Agalakova et al. 2005). They have also demonstrated the role of ouabain as a neuro-hormone by intra-hippocampal administration of ouabain and demonstrating an increase in the plasma and urine concentration of MBG as well as increased natriuresis from this (Fedorova, Agalakova et al. 2005). Also it has been shown that the synthesis of these CTS occurs in the mammalian adrenal cells; however the specific metabolic steps in this biosynthesis are still unknown (Dmitrieva, Bagrov et al. 2000).

3. Signaling though the sodium pump

Signaling though the sodium pump has been studied extensively in the recent years and our knowledge about the process has considerably increased. It is well known that there is more than just the 'classical enzymatic inhibition' causing increases in cytosolic sodium (Jaitovich and Bertorello 2010). One concern is that the circulating levels of CTS seen in pathological conditions do not appear to cause extensive inhibition of the pump in vitro and in vivo (Bagrov, Shapiro et al. 2009). In fact, the growth regulatory effects of CTS are seen even at nano and sub-nano molar concentrations, which do not cause any demonstrable inhibition of the pump activity (Aydemir-Koksoy, Abramowitz et al. 2001; Aydemir-Koksoy and Allen 2001; Saunders and Scheiner-Bobis 2004; Khundmiri, Metzler et al. 2006; Qiu, Gao et al. 2007). Another concern is that it has been difficult if not impossible to demonstrate changes in cytosolic sodium caused by physiological and even pharmacological concentrations of CTS. Perhaps more troubling, small increases in the cytosolic sodium levels caused by pump inhibition would be expected to minimize effects on net Na/K-ATPase activity by mass action as cytosolic Na is generally maintained at concentrations where it can actually regulate pump activity. Last but most significantly, sodium ionophores do not cause the biological effects of CTS (Liu, Tian et al. 2000; Oweis, Wu et al. 2006).

While the classical pathway of pump inhibition may still explain some of the effects of CTS, a novel signal cascade involving the Na/K-ATPase residing in specific membrane environments has been proposed and documented by Xie and others (Li and Xie 2009). This research performed on neonatal rat cardiac myocytes showed that ouabain caused the Na/K ATPase to interact with neighboring membrane proteins and caused cytosolic cascades of signaling. The administration of ouabain to the cardiomyocytes caused an increase in reactive oxygen species (ROS) (Liu, Tian et al. 2000). It was seen from the experiments that first there was phosphorylation of Src and leading to the activation of Ras. This trans-activated the EGFR and triggered a signaling cascade that led to the production of ROS (Haas, Askari et al. 2000; Liu, Tian et al. 2000; Kometiani, Askari et al. 2001; Haas, Wang et al. 2002; Wang, Haas et al. 2004; Tian, Cai et al. 2006). Also it has been shown that these ROS were key in the signaling function of Na/K ATPase. The administration of N Acetyl Cysteine (NAC) or green tea extract which act as ROS quenchers blocked the gene transcription effects of CTS (Xie, Kometiani et al. 1999; Liu, Tian et al. 2000; Priyadarshi, Valentine et al. 2003; Elkareh, Kennedy et al. 2007). At present it is unclear as to how ROS effect downstream signaling. One possibility albeit unproven is that the Na/K ATPase itself may serve as a receptor for the ROS enhancing its sensitivity by conformational change. Further work in this exciting area is currently underway. Development of ROS in response to sodium pump signaling is shown in figure 2.

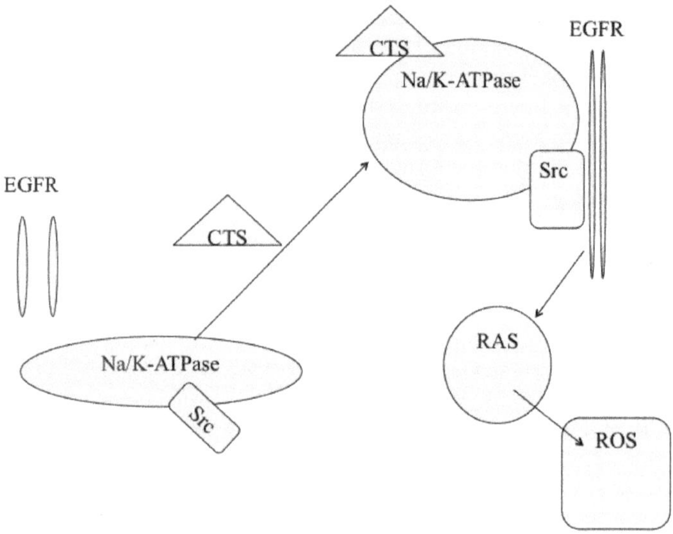

Fig. 2. Schematic showing how cardiotonic steroids (CTS) change the conformation of the Na/K-ATPase residing in caveolae or lipid rafts, allowing Src to transactivate the EGFR and cause signal transduction through RAS resulting in the generation of reactive oxygen species (ROS).

Several studies have shown that low concentrations of ouabain have stimulated tyrosine phosphorylation of several proteins in a variety of cells including cardiac myocytes, HeLa and LLC-PK1 cells (Kometiani, Li et al. 1998; Contreras, Shoshani et al. 1999; Haas, Askari et al. 2000; Aydemir-Koksoy, Abramowitz et al. 2001; Kometiani, Liu et al. 2005; Kotova, Al-Khalili et al. 2006; Kotova, Galuska et al. 2006). Importantly the addition of tyrosine kinase inhibitors like herbimycin A and genistein, blocked ouabain induced tyrosine phosphorylation and subsequently the downstream effects in these cultured cells (Haas, Askari et al. 2000; Aydemir-Koksoy, Abramowitz et al. 2001). Tyrosine phosphorylation can occur in one of two ways, either by activation of tyrosine kinases or by inhibition of tyrosine phosphatases or a combination of both. The Na/K ATPase does not have intrinsic tyrosine kinase activity. It is interesting that even though the alpha subunit has a phosphatase activity, preliminary studies suggest that it does not have significant tyrosine phosphatase activity (Li and Xie 2009). However, it has clearly been shown that ligands extrinsic to the Na/K-ATPase signal cascade can stimulate tyrosine kinase activity by employing receptors without any intrinsic tyrosine kinase activity (Ihle and Kerr 1995; McGarrigle and Huang 2007). One such demonstrated pathway is the G protein coupled receptors (GPCRs) that employ the Src family of kinases (McGarrigle and Huang 2007). It was hence postulated that the Src family of kinases could play a role in the ouabain induced tyrosine phosphorylation (McGarrigle and Huang 2007).

Studies done by Haas et al. have indeed shown that Src is involved in the phosphorylation of proteins in CTS signaling. These studies showed that ouabain caused stimulation of Src in cardiac myocytes as well as LLC-PK1 cells. Inhibition of Src blocked the ouabain-induced phosphorylation and abolished the downstream signaling including the activation of ERK (Haas, Askari et al. 2000; Haas, Wang et al. 2002). Furthermore there is sufficient evidence for the fact the Na/K ATPase interacts with Src and forms a functional receptor complex. These workers observed that the pump and Src could be co-localized in the caveolar fractions in several different types of cells. Also immunofluorescence showed the co-localization of these two in the plasma membrane. Both the proteins could also be co-immunoprecipitated by using antibodies to either alpha 1 and to Src. Fluorescence resonance energy transfer (FRET) has also shown these two proteins to be in close proximity (Liu, Mohammadi et al. 2003; Wang, Haas et al. 2004; Liang, Cai et al. 2006; Tian, Cai et al. 2006). They have also showed that the interaction between the Na/K ATPase and Src keeps Src in an inactive state. It was seen that when ouabain binds to the sodium pump it reduced the binding of the Src Kinase domain. This freeing of the Src kinase domain possibly results in the activation of the Na/K ATPase associated Src kinase (Tian, Cai et al. 2006). Additionally experiments were done to see if the loss or knockdown of Na/K ATPase would release the interacting Src and increase in tyrosine kinase activity. Graded knockdown of LLC-PK1 cells with alpha 1 specific siRNA was achieved and Src activity was studied. It was seen that the knockdown of the pump resulted in an increase in basal Src activity in an alpha 1 amount dependent manner. Tyrosine phosphorylation of several protein molecules was also increased secondary to this. Moreover stimulation of these cells with ouabain failed to stimulate Src and ERK 1 and 2 any further. When these knockdown cells were rescued with rat alpha 1, it restored Src to its basal levels and allowed for stimulation of the complex at higher levels of Ouabain as would be expected with the differences in sensitivity of rat versus pig alpha 1 (Liang, Cai et al. 2006).

It is also known that the binding of ouabain to the receptor complex leads to the recruitment and transactivation of the EGFR. This was due to the Src dependent phosphorylation of the EGFR at sites other than the major auto-phosphorylation site Y1173. The transactivated EGFR in turn recruited Shc to the complex and resulted in the activation of the Ras/Raf/MEK/ERK cascade (Haas, Askari et al. 2000; Aydemir-Koksoy, Abramowitz et al. 2001; Haas, Wang et al. 2002; Kotova, Al-Khalili et al. 2006). Further studies have shown that once the Src Na/K ATPase complex has been activated it leads to the synthesis of ROS, which has been thought of as a second messenger. It has been demonstrated by Xie and coworkers that exposure of myocytes to ouabain causes a rapid increase in the generation of ROS. These ROS were demonstrated with the help of a fluorescence dye CMDCF. The generation of the ROS was prevented by pre-treatment of the cells to anti-oxidants such as N Acetyl Cysteine (NAC) and Vitamin E. By studying the blockade of the downstream signaling it was seen that ROS is involved with the signaling causing stimulation of Ras, activation of p42/44 mitogen-activated protein kinases, induction of genes for skeletal muscle actin and atrial natriuretic peptide and the activation and translocation of the transcription factor NF-κB among several other effects (Xie, Kometiani et al. 1999). Since a lot of these are calcium dependent steps further experiments were done to see if the ROS production was calcium dependent as well. Ouabain caused the production of ROS in myocytes that were stimulated in culture media that were calcium deficient. This indicated that the production of ROs was calcium independent and possibly the increases in calcium was due to a parallel mechanism from the inhibition of the sodium pump activity (Liu, Tian et al. 2000)

Sites of generation and targets of ROS are currently being worked out, with clues in favor of Ras activation induced mitochondrial production (Liu, Tian et al. 2000)however other components of the downstream signaling including the involvement of PLC, PI3K and PKC have been established. Src activation led to the stimulation of PLC gamma and subsequently the activation of PKC and PI3 mediated calcium signaling. Moreover it was seen that ouabain also stimulates PI3K which works with PKC to cause endocytosis of this sodium pump complex. This probably is the explanation for how the signal transduction is eventually terminated. (Tian, Liu et al. 2003; Liu, Liang et al. 2005; Yuan, Cai et al. 2005; Pierre, Yang et al. 2007; Chen, Cai et al. 2008; Elkareh, Periyasamy et al. 2009).

This signaling pathway may link to Bricker's concept of CTS as a natriuretic hormone. Specifically, our group has noted that CTS induce endocytosis of the Na/K-ATPase in kidney tissues. In chronically salt loaded Sprague-Dawley rats, renal MBG excretion was significantly elevated and anti-MBG antibody reduced natriuresis and restored sodium pump activity in the renal cortex (Periyasamy, Liu et al. 2005). The same study demonstrated that in addition to the direct inhibition of the Na/K-ATPase, MBG is capable to exhibit its natriuretic via internalization of the sodium pump in the proximal tubule (Periyasamy, Liu et al. 2005). The endocytosis of the proximal tubular Na/K-ATPase induced by CTS has been shown to proceed through clathrin coated pits and require PI3K activation as well as the plasmalemmal pump being in the context of caveolae as well as signaling through the Src-EGFR pathway (Liu, Kesiry et al. 2004; Liu, Liang et al. 2005). Further work demonstrated that CTS could induce decreases in the apical expression of one of the plasma membrane Na^+/H^+ exchanger, NHE3 (Oweis, Wu et al. 2006; Liu and Shapiro 2007). Taken together, these data suggest that increases in the circulating levels of MBG accompany salt loading, which, in turn, may induce decreases in both basolateral and apical sodium transport in the proximal tubule.

4. Uremic cardiomyopathy

It is a well-known fact that cardiovascular mortality accounts for more that 50% of all deaths in patients with renal failure. It is seen that this mortality is more attributed to cardiac failure and sudden cardiac death than coronary events (Sarnak, Levey et al. 2003; Weiner, Tighiouart et al. 2004). Available data also suggests that pre end stage renal disease (ESRD) patients have cardiac mortality rates very similar to that of ESRD patients (Stack and Bloembergen 2001; Paparello, Kshirsagar et al. 2002; Sarnak 2003; Sarnak, Levey et al. 2003). Echocardiography has shown that diastolic dysfunction and LVH are both very common in ESRD patients on dialysis and other patients with chronic kidney disease (Harnett, Parfrey et al. 1988; Mitsnefes, Daniels et al. 2001; Stack and Saran 2002). Systolic dysfunction in these patients is less uniformly demonstrable (Raj, D'Mello et al. 1997) and it has been shown that development of LVH may be a predictor of higher mortality in dialysis patients (Nakazato, Kawada et al. 2002; Tyralla and Amann 2003) as this correlates with the development of cardiac arrhythmias.

Of late myocardial fibrosis that was described in uremia as early as 1943 by Rossle and then described again by Ritz et al. seems to play a very important role in the pathogenesis (Mall, Huther et al. 1990). It has been shown by the same group that the fibrosis occurred early after subtotal nephrectomy without myocardial necrosis suggesting a reactive fibrosis rather than a reparative fibrosis. It was seen that the interstitial volume density increased at the expense of capillary volume and this caused the swelling of the cytoplasm and nuclei of the interstitial cells where as the endothelial cells remained unchanged (Mall, Rambausek et al. 1988). The cardiac fibrosis can explain the abnormalities in the left ventricular compliance causing diastolic dysfunction as well as inhomogeneity in the electrical conduction causing arrhythmias. The factors thought to be involved in the genesis of myocardial fibrosis and LVH include anemia, hypertension, hyperparathyroidism, cardiotonic steroids, oxidative stress and the activation of the RAS aldosterone system.

Of the above-mentioned factors anemia seems to be the weakest to be implicated in uremic cardiomyopathy. Only a very modest improvement in LVH to the tune of 10-20% has been seen with sustained increases in hematocrit (Foley, Parfrey et al. 2000). Also the LVH seen is concentric in nature which is not what would be expected with anemia (Harnett, Parfrey et al. 1988). Interestingly erythropoietin therapy worsened LVH possibly because of worsening BP control (Minagawa, Hirano et al. 1994).

Among the several implicated factors hypertension seems to be the factor in chronic renal failure that is best linked to LVH (Huting and Alpert 1992; Morduchowicz, Zabludowski et al. 1993; Harnett and Parfrey 1994). Although there is sufficient evidence to prove that hypertension causes LVH, it does not account for the frequency and severity of LVH seen in ESRD patients (Huting and Alpert 1992; Foley and Parfrey 1998; Nishikimi, Minami et al. 2001). Hence this points to the presence of other factors in the pathogenesis. However hypertension must be aggressively pursued in patients with renal failure as treatment has resulted in a modest amelioration of LVH (Dyadyk, Bagriy et al. 1997).

It also seems that the activation of the renin angiotensin aldosterone axis seems to be a factor independent of hypertension. Experimental studies by Diez et al. and Ritz et al. have shown that the activation of this system in involved in the genesis of cardiac fibrosis (Amann, Simonaviciene et al. 2001; Diez, Lopez et al. 2001; Diez 2004; Gonzalez, Lopez et al. 2004). In conjunction with this Pirola et al. have also shown that angiotensin II also stimulated the release of PTH (Pirola, Wang et al. 1993; Okano, Wu et al. 1994) and in the next section we will discuss how PTH seems to be an important factor in causing fibrosis and LVH. It has been shown that treatment with ACE inhibitors causes regression of LVH independent of hypotensive effects (Cannella, Paoletti et al. 1997; Dyadyk, Bagriy et al. 1997; Vlahakos, Hahalis et al. 1997). This lends more credibility to the idea that cardiac fibrosis may be an important factor in the pathogenesis of uremic cardiomyopathy.

Hyperparathyroidism has been proposed to be a factor as it causes abnormalities in cardiac energy metabolism and growth. Calcium ions are very important for the myocardial excitation contraction coupling and the cardiac contraction and relaxation. The release of calcium from the sarcoplasmic reticulum is the key step in the initiation of the coupling. Dissociation and sequestration of the calcium by an energy dependent pump like SERCA produces relaxation. The intracellular calcium homeostasis seems to be maintained by the membrane bound Na/Ca exchanger and SERCA which in turn is dependent on Na/K ATPase and Na/H exchanger (Morgan 1991). Both parathyroid hormone (PTH) and Parathyroid hormone related peptide (PTHrP) have been shown to acutely increase the force of contraction in isolated beating rat cardiac myocytes (Wang, Wu et al. 1993; Smogorzewski 1995). PTH excess in uremic patients has also been shown to increase cytosolic calcium levels that were correlated with the plasma PTH concentrations. These were also shown to be corrected with parathyroidectomy (PTX) (Raine, Bedford et al. 1993). Even though increased calcium entry has been thought to be the most important step in sustaining high intra myocyte calcium concentrations reductions in the NA/K ATPase and Na/H exchange rates suggesting impaired calcium extrusion may contribute to altered cellular calcium homeostasis (Smogorzewski 1995). Parathyroid hormone (PTH) now is known to cause increased endocytosis of Na/K ATPase and this may amplify CTS mediated signaling through the sodium pump (Khundmiri, Bertorello et al. 2004). Baczynski el al. have also reported that there is uncoupling of the oxidative phosphorylation and inhibited myocardial energy production in isolated myocardial mitochondria which may further this problem (Baczynski, Massry et al. 1985).

In humans with ESRD the presence of secondary hyperparathyroidism has been shown to be associated with increased myocardial calcium content and impaired systolic and diastolic functions. However these changes have not consistently been seen to improve with PTX suggesting that in the long term these changes induced by PTH become irreversible or there are other factors contributing to the myocardial dysfunction that are more important than just PTH excess (Drueke, Fauchet et al. 1980; Rostand, Sanders et al. 1988; Coratelli, Buongiorno et al. 1989; Ohara, Hiramatsu et al. 1995; Rostand and Drueke 1999). In reference to this the presence of 1,25 (OH)2 D3 receptors have been confirmed on the myocardial cells and the administration of Vitamin D in ESRD patients seems to correct the cardiac dysfunction either by correcting the excessive secretion of PTH or by a Vitamin D dependent process in the cardiac cells (Coratelli, Petrarulo et al. 1984; Shane, Mancini et al. 1997).

Our group has focused attention on CTS in the pathogenesis of uremic cardiomyopathy. Along with acute impairment of relaxation in normal adult rat cardiomyocytes when exposed to MBG (Periyasamy, Chen et al. 2001) experimental chronic renal failure induced in rats by 5/6th nephrectomy (Kennedy, Elkareh et al. 2008) causes a cardiomyopathy that is very similar to clinical chronic renal failure. It has been observed that LVH develops quite early and this is accompanied by impaired myocyte relaxation causing diastolic dysfunction. It seems that this impaired relaxation is associated with a significant down regulation of SERCA2a mRNA (Kennedy, Omran et al. 2003; Kennedy, Vetteth et al. 2006), which is known to be responsible for the rapid reduction of cytosolic calcium after systole (Bassani, Bassani et al. 1995; Bers, Bassani et al. 1996; Kennedy, Vetteth et al. 2006). Left ventricular catheterization in 5/6th nephrectomized rats at 4 weeks and calculation of dP/dT for relaxation indicated the presence of significant diastolic dysfunction (Kennedy, Vetteth et al. 2006). LVH was also demonstrated in these hearts by echocardiography as well as increases in heart weights and left ventricular end systolic volumes. There were also increases in the posterior wall thickness. Interestingly the LVH and diastolic dysfunction were also present in rats that were just infused MBG using an intra-peritoneal pump, and tended to resolve in animals immunized with an MBG-BSA conjugate that resulted in high titer specific response to MBG (Kennedy, Vetteth et al. 2006).

The animal studies done to reproduce the phenotype of cardiomyopathy by infusing with MBG so as to achieve plasma levels of MBG consistent with renal failure as well as induction of experimental renal failure by 5/6th nephrectomy, both interestingly revealed a significant amount of cardiac fibrosis in both the rat and the mouse. Also active immunization against the

MBG as discussed above as well as reduction of MBG levels by adrenalectomy prevented the onset of cardiac fibrosis seen in these animals. The heart tissue from these animals also showed evidence of activation of Na/K ATPase signaling as seen by increases in Src and MAPK phosphorylation. It was also demonstrated that there was significant increases in oxidant stress in the heart and other tissues (Kennedy, Vetteth et al. 2006). This noted fibrosis seems to play a significant role in the pathogenesis of uremic cardiomyopathy.

The above studies prompted in-vitro studies on fibroblast in order to see the effects of MBG and other CTS such as ouabain. It was seen that in fibroblast cultures grown to confluence there was increased proline incorporation as well as increased collagen production. There was also evidence of activation of Na/K ATPase signaling as there was increased Src and MAPK activation. Interestingly there was evidence of increases in oxidant stress and the scavenging of these ROS resulted in the inhibition of the Src pathway as well as prevented the increases in proline incorporation and collagen synthesis (Elkareh, Kennedy et al. 2007).

It has been further established that this fibrosis is dependent on the down regulation of Fli-1, which is a negative regulator of collagen synthesis (Czuwara-Ladykowska, Shirasaki et al. 2001). MBG was seen to induce decreases in Fli-1 expression in cardiac and renal fibroblasts, which was dependent on the nuclear translocation of PKC delta from the cytoplasm. This translocation seems to be necessary for the phosphorylation and degradation of the Fli-1 (Elkareh, Periyasamy et al. 2009). This is illustrated in figure 3.

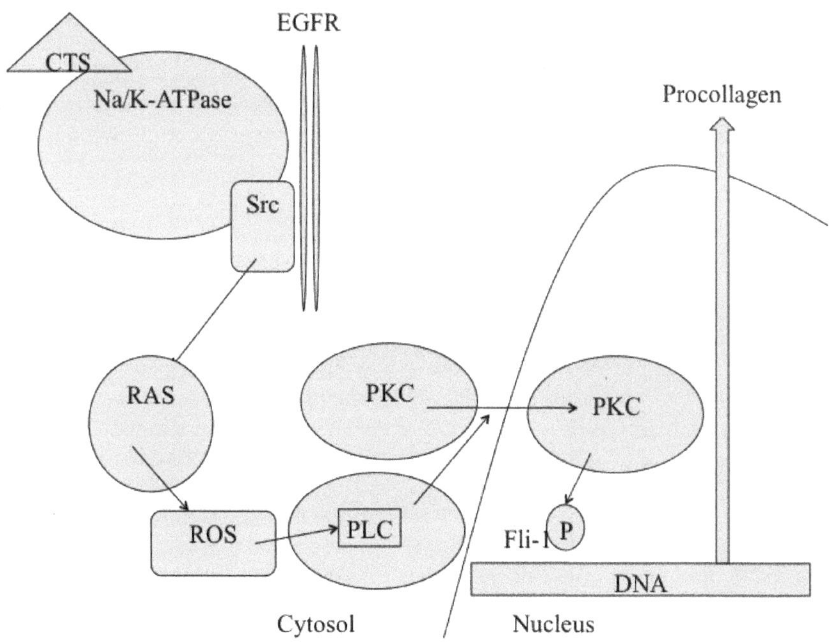

Fig. 3. Schematic showing how the signal cascade caused by cardiotonic steroids (CTS) causes the activation of phospholipase C (PLC) which then causes the translocation of protein kinase C (PKC, delta isoform) to the nucleus where it phosphorylates Fli-1. The phosphorylated Fli-1 is then rapidly degraded allowing for the disinhibition of procollagen synthesis and tissue fibrosis.

Since mineralocorticoid antagonists have been shown to ameliorate cardiac fibrosis, studies using spironolactone and canrenone have shown that both cause significant attenuation of fibrosis in-vivo as caused by experimental renal failure. Both these compounds also seemed to act as competitive inhibitors of CTS binding to Na/K ATPase and hence prevent MBG signaling (Tian, Shidyak et al. 2009). The role of CTS is thus clear in the pathogenesis of cardiac dysfunction with respect to calcium handling and the genesis of fibrosis.
The presence of oxidative stress in the ESRD patients has been well documented (Fiorillo, Oliviero et al. 1998; Tetta, Biasioli et al. 1999). Most of the reactive oxygen species are produced by the mitochondria and a dysfunction in the mitochondria has been discussed above. Oxidative stress has been well known to affect cardiovascular function, cause endothelial dysfunction and hence promote atherosclerosis as well as cause increases in sympathetic activity (Miyazaki, Matsuoka et al. 2000; Wolf 2000; Zanzinger and Czachurski 2000; Himmelfarb, Stenvinkel et al. 2002). Reactive aldehydes measured as carbonyl compounds can be formed as the end product of various oxidative reactions and have been shown to be elevated in uremia. These result in the formation of advanced glycation end products (AGE). These reactive aldehydes and AGE have been demonstrated in the pathogenesis of vascular dysfunction as well as fibrosis (Uchida 2000; Amann, Tornig et al. 2002). The interaction of the AGE with specific receptors have also shown to increase the production of IL-6 and thus increasing the production of CRP in the liver and thereby propagating inflammation (Himmelfarb, Stenvinkel et al. 2002). Increases in CRP have a strong negative correlation with the levels of plasma tocopherol as shown by Thevenin et al. (Nguyen-Khoa, Massy et al. 2001) further showing that antioxidants are decreased in inflammation. Importantly it has been shown that tocopherol decreased fibrosis in the hearts of nephrectomized rats (Amann, Tornig et al. 2002). Hence chronic oxidative stress and damage seems to be an important mechanism in the pathogenesis of chronic inflammation and uremic cardiomyopathy.

5. Conclusion

Chronic renal failure is complicated by a cardiomyopathy that is characterized by LVH and diastolic dysfunction. CTS such as MBG are found in higher concentrations in the plasma of such patients. It is clear form several studies that these CTS are involved via signaling through Na/K ATPase in causing cardiomyocyte hypertrophy, impairing relaxation and inducing fibrosis by increased collagen synthesis, which seems to be dependent on increased oxidant stress. Other major factors possibly involved in the pathogenesis of this cardiomyopathy include hyperparathyroidism, chronic oxidant stress and the activation of the RAS aldosterone system.
However mechanisms involving CTS and PTH and the interaction of the two systems seem to be emerging as the foremost candidate involved in the pathogenesis of uremic cardiomyopathy and may present prime targets for therapeutic interventions in the future.

6. References

Alsheikh-Ali, A. A., T. A. Trikalinos, et al. (2011). "Risk of arrhythmic and nonarrhythmic death in patients with heart failure and chronic kidney disease." *American heart journal* 161(1): 204-209 e201.

Amann, K., A. Simonaviciene, et al. (2001). "Blood pressure-independent additive effects of pharmacologic blockade of the renin-angiotensin and endothelin systems on progression in a low-renin model of renal damage." *Journal of the American Society of Nephrology : JASN* 12(12): 2572-2584.

Amann, K., J. Tornig, et al. (2002). "Effect of antioxidant therapy with dl-alpha-tocopherol on cardiovascular structure in experimental renal failure." *Kidney international* 62(3): 877-884.

Aydemir-Koksoy, A., J. Abramowitz, et al. (2001). "Ouabain-induced signaling and vascular smooth muscle cell proliferation." *The Journal of biological chemistry* 276(49): 46605-46611.

Aydemir-Koksoy, A. and J. C. Allen (2001). "Low concentrations of ouabain induce vascular smooth muscle cell proliferation." *Cellular and molecular biology* 47(2): 341-345.

Baczynski, R., S. G. Massry, et al. (1985). "Effect of parathyroid hormone on myocardial energy metabolism in the rat." *Kidney international* 27(5): 718-725.

Bagrov, A. Y. and O. V. Fedorova (1998). "Effects of two putative endogenous digitalis-like factors, marinobufagenin and ouabain, on the Na+, K+-pump in human mesenteric arteries." *Journal of hypertension* 16(12 Pt 2): 1953-1958.

Bagrov, A. Y., N. I. Roukoyatkina, et al. (1993). "Digitalis-like and vasoconstrictor effects of endogenous digoxin-like factor(s) from the venom of Bufo marinus toad." *Eur J Pharmacol* 234(2-3): 165-172.

Bagrov, A. Y., N. I. Roukoyatkina, et al. (1995). "Effects of two endogenous Na+,K(+)-ATPase inhibitors, marinobufagenin and ouabain, on isolated rat aorta." *Eur J Pharmacol* 274(1-3): 151-158.

Bagrov, A. Y., J. I. Shapiro, et al. (2009). "Endogenous cardiotonic steroids: physiology, pharmacology, and novel therapeutic targets." *Pharmacol Rev* 61(1): 9-38.

Bassani, R. A., J. W. Bassani, et al. (1995). "Relaxation in ferret ventricular myocytes: role of the sarcolemmal Ca ATPase." *Pflugers Archiv : European journal of physiology* 430(4): 573-578.

Bers, D. M., J. W. Bassani, et al. (1996). "Na-Ca exchange and Ca fluxes during contraction and relaxation in mammalian ventricular muscle." *Annals of the New York Academy of Sciences* 779: 430-442.

Bricker, N. S. and L. G. Fine (1978). "Uremia: formulations and expectations. The trade-off hypothesis: current status." *Kidney international. Supplement*(8): S5-8.

Cannella, G., E. Paoletti, et al. (1997). "Prolonged therapy with ACE inhibitors induces a regression of left ventricular hypertrophy of dialyzed uremic patients independently from hypotensive effects." *American journal of kidney diseases : the official journal of the National Kidney Foundation* 30(5): 659-664.

Chen, Y., T. Cai, et al. (2008). "Regulation of inositol 1,4,5-trisphosphate receptor-mediated calcium release by the Na/K-ATPase in cultured renal epithelial cells." *J Biol Chem* 283(2): 1128-1136.

Contreras, R. G., L. Shoshani, et al. (1999). "Relationship between Na(+),K(+)-ATPase and cell attachment." *Journal of cell science* 112 (Pt 23): 4223-4232.

Coratelli, P., E. Buongiorno, et al. (1989). "Pathogenetic aspects of uremic cardiomyopathy." *Mineral and electrolyte metabolism* 15(4): 246-253.

Coratelli, P., F. Petrarulo, et al. (1984). "Improvement in left ventricular function during treatment of hemodialysis patients with 25-OHD3." *Contributions to nephrology* 41: 433-437.

Croyle, M. L., A. L. Woo, et al. (1997). "Extensive random mutagenesis analysis of the Na+/K+-ATPase alpha subunit identifies known and previously unidentified amino acid residues that alter ouabain sensitivity--implications for ouabain binding." *European journal of biochemistry / FEBS* 248(2): 488-495.

Czuwara-Ladykowska, J., F. Shirasaki, et al. (2001). "Fli-1 inhibits collagen type I production in dermal fibroblasts via an Sp1-dependent pathway." *J Biol Chem* 276(24): 20839-20848.

de Wardener, H. E., E. M. Clarkson, et al. (1971). "Evidence for a hormone other than aldosterone which controls urinary sodium excretion." *Adv Nephrol Necker Hosp* 1: 97-111.

Diez, J. (2004). "Profibrotic effects of angiotensin II in the heart: a matter of mediators." *Hypertension* 43(6): 1164-1165.

Diez, J., B. Lopez, et al. (2001). "Clinical aspects of hypertensive myocardial fibrosis." *Current opinion in cardiology* 16(6): 328-335.

Dmitrieva, R. I., A. Y. Bagrov, et al. (2000). "Mammalian bufadienolide is synthesized from cholesterol in the adrenal cortex by a pathway that Is independent of cholesterol side-chain cleavage." *Hypertension* 36(3): 442-448.

Drueke, T., M. Fauchet, et al. (1980). "Effect of parathyroidectomy on left-ventricular function in haemodialysis patients." *Lancet* 1(8160): 112-114.

Dyadyk, A. I., A. E. Bagriy, et al. (1997). "ACE inhibitors captopril and enalapril induce regression of left ventricular hypertrophy in hypertensive patients with chronic renal failure." *Nephrology, dialysis, transplantation : official publication of the European Dialysis and Transplant Association - European Renal Association* 12(5): 945-951.

Elkareh, J., D. J. Kennedy, et al. (2007). "Marinobufagenin stimulates fibroblast collagen production and causes fibrosis in experimental uremic cardiomyopathy." *Hypertension* 49(1): 215-224.

Elkareh, J., S. M. Periyasamy, et al. (2009). "Marinobufagenin induces increases in procollagen expression in a process involving protein kinase C and Fli-1: implications for uremic cardiomyopathy." *Am J Physiol Renal Physiol* 296(5): F1219-1226.

Fedorova, O. V., N. I. Agalakova, et al. (2005). "Brain ouabain stimulates peripheral marinobufagenin via angiotensin II signalling in NaCl-loaded Dahl-S rats." *J Hypertens* 23(8): 1515-1523.

Fedorova, O. V., P. A. Doris, et al. (1998). "Endogenous marinobufagenin-like factor in acute plasma volume expansion." *Clinical and experimental hypertension* 20(5-6): 581-591.

Fedorova, O. V., I. A. Zhuravin, et al. (2007). "Intrahippocampal microinjection of an exquisitely low dose of ouabain mimics NaCl loading and stimulates a bufadienolide Na/K-ATPase inhibitor." *J Hypertens* 25(9): 1834-1844.

Fiorillo, C., C. Oliviero, et al. (1998). "Oxidative stress and antioxidant defenses in renal patients receiving regular haemodialysis." *Clinical chemistry and laboratory medicine : CCLM / FESCC* 36(3): 149-153.

Foley, R. N. and P. S. Parfrey (1998). "Cardiovascular disease and mortality in ESRD." *Journal of nephrology* 11(5): 239-245.

Foley, R. N., P. S. Parfrey, et al. (2000). "Effect of hemoglobin levels in hemodialysis patients with asymptomatic cardiomyopathy." *Kidney international* 58(3): 1325-1335.

Gonzalez, A., B. Lopez, et al. (2004). "Fibrosis in hypertensive heart disease: role of the renin-angiotensin-aldosterone system." *The Medical clinics of North America* 88(1): 83-97.

Graves, S. W. (1986). "Endogenous digitalis-like factors." *Critical reviews in clinical laboratory sciences* 23(3): 177-200.

Graves, S. W. and G. H. Williams (1987). "Endogenous digitalis-like natriuretic factors." *Annual review of medicine* 38: 433-444.

Haas, M., A. Askari, et al. (2000). "Involvement of Src and epidermal growth factor receptor in the signal-transducing function of Na+/K+-ATPase." *J Biol Chem* 275(36): 27832-27837.

Haas, M., H. Wang, et al. (2002). "Src-mediated inter-receptor cross-talk between the Na+/K+-ATPase and the epidermal growth factor receptor relays the signal from ouabain to mitogen-activated protein kinases." *J Biol Chem* 277(21): 18694-18702.

Hamlyn, J. M., M. P. Blaustein, et al. (1991). "Identification and characterization of a ouabain-like compound from human plasma." *Proc Natl Acad Sci U S A* 88(14): 6259-6263.

Harnett, J. D. and P. S. Parfrey (1994). "Blood pressure control and regression of LV hypertrophy in dialysis patients." *Contributions to nephrology* 106: 110-113.

Harnett, J. D., P. S. Parfrey, et al. (1988). "Left ventricular hypertrophy in end-stage renal disease." *Nephron* 48(2): 107-115.

Himmelfarb, J., P. Stenvinkel, et al. (2002). "The elephant in uremia: oxidant stress as a unifying concept of cardiovascular disease in uremia." *Kidney international* 62(5): 1524-1538.

Huting, J. and M. A. Alpert (1992). "Progression of left ventricular hypertrophy in end-stage renal disease treated by continuous ambulatory peritoneal dialysis depends on hypertension and hypercirculation." *Clinical cardiology* 15(3): 190-196.

Ihle, J. N. and I. M. Kerr (1995). "Jaks and Stats in signaling by the cytokine receptor superfamily." *Trends in genetics : TIG* 11(2): 69-74.

Jaitovich, A. and A. M. Bertorello (2010). "Salt, Na+,K+-ATPase and hypertension." *Life Sci* 86(3-4): 73-78.

Kawamura, A., J. Guo, et al. (1999). "On the structure of endogenous ouabain." *Proceedings of the National Academy of Sciences of the United States of America* 96(12): 6654-6659.

Kennedy, D., E. Omran, et al. (2003). "Effect of chronic renal failure on cardiac contractile function, calcium cycling, and gene expression of proteins important for calcium homeostasis in the rat." *Journal of the American Society of Nephrology : JASN* 14(1): 90-97.

Kennedy, D. J., J. Elkareh, et al. (2008). "Partial nephrectomy as a model for uremic cardiomyopathy in the mouse." *Am J Physiol Renal Physiol* 294(2): F450-454.

Kennedy, D. J., S. Vetteth, et al. (2006). "Central role for the cardiotonic steroid marinobufagenin in the pathogenesis of experimental uremic cardiomyopathy." *Hypertension* 47(3): 488-495.

Kennedy, D. J., S. Vetteth, et al. (2006). "Ouabain decreases sarco(endo)plasmic reticulum calcium ATPase activity in rat hearts by a process involving protein oxidation." *American journal of physiology. Heart and circulatory physiology* 291(6): H3003-3011.

Khundmiri, S. J., A. M. Bertorello, et al. (2004). "Clathrin-mediated endocytosis of Na+,K+-ATPase in response to parathyroid hormone requires ERK-dependent phosphorylation of Ser-11 within the alpha1-subunit." *The Journal of biological chemistry* 279(17): 17418-17427.

Khundmiri, S. J., M. A. Metzler, et al. (2006). "Ouabain induces cell proliferation through calcium-dependent phosphorylation of Akt (protein kinase B) in opossum kidney proximal tubule cells." *American journal of physiology. Cell physiology* 291(6): C1247-1257.

Kometiani, P., A. Askari, et al. (2001). "Downregulation of cardiac myocyte Na(+)-K(+)-ATPase by adenovirus-mediated expression of an alpha-subunit fragment." *American journal of physiology. Heart and circulatory physiology* 280(3): H1415-1421.

Kometiani, P., J. Li, et al. (1998). "Multiple signal transduction pathways link Na+/K+-ATPase to growth-related genes in cardiac myocytes. The roles of Ras and mitogen-activated protein kinases." *The Journal of biological chemistry* 273(24): 15249-15256.

Kometiani, P., L. Liu, et al. (2005). "Digitalis-induced signaling by Na+/K+-ATPase in human breast cancer cells." *Molecular pharmacology* 67(3): 929-936.

Komiyama, Y., X. H. Dong, et al. (2005). "A novel endogenous digitalis, telocinobufagin, exhibits elevated plasma levels in patients with terminal renal failure." *Clin Biochem* 38(1): 36-45.

Kotova, O., L. Al-Khalili, et al. (2006). "Cardiotonic steroids stimulate glycogen synthesis in human skeletal muscle cells via a Src- and ERK1/2-dependent mechanism." *The Journal of biological chemistry* 281(29): 20085-20094.

Kotova, O., D. Galuska, et al. (2006). "Metabolic and signaling events mediated by cardiotonic steroid ouabain in rat skeletal muscle." *Cellular and molecular biology* 52(8): 48-57.

Kreuz, J., F. Horlbeck, et al. (2011). "An impaired renal function: a predictor of ventricular arrhythmias and mortality in patients with nonischemic cardiomyopathy and heart failure." *Pacing and clinical electrophysiology : PACE* 34(7): 894-899.

Li, Z. and Z. Xie (2009). "The Na/K-ATPase/Src complex and cardiotonic steroid-activated protein kinase cascades." *Pflugers Archiv : European journal of physiology* 457(3): 635-644.

Liang, M., T. Cai, et al. (2006). "Functional characterization of Src-interacting Na/K-ATPase using RNA interference assay." *The Journal of biological chemistry* 281(28): 19709-19719.

Lingrel, J. B. (2010). "The physiological significance of the cardiotonic steroid/ouabain-binding site of the Na,K-ATPase." *Annual review of physiology* 72: 395-412.

Liu, J., R. Kesiry, et al. (2004). "Ouabain induces endocytosis of plasmalemmal Na/K-ATPase in LLC-PK1 cells by a clathrin-dependent mechanism." *Kidney Int* 66(1): 227-241.

Liu, J., M. Liang, et al. (2005). "Ouabain-induced endocytosis of the plasmalemmal Na/K-ATPase in LLC-PK1 cells requires caveolin-1." *Kidney Int* 67(5): 1844-1854.

Liu, J. and J. I. Shapiro (2007). "Regulation of sodium pump endocytosis by cardiotonic steroids: Molecular mechanisms and physiological implications." *Pathophysiology*.

Liu, J., J. Tian, et al. (2000). "Ouabain interaction with cardiac Na+/K+-ATPase initiates signal cascades independent of changes in intracellular Na+ and Ca2+ concentrations." *J Biol Chem* 275(36): 27838-27844.

Liu, L., K. Mohammadi, et al. (2003). "Role of caveolae in signal-transducing function of cardiac Na+/K+-ATPase." *American journal of physiology. Cell physiology* 284(6): C1550-1560.

Mall, G., W. Huther, et al. (1990). "Diffuse intermyocardiocytic fibrosis in uraemic patients." *Nephrology, dialysis, transplantation : official publication of the European Dialysis and Transplant Association - European Renal Association* 5(1): 39-44.

Mall, G., M. Rambausek, et al. (1988). "Myocardial interstitial fibrosis in experimental uremia--implications for cardiac compliance." *Kidney international* 33(4): 804-811.

McGarrigle, D. and X. Y. Huang (2007). "GPCRs signaling directly through Src-family kinases." *Science's STKE : signal transduction knowledge environment* 2007(392): pe35.

Mimura, M., H. Makino, et al. (1992). "Reduction of erythrocyte (Na(+)-K+) ATPase activities in non-insulin-dependent diabetic patients with hyperkalemia." *Metabolism: clinical and experimental* 41(4): 426-430.

Minagawa, T., T. Hirano, et al. (1994). "The effect of recombinant human erythropoietin (r-HuEPO) on left ventricular mass and left ventricular hemodynamics in hemodialysis patients." *Nippon Jinzo Gakkai shi* 36(8): 934-941.

Mitsnefes, M. M., S. R. Daniels, et al. (2001). "Changes in left ventricular mass in children and adolescents during chronic dialysis." *Pediatric nephrology* 16(4): 318-323.

Miyazaki, H., H. Matsuoka, et al. (2000). "Hemodialysis impairs endothelial function via oxidative stress: effects of vitamin E-coated dialyzer." *Circulation* 101(9): 1002-1006.

Mohmand, B., D. K. Malhotra, et al. (2005). "Uremic cardiomyopathy: role of circulating digitalis like substances." *Front Biosci* 10: 2036-2044.

Morduchowicz, G., J. Zabludowski, et al. (1993). "Ambulatory blood pressure monitoring assessment of blood pressure control in hypertension associated with chronic renal failure." *Nephrology, dialysis, transplantation : official publication of the European Dialysis and Transplant Association - European Renal Association* 8(10): 1169-1171.

Morgan, J. P. (1991). "Abnormal intracellular modulation of calcium as a major cause of cardiac contractile dysfunction." *The New England journal of medicine* 325(9): 625-632.

Nakazato, T., T. Kawada, et al. (2002). "Left ventricular hypertrophy was infrequent in patients starting dialysis after undergoing a strict blood pressure control in the pre-dialytic period." *Internal medicine* 41(11): 925-930.

Nguyen-Khoa, T., Z. A. Massy, et al. (2001). "Oxidative stress and haemodialysis: role of inflammation and duration of dialysis treatment." *Nephrology, dialysis, transplantation : official publication of the European Dialysis and Transplant Association - European Renal Association* 16(2): 335-340.

Nishikimi, T., J. Minami, et al. (2001). "Left ventricular mass relates to average systolic blood pressure, but not loss of circadian blood pressure in stable hemodialysis patients: an ambulatory 48-hour blood pressure study." *Hypertension research : official journal of the Japanese Society of Hypertension* 24(5): 507-514.

Ohara, N., K. Hiramatsu, et al. (1995). "Effect of parathyroid hormone on left ventricular diastolic function in patients with primary hyperparathyroidism." *Mineral and electrolyte metabolism* 21(1-3): 63-66.

Okamoto, S. (1988). "[Endogenous digitalis-like substance and Na-K-ATPase inhibitor in cardiovascular and renal disease]." *Nippon Naibunpi Gakkai zasshi* 64(1): 39-50.

Okano, K., S. Wu, et al. (1994). "Parathyroid hormone (PTH)/PTH-related protein (PTHrP) receptor and its messenger ribonucleic acid in rat aortic vascular smooth muscle cells and UMR osteoblast-like cells: cell-specific regulation by angiotensin-II and PTHrP." *Endocrinology* 135(3): 1093-1099.

Oweis, S., L. Wu, et al. (2006). "Cardiac glycoside downregulates NHE3 activity and expression in LLC-PK1 cells." *Am J Physiol Renal Physiol* 290(5): F997-1008.

Paparello, J., A. Kshirsagar, et al. (2002). "Comorbidity and cardiovascular risk factors in patients with chronic kidney disease." *Seminars in nephrology* 22(6): 494-506.

Periyasamy, S. M., J. Chen, et al. (2001). "Effects of uremic serum on isolated cardiac myocyte calcium cycling and contractile function." *Kidney international* 60(6): 2367-2376.

Periyasamy, S. M., J. Liu, et al. (2005). "Salt loading induces redistribution of the plasmalemmal Na/K-ATPase in proximal tubule cells." *Kidney Int* 67(5): 1868-1877.

Pierre, S. V., C. Yang, et al. (2007). "Ouabain triggers preconditioning through activation of the Na+,K+-ATPase signaling cascade in rat hearts." *Cardiovasc Res* 73(3): 488-496.

Pirola, C. J., H. M. Wang, et al. (1993). "Angiotensin II regulates parathyroid hormone-related protein expression in cultured rat aortic smooth muscle cells through transcriptional and post-transcriptional mechanisms." *The Journal of biological chemistry* 268(3): 1987-1994.

Priyadarshi, S., B. Valentine, et al. (2003). "Effect of green tea extract on cardiac hypertrophy following 5/6 nephrectomy in the rat." *Kidney Int* 63(5): 1785-1790.

Qiu, J., H. Q. Gao, et al. (2007). "Proteomics analysis of the proliferative effect of low-dose ouabain on human endothelial cells." *Biological & pharmaceutical bulletin* 30(2): 247-253.

Raine, A. E., L. Bedford, et al. (1993). "Hyperparathyroidism, platelet intracellular free calcium and hypertension in chronic renal failure." *Kidney international* 43(3): 700-705.

Raj, D. S., S. D'Mello, et al. (1997). "Left ventricular morphology in chronic renal failure by echocardiography." *Renal failure* 19(6): 799-806.

Rostand, S. G. and T. B. Drueke (1999). "Parathyroid hormone, vitamin D, and cardiovascular disease in chronic renal failure." *Kidney international* 56(2): 383-392.

Rostand, S. G., C. Sanders, et al. (1988). "Myocardial calcification and cardiac dysfunction in chronic renal failure." *The American journal of medicine* 85(5): 651-657.

Sarnak, M. J. (2003). "Cardiovascular complications in chronic kidney disease." *American journal of kidney diseases : the official journal of the National Kidney Foundation* 41(5 Suppl): 11-17.

Sarnak, M. J., A. S. Levey, et al. (2003). "Kidney disease as a risk factor for development of cardiovascular disease: a statement from the American Heart Association Councils on Kidney in Cardiovascular Disease, High Blood Pressure Research, Clinical Cardiology, and Epidemiology and Prevention." *Hypertension* 42(5): 1050-1065.

Saunders, R. and G. Scheiner-Bobis (2004). "Ouabain stimulates endothelin release and expression in human endothelial cells without inhibiting the sodium pump." *European journal of biochemistry / FEBS* 271(5): 1054-1062.

Shane, E., D. Mancini, et al. (1997). "Bone mass, vitamin D deficiency, and hyperparathyroidism in congestive heart failure." *The American journal of medicine* 103(3): 197-207.

Smogorzewski, M. (1995). "PTH, chronic renal failure and myocardium." *Mineral and electrolyte metabolism* 21(1-3): 55-62.

Stack, A. G. and W. E. Bloembergen (2001). "A cross-sectional study of the prevalence and clinical correlates of congestive heart failure among incident US dialysis patients." *American journal of kidney diseases : the official journal of the National Kidney Foundation* 38(5): 992-1000.

Stack, A. G. and R. Saran (2002). "Clinical correlates and mortality impact of left ventricular hypertrophy among new ESRD patients in the United States." *American journal of kidney diseases : the official journal of the National Kidney Foundation* 40(6): 1202-1210.

Stokes, G. S., D. Willcocks, et al. (1986). "Measurement of circulating sodium-pump inhibitory activity in uraemia and essential hypertension." *Journal of hypertension. Supplement : official journal of the International Society of Hypertension* 4(6): S376-378.

Sweadner, K. J. (1989). "Isozymes of the Na+/K+-ATPase." *Biochim Biophys Acta* 988(2): 185-220.

Takahashi, H., M. Nishimura, et al. (1989). "[Endothelin and endogenous digitalis-like substance in cardiovascular regulation: a review]." *Rinsho byori. The Japanese journal of clinical pathology* 37(10): 1103-1113.

Tetta, C., S. Biasioli, et al. (1999). "An overview of haemodialysis and oxidant stress." *Blood purification* 17(2-3): 118-126.

Tian, J., T. Cai, et al. (2006). "Binding of Src to Na+/K+-ATPase forms a functional signaling complex." *Mol Biol Cell* 17(1): 317-326.

Tian, J., J. Liu, et al. (2003). "Involvement of mitogen-activated protein kinases and reactive oxygen species in the inotropic action of ouabain on cardiac myocytes. A potential role for mitochondrial K(ATP) channels." *Mol Cell Biochem* 242(1-2): 181-187.

Tian, J., A. Shidyak, et al. (2009). "Spironolactone attenuates experimental uremic cardiomyopathy by antagonizing marinobufagenin." *Hypertension* 54(6): 1313-1320.

Tyralla, K. and K. Amann (2003). "Morphology of the heart and arteries in renal failure." *Kidney international. Supplement*(84): S80-83.

Uchida, K. (2000). "Role of reactive aldehyde in cardiovascular diseases." *Free radical biology & medicine* 28(12): 1685-1696.

Vlahakos, D. V., G. Hahalis, et al. (1997). "Relationship between left ventricular hypertrophy and plasma renin activity in chronic hemodialysis patients." *Journal of the American Society of Nephrology : JASN* 8(11): 1764-1770.

Wang, H., M. Haas, et al. (2004). "Ouabain assembles signaling cascades through the caveolar Na+/K+-ATPase." *J Biol Chem* 279(17): 17250-17259.

Wang, R., L. Wu, et al. (1993). "The changes in contractile status of single vascular smooth muscle cells and ventricular cells induced by bPTH-(1-34)." *Life sciences* 52(9): 793-801.

Weiner, D. E., H. Tighiouart, et al. (2004). "Chronic kidney disease as a risk factor for cardiovascular disease and all-cause mortality: a pooled analysis of community-based studies." *Journal of the American Society of Nephrology : JASN* 15(5): 1307-1315.

Wolf, G. (2000). "Free radical production and angiotensin." *Current hypertension reports* 2(2): 167-173.

Xie, Z., P. Kometiani, et al. (1999). "Intracellular reactive oxygen species mediate the linkage of Na+/K+-ATPase to hypertrophy and its marker genes in cardiac myocytes." *J Biol Chem* 274(27): 19323-19328.

Yuan, Z., T. Cai, et al. (2005). "Na/K-ATPase tethers phospholipase C and IP3 receptor into a calcium-regulatory complex." *Mol Biol Cell* 16(9): 4034-4045.

Zanzinger, J. and J. Czachurski (2000). "Chronic oxidative stress in the RVLM modulates sympathetic control of circulation in pigs." *Pflugers Archiv : European journal of physiology* 439(4): 489-494.

Part 3

Takotsubo Cardiomyopathy

11

Takotsubo Cardiomyopathy

Abdul Moiz Hafiz[1], M. Fuad Jan[2], Timothy E. Paterick[2], Suhail Allaqaband[2] and A. Jamil Tajik[2]

[1]Winthrop-University Hospital, Mineola, New York,
[2]Aurora Cardiovascular Services, Aurora Sinai/Aurora St. Luke's Medical Centers, University of Wisconsin School of Medicine and Public Health, Milwaukee, Wisconsin, USA

1. Introduction

Since the first report in 1990, takotsubo cardiomyopathy (TTC) has been increasingly recognized as a novel form of nonischemic acute cardiomyopathy. It is an important differential in diagnosis of acute coronary syndrome (ACS) due to its similar presentation. However, it distinguishes itself from an ACS in the fact that regional wall motion abnormalities extend beyond a single coronary vascular bed and are reversible, and epicardial coronary occlusion is absent (1).

In TTC, left ventricular (LV) dysfunction can be remarkably depressed but recovers within a few weeks (2) in the vast majority of patients. This syndrome has been described by more than 75 individual descriptive names in the literature, emphasizing those disease features that were most impressive to individual investigators (3) (Table 1).

Increased awareness about this syndrome has led to its incorporation into the American Heart Association classification of reversible cardiomyopathies (4,5). Pathogenesis of this syndrome is still not well understood, although physical and emotional stressors and mediation by pathologic sympathetic myocardial stunning are believed to play key roles. However, in an important minority of patients, a detailed personal history does not elicit an antecedent event (3).

Apical ballooning	
	Apical ballooning syndrome
	Acute left ventricular apical ballooning syndrome
	Left ventricular apical ballooning syndrome
	Transient left ventricular apical ballooning syndrome
	Primary apical ballooning
	Transient apical ballooning
	Transient apical ballooning syndrome
	Transient cardiac apical ballooning syndrome
	Transient left apical ballooning syndrome
	Transient cardiac ballooning
	Left apical ballooning syndrome
	Acute apical ballooning syndrome

Cardiac apical ballooning syndrome
Apical ballooning
Apical ballooning without apical ballooning
Apical ballooning cardiomyopathy
Reversible apical ballooning of left ventricle
Left ventricular ballooning syndrome
Midventricular variant of transient apical ballooning
Midventricular ballooning syndrome
Transient left ventricular mid-portion ballooning
Transient midventricular ballooning
Transient midventricular ballooning cardiomyopathy
Transient left ventricular nonapical ballooning
Reverse or inverted left ventricular apical ballooning syndrome
Inverted left ventricular apical ballooning syndrome
Transient basal ballooning
Tako-tsubo
Takotsubo cardiomyopathy
Takotsubo-like cardiomyopathy
Takotsubo syndrome
Takotsubo disease
Takotsubo left ventricular dysfunction
Takotsubo-like left ventricular dysfunction
Takotsubo-like transient biventricular dysfunction
Takotsubo-like transient left ventricular ballooning
Takotsubo-shaped cardiomyopathy
Takotsubo-shaped hypokinesia of left ventricle
Takotsubo-type cardiomyopathy
Takotsubo transient left ventricular apical ballooning
Midventricular takotsubo cardiomyopathy
Midventricular form of takotsubo cardiomyopathy
Inverted takotsubo contractile pattern
Inverted takotsubo cardiomyopathy
Inverted takotsubo pattern
Atypical takotsubo cardiomyopathy
Reverse takotsubo syndrome
Atypical basal type takotsubo cardiomyopathy
Stress cardiomyopathy
Acute stress cardiomyopathy
Human stress cardiomyopathy
Acute and reversible cardiomyopathy provoked by stress
Stress-induced cardiomyopathy
Stress-induced takotsubo cardiomyopathy
Stress-induced apical ballooning syndrome
Stress-related left ventricular dysfunction
Stress-related cardiomyopathy
Stress-related cardiomyopathy syndrome

Stress takotsubo cardiomyopathy
Emotional stress-induced ampulla cardiomyopathy
Midventricular stress cardiomyopathy
Atypical transient stress-induced cardiomyopathy
Stress-induced myocardial stunning
Emotional stress-induced takotsubo cardiomyopathy
Stress-associated catecholamine-induced cardiomyopathy
Neurogenic stress syndrome
Other
Neurogenic stunned myocardium
Adrenergic cardiomyopathy
Broken heart syndrome
Ampulla cardiomyopathy
Ampulla-shaped cardiomyopathy
"Chestnut-shaped" transient regional left ventricular hypokinesia
Ball-shaped spherical dilation of left ventricular apex
The artichoke heart
Transient midventricular akinesia
Transient antero-apical dyskinesia

Reproduced from Sharkey et al. Why not just call it tako-tsubo cardiomyopathy: a discussion of nomenclature. J Am Coll Cardiol 2011;57:1496-1497, with permission from Elsevier.

Table 1. Names Tabulated From Published Reports

2. History

In 1990, Sato and colleagues (6) first described a reversible cardiomyopathy as "tako-tsubo-like left ventricular dysfunction." One year later, Dote and colleagues (7) reported 5 patients with a novel, acute cardiac condition characterized by distinctive regional left ventricular LV systolic dysfunction and transient LV apical ballooning in the absence of significant coronary artery disease. Other Japanese investigators were intrigued by the unusual end-systolic shape of the LV, which resembled the "tako-tsubo," (a fisherman's pot with a round bottom and narrow neck used for trapping octopuses) (2,8,9) (Figure 1). Consequently, the term takotsubo was introduced to describe a new cardiomyopathic syndrome characterized by reversible LV systolic dysfunction (3). Many reports were published from different countries afterwards, and it was first reported in the United States in 2004 (5). A search for the term "takotsubo cardiomyopathy" in MEDLINE returned 1,090 articles (Figure 2).

3. Epidemiology

A few case reports were published prior to 2000, but the recognition of takotsubo cardiomyopathy has increased gradually since 2001, and this condition probably accounts for 1% to 2% of all cases of suspected acute myocardial infarction (MI) (10,11). Given the relatively recent recognition of TTC, epidemiology of this condition is still emerging. TTC is reported to occur predominantly in postmenopausal women (82-100%) (12) soon after exposure to sudden, unexpected emotional or physical stress. Kushiro and colleagues reported CD36 deficiency in a patient with stress-induced cardiomyopathy (13), suggesting an association between this entity and certain genetic profiles. This observation has led to the speculation that TTC might have a genetic component as described in a report by Cherian and colleagues (14).

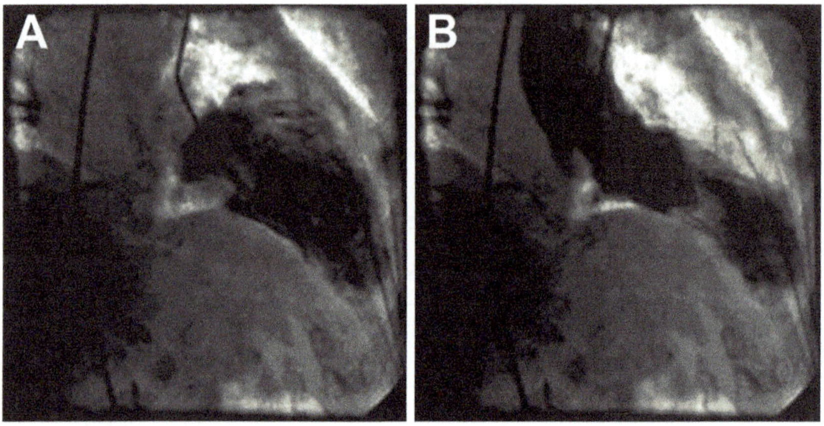

Fig. 1. Left ventriculograms obtained in a 65-year-old female who presented with acute shortness of breath. Panel A is a right anterior oblique (RAO) view of the left ventricle in the diastolic frame. Panel B is the RAO view of the left ventricle in the systolic frame. Note the dilated apical and akinetic outpouching of the left ventricle in Panel B. The coronaries in this patient were normal, consistent with the diagnosis of takotsubo cardiomyopathy.

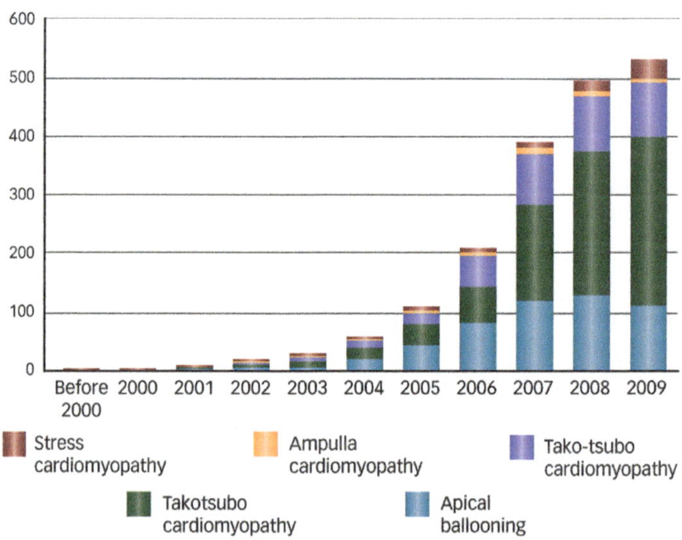

Fig. 2. Increase in the number of publications on MEDLINE® concerning takotsubo cardiomyopathy. (Originally published in *Asia-Pacific Cardiology* 2011;3:60-3. ©Touch Briefings. Reprinted with permission.)

4. Clinical presentation

4.1 The patient

TTC has characteristically been reported in women, with a median age varying from 61 to 76 years in prior case series (2,9,11,15-21). All large-cohort reports of TTC have shown that most patients presenting with the syndrome are postmenopausal women (5). However, it has also been reported in men and patients <50 years (1,3,15,16) and even in a 2-year-old girl (22). In the first large Japanese series describing TTC, 76 patients were women, 12 were men, and the median age was 67 ± 13 years (2).

4.2 The triggering event

Different stresses prior to presentation have been reported to trigger TTC, but the common theme is a sudden physical or emotional stress. The numerous events precipitating TTC are depicted in Table 2. Recurrence of TTC has also been rarely reported with similar or different triggering events (recurrence range, 0 to 8%) (23). TTC has been reported to be associated with pheochromocytoma (24-27) and subarachnoid hemorrhage (28-31) in some published reports.

Emotional stress	
	Death or severe illness or injury of a family member, friend, or pet
	Receiving bad news—diagnosis of a major illness, daughter's divorce, spouse leaving for war
	Severe argument
	Public speaking
	Involvement with legal proceedings
	Financial loss—business, gambling
	Car accident
	Surprise party
	Move to a new residence
Physical stress	
Non-cardiac surgery or procedure—cholecystectomy, hysterectomy	
	Severe illness—asthma or chronic obstructive airway exacerbation, connective tissue disorders, acute cholecystitis, pseudomembranous colitis
	Severe pain—fracture, renal colic, pneumothorax, pulmonary embolism
	Recovering from general anesthesia
	Cocaine use
	Opiate withdrawal
	Stress test—dobutamine stress echo, exercise sestamibi
	Thyrotoxicosis

Reproduced from Prasad et al. Apical ballooning syndrome (Tako-Tsubo or stress cardiomyopathy): A mimic of acute myocardial infarction. Am Heart J 2008;155:408-17, with permission from Elsevier.

Table 2. Stressors Reported to Trigger Takotsubo Cardiomyopathy

4.3 The syndrome

The characteristic clinical syndrome is acute LV dysfunction (10). Patients usually present with typical chest pain (70-90%) and dyspnea (20%) (10); other less common presentations include syncope (12), pulmonary edema and cardiac arrest. Dynamic electrocardiographic changes and elevated cardiac biomarkers (reflecting acute myocardial injury) are usually present. Coronary angiography, however, does not reveal any evidence of epicardial coronary obstruction. Left ventriculography (Figure 1) reveals LV dysfunction and wall motion abnormalities affecting apical and, frequently, midventricular myocardium but sparing the basal myocardium, changes which resemble a flask with a narrow neck and a round bottom shaped like the Japanese octopus trap "*tako-tsubo*" (32). Symptoms can be severe and lead to death in 2% of patients (3). Song and colleagues reported 32% (n=16) of their patients with TTC (n=50) presented with cardiogenic shock as initial presentation (33). Table 3 shows clinical features in a prior published series (10).

4.4 Electrocardiography

Most common electrocardiographic changes reported in TTC are ST-segment elevations in precordial leads (10) on admission (range, 46-100% of patients) (12). Subsequent deep symmetrical T-wave inversion in multiple leads and Q-wave formation (range, 6-31% of patients) (12) also are frequently found (10). Also present may be QT interval prolongation (5) (range, 450-501 ms) (12). The combination of clinical symptoms and electrocardiographic changes at patient's initial presentation makes differentiation of TTC from ACS very difficult. A typical electrocardiogram obtained in one of our patients at presentation and 48 hours later is shown in Figure 3.

4.5 Cardiac biomarkers

Most patients present with elevated cardiac biomarkers and have a modest peak in levels within 24 hours (15,19,34), but levels are markedly lower than would be anticipated on the basis of the extent of wall motion abnormalities and electrocardiogram findings (1).

4.6 Left ventriculography

Diagnosis of TTC is frequently made in the cardiac catheterization laboratory during left ventriculography as the patients are initially triaged as an ACS and are referred for urgent or emergency coronary angiography (35). Left ventriculography (Figure 4) reveals the classic appearance of left ventricle with dilated apex and akinetic apical or midventricular walls (or both) and a hypercontractile basal segment. However, more variants of TTC have been reported with diversity in patterns of regional LV systolic dyssynergy. Singh and colleagues (36) reported a series of 107 patients (age=66 ± 14 years, n=99 females) and observed the regional contractility phenotypes shown in Table 4. A study by Kurowski and colleagues (n=35 patients) identified 60% of patients to be typical (apical) and 40% to be atypical (midventricular) variants (11). Subclassifying TTC variants with different names should be avoided as it can lead to more confusion (3). The proposed alternate names - "transient ballooning syndrome" (37) or "transient stress-induced left ventricular dysfunction syndrome" - seem to capture the essential features of the disease, though takotsubo cardiomyopathy remains the most widely used.

	Tsuchihashi et al	Kurowski et al	Kurisu et al	Sharkey et al	Wittstein et al	Inoue et al	Sato et al	Bybee et al	Yoshida et al	Akashi et al
Subjects, n	88	35	30	22	19	18	16	16	15	13
Country	Japan	Germany	Japan	U.S.	U.S.	Japan	Japan	U.S.	Japan	Japan
Series, type	Retro	Pro	Retro	Pro	Pro	Retro	Retro	Pro	Pro	Pro
Age, y	67 ± 13	72 ± 9	70 ± 8	65 ± 13	61 ± 15	76 ± 8	71 ± 9	71 ± 12	72 ± 7	73 ± 10
Women, %	86	94	93	91	95	94	94	100	80	85
Preceding emotional stressor, %	20	42	17	86	100	11	...	38	40	31
Preceding stressor, %	43	42	17	14	...	39	100	4	40	69
Chest pain, %	67	...	67	91	95	72	100	69	87	54
ST-segment elevation, %	90	69	100	59	11	100	56	81	87	92
ST-segment elevation in precordial leads, %	85	...	97	59	...	100	...	81	...	92
Q waves, %	27	...	...	45	37	56†	...	31	7	...
Mean QTc, ms	...	...	...	...	542*	...	...	501 ± 55	508*	...
Elevation in cardiac enzynme leads, %	56	...	...	...	...	...	56	100	...	85
Initial average LVEF	0.41 ± 0.11	0.5 ± 0.13	0.49 ± 0.12	0.29 ± 0.09	0.20*	...	0.49 ± 0.04	0.4	0.43 ± 0.08	0.42 ± 0.10
Follow-up LVEF	0.64 ± 0.10	0.68 ± 0.12	0.69 ± 0.12	0.63 ± 0.06	0.60*	...	0.66 ± 0.03	0.6	0.76 ± 0.01	0.65 ± 0.08
Time of recovery, d	...	...	11.3 ± 4.3	24 ± 29	21*	...	17.7	8	11 ± 4	17 ± 7
Initial Forrester subset	...	...	...	...	...	...	...	...	...	1.9 ± 0.3
Pulmonary edema, %	22	...	3	0	16	28	6	44	...	0
Coronary stenosis >50%, %	0	0	0	0	5	0	0	0	...	0
Angiographically normal coronary arteries, %	...	0	33	100	95	100	100	25	100	100
Spontaneous multivessel spasm, %	0	0	10	...	0	0	0	0	0	0
Provacable multivessel spasm, n/ n (%)	5/ 48 (10)	...	6/ 14 (43)	...	...	...	0/ 6 (0)	...	1/ 6 (17)	0/ 11 (0)
Transient intraventricular pressure gradient, %	18	...	...	23	...	...	...	13	14	...
In-hospital mortality, %	1	3 (9)	0	0	0	6	0	0	0	8
Documented recurrence, n/ n (%)	2/ 72 (3)	2 (6)	0	2/ 22 (9)	0	...	...	1/ 16 (6)	...	0

LVEF indicates left ventricular ejection fraction; Retro, retrospective; Pro, prospective. Values are expressed as mean ± SD when appropriate.
*Median.
†In precordial leads.
Adapted from Gianni et al. Apical ballooning syndrome or takotsubo cardiomyopathy: a systematic review. Eur Heart J 2006;27:1523–1529, with permission from Oxford University Press.

Table 3. Patient Clinical and Laboratory Characteristics

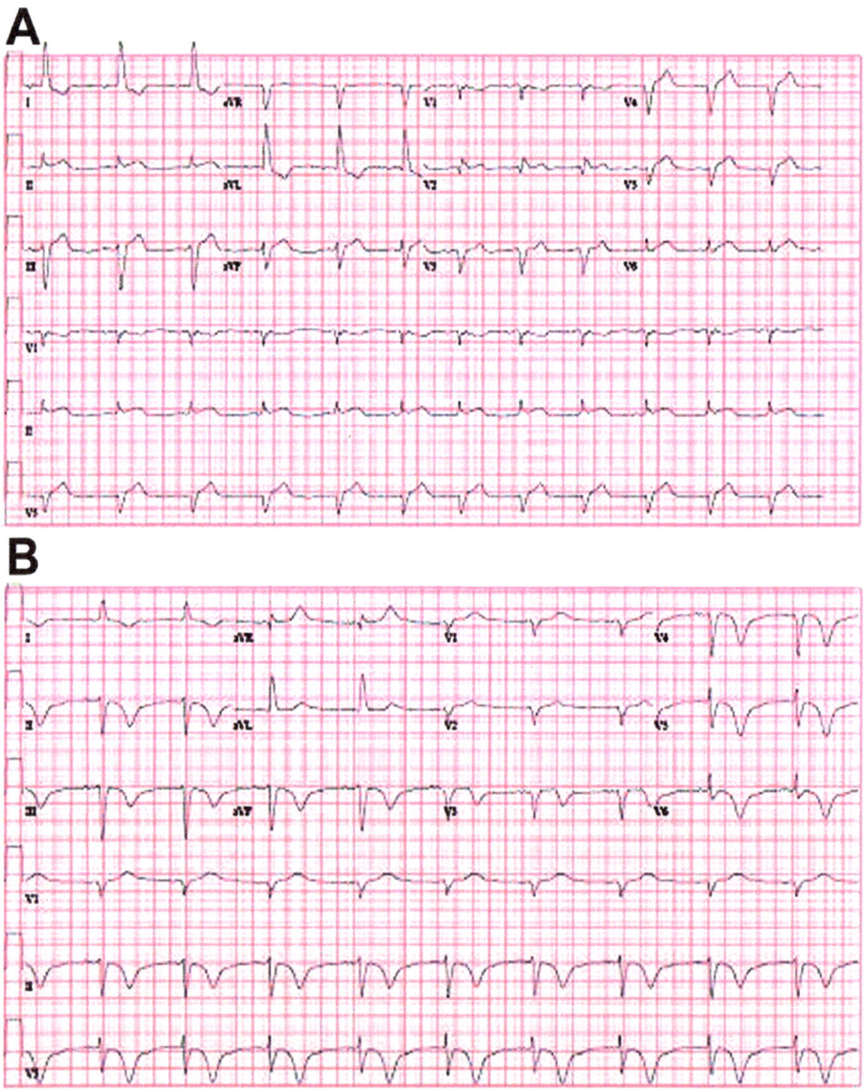

Fig. 3. Electrocardiogram (ECG) changes in one of our patients with takotsubo cardiomyopathy. Panel A: ECG at presentation revealed a 1-mm elevation in V3 and V4 and a new-onset left bundle branch block. Panel B: ECG at 48 hours after presentation revealed T-wave abnormalities in multiple leads.

Posterobasal	1%
Basal + midventricular	1%
Diaphragmatic	2%
Localized apical	2%
Anterolateral	11%
Complete midventricular	29%
Classical takotsubo cardiomyopathy	54%

Data compiled from Singh et al.[36]

Table 4. Variants of Takotsubo Cardiomyopathy[36]

4.7 Coronary angiography

Coronary angiography on presentation fails to reveal any coronary obstruction or acute plaque rupture. However, patients with coronary artery disease can develop TTC. Kurisu and colleagues (38) reported 10% of patients in their series of takotsubo patients (total patients=97) had >75% coronary artery obstruction in a major coronary vessel, though coronary stenosis is uncommon in patients presenting with TTC (1), and absence of an acute coronary artery syndrome is a diagnostic criterion for diagnosis of TTC.

4.8 Echocardiography

Echocardiography also plays a pivotal role in the diagnosis of TTC. This is particularly so given the ability to rapidly perform bedside echocardiography with echo-Doppler imaging. Accurate evaluation by echocardiography, particularly after coronary evaluation by catheterization, can assist in further defining the diagnosis, particularly, when echocardiography repeated after few days to weeks shows complete normalization of regional wall motion abnormalities and LV ejection fraction. Typically, TTC appears like an evolving acute anterior wall myocardial infarction (MI) with akinesia of the apex, apical anterior wall and septum (Figure 5). Left ventricular outflow tract obstruction, a transient phenomenon in TTC, can also be recognized by echocardiography.

In contemporary clinical practice, three-dimensional speckle tracking echocardiography (3D-STE) can be used to assess myocardial mechanical function. It permits the calculation of complex myocardial mechanical parameters such as strain and strain rate, rotation, torsion, as well as LV volume and ejection fraction in three dimensions within minutes. It has been validated against sonomicrometry, magnetic resonance imaging (MRI) tagging, and found to be more accurate and reproducible than two-dimensional speckle tracking echocardiography (2D-STE). We have observed that the global longitudinal, circumferential and radial strains are all decreased significantly in acute anterior wall myocardial infarction and TTC in the acute phase. However, regional circumferential and radial strains at mid and apical LV are significantly lower in TTC patients than in acute anterior wall MI.

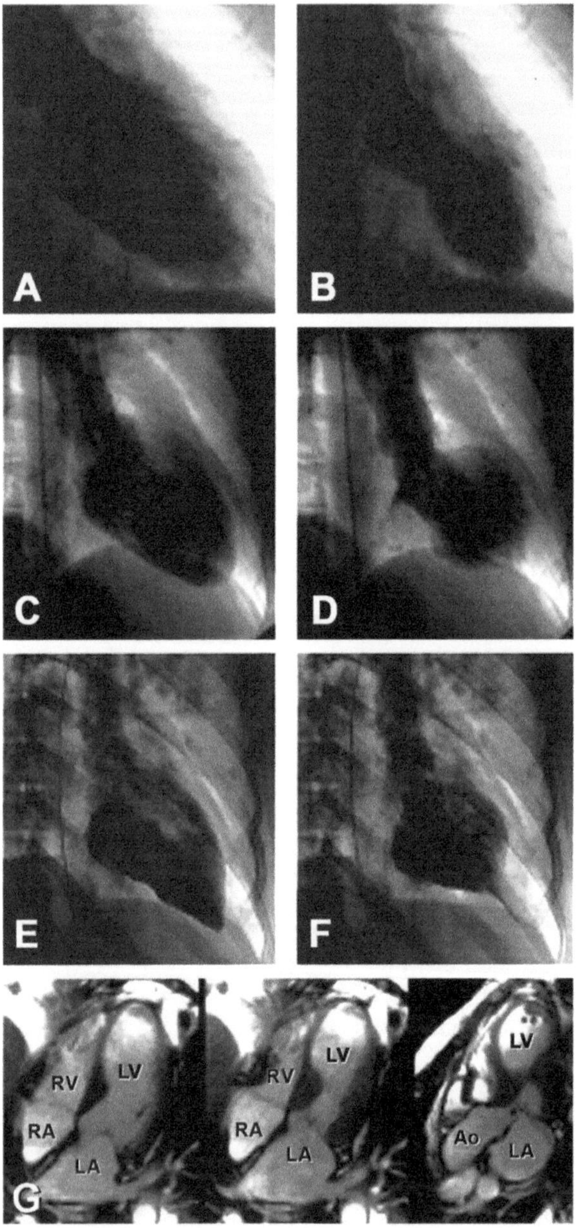

Fig. 4. Radiograph of the left ventricle. (A) Left ventriculogram in diastole. (B) Left ventriculogram in systole shows preserved contraction of the base of the ventricle and apical ballooning. (C) Right anterior oblique view in diastole. (D) Right anterior oblique view in systole. Note the hypercontractility of the basal and apical segments and ballooning of the midventricular segments. (E) After methamphetamine use in end-diastole. (F) After

methamphetamine use in end-systole. Basal segments are akinetic, the papillary level shows normal contractility, and the apex is hypercontractile. (G) Cardiac magnetic resonance image. Hypotension may be due to dynamic outflow tract obstruction caused by hyperkinesis of the basal left ventricle segments and systolic anterior motion of the mitral valve. Four-chamber, steady-state, free-precession image: end-diastole (left) and end-systole (center) show left and right ventricular apical akinesis. (Right) Three-chamber image in systole shows systolic anterior motion of the mitral leaflets (*) with dynamic left ventricular outflow tract obstruction; left ventricular apical mass consistent with thrombus (**). Ao = aorta; LA = left atrium; LV = left ventricle; RA = right atrium; RV = right ventricle. (Panels A and B are adapted from Hurst et al. Takotsubo cardiomyopathy: A unique cardiomyopathy with variable ventricular morphology. JACC: Cardiovascular Imaging 2010;3:641-9, with permission from Elsevier. Panels C and D are adapted from Hurst et al. Transient midventricular ballooning syndrome: a new variant. J Am Coll Cardiol 2006;48:579-83, with permission from Elsevier. Panels E and F are adapted from Reuss et al. Isolated left ventricular basal ballooning phenotype of transient cardiomyopathy in young women. Am J Cardiol 2007;99:1451-3, with permission from Elsevier. Panel G is adapted from Syed et al. Apical ballooning syndrome or aborted acute myocardial infarction? Insights from cardiovascular magnetic resonance imaging. Int J Cardiovasc Imaging 2008;24:875-82, with permission from Springer.)

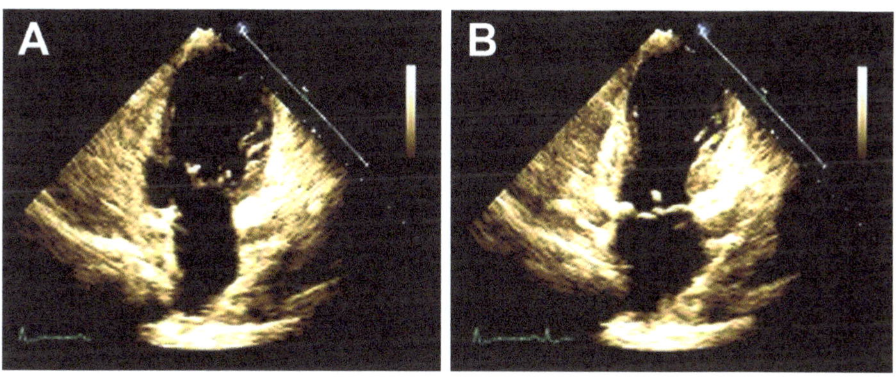

Fig. 5. Two-chamber view of the left ventricle, obtained in diastole (Panel A) and systole (Panel B), in a 56-year-old female who presented to the hospital in florid pulmonary edema after witnessing a car accident. Panel B demonstrates the akinetic and balloon apex in systole with a hypercontractile base, a classic variant of takotsubo cardiomyopathy.

4.9 Cardiac magnetic resonance imaging

Cardiac magnetic resonance imaging may be helpful in differentiating TTC from MI and myocarditis. TTC is characterized by the absence of delayed gadolinium enhancement, whereas MI is characterized by subendocardial delayed hyperenhancement and myocarditis is characterized by patchy delayed hyperenhancement (39-41). Cardiac magnetic resonance can also demonstrate the typical bulging of the LV apex and hypercontractile function of the base with accurate rendering of the LV stroke volume. It can also demonstrate the presence of LV thrombus in akinetic apex (Figure 6).

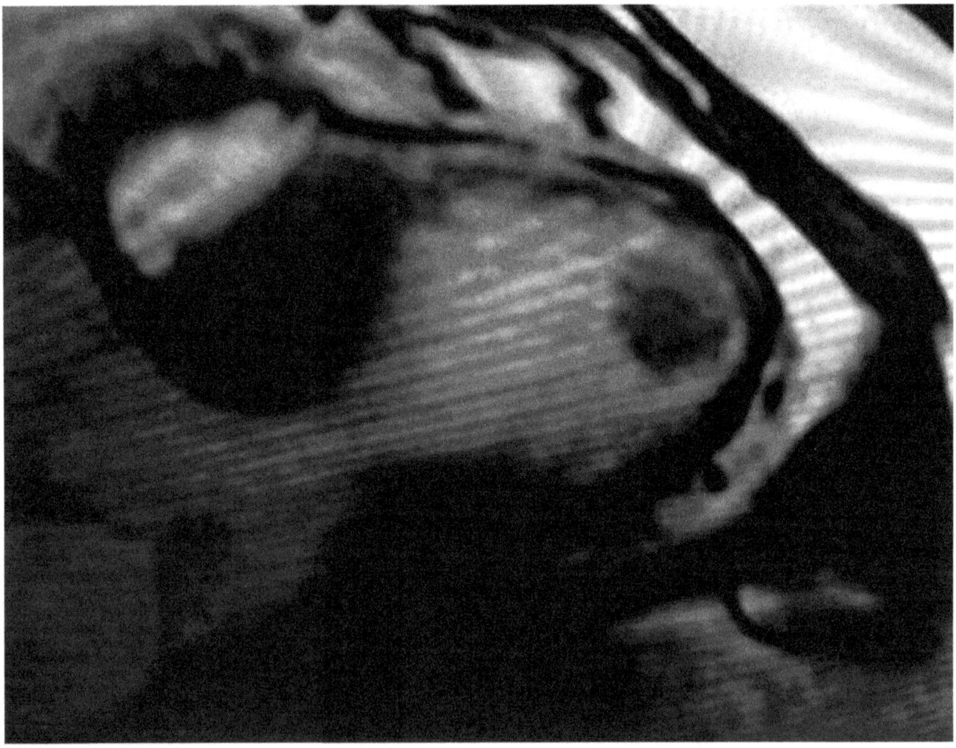

Fig. 6. Two-chamber Fast Imaging Employing Steady-State Acquisition (FIESTA) motion sensing in a 76-year-old female who presented to the hospital with chest pain and shortness of breath after witnessing an acute asthma attack in her grandchild. The figure demonstrates left ventricular apical bulging and a hypercontractile base with a 1.5 × 1.5-cm thrombus within the left ventricular apex.

4.10 Clinical outcome and prognosis

A complete recovery of LV wall motion abnormalities is a hallmark of this syndrome in virtually all patients (2,15,16,35). Recovery time varies, from as short as several days to as long as 4-8 weeks, and is a requirement for the diagnosis (15). The diagnostic criteria are summarized in Table 5.

1. Transient hypokinesis, akinesis, or dyskinesis of the left ventricular mid-segments with or without apical involvement; the regional wall motion abnormalities extend beyond a single epicardial vascular distribution; a stressful trigger is often, but not always, present.*
2. Absence of obstructive coronary disease or angiographic evidence of acute plaque rupture. †
3. New electrocardiographic abnormalities (either ST-segment elevation and/or T-wave inversion) or modest elevation in cardiac troponin.
4. Absence of:
   Pheochromocytoma
   Myocarditis

In both of the above circumstances, the diagnosis of takotsubo cardiomyopathy should be made with caution, and a clear stressful precipitating trigger must be sought.

*There are rare exceptions to these criteria such as those patients in whom the regional wall motion abnormality is limited to a single coronary territory.

†It is possible that a patient with obstructive coronary atherosclerosis may also develop takotsubo cardiomyopathy. However, this is very rare in our experience and in the published literature, perhaps because such cases are misdiagnosed as an acute coronary syndrome.

Reproduced from Prasad et al. Apical ballooning syndrome (Tako-Tsubo or stress cardiomyopathy): A mimic of acute myocardial infarction. Am Heart J 2008;155:408-17, with permission from Elsevier.

Table 5. Proposed Mayo Clinic Criteria for Takotusbo Cardiomyopathy

The overall prognosis of TTC appears to be favorable in patients who survive the initial acute phase of heart failure. In-hospital mortality has been reported between 0 and 8% (12). Reported complications associated with TTC are left heart failure with and without pulmonary edema, cardiogenic shock, dynamic intraventricular obstruction with left ventricular intracavitary pressure gradient generation, mitral regurgitation resulting from chordal tethering as well as systolic anterior motion of the mitral valve apparatus, ventricular arrhythmias, LV mural thrombus formation, left ventricular free-wall rupture and death (12). Cardiogenic shock (6.5%), congestive heart failure (3.8%) and ventricular tachycardia (1.6%) are other known complications, while ventricular fibrillation, LV mural thrombus formation, ventricular septal defect, LV free wall rupture and pneumothorax have infrequently been reported (12,37).

Recently, Madhavan and colleagues (42) have proposed the "Mayo Clinic Risk Score" system for acute heart failure in TTC (Table 6). The scoring system was developed to predict which patients with TTC are at risk of developing systolic heart failure. Presence of 1, 2 and 3 points was associated with 28%, 58% and 85% risk of acute heart failure.

Risk Factor	Score
Age > 70 years	1
Presence of physical stressor	1
Ejection fraction < 40%	1

Table 6. Proposed Mayo Clinic Risk Scoring System of Acute Heart Failure in Takotsubo Cardiomyopathy

5. Pathogenesis

The aphorism "a broken heart" is well known to be associated with emotional stress by the lay person. Association of TTC with acute emotional and physical stress lends a scientific basis for this observation. But the exact underlying mechanism still proves elusive. Due to the recent recognition of TTC and its low incidence of diagnosis, as mentioned earlier, only a relatively small number of patients have been studied in a few published series. No large studies have confirmed the etiology of TTC (43). A rapidly accumulating body of evidence has led to very interesting insights into the possible pathophysiology of TTC. Most current hypotheses are based on cathecholamine surges in the setting of acute emotional or physical stress leading to catecholamine-related cardiac toxic effects (32,44-49) and was first suggested by Wittstein and colleagues (16). In this section we examine various advancements in understanding TTC pathophysiology.

5.1 Obstruction of the left ventricular outflow tract

Early investigators observed left ventricular outflow tract (LVOT) obstruction in some patients presenting with TTC. Villarreal and colleagues hypothesized that patients with a sigmoid interventricular septum, small LVOT, reduced LV volume (primarily elderly women) and an abnormal orientation of a slack mitral apparatus have a geometric predisposition to dynamic LVOT obstruction, which may manifest in the setting of intense adrenergic stimulation or hypovolemia (50,51). Elderly females seem to have a higher incidence of basal septal thickening (52), and this could become a substrate for LVOT obstruction leading to severe, transient midcavity obstruction in the setting of a cathecholamine surge (53). LVOT obstruction may cause or worsen hypotension due to LV systolic dysfunction by contributing to significant mitral regurgitation secondary to systolic anterior motion of mitral valve and dynamic LVOT obstruction (54). Presence of LVOT may change the management of TTC patients and is detailed in the treatment section of this chapter. However, incidence of LVOT obstruction in patients presenting with TTC in various studies has varied from 11-25% of patients (12,52,55) and is not observed in all patients. Its role in the pathogenesis of TTC is unclear, and it remains uncertain if LVOT obstruction is a cause or a consequence of TTC (49).

5.2 Vasospasm of epicardial coronary arteries hypothesis

Clinical presentation of TTC bears close resemblance to an acute MI. Therefore, early hypotheses speculated that an ischemic event triggered by transient coronary plaque rupture (56) or reversible coronary vessel spasm (7) was responsible for "stunning" the ventricle. A few authors reported finding a long left anterior descending artery (LAD) that wrapped around the apex in their patients presenting with TTC, and it was hypothesized that transient obstruction of epicardial blood flow to the left ventricle in a given coronary bed may lead to the regional akinesis or "ballooning" typically observed in TTC. However, there are multiple problems with such an explanation. For one, the aforementioned coronary artery anatomy is not found on coronary angiography in all patients presenting with TTC. Secondly, spontaneous coronary vasospasm has been reported in only 2% of patients with TTC (12). Furthermore, an acute coronary vessel-obstructing lesion has not been described in patients with TTC immediately after presentation (57) and has been proposed as an exclusion criterion (35) for TTC diagnosis. Thirdly, as mentioned earlier, there are reports of numerous phenotypes of TTC that present with regional hypokinesis that encompasses territories of the left ventricle not supplied by a single vessel (35). Fourthly, histological examination of cardiac tissue in patients with acute MI reveals polymorphonuclear inflammation, whereas TTC is associated with an interstitial mononuclear inflammatory response and considerable increase in extracellular matrix protein and contraction band necrosis—a unique form of myocyte injury characterized by hypercontracted sarcomeres and dense eosinophilic transverse bands associated with catecholamine-excess states like pheochromocytoma and subarachnoid hemorrhage (16,49). Finally, provocative tests with infusion of ergometrine or acetylcholine for inducible coronary vasospasm in patients with TTC were only positive in 28.6% of patients (55) and 27.6% of patients (58) in two published series, respectively. These equivocal results combined with the factors mentioned above make obstruction of blood flow in epicardial coronary vessels seem less likely to explain the pathophysiology of TTC.

5.3 Coronary microvascular blood flow abnormalities

Several investigators (11,19,59) have suggested microvascular dysfunction to be a potential pathophysiologic mechanism in TTC. Kume and colleagues demonstrated microcirculation disturbances in patients with TTC by use of Doppler flow-wire assessment (60). Other investigators have used TIMI (Thrombolysis in Myocardial Infarction) frame counts to assess coronary blood flow. Using this technique, Kurisu (59) and colleagues found significantly higher frame counts in TTC compared to a control group. Bybee and colleagues (19) also found abnormal TIMI frame counts in one or more major epicardial vessels in patients with TTC in their published series. These findings suggest that microvascular integrity in TTC is impaired in all coronary arteries in many patients, and the microvascular dysfunction in LAD is comparable to that of patients with acute anterior ST-segment elevation myocardial infarction after recanalization of the infarct-related artery.

Nuclear studies with single-photon emission tomography (SPET) and fluorodeoxyglucose positron emission tomography (FDG-PET) were performed by Kurowski (11) in their patients with TTC and revealed that myocardial glucose metabolism was more affected than perfusion. The authors concluded that this "inverse mismatch" pattern is similar to that seen in postischemic "stunned" myocardium (61).

These findings indicate that diffuse coronary microvascular dysfunction is present in patients with TTC. However, whether this is an effect or cause of this syndrome is unclear (10). This type of microvascular dysfunction, however, can be a result of a surge in catecholamine secretion, which is described in detail later in this chapter.

5.4 Catecholamine-induced acute myocardial stunning hypothesis

5.4.1 Alterations in calcium handling

Akashi and colleagues were the first to report elevated serum catecholamine levels in patients with TTC (62). Wittstein and colleagues (16) later reported supraphysiologic levels of plasma catecholamines in their series (n=19 patients), which reported plasma levels of epinephrine, norepinephrine and dopamine in patients with TTC to be 2-3 times higher than those of patients with Killip class III MI and 7-32 times higher than the published normal values (63). They also noted higher levels of both neuronal (dihydroxyphenylglycol, dihydroxyphenylglycol and dihydroxyphenylacetic acid) and extraneuronal catecholamines (metanephrine, normetanephrine and neuropeptide Y). In Wittstein's series, the plasma cathecholamine levels trended downward by day 7-9 but still remained elevated. They concluded that TTC was associated with activation of adrenomedullary hormonal system and enhanced sympathoneural activity. Similarly, administration of epinephrine at suprapharmacological doses led to induction of stress cardiomyopathy in two cases (64,65). Several investigators (16,32,66) have suggested direct myocardial stunning as a result of the catecholamine surges. Such a stunning could possibly explain the findings in TTC. Catecholamine-overload state is associated with the following histologic changes: 1.) increased production of extracellular matrix leading to a rapid increase in fibrosis; 2.) contraction band necrosis; and 3.) mild neutrophil infiltration (44). There is increased production of oxygen-derived free radicals (67) that interfere with sodium and calcium transporters, resulting in myocyte dysfunction through increased transsarcolemmal calcium influx and cellular calcium overload (68). Mori and colleagues (69) demonstrated that apical myocardium has a higher concentration of beta-adrenoceptors with a concentration gradient decreasing from apex to base. This could explain the enhanced responsiveness to sympathetic stimulation potentially making the apex more vulnerable to sudden surges in circulating catecholamine levels and, thus, could explain the typical phenotype most commonly found in TTC patients (16).

Investigators have noted disturbance of the calcium regulatory system in stress-induced cardiomyopathy. Some animal models have been shown to describe altered expression of the calcium regulatory system protein genes by supraphysiological levels of catecholamines (70,71) (Figure 7).

Sarcolipin regulates sarcoplasmic/endoplasmic reticulum calcium ATPase2 (SERCA) by lowering its affinity for calcium. Elevated catecholamines in TTC cause increased expression of sarcolipin in the acute phase, leading to reduced affinity of SERCA2 for calcium (49,72,73). Elevated levels of catecholamines also lead to reduced expression of SERCA2 messenger RNA levels through intense G-protein-stimulated β1 and β2 adrenergic receptor signaling in animal models (74). The G-protein-stimulated β1-adrenergic receptor and α1-adrenergic receptor can directly modulate SERCA2 gene expression (via cyclic AMP-responsive element binding protein 1 and calcineurin-nuclear factor of activated T cells signaling pathways) (75). Excessive adrenergic signaling could thus explain the cardiotoxicity observed in patients with stress cardiomyopathy from cardiomyocytes calcium overload, mitochondrial calcium overload, reactive oxygen species production and oxidative stress (32,49). However, there is no evidence to suggest that alterations in expression of calcium-handling proteins are responsible for the acute deleterious effects of TTC (49).

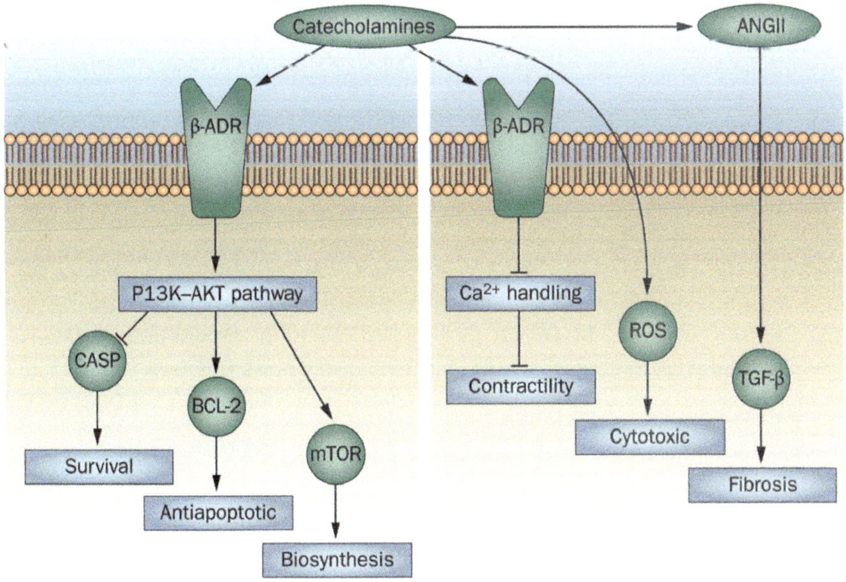

Fig. 7. The pathomechanistic concept of stress cardiomyopathy. Overexpression of catecholamines following a stress event leads to a number of changes that can have either protective or adverse effects. Abbreviations: β-ADR, β-adrenergic receptor; ANGII, angiotensin II; CASP, caspase; mTOR, mammalian target of rapamycin; PI3K–AKT, phosphatidylinositol 3 kinase–AKT; ROS, reactive oxygen species; TGF-β, transforming growth factor β. Reproduced from Nef et al. Mechanisms of stress (Takotsubo) cardiomyopathy. Nat Rev Cardiol 2010;7:187–193, with permission from Nature Publishing Group.

5.4.2 Stimulus trafficking

5.4.2.1 Stimulus trafficking causes negative inotropism

Human ventricular cardiomyocytes have two types of β-adrenergic receptors (AR), β1 and β2, but the concentration of β2 is higher than β1 (4:1) (76). At physiological and elevated concentrations, norepinephrine and epinephrine act via β1-AR exerting positive inotropic and lusitropic responses through coupling with the Gs protein family. Epinephrine has higher affinity for β2-AR and activates the Gs protein family, causing positive inotropic response. However, at supraphysiological levels, epinephrine stimulates a negative inotropic effect (77) by causing a switch from β2-AR Gs protein signaling to β2-AR Gi protein signaling (78), a process called stimulus trafficking (32). Intense activation of the β1-AR Gs protein and β2-AR Gs protein pathways is thought to initiate the switch in signal trafficking from β2-AR Gs protein to β2-AR Gi protein coupling (79). The Gi protein pathway exerts a negative inotropic effect through multiple pathways (32).

After the surge in epinephrine levels has cleared from the circulation, negative inotropy-causing β2-ARs that are coupled to Gi proteins either switch back to Gs protein coupling or are internalized and degraded, enabling cardiomyocytes to recover their inotropic function.

This sequence of events would explain the reported recovery of ventricular function in individuals with stress cardiomyopathy (32).

5.4.2.2 Typical TTC phenotype explained by stimulus trafficking

In human hearts, the density of the sympathetic nerve endings is approximately 40% greater at the base compared to the apex (80), whereas the concentration of β-ARs is higher in the apical myocardium (69). It has been proposed that the concentration of β-ARs in the apical myocardium is increased to compensate for the decrease in the direct sympathetic innervation, thereby maintaining a balanced responsiveness of the ventricle-to-sympathetic drive (32). Thus, the apex might be more sensitive and responsive to circulating catecholamines. An increasing density of β2-ARs from the base to the apex could explain the regional difference in response to high catecholamine levels, with circulating epinephrine having a greater influence on apical function, relative to basal function.

5.5 Atypical phenotype

Certain factors can influence the local epinephrine concentration in the myocardium. A study in rabbits demonstrated conversion of norepinephrine to epinephrine by phenylethanolamine N-methyltransferase in the ventricular myocardium (81). Thus, regional differences in epinephrine concentrations can play a role in responsiveness of the myocardium to catecholamines and could explain atypical phenotypes observed in some TTC patients (32).

5.6 Female predominance related to hormones

Some investigators have suggested reduction of estrogen levels in postmenopausal females to be one of the underlying factors of TTC.

Estrogen receptors are expressed on cardiomyocytes (82), thus cardiomyocyte function could be directly affected by estrogen levels. Estrogen has also been shown to significantly suppress SERCA2 expression in ovariectomized rats compared to controls, thus altering cardiac myocyte sarcoplasmic reticulum calcium uptake (83). In the latter study, investigators noted that estrogen and progesterone supplementations were equally effective in preventing changes in ovariectomized hearts.

Men rarely develop stress cardiomyopathy yet are physiologically estrogen-deficient, which suggests that this syndrome is not due to ovarian hormone deficiency. However, effects of hormone deficiency on contractility in the presence of excessive catecholamine levels need further clarification (49).

5.7 Possible familial link

Burgdorf and colleagues (84) recently reported a series of 144 patients with TTC (107 typical cases and 34 atypical cases) in which 26 patients were known to have cancer, while 7 patients were newly diagnosed with cancer. On basis of this observation, they proposed that an association between cancer and TTC cannot be excluded and that patients diagnosed with TTC should undergo screening for cancer. While there might be an association, one possible confounder could be the neurally mediated hypothesis of stress associated with learning about the diagnosis of cancer.

6. Treatment

TTC is a self-limiting syndrome; cardiac function returns to pre-TTC levels within a few weeks and patients carry a favorable prognosis (2). However, patients require standard supportive treatment during the acute phase. This treatment is similar to a congestive heart failure treatment regimen with diuretics and vasodilators (16). Vasopressors and beta-agonists should be avoided due to catecholamine-surplus state. Also, epinephrine administered may drive further β2-AR, Gi protein-mediated negative inotropism (32). Use of β-blockers should be carefully considered as some β-blockers can also cause stimulus trafficking of β2-ARs to Gi protein coupling (85), which, in the acute phase of TTC, can lead to further suppression of LV function. However, in the long term, β2-AR/Gi coupling may enhance the ability of β-blockers to protect and improve the function of the failing heart (85). Mechanical circulatory support in patients with intraaortic balloon counter pulsation (IABP) is appropriate to avoid vasopressor support in these patients (16). Administration of intravenous calcium or levosimendan (a calcium-sensitizing agent) has also been suggested as the inotrope of choice in TTC patients (86,87), but has not been clinically validated in any major study. Some investigators have used it to avoid IABP in TTC patients (88). In patients with moderate to severe hemodynamic compromise and echocardiographic evidence of significant LVOT obstruction (with a dynamic gradient possibly accompanied by systolic anterior motion of mitral valve), both IABP counter pulsation and inotropes are relatively contraindicated because they could worsen the dynamic gradient and thereby further jeopardize cardiac function (54,89); treatment should instead be more conservative with careful fluid management to avoid excessive preload reduction, β-blockers if tolerated (to increase diastolic filling time and thus end-diastolic volume) and occasionally peripheral vasoconstrictors (54,90,91). Finally, in patients with life-threatening acute left ventricular failure, temporary use of a LV assist device may be required (32).

7. Conclusion

Takotsubo cardiomyopathy is a unique form of transient nonischemic stress-induced cardiomyopathy. A well-recognized syndrome now, two decades after its first reported case, it is also being reported in populations other than postmenopausal women. Even though apical ballooning phenotype is the most common and typical presentation, much confusion has resulted from various nomenclatures being used for different presentations of this syndrome. The underlying mechanism is not fully understood but could be common and explained by changes in molecular pathways like *stimulus trafficking* under supraphysiological levels of catecholamines, and influenced by hormonal status. Clinical history, electrocardiogram and diagnostic imaging with coronary angiography and/or cardiac magnetic resonance imaging that establishes typical phenotypic features of the disease in absence of significant obstructive coronary artery disease are essential for diagnosis and to differentiate it from an acute myocardial infarction. Management focuses on supportive care in the acute phase, while avoiding vasopressor medications. Mortality is low if patients survive the initial critical period and, by definition, they go on to have a full recovery. Recurrence has been reported but is rare. More studies are needed to fully understand the underlying mechanisms.

8. References

[1] Hurst RT, Prasad A, Askew JW 3rd, Sengupta PP, Tajik AJ. Takotsubo cardiomyopathy: a unique cardiomyopathy with variable ventricular morphology. *JACC Cardiovasc Imaging* 2010;3:641-9.

[2] Tsuchihashi K, Ueshima K, Uchida T, Oh-mura N, Kimura K, Owa M, Yoshiyama M, Miyazaki S, Haze K, Ogawa H, Honda T, Hase M, Kai R, Morii I; Angina Pectoris-Myocardial Infarction Investigations in Japan. Transient left ventricular apical ballooning without coronary artery stenosis: a novel heart syndrome mimicking acute myocardial infarction. Angina Pectoris-Myocardial Infarction Investigations in Japan. *J Am Coll Cardiol* 2001;38:11-8.

[3] Sharkey SW, Lesser JR, Maron MS, Maron BJ. Why not just call it tako-tsubo cardiomyopathy: a discussion of nomenclature. *J Am Coll Cardiol* 2011;57:1496-7.

[4] Maron BJ, Towbin JA, Thiene G, Antzelevitch C, Corrado D, Arnett D, Moss AJ, Seidman CE, Young JB; American Heart Association; Council on Clinical Cardiology, Heart Failure and Transplantation Committee; Quality of Care and Outcomes Research and Functional Genomics and Translational Biology Interdisciplinary Working Groups; Council on Epidemiology and Prevention. Contemporary definitions and classification of the cardiomyopathies: an American Heart Association Scientific Statement from the Council on Clinical Cardiology, Heart Failure and Transplantation Committee; Quality of Care and Outcomes Research and Functional Genomics and Translational Biology Interdisciplinary Working Groups; and Council on Epidemiology and Prevention. *Circulation* 2006;113:1807-16.

[5] Kapoor D, Bybee KA. Stress cardiomyopathy syndrome: a contemporary review. *Curr Heart Fail Rep* 2009;6:265-71.

[6] Sato H, Tateishi H, Uchida T. Takotsubo-type cardiomyopathy due to multivessel spasm. In: Kodama K, Haze K, Hon M, editors. *Clinical Aspect of Myocardial Injury: From Ischemia to Heart Failure.* Tokyo, Japan: Kagakuhyouronsha; 1990. p. 56–64.

[7] Dote K, Sato H, Tateishi H, Uchida T, Ishihara M. Myocardial stunning due to simultaneous multivessel coronary spasms: a review of 5 cases. *J Cardiol* 1991;21:203-14.

[8] Kawai S, Suzuki H, Yamaguchi H, Tanaka K, Sawada H, Aizawa T, Watanabe M, Tamura T, Umawatari K, Kawata M, Nakamura T, Yamanaka O, Okada R. Ampulla cardiomyopathy ('Takotusbo' cardiomyopathy)--reversible left ventricular dysfunction: with ST segment elevation. *Jpn Circ J* 2000;64:156-9.

[9] Kurisu S, Sato H, Kawagoe T, Ishihara M, Shimatani Y, Nishioka K, Kono Y, Umemura T, Nakamura S. Tako-tsubo-like left ventricular dysfunction with ST-segment elevation: a novel cardiac syndrome mimicking acute myocardial infarction. *Am Heart J* 2002;143:448-55.

[10] Akashi YJ, Goldstein DS, Barbaro G, Ueyama T. Takotsubo cardiomyopathy: a new form of acute, reversible heart failure. *Circulation* 2008;118:2754-62.

[11] Kurowski V, Kaiser A, von Hof K, Killermann DP, Mayer B, Hartmann F, Schunkert H, Radke PW. Apical and midventricular transient left ventricular dysfunction syndrome (tako-tsubo cardiomyopathy): frequency, mechanisms, and prognosis. *Chest* 2007;132:809-16.

[12] Bybee KA, Kara T, Prasad A, Lerman A, Barsness GW, Wright RS, Rihal CS. Systematic review: transient left ventricular apical ballooning: a syndrome that mimics ST-segment elevation myocardial infarction. *Ann Intern Med* 2004;141:858-65.

[13] Kushiro T, Saito F, Kusama J, Takahashi H, Imazeki T, Tani S, Kikuchi S, Imai S, Matsudaira K, Watanabe I, Hino T, Sato Y, Nakayama T, Nagao K, Kanmatsuse K. Takotsubo-shaped cardiomyopathy with type I CD36 deficiency. *Heart Vessels* 2005;20:123-5.

[14] Cherian J, Angelis D, Filiberti A, Saperia G. Can takotsubo cardiomyopathy be familial? *Int J Cardiol* 2007;121:74-5.

[15] Sharkey SW, Lesser JR, Zenovich AG, Maron MS, Lindberg J, Longe TF, Maron BJ. Acute and reversible cardiomyopathy provoked by stress in women from the United States. *Circulation* 2005;111:472-9.

[16] Wittstein IS, Thiemann DR, Lima JA, Baughman KL, Schulman SP, Gerstenblith G, Wu KC, Rade JJ, Bivalacqua TJ, Champion HC. Neurohumoral features of myocardial stunning due to sudden emotional stress. *N Engl J Med* 2005;352:539-48.

[17] Inoue M, Shimizu M, Ino H, Yamaguchi M, Terai H, Fujino N, Sakata K, Funada A, Tatami R, Ishise S, Kanaya H, Mabuchi H. Differentiation between patients with takotsubo cardiomyopathy and those with anterior acute myocardial infarction. *Circ J* 2005;69:89-94.

[18] Sato M, Fujita S, Saito A, Ikeda Y, Kitazawa H, Takahashi M, Ishiguro J, Okabe M, Nakamura Y, Nagai T, Watanabe H, Kodama M, Aizawa Y. Increased incidence of transient left ventricular apical ballooning (so-called 'Takotsubo' cardiomyopathy) after the mid-Niigata Prefecture earthquake. *Circ J* 2006;70:947-53.

[19] Bybee KA, Prasad A, Barsness GW, Lerman A, Jaffe AS, Murphy JG, Wright RS, Rihal CS. Clinical characteristics and thrombolysis in myocardial infarction frame counts in women with transient left ventricular apical ballooning syndrome. *Am J Cardiol* 2004;94:343-6.

[20] Yoshida T, Hibino T, Kako N, Murai S, Oguri M, Kato K, Yajima K, Ohte N, Yokoi K, Kimura G. A pathophysiologic study of tako-tsubo cardiomyopathy with F-18 fluorodeoxyglucose positron emission tomography. *Eur Heart J* 2007;28:2598-604.

[21] Akashi YJ, Musha H, Kida K, Itoh K, Inoue K, Kawasaki K, Hashimoto N, Miyake F. Reversible ventricular dysfunction takotsubo cardiomyopathy. *Eur J Heart Fail* 2005;7:1171-6.

[22] Schoof S, Bertram H, Hohmann D, Jack T, Wessel A, Yelbuz TM. Takotsubo cardiomyopathy in a 2-year-old girl: 3-dimensional visualization of reversible left ventricular dysfunction. *J Am Coll Cardiol* 2010;55:e5.

[23] Hafiz AM, Jan F, Allaqaband S. The near fatal crossing: a rare recurrence of takotsubo cardiomyopathy in a 66-year-old woman. *Internet Journal of Cardiology* 2009;7.

[24] Takizawa M, Kobayakawa N, Uozumi H, Yonemura S, Kodama T, Fukusima K, Takeuchi H, Kaneko Y, Kaneko T, Fujita K, Honma Y, Aoyagi T. A case of transient left ventricular ballooning with pheochromocytoma, supporting pathogenetic role of catecholamines in stress-induced cardiomyopathy or takotsubo cardiomyopathy. *Int J Cardiol* 2007;114:e15-7.

[25] Gujja KR, Aslam AF, Privman V, Tejani F, Vasavada B. Initial presentation of pheochromocytoma with Takotsubo cardiomyopathy: a brief review of literature. *J Cardiovasc Med* (Hagerstown) 2010;11:49-52.
[26] Rossi AP, Bing-You RG, Thomas LR. Recurrent takotsubo cardiomyopathy associated with pheochromocytoma. *Endocr Pract* 2009;15:560-2.
[27] Sanchez-Recalde A, Costero O, Oliver JM, Iborra C, Ruiz E, Sobrino JA. Images in cardiovascular medicine. Pheochromocytoma-related cardiomyopathy: inverted Takotsubo contractile pattern. *Circulation* 2006;113:e738-9.
[28] Santana-Cabrera L, Escot CR, Medina Gil JM, Ortiz CP. Takotsubo Cardiomyopathy Associated with Acute Subarachnoid Hemorrhage. *J Emerg Med* 2010 Oct 6. [Epub ahead of print]
[29] Kittisupamongkol W. Takotsubo cardiomyopathy in subarachnoid hemorrhage. *Int J Cardiol* 2010;144:324; author reply 325.
[30] Das M, Gonsalves S, Saha A, Ross S, Williams G. Acute subarachnoid haemorrhage as a precipitant for takotsubo cardiomyopathy: a case report and discussion. *Int J Cardiol* 2009;132:283-5.
[31] Ono Y, Kawamura T, Ito J, Kanayama S, Miura T, Kikuchi F. Ampulla (takotsubo) cardiomyopathy associated with subarachnoid hemorrhage worsening in the late phase of vasospasm--case report. *Neurol Med Chir* (Tokyo) 2004;44:72-4.
[32] Lyon AR, Rees PS, Prasad S, Poole-Wilson PA, Harding SE. Stress (Takotsubo) cardiomyopathy--a novel pathophysiological hypothesis to explain catecholamine-induced acute myocardial stunning. *Nat Clin Pract Cardiovasc Med* 2008;5:22-9.
[33] Song BG, Park SJ, Noh HJ, Jo HC, Choi JO, Lee SC, Park SW, Jeon ES, Kim DK, Oh JK. Clinical characteristics, and laboratory and echocardiographic findings in takotsubo cardiomyopathy presenting as cardiogenic shock. *J Crit Care* 2010;25:329-35.
[34] Desmet WJ, Adriaenssens BF, Dens JA. Apical ballooning of the left ventricle: first series in white patients. *Heart* 2003;89:1027-31.
[35] Prasad A, Lerman A, Rihal CS. Apical ballooning syndrome (Tako-Tsubo or stress cardiomyopathy): a mimic of acute myocardial infarction. *Am Heart J* 2008;155:408-17.
[36] Singh NK, Rumman S, Mikell FL, Nallamothu N, Rangaswamy C. Stress cardiomyopathy: clinical and ventriculographic characteristics in 107 North American subjects. *Int J Cardiol* 2010;141:297-303.
[37] Bielecka-Dabrowa A, Mikhailidis DP, Hannam S, Rysz J, Michalska M, Akashi YJ, Banach M. Takotsubo cardiomyopathy--the current state of knowledge. *Int J Cardiol* 2010;142:120-5.
[38] Kurisu S, Inoue I, Kawagoe T, Ishihara M, Shimatani Y, Nakama Y, Maruhashi T, Kagawa E, Dai K, Matsushita J, Ikenaga H. Prevalence of incidental coronary artery disease in tako-tsubo cardiomyopathy. *Coron Artery Dis* 2009;20:214-8.
[39] Madhavan M, Prasad A. Proposed Mayo Clinic criteria for the diagnosis of Tako-Tsubo cardiomyopathy and long-term prognosis. *Herz* 2010 Jun 3. [Epub ahead of print]
[40] Mitchell JH, Hadden TB, Wilson JM, Achari A, Muthupillai R, Flamm SD. Clinical features and usefulness of cardiac magnetic resonance imaging in assessing

myocardial viability and prognosis in Takotsubo cardiomyopathy (transient left ventricular apical ballooning syndrome). *Am J Cardiol* 2007;100:296-301.

[41] Deetjen AC, Conradi G, Mollmann S, Rad A, Hamm CW, Dill T. Value of gadolinium-enhanced magnetic resonance imaging in patients with Tako-Tsubo-like left ventricular dysfunction. *J Cardiovasc Magn Reson* 2006;8:367-72.

[42] Madhavan M, Rihal CS, Lerman A, Prasad A. Acute heart failure in apical ballooning syndrome (TakoTsubo/stress cardiomyopathy): clinical correlates and Mayo Clinic risk score. *J Am Coll Cardiol* 2011;57:1400-1.

[43] Tarkin JM, Khetyar M, Kaski JC. Management of Tako-tsubo syndrome. *Cardiovasc Drugs Ther* 2008;22:71-7.

[44] Nef HM, Möllmann H, Kostin S, Troidl C, Voss S, Weber M, Dill T, Rolf A, Brandt R, Hamm CW, Elsässer A. Tako-Tsubo cardiomyopathy: intraindividual structural analysis in the acute phase and after functional recovery. *Eur Heart J* 2007;28:2456-64.

[45] Nef HM, Möllmann H, Elsässer A. Tako-tsubo cardiomyopathy (apical ballooning). *Heart* 2007;93:1309-15.

[46] Nef HM, Möllmann H, Troidl C, Kostin S, Voss S, Hilpert P, Behrens CB, Rolf A, Rixe J, Weber M, Hamm CW, Elsässer A. Abnormalities in intracellular Ca2+ regulation contribute to the pathomechanism of Tako-Tsubo cardiomyopathy. *Eur Heart J* 2009;30:2155-64.

[47] Nef HM, Möllmann H, Hilpert P, Troidl C, Voss S, Rolf A, Behrens CB, Weber M, Hamm CW, Elsässer A. Activated cell survival cascade protects cardiomyocytes from cell death in Tako-Tsubo cardiomyopathy. *Eur J Heart Fail* 2009;11:758-64.

[48] Akashi YJ, Nef HM, Möllmann H, Ueyama T. Stress cardiomyopathy. *Annu Rev Med* 2010;61:271-86.

[49] Nef HM, Möllmann H, Akashi YJ, Hamm CW. Mechanisms of stress (Takotsubo) cardiomyopathy. *Nat Rev Cardiol* 2010;7:187-93.

[50] Villareal RP, Achari A, Wilansky S, Wilson JM. Anteroapical stunning and left ventricular outflow tract obstruction. *Mayo Clin Proc* 2001;76:79-83.

[51] Fefer P, Chelvanathan A, Dick AJ, Teitelbaum EJ, Strauss BH, Cohen EA. Takotsubo cardiomyopathy and left ventricular outflow tract obstruction. *J Interv Cardiol* 2009;22:444-52.

[52] El Mahmoud R, Mansencal N, Pilliére R, Leyer F, Abbou N, Michaud P, Nallet O, Digne F, Lacombe P, Cattan S, Dubourg O. Prevalence and characteristics of left ventricular outflow tract obstruction in Tako-Tsubo syndrome. *Am Heart J* 2008;156:543-8.

[53] Merli E, Sutcliffe S, Gori M, Sutherland GG. Tako-Tsubo cardiomyopathy: new insights into the possible underlying pathophysiology. *Eur J Echocardiogr* 2006;7:53-61.

[54] Shah BN, Curzen NP. Dynamic left ventricular outflow tract obstruction and acute heart failure in tako-tsubo cardiomyopathy. *J Am Coll Cardiol* 2011;58:1195-6.

[55] Gianni M, Dentali F, Grandi AM, Sumner G, Hiralal R, Lonn E. Apical ballooning syndrome or takotsubo cardiomyopathy: a systematic review. *Eur Heart J* 2006;27:1523-9.

[56] Ibanez B, Choi BG, Navarro F, Farre J. Tako-tsubo syndrome: a form of spontaneous aborted myocardial infarction? *Eur Heart J* 2006;27:1509-10.

[57] Desmet W. Dynamic LV obstruction in apical ballooning syndrome: the chicken or the egg. *Eur J Echocardiogr* 2006;7:1-4.

[58] Pilgrim TM, Wyss TR. Takotsubo cardiomyopathy or transient left ventricular apical ballooning syndrome: A systematic review. *Int J Cardiol* 2008;124:283-92.

[59] Kurisu S, Inoue I, Kawagoe T, Ishihara M, Shimatani Y, Nishioka K, Umemura T, Nakamura S, Yoshida M, Sato H. Myocardial perfusion and fatty acid metabolism in patients with tako-tsubo-like left ventricular dysfunction. *J Am Coll Cardiol* 2003;41:743-8.

[60] Kume T, Akasaka T, Kawamoto T, Watanabe N, Yoshitani H, Akiyama M, Koyama Y, Neishi Y, Tsukiji M, Yoshida K. [Relationship between coronary flow reserve and recovery of regional left ventricular function in patients with tako-tsubo-like transient left ventricular dysfunction]. *J Cardiol* 2004;43:123-9.

[61] Trevi GP, Sheiban I. Chronic ischaemic ('hibernating') and postischaemic ('stunned') dysfunctional but viable myocardium. *Eur Heart J* 1991;12 Suppl G:20-6.

[62] Akashi YJ, Nakazawa K, Sakakibara M, Miyake F, Koike H, Sasaka K. The clinical features of takotsubo cardiomyopathy. *QJM* 2003;96:563-73.

[63] Goldstein DS, Eisenhofer G, Kopin IJ. Sources and significance of plasma levels of catechols and their metabolites in humans. *J Pharmacol Exp Ther* 2003;305:800-11.

[64] Volz HC, Erbel C, Berentelg J, Katus HA, Frey N. Reversible left ventricular dysfunction resembling Takotsubo syndrome after self-injection of adrenaline. *Can J Cardiol* 2009;25:e261-2.

[65] Litvinov IV, Kotowycz MA, Wassmann S. Iatrogenic epinephrine-induced reverse Takotsubo cardiomyopathy: direct evidence supporting the role of catecholamines in the pathophysiology of the "broken heart syndrome." *Clin Res Cardiol* 2009;98:457-62.

[66] Khullar M, Datta BN, Wahi PL, Chakravarti RN. Catecholamine-induced experimental cardiomyopathy--a histopathological, histochemical and ultrastructural study. *Indian Heart J* 1989;41:307-13.

[67] Singal PK, Kapur N, Dhillon KS, Beamish RE, Dhalla NS. Role of free radicals in catecholamine-induced cardiomyopathy. *Can J Physiol Pharmacol* 1982;60:1390-7.

[68] Bolli R, Marbán E. Molecular and cellular mechanisms of myocardial stunning. Physiol Rev 1999;79:609-34.

[69] Mori H, Ishikawa S, Kojima S, Hayashi J, Watanabe Y, Hoffman JI, Okino H. Increased responsiveness of left ventricular apical myocardium to adrenergic stimuli. *Cardiovasc Res* 1993;27:192-8.

[70] Stein B, Bartel S, Kirchhefer U, Kokott S, Krause EG, Neumann J, Schmitz W, Scholz H. Relation between contractile function and regulatory cardiac proteins in hypertrophied hearts. *Am J Physiol* 1996;270(6 Pt 2):H2021-8.

[71] Boluyt MO, Long X, Eschenhagen T, Mende U, Schmitz W, Crow MT, Lakatta EG. Isoproterenol infusion induces alterations in expression of hypertrophy-associated genes in rat heart. *Am J Physiol* 1995;269(2 Pt 2):H638-47.

[72] Babu GJ, Bhupathy P, Petrashevskaya NN, Wang H, Raman S, Wheeler D, Jagatheesan G, Wieczorek D, Schwartz A, Janssen PM, Ziolo MT, Periasamy M. Targeted overexpression of sarcolipin in the mouse heart decreases sarcoplasmic reticulum calcium transport and cardiac contractility. *J Biol Chem* 2006;281:3972-9.

[73] Asahi M, Otsu K, Nakayama H, Hikoso S, Takeda T, Gramolini AO, Trivieri MG, Oudit GY, Morita T, Kusakari Y, Hirano S, Hongo K, Hirotani S, Yamaguchi O, Peterson A, Backx PH, Kurihara S, Hori M, MacLennan DH. Cardiac-specific overexpression of sarcolipin inhibits sarco(endo)plasmic reticulum Ca2+ ATPase (SERCA2a) activity and impairs cardiac function in mice. *Proc Natl Acad Sci U S A* 2004;101:9199-204.

[74] Linck B, Bokník P, Baba HA, Eschenhagen T, Haverkamp U, Jäckel E, Jones LR, Kirchhefer U, Knapp J, Läer S, Müller FU, Schmitz W, Scholz H, Syska A, Vahlensieck U, Neumann J. Long-term beta adrenoceptor-mediated alteration in contractility and expression of phospholamban and sarcoplasmic reticulum Ca(++)-ATPase in mammalian ventricle. *J Pharmacol Exp Ther* 1998;286:531-8.

[75] Lipskaia L, Lompré AM. Alteration in temporal kinetics of Ca2+ signaling and control of growth and proliferation. *Biol Cell* 2004;96:55-68.

[76] Port JD, Bristow MR. Altered beta-adrenergic receptor gene regulation and signaling in chronic heart failure. *J Mol Cell Cardiol* 2001;33:887-905.

[77] Heubach JF, Ravens U, Kaumann AJ. Epinephrine activates both Gs and Gi pathways, but norepinephrine activates only the Gs pathway through human beta2-adrenoceptors overexpressed in mouse heart. *Mol Pharmacol* 2004;65:1313-22.

[78] Heubach JF, Blaschke M, Harding SE, Ravens U, Kaumann AJ. Cardiostimulant and cardiodepressant effects through overexpressed human beta2-adrenoceptors in murine heart: regional differences and functional role of beta1-adrenoceptors. *Naunyn Schmiedebergs Arch Pharmacol* 2003;367:380-90.

[79] Zamah AM, Delahunty M, Luttrell LM, Lefkowitz RJ. Protein kinase A-mediated phosphorylation of the beta 2-adrenergic receptor regulates its coupling to Gs and Gi. Demonstration in a reconstituted system. *J Biol Chem* 2002;277:31249-56.

[80] Kawano H, Okada R, Yano K. Histological study on the distribution of autonomic nerves in the human heart. *Heart Vessels* 2003;18:32-9.

[81] Kuroko Y, Yamazaki T, Tokunaga N, Akiyama T, Kitagawa H, Ishino K, Sano S, Mori H. Cardiac epinephrine synthesis and ischemia-induced myocardial epinephrine release. *Cardiovasc Res* 2007;74:438-44.

[82] Grohé C, Kahlert S, Löbbert K, Stimpel M, Karas RH, Vetter H, Neyses L. Cardiac myocytes and fibroblasts contain functional estrogen receptors. *FEBS Lett* 1997;416:107-12.

[83] Bupha-Intr T, Wattanapermpool J. Regulatory role of ovarian sex hormones in calcium uptake activity of cardiac sarcoplasmic reticulum. *Am J Physiol Heart Circ Physiol* 2006;291:H1101-8.

[84] Burgdorf C, Nef HM, Haghi D, Kurowski V, Radke PW. Tako-tsubo (stress-induced) cardiomyopathy and cancer. *Ann Intern Med* 2010;152:830-1.

[85] Harding SE, Gong H. beta-adrenoceptor blockers as agonists: coupling of beta2-adrenoceptors to multiple G-proteins in the failing human heart. *Congest Heart Fail* 2004;10:181-5; quiz 186-7.

[86] Padayachee L. Levosimendan: the inotrope of choice in cardiogenic shock secondary to takotsubo cardiomyopathy? *Heart Lung Circ* 2007;16 Suppl 3:S65-70.

[87] De Santis V, Vitale D, Tritapepe L, Greco C, Pietropaoli P. Use of levosimendan for cardiogenic shock in a patient with the apical ballooning syndrome. *Ann Intern Med* 2008;149:365-7.

[88] Antonini M, Stazi GV, Cirasa MT, Garotto G, Frustaci A. Efficacy of levosimendan in Takotsubo-related cardiogenic shock. *Acta Anaesthesiol Scand* 2010;54:119-20.

[89] Brown ML, Abel MD, Click RL, Morford RG, Dearani JA, Sundt TM, Orszulak TA, Schaff HV. Systolic anterior motion after mitral valve repair: is surgical intervention necessary? *J Thor Cardiovasc Surg* 2007;133:136-43.

[90] Madhavan M, Pislaru SV, Prasad A. Reply. *J Am Coll Cardiol* 2011;58:1196.

[91] Kyuma M, Tsuchihashi K, Shinshi Y, Hase M, Nakata T, Ooiwa H, Abiru M, Hikita N, Adachi T, Shoji T, Fujise Y, Shimamoto K. Effect of intravenous propranolol on left ventricular apical ballooning without coronary artery stenosis (ampulla cardiomyopathy): three cases. *Circ J* 2002;66:1181-4.

12

Pathology of Takotsubo (Ampulla) Cardiomyopathy

Sachio Kawai
Department of Cardiology, Juntendo University School of Medicine, Tokyo, Japan

1. Introduction

Takotsubo (ampulla) cardiomyopathy is characterized by slight to moderate elevation of cardiac enzymes. It is reasonable to think that the elevated levels are evidence of myocardial damage (cardiac-specific enzymes are released from the cytoplasm of damaged cardiac myocytes into extracellular fluid). Thus, it is problematic to consider takotsubo cardiomyopathy as (neurogenic) stunned myocardium, because stunned myocardium is defined as a state without histopathological changes observable by light microscopy.[1] In the study, I will describe histological findings in autopsied cases in Japan and histopathological findings of endomyocardial biopsy cases with a literature review.

2. Autopsied cases

Nine Japanese autopsied cases were studied, with the permission of relevant institutions. We examined their histopathological changes, findings in transverse tissue sections by site (near the left ventricular apex and base) and by layer (relative damage by depth of ventricular myocardium), and differences in lesions.[2] Table 1 shows the age, sex, underlying diseases, trigger event, and symptoms of the cases.[3]

Case 2. A 66-year-old woman was admitted to the hospital with paralysis and brain infiltration by Hodgkin's lymphoma. Her symptoms improved with steroid therapy and radiation therapy. There was no clear trigger event. She developed sudden bradycardia, hypotension, and extensive ST-segment elevation. She underwent intravenous infusion of 2 mg epinephrine, and subsequently developed chest pain. The patient had a normal coronary angiogram, extensive hypokinesis mainly in the apical segment, and hyperkinesis of the basal segment. Creatinine kinase level increased to 169 U/l at a maximum. There was no pulmonary congestion, but severe hypoxemia continued and the patient died on the fourth day of illness.[4] Autopsy showed neither significant coronary artery stenosis nor significant fibrosis in the ventricular transverse sections near the apical or basal segment. The ventricular wall were thickened; 15.2 mm in the basal anterior wall, 13.8 mm in the basal lateral wall, 13.2 mm in the basal posterior wall, 17.5 mm in the basal interventricular septum, 10.0 mm in the apical anterior wall, 13.0 mm in the apical lateral wall, 10.2 mm in the apical posterior wall, and 8.0 mm in the apical interventricular septum. Histologically, there was disseminated or diffuse damage to the cardiac myocytes, and extensive damage was observed from the inner to outer layer. In general, pathological changes were myocyte damage, degeneration, lysis, or loss occurring in an individual myocyte or several myocytes. Some cases had lesions concentrated on specific muscle bundles and other cases had disseminated lesions (Figure 1, upper left). In addition, higher degree of cell infiltration was seen at sites with more severely damaged myocardium (Figure 1, lower left).

Cases	Underlying Disorders	Trigger Event	Initial Symptoms	Duration (cause of death)
61 F	RA, pneumonia	Septic shock	Syncope	2 days (sepsis)
66 F	Hodgkin, HT,	Epinephrine injection	Syncope	4 days (dyspnea)
75 M	Anorexia	Pneumonia	Pulmo. edema	20 days (pneumonia)
77 M	DM, CRF, Multiple myeloma	Leg ulcer	Chest pain	19 days (sepsis)
81 F	RA, HT	Pneumonia	Dyspnea	21 days (pulmo.hemo.)
81 F	Pneumonia	Dyspnea	Dyspnea	3 days (ARDS)
82 F	Bronchial asthma	Unknown	Syncope	20 days (sepsis)
83 F	HT	None	Palpitation	5 days (tamponade)
84 F	None	None	Chest pain	4 days (tamponade)

This table shows autopsied patients. The patients were composed of seven elderly females and two males aged 61 to 84 years. They had several serious underlying disorders and some patients had trigger events such as septic shock, injection of epinephrine, pneumonia. Initial symptoms were syncope or pulmonary edema, dyspnea or chest pain. They died from sepsis, respiratory failure, pneumonia, pulmonary hemorrhage, or cardiac tamponade. The duration of takotsubo cardiomyopathy ranged from 2 to 21 days.

Table 1. Autopsied cases

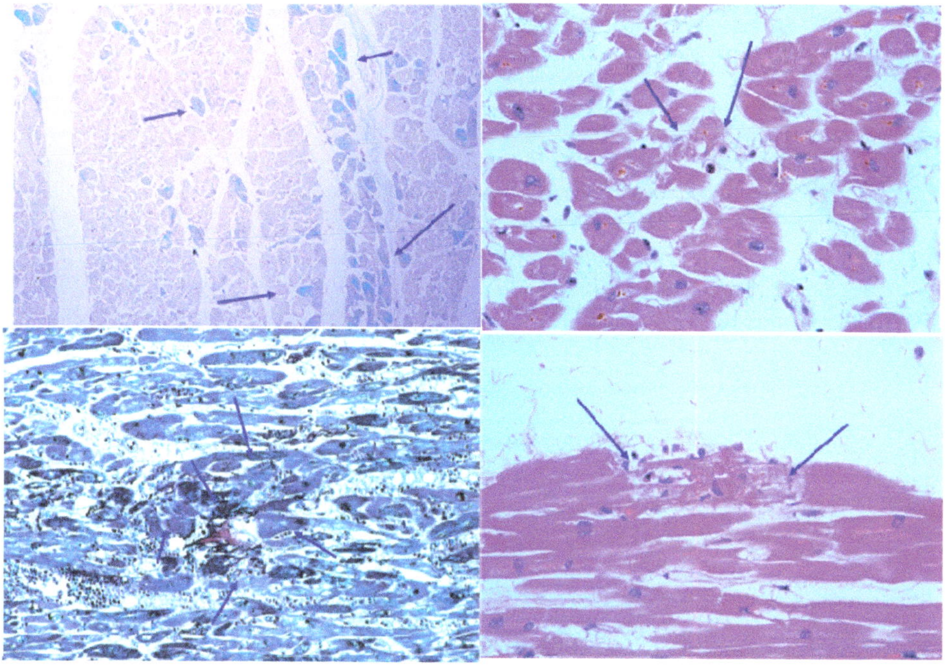

Upper left: Damaged individual myocytes or a group of myocytes had increased eosinophil staining. Inner layer of the base: Luxol fast blue stain, x 200. (Case 2 : 66y-o, Female)

Lower left: Middle layer of the apex: Phosphoptungstic acid hematoxylin stain, x 200. (Case 2 : 66y-o, Female)

Upper right: Injured cardiac myocytes are removed by infiltrated macrophages. Apical anterior, middle layer. Hematoxylin and eosin (H&E) stain, x 400. (Case 5 : 81Y-o, Female)

Lower right: Myocardial damage was observed even in the epicardial aspect which was difficult to explain by disorder of coronary circulation. Apical posterior, external layer. H&E stain, x 400. (Case 5 : 81Y-o, Female)

Fig. 1. Pathology of takotsubo cardiomyopathy

Case 5. An 81-year-old woman had chronic rheumatoid arthritis. She also had hypertension. She was admitted to the hospital due to pneumonia. Pneumonia was resistant to treatment. On the tenth day of hospitalization, she developed dyspnea after walking to the bathroom. Electrocardiography showed ST-segment elevation in leads I, II, aVL, and V2-6. Her blood pressure was 80 mm Hg and she went into shock. Emergency coronary angiography showed basal hyperkinesis, apical ballooning, and apical hypokinesis but no significant stenosis. Pulmonary artery wedge pressure was 20 mm Hg and the creatinine kinase level was 296 U/l. The patient developed acute respiratory distress syndrome and died on the eleventh day of hospitalization (second day of Takotsubo cardiomyopathy).[5] Histologically, a group of myocytes showed an increase in eosinophil staining, contraction band formation, necrosis, and rupture. Damaged individual myocytes were ingested by infiltrated macrophages (Figure 1, upper right). Myocardial damage was also seen in the epicardial aspect which was difficult to explain by disorder of coronary circulation (Figure 1, lower right).

Case 8. An 83-year-old woman was suspected as fulminant myocarditis. There was ST-segment elevation in leads II, III, aVF, and V2-6. The patient had extensive akinesis of the left ventricular apex and hyperkinesis of the base. Emergency coronary angiography showed no stenosis. Endomyocardial biopsy showed myocardial degeneration and necrosis, and inflammatory cell infiltration. The patient was diagnosed as fulminant myocarditis. She underwent intra-aortic balloon pumping, steroid pulse therapy, and percutaneous cardiopulmonary support. The patient died on the sixth day. Autopsy revealed an enlarged heart weighing 540 g and cardiac tamponade of 310 ml. The microscopic findings indicated myocardial damage consistent with other takotsubo cardiomyopathy cases and extensive and severe secondary cell infiltration (Figure 2). Interstitial cell infiltration was prominent and concentrated in areas with severe myocardial damage. Secondary findings included hemorrhage in the epicardial adipose tissue at the pulmonary arterial root and amyloid deposition.

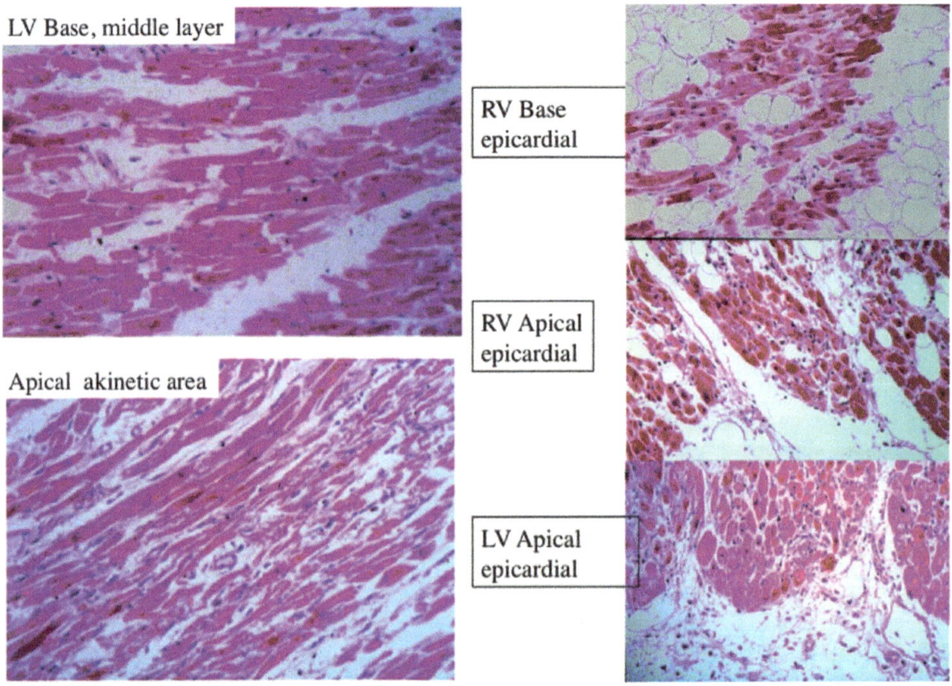

Marked segmentation of myocytes was observed in the middle layer of the hyperkinetic basal left ventricle (**lower left**). Damaged cells had undergone atrophy and lysis in the akinetic apical segment (lower left). There were similar lesions in the right ventricle. Segmentation was seen even in myocytes which were sparse in the adipose tissue in the basal outer layer (**upper right**). In the right ventricle in the apical aspect (**middle right**), there were marked myocyte injuries and lysis and interstitial cell infiltration in addition to segmentation. Similarly, when the apical left ventricle in the epicardial aspect (**lower right**) was examined, there was myocyte damage near the epicardial aspect and cell infiltration into the epicardium. Myocardial tissue: H&E stain, x200.

Fig. 2. Autopsied case: 83-year-old woman suspected of fulminant myocarditis

Figure 3 shows single myocyte lesions in the left ventricle in other cases. In this figure, two injured myocytes were observed. The myocardial injury did not extended to the adjacent myocytes.

3. Right ventricular lesion

When more detailed microscopic examinations were performed, there were also right ventricular lesions (Figure 4).

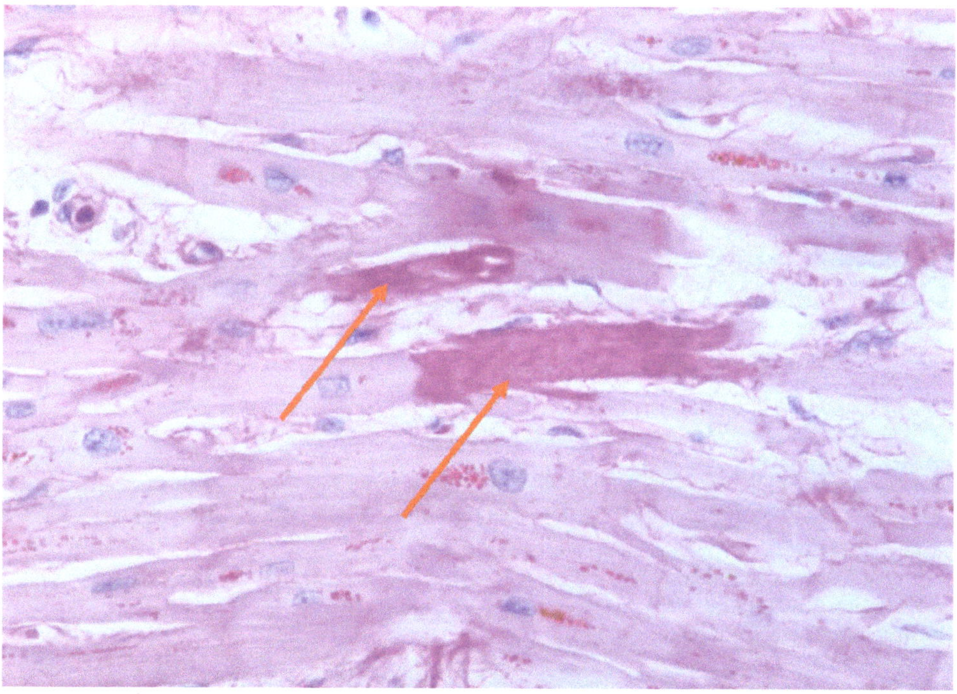

In this figure, two injured myocytes were observed (**red arrows**). The myocardial injury did not extended to the adjacent myocytes. Periodic acid Schiff reaction, x1000.

Fig. 3. Single myocyte lesions

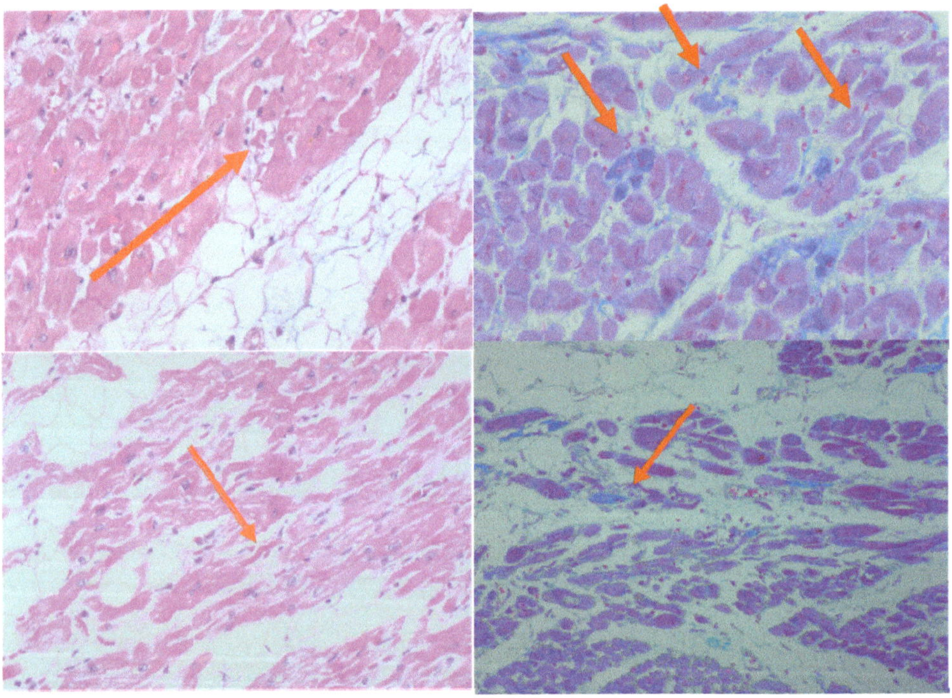

Upper left: 81 y-o, apical region, H&E stain, x 200
Lower left: 66 y-o, H&E stain, x 200
Upper right: 81 y-o, apical. H&E stain, x 200
Lower right: 84 y-o, H&E stain, x 300

Fig. 4. Right ventricular lesions

4. Morphometrical studies

The number of damaged myocytes relative to the number of myocytes comprising the ventricular wall (layer) were examined in the transverse section specimens of the ventricular apex and base. The transverse section specimen were scanned under high power view along two perpendicular lines (Figure 5). Increased eosinophilic staining (azan-blue stained degeneration), segmentation,[7] myofibrillar agglomeration with disrupted cross striation structure, and myofibrillar degeneration, lysis, and loss (showing fragmentation) were counted as the damaged myocytes. The myocytes with normal cross striation structure were not considered as damaged cells. The damaged myocytes to the number of the myocytes comprising the ventricular wall was calculated. This ratio (in percentage) was significantly higher in the apical segment at 13.5% than in the basal segment at 5.3% (Table 2) .

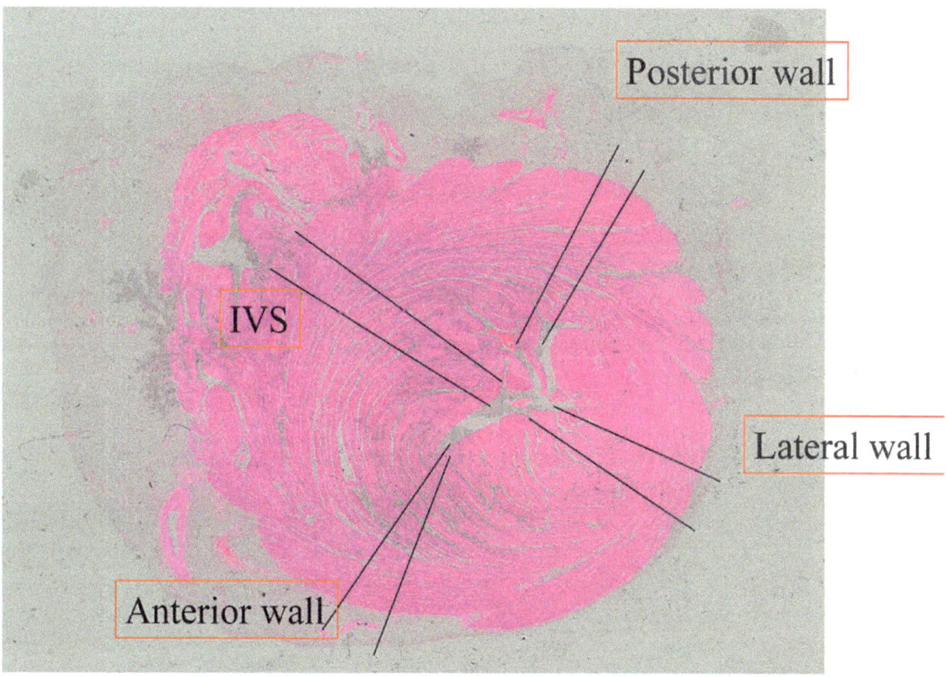

Autopsy study: The number of myocardial cells comprising the compact layer of the ventricular wall and the numbers of the damaged myocytes were counted as follows. Two sampling lines perpendicular to the compact layer were drawn from the outer to the inner layers, and the numbers of the normal myocardial cells and the damaged myocytes intersecting the lines were determined employing an image analyzer. The mean values were determined at 4 sites on the transverse section: the anterior, lateral and, posterior walls of the left ventricle, the middle-portion of the interventricular septum. Transverse sections from the cardiac base and the apical segment were scanned.

Fig. 5. Percentage of the injured myocytes (morphometrical measurement)

Cases	Apical section					Basal section				
	A	L	P	IVS	mean (%)	A	L	P	IVS	mean
61F	10.0	11.4	10.3	10.3	10.5	3.5	5.2	6.5	5.1	5.1
66F	10.9	6.2	2.3	8.8	7.1	3.0	4.3	2.5	2.0	3.0
75M	14.3	12,0	12.2	12.0	12.6	3.2	5.4	5.8	5.1	4.9
77M	9.3	11.9	7.2	6.5	6.3	3.2	4.3	2.8	2.7	3.3
81F	10.7	12.0	8.0	10.1	10.2	3.5	5.4	4.4	5.0	4.6
81F	16.8	17.0	18.3	14.7	16.7	5.4	5.7	4.7	5.0	5.2
82F	14.5	17.1	12.6	12.6	13.9	7.8	8.0	6.2	4.7	6.7
83F	15.8	19.8	29.6	33.1	23.6	9.5	5.8	5.3	9.8	7.6
84F	23.0	20.0	21.7	17.9	20.7	10.1	17.1	19.6	12.0	14.7
mean					13.5					6.4

A: anterior wall, L: lateral wall, P: posterior wall, IVS: interventricular septum

Percentage of damaged myocytes to the number of the myocytes comprising the ventricular wall was tabled in this slide.
The left-sided figures were percentages of the damaged myocytes in the apical portion. The figures of the right were those from the basal segments. Percentages of the damaged myocytes in Takotsubo cardiomyopathy were relatively small compared to those of injured myocytes in patients with myocardial infarction. There is significant difference in the distribution of the myocardial lesion between cardiac base and the apical region. Percentages of the damaged myocytes were higher in the apical area than in the basal segment.

Table 2. Percentage of relative myocardial damage

Transverse sections of the left ventricular anterior wall were examined near the base and apex (myocardial transverse sections observed from the epicardial and endocardial aspects). A light microscope was used with a grid in the eyepiece (42-point "Weibel" test grid) to measure the relative density of capillaries. In the 21-line segments in the test grid, the number of capillaries was counted in each of 10 fields of view. The relative density of capillaries was 7.1 ± 1.01 in the base and 6.5 ± 0.96 in the apex, indicating no significant difference. These densities could not explain the difference in damaged myocytes by site or the difference in wall motion by site.

5. Relative injury score

Percentage of damaged myocytes to the number of the myocytes comprising the ventricular wall is tabled in the Table 3. The upper figures are percentages of the damaged myocytes in the basal portion. The lower figures were those from the apical segments. Percentages of the damaged myocytes in Takotsubo cardiomyopathy were relatively small compared to those of injured myocytes in patients with myocardial infarction. There is a significant difference in the distribution of the myocardial lesion between the cardiac base and the apical region. Percentages of the damaged myocytes were higher in the apical area than in the basal segment. The damage was particularly severe in the trabeculae carneae of the anterior wall (by site) and the subendocardium (by layer) .

Basal	Anterior	Lateral	Posterior	Septal	
Subendocardium	21.2%	21.1%	22.3%		21.6%
Inner layer	24.0%	22.6%	23.2%	19.2%	22.2%
Middle layer	22.1%	24.8%	24.5%	21.8%	23.3%
Outer layer	17.6%	18.3%	15.0%	19.7%	17.7%
	21.2%	21.7%	21.3%	20.2%	

Apical	Anterior	Lateral	Posterior	Septal	
Subendocardium	33.5% **	21.5%	24.5%		26.5%
Inner layer	29.4%	27.1%	23.8%	26.5%	26.7%*
Middle layer	33.3% *	28.9%	23.8%	29.3%	28.8%*
Outer layer	24.8% *	22.8%	21.2%*	26.5%*	23.8%
	30.2%*	25.1%	23.3%*	27.4%*	

*:p<0.05, **p<0.01

Percentage of damaged myocytes to the number of the myocytes in the several layers (the subendocardium and trabeculla layers, the inner layers, the middle layers and the outer layers of the anterior, the lateral, the posterior wall and the interventricular septum) was tabled in the Table 3. The upper figures were percentages of the damaged myocytes in the basal portion. The lower figures were those from the apical segments. There is a significant difference in the distribution of the myocardial lesion between the cardiac base and the apical region. Percentages of the damaged myocytes were higher in the apical area than in the basal segment. The damage was particularly severe in the trabeculae carneae of the anterior wall (by site) and the subendocardium (by layer) .

Table 3. Relative Injury Score

6. Summary of cardiac autopsy findings

Clear myocardial lesions were observed in takotsubo cardiomyopathy cases. Epicardial lesions were observed (Figure 1, lower right) which are uncommon in ischemia. Right ventricular lesions were also observed (Figure 4). The myocardial lesions were characterized mainly by individual myocytes or a group of myocytes with increased eosinophil staining , contraction band formation, necrosis, and rupture. The basis of the lesion was a damaged individual myocyte (Figure 3) and aggregation of these damaged myocytes (Figure 1, upper left. If individual myocyte damage occurs due to disorder of microcirculatory units composing the intramyocardial circulatory system,[8] it is difficult to explain pathological changes of takotsubo cardiomyopathy as intramyocardial circulatory disorder.

The extension of lesion was near circumferential within the same ventricle and it tended to be prominent from the mid-portion to apex of the ventricle. In histological measurement, the proportion of damaged myocytes was higher in the apex than the base (mid-portion).

Damage was prominent in the apical inner and middle layers (by ventricular myocardial layer) and in the anterior wall, posterior wall, and septum (by site). The damage was particularly severe in the trabeculae carneae of the anterior wall (by site) and subendocardium (by layer) (Table 3). These results indicate that it might be possible to depict predilection sites by MRI with delayed gadolinium enhancement.[9]

Autopsy cases with myocardial diseases were reported in the regional meetings of the Japanese Circulation Society. There have been many recent reports such as on a 77-year-old woman with myocardial infarction-like electrocardiographic pattern during the course of malabsorption syndrome[10] and on an 84-year-old woman who died from cardiac rupture[11] (four days after the onset, cardiac arrest occurred due to cardiac rupture). In the Circulation Journal, Sacha et al.[12] stated the case of Ohara et al.[13] in the same journal as the first autopsy case [of takotsubo cardiomyopathy] and their own case was the second one. However, this information is not accurate. There were previously reported autopsy cases in the journals Heart and Respiration & Circulation. There were reports of takotsubo cardiomyopathy itself by Kumamoto et al.,[14] Sasa et al.,[15] and Tokioka et al.[16] Thus, there were already reports of takotsubo cardiomyopathy as a phenomenon, and autopsy cases were published in a journal[17] before that of Ohara et al. Thus, Sacha et al. should have been advised to revise the information in the peer review.

7. Case presentation of endomyocardial biopsy

Table 4 shows 15 cases of endomyocardial biopsy for which relevant institutions provided approval for microscopic examination. The cases are listed in the order of number of days from onset to biopsy.

8. Case biopsied on the day of onset (Case 2)

The patient was an 82-year-old woman who had undergone uterine myomectomy at age 48. She developed sudden pharyngeal discomfort. There was ST-segment elevation in leads II, III, aVF, and V2-6. Echocardiography showed diffuse hypokinesis except in the base. Ventriculography revealed hyperkinesis of the base and balloon-like enlargement of the apex. She was suspected of myocarditis and underwent biopsy. Her condition improved on the 26th day of illness. Biopsy showed slight increase in young connective tissue and infiltration of cells, including polymorphonuclear leukocytes (Figure 6, upper left).

9. Case thought to have a ventricular aneurysm (Case 7)

The patient was a 69-year-old man with no contributory medical history. He became lost in the mountains while gathering edible wild plants and was rescued 7 hours later. He experienced shortness of breath thereafter and had pleural effusion 18 days later. Coronary angiography revealed 90% occlusion in #11 and complete occlusion in peripheral #12. There was also unexplainable severe left ventricular asynergy and an apical mural thrombus. Biopsy showed cell-rich fibrosis. One week later, his condition improved except in the circumflex branch and apical regions. He underwent resection of a ventricular aneurysm 2.5 months later. Histologically, ventricular aneurysm was endocardial fibroelastosis. There was also a full-thickness loss of myocytes, leaving only a small amount of remaining myocytes in the inner layer, and fibrosis with flaccidity (Figure 6, lower left).

Case Number	Gender/Age	Underlying disorders	Trigger event	Symptoms	Day of biopsy	Biopsy pathology
1	F/71	Premature ventricular contraction, Hypertension	Status after sigmoid colon surgery, Dehydration, Cessation of beta blocking agent	Chest pain	1	Cell infiltrations, myocardial depletion
2	F/82	Neurosis	None	Anorexia, throat discomfort	1	Small round cell infiltration (including polymorphonuclear leukocytes), myocyte injury
3	F/64	pulmonary fibrosis	Attempted suicide, Near drowning	Dyspnea	4	Small round cell infiltration
4	F/75	None	None	Dyspnea, chest discomfort	5	Myocardial depletion, slight fibrosis with lymphocyte infiltration
5	M/48	hypertension	none	Sudden chest pain	5	Focal depletion, myocardial fibrosis
					30	Focal, patchy fibrosis
6	F/63	Angina pectoris	Emotional stress	Palpitation, Dyspnea, chest and back pain	10	Myocardial fibrosis, myocardial depletion, fibrocellular proliferation
7	M/69	None	distress in the mountain	Pleural effusion	11	Cell-rich fibrosis, Focal depletion, small round cell infiltration
					3 months	Fibrous ventricular aneurysm
8	F/68	Paf, HT, AP, AR severe	None	Syncope, cough	12	Myocardial fibrosis with mild cell infiltrates
9	F/60	Hypertension	None	Cough, Dyspnea, preshock	15	Focal fibrosis, interstitial edema
10	F/59	Hypertension, Hyperlipidemia	Memorial service for her grandmother	Chest pain	17	Focal myocardial depletion, increase of connective tissue with cell infiltration
11	F/57	Sarcuidosis, hyperlipemia	Quarrel with neighbour	Chest pain	20	Intermysial fibrosis, edema, sight cell infiltrates
12	F/76	Diabetes mellitus	None	Dyspnea	22	Myocardial depletion cell-rich, fibrosis, replacemntal
13	F/76	Status after mammary cancer, cataracta	Admission of her husband, stress from common cold	chest pain	23	old perivascular fibrosis, slight cell infiltrates
14	M/53	Heavy drinker, Acute renal failure	Hypotension, Hemofiltration, Dopamine	Dyspnea	26	Patchy fibrosis, myocardial depletion, cell infiltration
15	F/74	pulmonary tuberculosis	Quarrel with neighbour for 6 months	Sudden chest pain	28	Perimyocardial fibrosis

This table shows 15 cases received biopsy or myocardial resection. Table was listed according to the day of biopsy; from 1st day to 28th day. Case 5 and case 7 had two samples. They received serial biopsy or aneurysmectomy.

Six patients had no trigger event, and seven patients' symptoms were not chest pain. Cases in early phase, from 1st day to 4th day biopsy, showed cell infiltration, myocardial depletion, and myocardial injury. Cases in late phase that is 12th day or later, showed focal fibrosis.

Table 4. Endomyocardial biopsy cases

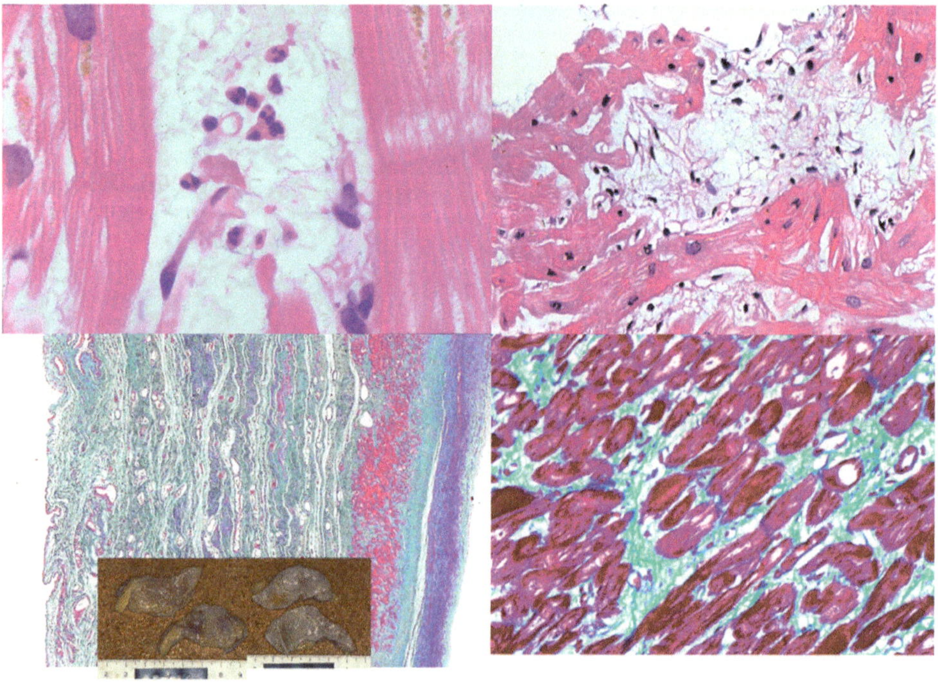

Upper left: Case biopsied on the day of onset (Case 2), biopsy showed slight increase in young connective tissue and infiltration of cells, including polymorphonuclear leukocytes .
Lower left: Case thought to have a ventricular aneurysm (Case 7), histologically, ventricular aneurysm was endocardial fibroelastosis. There was also a full-thickness loss of myocytes, leaving only a small amount of remaining myocytes in the inner layer, and fibrosis with flaccidity.
Upper right: Case with serial biopsies (Case 5 the biopsy on the fifth day), there was loss of myocytes and increase in young connective tissue rich in cellular elements
Lower right: Case with serial biopsies (Case 5 the biopsy one month later), mature connective tissue was observed in the myocardium.

Fig. 6. Pathology of endomyocardial biopsy

10. Case with serial biopsies (Case 5)

The patient was a 48-year-old man who had hypertension since 1996 for which he was treated by a calcium channel blocker. At 4 AM on September 5, 1998, he suddenly experienced chest pain which lasted 20 minutes. He developed mild chest pain at 5 PM and admitted to the hospital at 9 PM. His white blood cell count was moderately elevated at 16000. Electrocardiography revealed no abnormality but echocardiography revealed extensive asynergy mainly in the apex. Emergency cardiac catheterization was performed while nitrate was administered. Coronary angiography was normal, but left ventriculography showed takotsubo-like ballooning. The patient complained of severe chest pain during the procedure. For the first time, the patient showed ST-segment elevation of 6 mm in the precordial lead. When coronary angiography was performed again, no abnormality was observed and coronary blood flow indicated a hyperdynamic state. The patient underwent a conservative treatment and his symptoms improved after a few hours. A giant negative T-wave was subsequently observed, but left ventriculography showed a tendency for improvement one month later. Biopsy was performed on the fifth day, and there was loss of myocytes and increase in young connective tissue rich in cellular elements (Figure 6, upper right). Mature connective tissue was observed in the biopsy one month later (Figure 6, lower right).

11. Summary of biopsy findings

The trigger was assumed to be emotional stress in 8 cases. The initial symptom was chest pain in 7 cases and dyspnea in 6 cases. Ventricular outflow tract obstruction was seen in 2 cases. Histological findings included focal fibrosis, cell infiltration including of polymorphonuclear leukocytes, and loss of myocytes. It was speculated that early cell infiltration was followed by changes over time, including loss of myocytes and focal fibrosis. Ventricular aneurysm was seen as a sequela in some cases.

12. Discussion

If cardiac enzyme levels are elevated, it is easy to speculate that myocardial tissue damage has developed. However, only a small percentage of cases undergoes endomyocardial biopsy. Kurisu et al.[18] characterized their findings of 3 cases that underwent endomyocardial biopsy as focal myocytolysis, mild mononuclear cell infiltration, and a slightly increased amount of connective tissue. For 5 cases that underwent endomyocardial biopsy, Akashi et al.[19] described the following findings suggestive of (chronic) myocarditis: lymphocytic infiltration, interstitial fibrosis, myocyte atrophy, and fatty infiltration. Gianni et al.[20] examined 15 cases in 4 papers and stated that there were no biopsy findings of myocarditis. Yoshida et al.[21] examined 9 cases that underwent endomyocardial biopsy. They found 4 cases with myocardial fibrosis, 3 cases with mononuclear cell infiltration, and 4 cases with contraction-band necrosis. However, none of the cases had significant inflammatory infiltrates or necrosis of myocytes. Pilgrim and Wyss[22] reviewed 5 reports including that of Kawai et al.[23] and described characteristics of focal loss of myocytes, contraction-band necrosis, interstitial fibrosis, and mild cell infiltration. For 5 cases that underwent biopsy, Von Korn et al.[24] found cell infiltration in 2 cases that satisfied the Dallas criteria. Wani et al.[25] found deposition of periodic-acid Schiff-positive material, fibrosis, enlargement, and lymphocyte and granulocyte infiltration. However, they ruled out myocarditis. Matsuyama et al.[26] performed an autopsy in a case of amyotrophic lateral sclerosis with takotsubo cardiomyopathy. They found disseminated areas of focal fibrosis and vacuolar degeneration of the myocytes.

Otsubo et al.[27] and Nef et al.[28] reported on findings from biopsies performed at the acute and recovery phases. In the acute phase, they found myocyte hypertrophy, glycogen granules of various sizes, contractile protein, disorder of the cytoskeleton, and increased extracellular matrix. However, they did not find oncocytic necrosis or apoptosis. The damage was completely resolved in a biopsy performed at the recovery phase. They concluded that morphological changes in takotsubo cardiomyopathy were caused by the disorder of microcirculation (due to excessive catecholamine) and direct myocardial damage by catecholamine.

There are a relatively large number of reports on myocarditis mimicking takotsubo cardiomyopathy.[29,30] Kubo et al.[31] also reported on a case of acute myocarditis diagnosed as takotsubo cardiomyopathy. A lesion of takotsubo cardiomyopathy can be morphologically similar to catecholamine cardiomyopathy and stress-induced cardiomyopathy.[32] Immediate changes in lesions of catecholamine cardiomyopathy are angioedema and interstitial edema. There are also loss of cross striation, vacuolization, and lipid droplets (disruption of myofibrils in electron microscopy). The change that occurs in a few hours is interstitial edema. Polymorphonuclear leukocyte infiltration also occurs followed by mononuclear cell infiltration. There are Antischkow cells near the blood vessels and arteriolar fibrinoid degeneration. (There was also contraction-band increase and disruption of sarcomere structure in electron microscopy.) The following are observed on the third day: focal necrosis (lysis of myofibrils), and cell infiltration of histocytes, lymphocytes, and sometimes plasma cells. The following are seen after a few weeks: removal of necrosed myocytes by macrophage, resolution of acute inflammatory response, and replacement fibrosis. Inflammation is seen depending on how much time had passed.[33] Early infiltration of polymorphonuclear leukocytes occurs in catecholamine cardiomyopathy, unlike infarction, and the key to its diagnosis is also a focal lesion.

In takotsubo cardiomyopathy, the following should be noted in the evaluation of microcirculation disorder.[34] Many cases of cardiomyopathy are elderly with non-specific arteriolosclerosis in the myocardium (Figure 7) which occurs with aging.

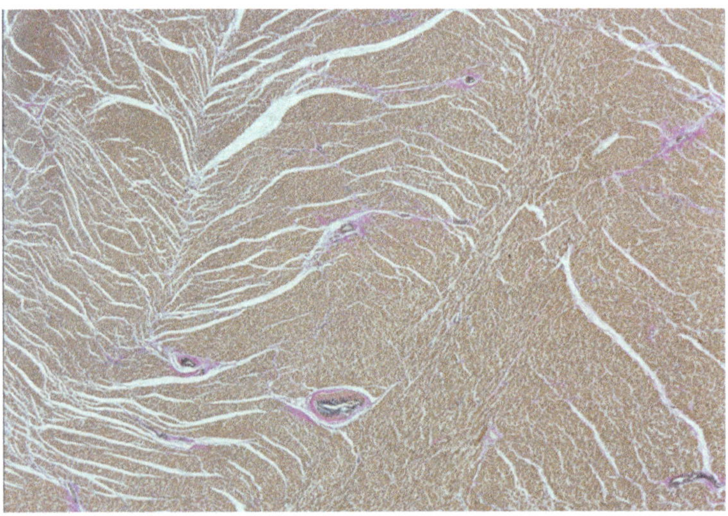

Arteriolosclerosis in the myocardium was observed frequently. Elastica van-Geison stain, x 20

Fig. 7. Autopsied case of takotsubo cardiomyopathy: histology of the interventricular septum

13. Conclusion

There was a clear myocardial lesion in takotsubo cardiomyopathy. The myocardial lesions are characterized mainly by individual myocytes or a group of myocytes with increased eosinophil staining, contraction band formation, necrosis, and rupture. The basis of the lesion is a damaged individual myocyte and aggregation of these damaged myocytes. It is speculated that early cell infiltration occurs followed by changes over time, including loss of myocytes and focal fibrosis.

14. Acknowledgements

I would like to express our appreciation to the following individuals for kindly supplying the tissues: Drs.Hiromasa Suzuki and Atsushi Yamada of Juntendo University School of Medicine, Dr. Koshi Mawatari of Kagoshima Seikyo Hospital, Dr.Toshio Shimada of Shimane Medical University (presently Shizuoka General Hospital), Drs. Hitoshi Sawada and Tadanori Aizawa of Cardiovascular Institute Hospital, Drs. Hironori Murakami and Nagisa Hanawa of Teine Keijinkai Hospital, Dr. Kasumi Takemura of the Kyoto Department of Cardiology at Prefectural Yosanoumi Hospital (Second Department of Medicine, Kyoto Prefectural University of Medicine), Dr. Osamu Yamanaka of International Goodwill Hospital (presently Poula Clinic), Dr. Nobuhiro Kotani of Shimane Medical University (presently Clinical Laboratory, Hamada Medical Center), Dr. Tsutomu Tamura of Itabashi Chuo Medical Center, Dr. Masafumi Watanabe of the Department of Cardiovascular Medicine at the University of Tokyo 、Drs. Masahito Kawada and Tetsuya Nakamura of National Hospital Organization Kobe Medical Center, and Dr. Hiroshi Matsushita of Toranomon Hospital.

15. References

[1] Kloner RA, Przyklen K, Patel B: Altered myocardial states. The stunned and hibernating myocardium. Am J Med 1989; 86 (Suppl 1A):14-22.

[2] Kawai S, Suzuki H, Yamaguchi H, Kawada M, Nakamura T, Nishiyama S, Monomura S, Matsushita H: [Autopsy findings of takotsubo cardiomyopathy.] Study report of the study group of idiopathic cardiomyopathy sponsored by the Health and Welfare Ministry. 106-109, March 2003. (in Japanese)

[3] Kawai S, Yamaguchi H, Suzuki H: [Pathology of takotsubo cardiomyopathy.] Heart View 8(2):159-166, 2004. (in Japanese)

[4] Anzai H, Komiyama N, Kinoshita N, et al.: [Case of stunned myocardium caused by overdose of epinephrine.] Kokyu to Junkan 44(2):199-204, 1996. (in Japanese)

[5] Kawada M, Okada T, Shimizu M, et al.: [An autopsy case of cardiac dysfunction of unknown origin associated with severe pneumonia.] Heart 31(5):337-343, 1999. (in Japanese)

[6] Kotani N, et al.: [Takotsubo-type fulminant myocarditis: a case report [abstract].] Jpn Circ J 64(S2):826, 2000. (in Japanese)

[7] Batsakis JG : Degenerative lesions of the heart. In Gould SE ed. "Pathology of the Heart and Blood Vessels, Third Edition.", Charles C Thomas, Springfield, Illinois, 480-521.

[8] Kaneko N: [A study on the basic structure and specific function of microcirculatory system in the human heart] Journal of Tokyo Women's Medical University 51(11):1574-92, 1981. (in Japanese)
[9] Rolf A, Nef HM, Möllmann H, Troidl C, Voss S, Conradi G, Rixe J, Steiger H, Beiring K, Hamm CW, Dill T.:Immunohistological basis of the late gadolinium enhancement phenomenon in tako-tsubo cardiomyopathy. Eur Heart J 30:1635-164,2009.
[10] Tsuneoka T, et al.: [Myocardial infarction-like electrocardiographic pattern during the course of malabsorption syndrome: an autopsy case [abstract].] Jpn Circ J 58(S2) :651, 1994. (in Japanese)
[11] Hirata Y: [A case of stunned myocardium with takotsubo-like left ventricular asynergy which developed cardiac rupture [abstract].] Jpn Circ J 63(S2):760, 1999. (in Japanese)
[12] Sacha J, Maselko J, Wester A, Szudrowicz Z, Pluta W. Left ventricular apical rupture caused by takotsubo cardiomyopathy -comprehensive pathological heart investigation. Circ J 2007;71:982-985.
[13] Ohara Y, Hiasa Y, Hosokawa, S et al: Left Ventricular Free Wall Rupture in Transient Left Ventricular Apical Ballooning. Circ J 65:621-623,2005
[14] Kuramoto K, Matsushita S, Murakami M: Acute reversible myocardial infarction after blood transfusion in the aged. Jpn Heart J 18:191-201,1977.
[15] Sasa H, Tsuboi H, Sone T, et al.: [Clinical significance of transient myocardial infarction-like electrocardiographic pattern in postoperative cases.] Heart 15:669-678, 1983. (in Japanese)
[16] Tokioka M, Miura H, Masaoka Y, et al.: [Transient appearance of asynergy on the echocardiogram and electrocardiographic changes simulating acute myocardial infarction following non-cardiac surgery.] J Cardiography 15:639-653, 1983. (in Japanese)
[17] Kawai S: [Takotsubo (ampulla, or amphora) cardiomyopathy.] Kokyu to Junkan 48(12):1237-1248,2000. (in Japanese)
[18] Kurisu S, Sato H, Kawagoe T, Ishihara M, Shimatani Y, Nishioka K, Kono Y, Umemura T, Nakamura S: Tako-tsubo-like left ventricular dysfunction with ST-segment elevation: a novel cardiac syndrome mimicking acute myocardial infarction. Am Heart J. 2002;143:448-55.
[19] Akashi Y. J., Nakazawa K., Sakakibara M., Miyake F., Koike H., Sasaka K.: The clinical features of takotsubo cardiomyopathy. Q J Med 2003; 96: 563-573.
[20] Gianni M, Dentali F, Grandi AM, Sumner G, Hiralal R, Lonn E. : Apical ballooning syndrome or takotsubo cardiomyopathy: a systematic review. Eur Heart J. 2006;27(13):1523-9.
[21] Yoshida T, Hibino T, Kako N, Murai S, Oguri M, Kato K, Yajima K, Ohte N, Yokoi K , Kimura G. :A pathophysiologic study of tako-tsubo cardiomyopathy with F-18 fluorodeoxyglucose positron emission tomography. Eur Heart J (2007) 28:2598–2604.

[22] Pilgrim TM, Wyss TR: Takotsubo cardiomyopathy or transient left ventricular apical ballooning syndrome: a systematic review. Int J Cardiol 2007;124; 283-292.
[23] Kawai S, Suzuki H, Yamaguchi H, Tanaka K, Sawada H, Aizawa T, Watanabe M, Tamura T, Mawatari K, Kawada M, Nakamura T, Yamanaka O, Okada R. Ampulla cardiomyopathy (Takotsubo cardiomyopathy) -reversible left ventricular dysfunction with ST segment elevation- Jpn Circ J 2000;64:156-159.
[24] von Korn H, Yu J, Lotze U, Ohlow MA, Huegl B, Schulte W, Haberl K, Wagner A, Gruene S, Lauer B. : Tako-Tsubo-like cardiomyopathy: specific ECG findings, characterization and clinical findings in a European single center. Cardiology. 2009;112 (1):42-8.
[25] Wani S, Glatz K, Suter Y, Jamshidi P, Erne P. "Apical ballooning"-what is the cause? J Invasive Cardiol 2008;20:599-602.
[26] Matsuyama T, Sasagasako N, Koike A, Matsuura M, Koga T, Kawajiri M, Oyagi Y, Iwaki T, Kira J: [An autopsy case of amyotrophic lateral sclerosis with ampulla cardiomyopathy.] Clin Neurol 2008;48(4):249-54. (in Japanese)
[27] Ohtsubo M, Sakai H, Takano H, Kon H, Okamoto K, Yoshida N, Fujita M.[Atypical takotsubo cardiomyopathy with preservation of apical contraction: a case report including pathological findings.] J Cardiol 2005;46:237-242. (in Japanese)
[28] Nef HM, Möllmann H, Kostin S, Troidl C, Voss S, Weber M, Dill T, Rolf A, Brandt R, Hamm CW, Elsässer A. Tako-Tsubo cardiomyopathy: intraindividual structural analysis in the acute phase and after functional recovery. Eur Heart J 2007;28:2456-2464.
[29] Kawakami H, Matsuoka H, Koyama H, et al.: [A case of "Takotsubo" like cardiomyopathy due to acute myocarditis.] Respiration & Circulation 46:913-917, 1998. (in Japanese)
[30] Caforio AL, Tona F, Vinci A, Calabrese F, Ramondo A, Cacciavillani L, Corbetti F, Leoni L, Thiene G, Iliceto S, Angelini A. : Acute biopsy-proven lymphocytic myocarditis mimicking Takotsubo cardiomyopathy. Eur J Heart Fail. 2009;11:428-31.
[31] Kubo K, Ishibashi I, Miyazaki Y, Sakai Y, Matsuno K, Namikawa S, Sano M, Yamaoka T, Ono M, Kawana H: [An autopsy case of acute myocarditis that was diagnosed antemortem as takotsubo cardiomyopathy.] Heart 41:1222-1226, 2009. (in Japanese)
[32] Kassim TA, Clarke DD, Mai VQ, Clyde PW, Mohamed Shakir KM.: Catecholamine-induced cardiomyopathy. Endocr Pract. 2008;14(9):1137-49.
[33] Kawai S, Hashimoto K: [Catecholamine myocarditis.] Japanese Journal of Clinical Medicine 38 (fall special edition), Internal Medicine to Pathology 3680-3685, 1980. (in Japanese)

[34] Kume T, Akasaka T, Kawamoto T, Yoshitani H, Watanabe N, Neishi Y, Wada N, Yoshida K.：Assessment of coronary microcirculation in patients with Takotsubo-like left ventricular dysfunction。Circ J 69：934-9,2005

13

Stress-Induced Cardiomyopathy: Clinical Observations

Jun-Won Lee[1], Hyun-Kyo Lim[2], Jang-Young Kim[1] and Sungwoo Ryoo[3]
[1]*Division of Cardiology, Department of Internal Medicine,*
[2]*Department of Anesthesiology and Pain Medicine,*
Yonsei University Wonju College of Medicine, Wonju
[3]*Division of Biology, Kangwon National University, Chuncheon*
Korea

1. Introduction

Stress-induced cardiomyopathy has achieved global notoriety in only 20 years since it was introduced as "Takotsubo cardiomyopathy" (which means "octopus trap" in Japanese) (Dote et al., 1991). It is also known as "left ventricular apical ballooning", "ampulla cardiomyopathy" and "broken heart syndrome". Stress-induced cardiomyopathy is associated with typical electrocardiographic findings and severe chest pain suggesting ST-segment elevation myocardial infarction (STEMI). However, emergency coronary angiography usually does not show significant stenosis or definite flow limitation. In general, left ventricular ejection fraction (LVEF) is markedly depressed and is recovered within the normal range within 1–2 weeks. Most cases have a good outcome and some may not even need further medical therapy if the underlying the cause is uncovered. Several hypotheses have been proposed but the pathophysiologic mechanism is incompletely understood. Here we discuss the clinical findings, diagnostic modalities, possible pathophysiologic mechanisms, prognosis and management of stress-induced cardiomyopathy.

2. History of reporting of stress-induced cardiomyopathy

In 1980, strong evidences implying stress-induced cardiomyopathy were reported via the autopsies of homicidal victims (Cebelin & Hirsch, 1980). They found pathognomonic findings of contraction band necrosis in 11 patients who had died due to a physical assault without internal injuries. One case report revealed that severe emotional stress could bring about deterioration of cardiac function which developed into pulmonary edema (Anon, 1986). Echocardiographic studies demonstrated that left ventricular wall motion abnormalities and myocardial damage could be accompanied by subarachnoid hemorrhage (Pollick et al., 1988). This pioneering work inspired other investigators, who discovered that LVEF and regional wall motion abnormalities were significant predictors of death in patients with subarachnoid hemorrhage (Sugimoto et al., 2008). Reversible left ventricular dysfunction induced by excessive catecholamine surges in pheochromocytoma was also reported (Iga et al., 1989). This finding suggested that catecholamines at high concentrations can directly damage the myocardium.

Stress-induced cardiomyopathy was termed "Takotsubo cardiomyopathy" by Japanese cardiologists in 1991 (Dote et al., 1991). Advances in diagnostic imaging and emergency coronary angiography have contributed to increased recognition of stress-induced cardiomyopathy, and increasing numbers of reports have been published since then.

3. Clinical observations: Single-center experiences

We reported retrospective data of 39 patients diagnosed with stress-induced cardiomyopathy during 5 years in a single center (Lee, J.W. et al., 2010). Our results showed differences from other reports. In our study, 69% of patients were female, and the mean age was 61.3 ± 16.1 years. The most frequent symptom at initial presentation was dyspnea (46%) rather than chest pain (26%). Emotional stress was found in only 15% of subjects. The main triggering factors were physical stress associated with illness (59%), procedure-related complications (8%) and trauma (8%). Initial electrocardiography revealed T-wave inversion (46%), ST-segment elevation (28%) and ST-segment depression (5%). LVEF was recovered from 45 ± 16% upon hospital admission to 61 ± 13% upon hospital discharge. The level of B-type natriuretic peptide (BNP) was increased (745.4 ± 905.6 pg/mL) and 23 patients (59%) had elevated levels of highly-sensitive C-reactive protein (hs-CRP; 44 ± 61 mg/L) at initial presentation. The peak level of creatine kinase-MB (CK-MB) fraction and troponin I showed mild elevation (15.6 ± 20.9 ng/mL and 6.8 ± 12.3 ng/mL, respectively)

Echocardiography was shown to be a useful tool to detect transient left ventricular outflow tract (LVOT) obstruction, apical thrombus on the site of apical ballooning, and unusual inverted-type (mid-ventricular) ballooning.

Three patients (8%) died due to pneumonia and 13 patients (33%) experienced cardiogenic shock. Inotropic agents were needed in 10 patients (26%) and 9 patients (23%) required mechanical ventilation. When we assessed the prognostic factors affecting adverse events such as death or shock, LVEF and hs-CRP levels were independent risk factors by multivariate logistic regression analyses (adjusted for age, sex, and other risk factors).

4. Clinical findings

In general, stress-induced cardiomyopathy is characterized by sudden chest pain or dyspnea, ST-segment elevation mimicking acute myocardial infarction (AMI) or deep T-wave inversion, elevated levels of cardiac enzymes or BNP and transient left ventricular systolic dysfunction. Post-menopausal women seem to be more vulnerable to this syndrome. The definition is continually evolving. There are some divergences of opinion on clinical situations and management.

4.1 Age and sex

The elderly seem to be the most vulnerable to stress-induced cardiomyopathy. The mean age for presentation was >60 years (Bybee et al., 2004). However, a case of stress-induced cardiomyopathy in a newborn after fetal distress was caused by the umbilical cord being twisted around the chest and neck (Greco, 2011). The youngest patient we treated was a 26-year-old female. Despite literature suggesting that the elderly are the most affected, recent case reports have shown the possibility of development of stress-induced cardiomyopathy in patients of any age.

The higher prevalence of females is a consistent finding in published series (Bybee et al., 2004). Nevertheless, the reason for this difference in prevalence between males and females is unknown. Stöllberger & Finsterer suggested two intriguing hypotheses (Stöllberger & Finsterer, 2011). The first hypothesis is that males have been biologically better protected against the stress-induced cardiotoxicity of catecholamines than females throughout the centuries. They suggested that males were exposed to more physical stress and developed various protecting mechanisms (Stöllberger & Finsterer, 2011, as cited in Silventoinen et al., 2001). The higher density of adrenergic receptors of cardiomyocytes in males may result in delayed saturation of receptors and improved protection against catecholamine storms (Stöllberger & Finsterer, 2011, as cited in Leibel et al., 1987). The second hypothesis is that males are biologically less resistant than females against the stress-induced cardiotoxicity of catecholamines. Males comprise 78.9% of sudden cardiac deaths (Fragkouli & Vouguiouklakis, 2010) and one of the risk factors for sudden unexplained death in epilepsy patients was being male (Monté et al., 2007). Large-scale cohort studies could provide answers for the age and sex predominance of stress-induced cardiomyopathy.

4.2 Initial presenting symptoms

The most common presenting symptoms of stress-induced cardiomyopathy are chest pain and dyspnea. Not all studies reported the initial symptoms (especially in the case of dyspnea). Nevertheless, chest pain was the cardinal symptom in 185 of 273 patients (67.8%) and dyspnea the second most common symptom in 40 of 225 patients (17.8%) (Gianni et al., 2006). Cardiogenic shock, severe arrhythmia, mental change or syncope may be the initial presentation. Some patients suffer from chest pain and dyspnea; the most frequent symptom of stress-induced cardiomyopathy in patients in our institution was dyspnea.

In our experience, patients with dyspnea had a longer stay in hospital, elevated levels of BNP and hs-CRP, and decreased initial LVEF, but these differences were not statistically significant (Lee, J.W. et al., 2011). A recent prospective study in a tertiary referral hospital demonstrated that chest pain was more frequently observed in the emotional stress group, whereas dyspnea was the presenting symptom in the physical stress group (acute illness and in-hospital surgery/procedure) (Lee, P.H. et al., 2010).

New imaging modalities contribute to the early diagnosis of stress-induced cardiomyopathy. Hence, the proportion of initial symptoms might shift from emotional stress to physical stress.

4.3 Triggering factors

Triggering factors preceding this syndrome are, in general, divided into "emotional stress" and "physical stress". A wide variety of emotional stressors have been reported, including panic, fear, anxiety, grief and anger (Prasad et al., 2008; Sharkey et al., 2010). These emotional stressors include immediate ("fight-or-flight") responses and/or sustained responses, which implies the involvement of protective mechanisms of the body via the stress system (neurohormonal interaction) (Balkin & Cohen, 2011).

Among physical stressors, pheochromocytoma, subarachnoid hemorrhage, exposure to catecholamine/beta-agonist drugs and procedure-related events are representative cases associated with catecholamine excess. Other physical stressors include hypoxia, infection, metabolic abnormalities, invasive procedures, and general anesthesia (Park et al., 2010; Prasad et al., 2008; Sharkey et al., 2010). Madhavan et al. suggested the importance of physical stress (Madhavan et al., 2011). They suggested that patients with physical stressors had significant underlying co-morbidities that may contribute to the development of heart failure. In addition, physical stressors such as postoperative status may be associated with a more sustained surge in catecholamines compared with emotional stress, which may be shortlived (Park et al., 2010).

4.4 Electrocardiographic findings

The most common abnormality on electrocardiography (ECG) is ST-segment elevation resembling STEMI (Prasad et al., 2008). T-wave inversion is usually observed at initial presentation and during the subacute phase. The proportion of ST-segment elevation and T-wave inversion was 208 of 255 patients (81.6%) and 160 of 249 patients (64.3%), respectively (Gianni et al., 2006). Q waves also could be detected in 63 of 198 patients (31.8%). T-wave inversion may resolve over 3–4 months but may occur as early as 4–6 weeks and, in some cases, be present beyond 1 year (Prasad et al., 2009, as cited in Kurisu et al., 2004 and Matsuoka et al., 2003).

One study tried to distinguish stress-induced cardiomyopathy from anterior wall myocardial infarction by simple and non-invasive ECG tests (Jim et al., 2009). They found that if extensive left ventricular dysfunction and precordial ST-segment elevation were observed, the absence of ST-segment depression, or the presence of ST-segment elevation in inferior leads (particularly II ≥ III) were suggestive of stress-induced cardiomyopathy. Lead II is the most sensitive and specific for the detection of stress-induced cardiomyopathy because it is relatively protected from the opposing effect of lateral wall ischemia.

4.5 Laboratory findings

The level of troponin I or troponin T and CK-MB fraction is slightly elevated from baseline reference values. BNP levels in plasma are also elevated to various degrees (Lee, J.W. et al., 2010 and Morel et al., 2009).

One case-control study provided a comprehensive analysis of stress hormone and cardiac biomarker profiles in stress-induced cardiomyopathy, and the values were compared with those from patients with STEMI (Madhavan et al., 2009). The major findings were that: (1) levels of BNP were higher in stress-induced cardiomyopathy despite less necrosis of myocytes, similar left ventricular dysfunction and comparable hemodynamics; (2) there was a marked elevation in levels of an inflammatory biomarker (hs-CRP) in a magnitude similar to that seen in patients with STEMI.

Inflammation may have a crucial role in stress-induced cardiomyopathy. Morel et al. demonstrated that inflammatory status was related to the initial impairment of LVEF and to the extent of neurohormonal activation (Morel et al., 2009). Other research teams demonstrated that patients who developed left ventricular apical ballooning due to severe physical stress in the Intensive Care Unit had a higher frequency of sepsis, cardiomegaly, pulmonary edema and hypotension (Park et al., 2005).

One recent prospective study showed that inflammatory mediators and platelet-activity markers could be used to distinguish stress-induced cardiomyopathy from myocardial infarction (Pirzer et al., 2011). Expression of the platelet-activation marker CD62P and plasma levels of interleukin-6 were significantly lower in patients with stress-induced cardiomyopathy compared with myocardial infarction at the time of hospital admission. Plasma levels of interleukin-7 were significantly elevated in patients with stress-induced cardiomyopathy compared with patients with myocardial infarction 2–4 days after hospital admission.

The plasma concentrations of catecholamines during the acute phase were 2-3-times higher than in patients with AMI and heart failure, and 20-times higher than in normal adults (Wittstein et al., 2005). Uchida et al. also observed elevated levels of plasma epinephrine and norepinephrine in patients with stress-induced cardiomyopathy (Uchida et al., 2010). The plasma half-life of epinephrine is only 3 min (Zeb et al., 2011, as cited in Ferreira & Vane, 1967), so measurement of catecholamines should be conducted at the time of symptom onset.

4.6 Left ventricular systolic dysfunction

Initial left ventricular systolic function is usually impaired upon hospital admission (mean LVEF, 20–49%) and, in general, resolves within days-to-weeks after initial presentation (mean period, 18 days) (Nef et al., 2010). Most patients achieve normal systolic function during hospitalization, but a few fail to reach the normal range (Sharkey et al., 2010). Moreover, a recent study revealed that absence of functional recovery within 1 week (ejection fraction <50%) was an independent factor associated with mortality (Lee, P.H. et al., 2010).

4.7 Co-morbidity

There are no reported associations between stress-induced cardiomyopathy and co-morbidity. Collective data from 14 studies reported a history of hypertension in 43% of patients (108/247), diabetes mellitus in 11% (53/217) and current or past smoking in 23% (23/100). Others include chronic obstructive pulmonary disease, asthma and malignancy.

One observational study showed that patients with stress-induced cardiomyopathy had significantly higher levels of high-density lipoprotein-cholesterol and lower levels of low-density lipoprotein-cholesterol and triglyceride compared with age- and sex-matched patients with myocardial infarction (Gaddam et al., 2011). Hyper-alpha-lipoproteinemia was noted in 2 patients. That study had a major limitation because the study population was small. However, a history of dyslipidemia should be assessed at initial presentation. This result adds evidence that the pathogenesis is not due to atherosclerotic narrowing of epicardial coronary arteries.

4.8 Preferred time of onset

The occurrence of major cardiovascular events is not randomly distributed over time but instead exhibits chronobiological patterns. Stress-induced cardiomyopathy also seems to exhibit a temporal variation of onset, with peaks during the morning and in the summer (Bossone et al., 2011). One study reported that the highest number of cases was found on Monday and the lowest on Saturday. This phenomenon might be because of stress and catecholamine release (Manfredini et al., 2010). However, conclusions are hard to reach because of the relatively small number of patients involved in this study.

5. Imaging modalities and implications

Several imaging tools are used for the diagnosis of stress-induced cardiomyopathy: coronary angiography with left ventriculography, echocardiography, cardiac magnetic resonance (CMR) and nuclear imaging. Each examination has its own diagnostic value and benefit. One should understand the advantages and disadvantages and select the most appropriate method for the purpose.

5.1 Coronary angiography

Coronary angiography is essential and the only way to rule out obstruction of coronary arteries (especially in cases of ST-segment elevation). The modified Mayo Clinic criteria to diagnose stress-induced cardiomyopathy demand the absence of obstructive coronary artery disease or angiographic evidence of acute rupture of plaques that could be responsible for the observed wall motion abnormalities. A recent report suggested the possible concurrence of coronary artery disease with stress-induced cardiomyopathy (Winchester et al., 2008). Hence, several cases might be excluded because of the presence of coronary artery disease. If coronary atherosclerotic changes are not significant and regional wall motional abnormalities extend beyond a single coronary artery, stress-induced cardiomyopathy should be suspected. The endocardial border can be readily detected by left ventriculography (Fig. 1).

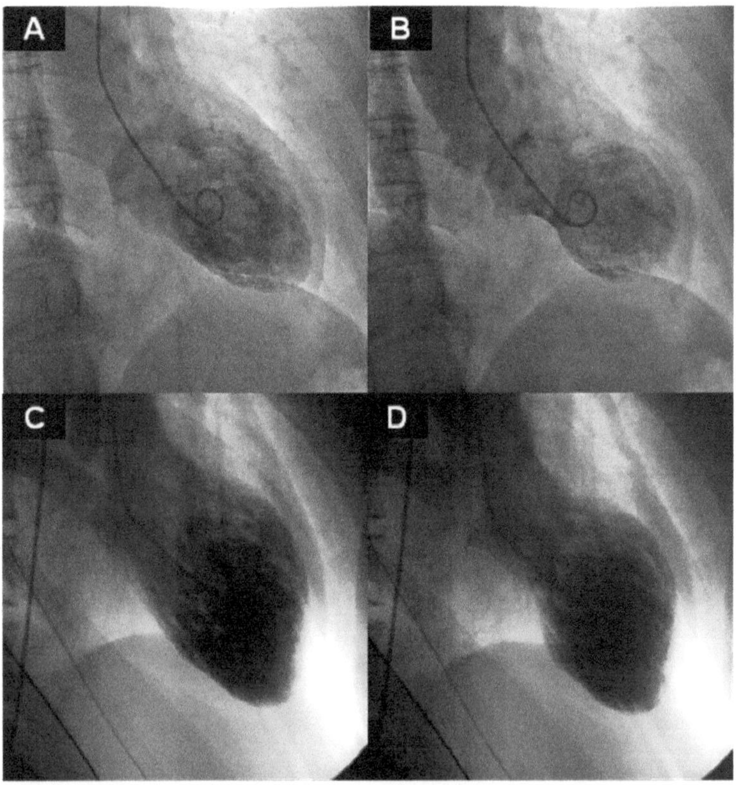

Fig. 1. Left ventriculography shows the typical pattern of apical ballooning with relative basal hypercontractility (A: end-diastole, B: end-systole) and inverted type of mid-ventricular ballooning with apical sparing (C: end-diastole, D: end-systole).

5.2 Echocardiography

Transthoracic echocardiography is the most important modality to distinguish this syndrome from AMI. It has many merits thanks to its non-invasiveness, portability, real-time accessibility, reproducibility and concurrent monitoring of anatomic and physiologic abnormalities (Lee, J.W. et al., 2011).

Echocardiography reveals the unique morphology of apical ballooning and the relative compensatory hypercontractiliy of the basal segments. One should closely observe two distinct features: (i) decrease in LVEF and (ii) (LVOT) obstruction. These factors are important to predict the severity and prognosis of stress-induced cardiomyopathy.

The decreased LVEF seen at hospital admission is a significant independent risk factor for death or cardiogenic shock (Lee, J.W. et al., 2010). The absence of recovery in left ventricular dysfunction within 1 week is also a powerful independent factor associated with mortality (Lee, P. H. et al., 2010).

Hypotensive events can be induced by dynamic LVOT obstruction, which results in the movement of the anterior mitral leaflets toward the interventricular septum in the systolic phase, so-called "systolic anterior motion" (SAM). Low cardiac output occurs as a result of reduced antegrade flow. This may occur in up to one-quarter of patients presenting with a septal bulge associated with SAM and mitral regurgitation (El Mahmoud et al., 2008). LVOT obstruction is a dynamic phenomenon depending on the hemodynamics at that time point, and thus echocardiography is a useful and readily accessible tool if unexplained hypotension or shock is observed.

Acute mitral regurgitation can be found in stress-induced cardiomyopathy. Mitral regurgitation seems to develop mainly due to displacement of the papillary muscle, which leads to impaired leaflet coaptation secondary to tethering. Parodi et al. suggested that mitral regurgitation accompanied by severe left ventricular dysfunction was a potent predictor of hemodynamic derangement leading to hazardous manifestations, including pulmonary edema and cardiogenic shock (Parodi et al., 2007).

Regional and global systolic function can be assessed and quantified by two-dimensional strain. This method is based on tracking the movement of stable acoustic patterns ("speckles") within the myocardium frame-by-frame throughout the cardiac cycle. Despite the general perception of basal hypercontractility, total longitudinal strain showed that systolic function in basal segments was decreased in one study (Heggemann et al., 2009).

Contrast echocardiography can be helpful in detection of the endocardial border (particularly if apical segments are difficult to evaluate because of poor image quality). Apical thrombus can be readily detected by contrast echocardiography. Contrast echocardiography can also demonstrate abnormalities in myocardial perfusion, which are indicative of microvascular dysfunction (Abdelmoneim, 2009). The normal myocardial perfusion pattern in the akinetic apex helps to discriminate stress-induced cardiomyopathy from anterior wall myocardial infarction.

Real-time three-dimensional imaging techniques and transesophageal echocardiography can give better information on volumetric change and anatomic abnormalities

5.3 CMR

CMR provides information on wall-motion abnormalities as well as myocardial viability. Contrast-enhanced CMR can identify myocardial inflammation through the presence of edema by T2-weighted images and/or myocardial tissue injury by late gadolinium enhancement (Schmalfuss, 2011). The special morphological pattern of late gadolinium uptake was reported recently for the first time (Avegliano et al., 2011). Early CMR (within 72 h of hospital admission) demonstrated mild enhancement of signals in the segments with abnormal contractility, which was clearly different from the segments with no signal enhancement and normal contractility. This special morphological pattern corresponded to localized inflammation and edema in the affected area, which could be related to slower gadolinium washout determined by interstitial edema and inflammation (and perhaps very small areas of necrosis). This pattern becomes normal after recovery from myocardial edema and contractility. The morphological pattern suggests that the pathophysiology is related to diffuse damage of the myocardium and the microcirculation rather than involvement of coronary epicardial vessels.

5.4 Nuclear imaging

Single-photon emission computed tomography (SPECT) shows perfusion defects in the affected segment beyond single coronary distribution. Imaging also showed that the perfusion defect was slightly smaller in extent compared with the distribution of the wall-motion defect in one study (Skovgaard et al., 2010). Fluorine 18 fluorodeoxyglucose positron emission tomography in the acute phase showed reduced (but not absent) glucose uptake in almost the entire left ventricle, indicating viable tissue. The myocardial glucose uptake 3 months later was evenly distributed in the affected areas.
The findings of ^{123}I-meta-iodobenzylguanidine myocardial scintigraphy depicted a unique pattern of ventricular asynergy and suggested the existence of cardiac sympathetic hyperactivity (Akashi et al., 2004). Conversely, Skovgaard et al. could not find signs of cardiac sympathetic dysfunction as evidenced by a normal and unchanged washout rate (Skovgaard et al., 2010). However, they demonstrated the interesting finding of increased uptake in the lung, which was shown in chronic heart failure.
The findings from these nuclear imaging studies provide possible evidence of coronary microvascular dysfunction.

6. Mechanisms of stress-induced cardiomyopathy

The mechanisms of stress-induced cardiomyopathy are incompletely understood. However, a growing body of evidence could explain the possible mechanism and pathophysiology. A proposed mechanism of stress-induced cardiomyopathy is summarized in Fig. 2.

6.1 Brain–heart connection

Although the heart has an intrinsic capacity to maintain homeostasis, it is always ready to recognize extrinsic stimuli through brain–heart connections and can elicit an appropriate response for physiological demands. This protective process is called the "stress system". The main central effectors of the stress system are highly interconnected and include hypothalamic corticotropin-releasing hormone and locus ceruleus-derived norepinephrine (Chrousos, 2009, as cited in Charmandari et al., 2005 and Chrousos & Gold, 1992). The principal peripheral effectors are glucocorticoids, which are regulated by the hypothalamic–pituitary–adrenal axis, and the catecholamines norepinephrine and epinephrine, which are regulated by the systemic and adrenomedullary sympathetic nervous systems (Chrousos, 2009). A functional positive feedback loop is formed by hypothalamic corticotrophin-releasing hormone and brainstem locus ceruleus-norepinephrine systems (Chrousos, 2007). The locus ceruleus also participates in a feedback loop with the adrenal medulla and the limbic system. The adrenal gland secretes epinephrine, which stimulates the locus ceruleus. Norepinephrine is released consecutively by this stimulus, which then sends signals to the hipppocampus and amygdala. The latter can re-stimulate the locus ceruleus in sequence (Soufer, 2002).

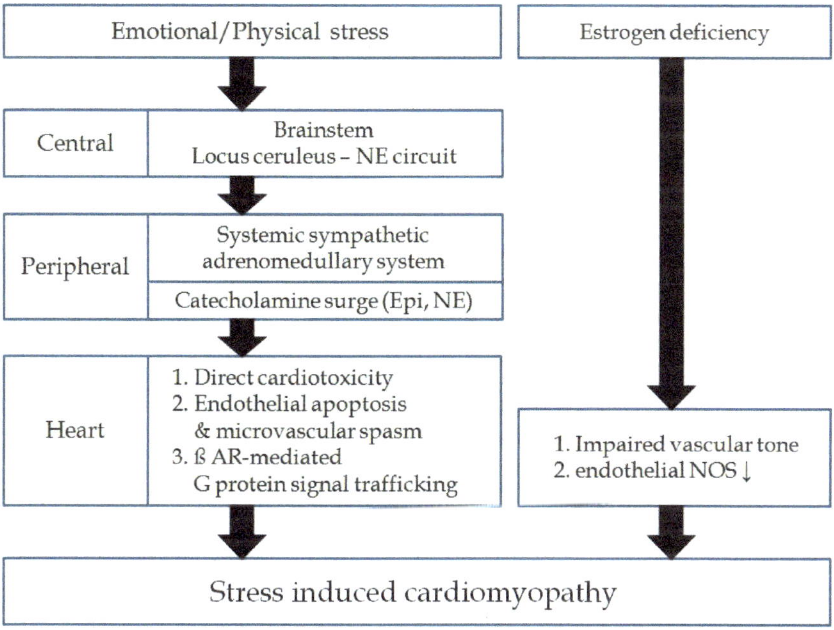

Fig. 2. Proposed mechanism of stress-induced cardiomyopathy. NE, norepinephrine; Epi, epinephrine; AR, adrenoreceptor; NOS, nitric oxide synthase.

Incessant emotional and/or physical stimuli may activate and sustain positive feedback stress response systems and result in marked elevation of plasma catecholamine levels in patients with stress-induced cardiomyopathy (Balkin & Cohen, 2011).

6.2 Catecholamine excess

Several situations that could induce sympathetic activation have suggested that cardiac dysfunction might be closely related to catecholamine excess. Subarachnoid hemorrhage and pheochromocytoma are typical examples (Kono et al., 1994; Pollick et al., 1988; Scott & Gutterman, 1995). Catecholamines could contribute to myocardial stunning in the absence of relevant myocardial perfusion abnormalities at rest (Morel et al., 2009). With respect to stress-induced cardiomyopathy, the possible contribution of catecholamines can be summarized into three components; (1) direct toxicity of norepinephrine/epinephrine and their metabolites; (2) adrenergic stimuli with spasm of the epicardial coronary artery and/or microvasculature; and (3) ß-adrenoreceptor-mediated stimulus-dependent G-protein stimulus trafficking.

6.2.1 Catecholamine toxicity

Proof of direct catecholamine-induced cardiotoxicity has been known since the mid-1970s. Early investigations showed that intravenous injection catecholamines in rats could affect morphological change on the cardiomyocyte plasma membrane (the "sacolemma") (Balkin & Cohen, 2011, as cited in Rona et al., 1975 & Boutet et al., 1976). When they injected catecholamines, the extracellular macromolecular tracer horseradish peroxidase became localized to intracellular compartments, which was retained in the extracellular environment in a normal physiological state.

The synthetic catecholamine isoproterenol was shown to increase myocardial Ca^{2+} content and depress cardiac sarcolemmal ATP-dependent Ca^{2+} uptake, Ca^{2+}-stimulated ATPase activity and Na^{+}-dependent Ca^{2+} accumulation in experimental hearts (Tappia, 2001). Those authors also demonstrated that similar findings were seen in isolated rat hearts perfused with the catecholamine oxidation product adrenochrome, (10–25 µg/mL).

These findings suggested that catecholamine and the oxidative stress that they cause result in the development of intracellular Ca^{2+} overload, heart dysfunction and subsequent myocardial death.

6.2.2 Catecholamine and microvascular spasm

The α1-adrenoreceptor is located in smooth muscle cells, which causes vasoconstriction in blood vessels (including the epicardial coronary artery). However, provocation tests using infusions of ergonovine or acetylcholine induced multivessel spasm in only 28% of patients with documented stress-induced cardiomyopathy (Gianni et al., 2006). This finding is insufficient to explain the underlying mechanism of stress-induced cardiomyopathy.

Microvascular spasm by catecholamine-induced sympathetic stimulation can alter the oxygen delivery of the myocardium, which develops localized contractile dysfunction within seconds. If blood flow is restored before myocardial damage, cardiac function can recover. This phenomenon is termed "stunned" or "hibernating" myocardium (Heusch & Schulz, 1996). It may take days or weeks for such cardiac dysfunction to recover.

As mentioned above, contrast echocardiographic perfusion imaging, CMR and nuclear imaging provide evidences of coronary microvascular dysfunction. Uchida et al. investigated the hypothesis that coronary microvessel apoptosis could be the missing link between stress and stress induced cardiomyopathy (Uchida et al., 2010). Plasma catecholamines, thrombolysis in myocardial infarction (TIMI) coronary flow grade and myocardial perfusion grade, and apoptosis of coronary microvessels in the biopsied myocardial specimens by terminal deoxynucleotidyl transferase-mediated nick end-labeling (TUNEL) were examined in 8 female patients with stress-induced cardiomyopathy. They found elevated levels of plasma epinephrine and norepinephrine, delayed myocardial perfusion without flow disturbance in the epicardial coronary arteries, focal myocardial necrosis, as well as extensive apoptosis of coronary microvessels in arterioles, venules and capillaries.

Reactive hyperemia as a parameter of endothelial function and vascular response to acute mental stress could be measured by peripheral arterial tonometry. Women with a history of stress-induced cardiomyopathy demonstrated impaired endothelium-dependent vasodilation, excessive vasoconstriction, and augmented sympathetic activation after experiencing acute mental stress compared with age-matched post-menopausal controls and patients with myocardial infarction (Martin et al., 2010).

In summary, it can be hypothesized that catecholamine-induced apoptosis of endothelial cells of coronary microvessels and the subsequent microvessel spasm which results in myocardial stunning by oxidative stress due to the ischemia–reperfusion mechanism leads to stress induced cardiomyopathy (Uchida et al., 2010).

6.2.3 ß-adrenoreceptor-mediated stimulus-dependent G-protein stimulus trafficking

ß-adrenoreceptors are members of one of the largest families of cell-surface signaling proteins called G-protein-coupled receptors (GPCRs). The main function of GPCRs is to convert extracellular stimuli into intracellular signals (Rosenbaum et al., 2009). Cardiac tissue has two subtypes of ß-adrenoreceptor: $ß_1$ and $ß_2$. The $ß_1$-adrenoreceptor stimulates only the G-αs protein. However, the $ß_2$-adrenoreceptor can activate two G proteins, G-αs and G-αi (part of the Gs and Gi heterotrimers, respectively), which differentially regulate adenylate cyclase. The latter generates cyclic adenosine monophosphate (cAMP), which activates protein kinase A (PKA) (Rosenbaum et al., 2009).

Specifically, in the heart, PKA phosphorylates the proteins involved in energy metabolism and excitation–contraction coupling. These include glycogen phosphorylase kinase, the L-type calcium channel, the sarcoplasmic reticulum membrane protein phospholamban, and cytoskeletal proteins. These phosphorylation events result in enhanced cardiac contractility (inotropy), accelerated cardiac relaxation (lusitropy), and increased heart rate (chronotropy) (Balkin & Cohen, 2011, as cited in Xiao, 2001 & Bers, 2002).

At physiological and elevated concentrations, norepinephrine, released from the sympathetic nerves, acts predominantly via the $ß_1$-adrenoreceptor on ventricular cardiomyocytes, exerting positive inotropic and lusitropic responses. Epinephrine also binds the $ß_1$-adrenoreceptor, but has a higher affinity for the $ß_2$-adrenoreceptor. At physiological concentrations, epinephrine binding to the $ß_2$-adrenoreceptor activates the Gs protein. At higher "supraphysiological" concentrations, epinephrine binds to the $ß_2$-adrenoreceptor and switches signaling from the Gs protein to the Gi protein, a process called "stimulus trafficking". This process results in negative inotropy, negative lusitropy and negative chronotropy. After the surge of epinephrine has finished, the $ß_2$-adrenoreceptor coupled to Gi proteins switches back to Gs protein coupling or is internalized and degraded, enabling cardiomyocytes to recover their inotropic function (Lyon et al., 2008).

6.3 Estrogen deficiency

Studies have shown that post-menopausal women are susceptible to stress-induced cardiomyopathy (Bybee et al., 2004). This strong female predominance has been strongly associated with estrogen deficiency. Indeed, ovariectomised rats without estradiol supplementation exposed to immobilization stress had reduced left ventricular systolic function and increased heart rate and blood pressure in comparison with rats that were supplemented with estradiol (Ueyama et al., 2007). They also demonstrated that chronic supplementation with estrogen attenuated stress-induced sympatho–adrenal outflow from the brain to the heart (indirect action on the nervous system) and upregulated cardioprotective substances such as atrial natriuretic peptide and heat shock protein 70 in the heart (direct action on the heart).

Estrogen has direct and indirect cardioprotective effects. The direct effect is rapid vasodilation primarily by activation of endothelial nitric oxide synthase (eNOS). The indirect long-term effect involves changes in the genetic expression of proteins that regulate vascular tone and the response to injury (Mendelsohn, 2002).

7. Prognosis and treatment

In most cases, the prognosis of stress-induced cardiomyopathy is good. Reported overall in-hospital mortality is 1.1% (Gianni et al., 2006), but the range varies to ~15–16% (Sharkey et al., 2010, and Lee, P.H. et al., 2010). The prevalence of complications was ~20%, including cardiogenic shock, acute heart failure, arrhythmias, intraventricular thrombus formation associated with distal embolization, left ventricular free wall rupture, recurrence, and even death (Bybee et al., 2004; Gianni et al., 2006; Zeb et al., 2010).

Acute systolic heart failure is the most common complication of stress-induced cardiomyopathy, and occurs in ~45% of patients (Madhavan et al., 2011). Madhavan et al. developed and validated a risk score that can be calculated at the time of presentation. Scores of 1, 2, and 3 points were associated with a risk of acute heart failure of 28%, 58%, and 85%, respectively. No specific therapy is required but, if needed, diuretics are used to improve pulmonary edema. Combined α- & ß-blockers may be advantageous, but the usefulness of these agents in combination should be evaluated in the future.

Cardiogenic shock may occur in the acute phase of stress-induced cardiomyopathy. Shock may be due to systolic dysfunction, or be secondary dynamic LVOT obstruction. Patients with systolic anterior motion or LVOT obstruction should not be exposed to inotropic agents even if there are in shock. Insertion of an intra-aortic balloon pump may be needed until the recovery of cardiac function is achieved.

Right ventricular involvement is relatively common and associated with lower LVEF, a longer duration of hospitalization, more complications (e.g., severe congestive heart failure), the use of an intra-aortic balloon pump, and cardiopulmonary resuscitation (Elesber et al., 2006). It has been reported that pleural effusion was more frequent in patients with stress-induced cardiomyopathy and was predictive of right ventricular dysfunction (Haghi et al., 2006).

One should keep in mind the possibility of intraventricular thrombus formation, which can be found not only in the left ventricle but also in the right ventricle and left atrial appendage (Buchholz et al., 2010; Haghi et al., 2008; Sharkey et al., 2010). Apical thrombus in the left ventricle carries a great risk of cerebrovascular accident and distal embolization during the recovery phase. Short-term use of anticoagulants and heparin as well as close follow-up echocardiography can protect against additional embolic events.

Arrhythmic complications include ventricular tachycardia, ventricular fibrillation, atrial fibrillation, atrioventricular block and sinus node dysfunction. The exact prevalence is unclear and no specific treatment has been developed. This issue needs more pooled data to assess the associations between stress-induced cardiomyopathy and arrhythmias (including conduction disorders).

The true prevalence of recurrence is not known, but only 3.5–5% of patients experienced recurrence in two studies (Gianni et al., 2006, and Sharkey et al., 2010).

Levosimendan has been suggested to be an ideal drug for patients with cardiogenic shock (Padayachee, 2007). Levosimendan is a non-catecholamine inotrope which sensitizes troponin C to calcium, leading to improved contractility. In addition, levosimendan does not compromise diastolic function. The opening of adenosine triphosphate-dependent potassium channels by levosimendan causes vasodilation. This decreases preload, afterload and pulmonary vascular resistance, and improves coronary perfusion. Further studies are required to determine the safety and efficacy of this agent before widespread use can be recommended.

8. Summary and conclusion

The development of stress-induced cardiomyopathy involves multiple interactions. Emotional and/or physical stressors activate the stress system via positive feedback loops and catecholamines are produced. Excessive amounts of catecholamines directly affect cardiomyocytes, induce apoptosis of endothelial cells of coronary microvessels with subsequent microvessel spasm and ß-adrenoreceptor-mediated stimulus-dependent G-protein stimulus trafficking. Estrogen deficiency makes the heart to vulnerable to stressors. Depending on the severity of cardiac involvement, various presentations can be seen. Diagnostic modalities should be chosen according to specific situations. Echocardiography is essential to monitor recovery or possible complications, and to plan further treatment. A growing body of evidence promises better understanding of stress-induced cardiomyopathy.

9. References

Abdelmoneim, S. S.; Mankad, S. V.; Bernier, M.; Dhoble, A.; Hagen, M. E.; Ness, S. A.; Chandrasekaran, K.; Pellikka, P. A.; Oh, J. K. & Mulvagh, S. L. (2009). Microvascular function in Takotsubo cardiomyopathy with contrast echocardiography: prospective evaluation and review of literature. *Journal of the American Society of Echocardiography*, Vol.22, No.11, pp. 1249-1255, ISSN 0894-7317

Akashi, Y. J.; Nakazawa, K.; Sakakibara, M.; Miyake, F.; Msha, H. & Sasaka, K. (2004). 123I-MIBG myocardial scintigraphy in patients with "takotsubo cardiomyopathy. *Journal of Nuclear Medicine*, Vol.45, No.7, pp. 1121-1127, ISSN 0161-5505

Anon. (1986). Case records of the Massachusetts General Hospital. Weekly clinicopathological exercises. Case 18-1986. A 44-year-old woman with substernal pain and pulmonary edema after severe emotional stress. *New England Journal of Medicine*, Vol.314, pp. 1240-1247

Avegliano, G.; Huguet, M.; Costabel, J. P.; Ronderos, R.; Bijnens, B.; Kuschnir, P.; Thierer, J.; Tobón-Gomez, C.; Martinez, G. O. & Frangi, A. (2011). Morphologic pattern of late gadolinium enhancement in Takotsubo cardiomyopathy detected by early cardiovascular magnetic resonance, *Clinical Cardiology*, Vol.34, No.3, pp. 178-182, ISSN 0160-9289

Balkin, D. M. & Cohen L. S. (2011). Takotsubo syndrome. *Coronary Artery Disease*, Vol.22, No.3, pp. 206-214, ISSN 0954-6928

Bers, D. M. (2002). Cardiac excitation-contraction coupling. *Nature*, Vol.415, No.6868, pp. 198-205, ISSN 0028-0836

Bossone, E.; Citro, R.; Eagle, K. A. & Manfredni, R. (2011). Tako-tsubo cardiomyopathy: is there a preferred time of onset? *Internal and Emergency Medicine*, Vol.6, No.3, pp. 221-226, ISSN 1828-0447

Boutet, M.; Huttner, I. & Rona, G. (1976). Permeability alteration of sarcolemmal membrane in catecholamin-induced cardiac muscle cell injury: in-vivo studies with fine structural diffusion tracer horseradish peroxidase. *Laboratory Investigation*, Vol.34, No.5, pp. 482-288, ISSN 0023-6837

Buchholz, S.; Ward, M. R.; Bhindi, R.; Nelson, G. I.; Figtree, G. A. & Grieve, S. M. (2010). Cardiac thrombi in stress (tako-tsubo) cardiomyopathy: more than an apical issue? *Mayo Clinic Proceedings*, Vol.85, No.9, pp. 863-864, ISSN 0025-6196

Bybee, K. A.; Kara, T.; Prasad, A.; Lerman, A.; Barsness, G. W.; Wright, R. S. & Rihal, C. S. (2004). Systematic review: transient left ventricular apical ballooning: a syndrome that mimics ST-segment elevation myocardial infarction. *Annals of Internal Medicine*, Vol.141, No.11, pp. 858-865, ISSN 0003-4819

Cebelin, M. S. & Hirsch, C. S. (1980) Human stress cardiomyopathy. Myocardial lesions in victims of homicidal assaults without internal injuries. *Human Pathology*, Vol.11, No.2, pp. 123-132, ISSN 0046-8177

Charmandari, E.; Tsigos, C. & Chrousos, G. P. (2005). Endocrinology of the stress response. *Annual Review of Physiology*, Vol.67, pp. 259-284, ISSN 0066-4278

Chrousos, G. P. & Gold, P. W. (1992). The concepts of stress and stress system disorders: overview of physical and behavioral homeostasis. *Journal of the American Medical Association*, Vol.267, No.9, pp. 1244-1252, ISSN 0098-7484

Chrousos, G. P. (2007). Organization and integration of the endocrine system. *Sleep Medicine Clinics*, Vol.2, No.2, pp. 125-145, ISSN 1556-407X

Chrousos, G. P. (2009). Stress and disorders of the stress system. *Nature Reviews Endocrinology*, Vol.5, No.7, pp. 374-381, ISSN 1759-5029

Dote, K.; Sato, H.; Tateishi, H.; Uchida, T. & Ishihara, M. (1991). Myocardial stunning due to simultaneous multivessel coronary spasms: a review of 5 cases. *Journal of Cardiology*, Vol.21, No.2, pp. 203-214, ISSN 0914-5087

El Mahmoud, R.; Mansencal, N.; Pilliére, R.; Leyer, F.; Abbou, N.; Michaud, P.; Nallet, O.; Digne, F.; Lacombe, P.; Cattan, S. & Dubourg, O. (2008). Prevalence and characteristics of left ventricular outflow tract obstruction in Tako-Tsubo syndrome. *American Heart Journal*, Vol.156, No.3, pp. 543-548, ISSN 0002-8703

Elesber, A. A.; Prasad, A.; Bybee, K. A.; Valeti, U.; Motiei, A.; Lerman, A.; Chandrasekaran, K. & Rihal, C. S. (2006). Transient cardiac apical ballooning syndrome: prevalence and clinical implications of right ventricular involvement. *Journal of the American College of Cardiology*, Vol.47, No.5, pp. 1082-1083, ISSN 0735-1097

Ferreira, S. H. & Vane, J. R. (1967). Half-lives of peptides and amines in the circulation. *Nature*, Vol.215, No.5107, pp. 1237-1240, ISSN 0028-0836

Fragkouli, K. & Vougiouklakis, T. (2010). Sudden cardiac death: an 11-year postmortem analysis in the region of Epirus, Greece. *Pathology - Research and Practice*, Vol.206, No.10, pp. 690-694, ISSN 0344-0338

Greco, C. A.; De, Rito, V.; Petracca, M.; Garzya, M.; Donateo, M. & Magliari, F. (2011). Takotsubo syndrome in a newborn. *Journal of the American Society of Echocardiography*, Vol.24, No.4, pp. 471.e5-e7, ISSN 0894-7317

Gianni, M.; Dentali, F.; Grandi, A. M.; Sumner, G.; Hiralal, R. & Lonn, E. (2006). Apical ballooning syndrome or takotsubo cardiomyopathy: a systematic review. *European Heart Journal*, Vol.27, No.13, pp. 1523-1529, ISSN 0195-668X

Haghi, D.; Athanasiadis, A.; Papavassiliu, T.; Suselbeck, T.; Fluechter, S.; Mahrholdt, H.; Borggrefe, M. & Sechtem, U. (2006). Right ventricular involvement in Takotsubo cardiomyopathy. *European Heart Journal*, Vol.27, No.20, pp.2433-2439, ISSN 0195-668X

Haghi, D.; Papavassiliu, T.; Heggemann, F.; Kaden, J. J.; Borggrefe, M. & Suselbeck, T. (2008). Incidence and clinical significance of left ventricular thrombus in tako-tsubo cardiomyopathy assessed with echocardiography. *Quarterly Journal of Medicine*, Vol.101, No.5, pp. 381-386, ISSN 1460-2393

Heggemann, F.; Weiss, C.; Hamm, K.; Kaden, J.; Süselbeck, T.; Papavassiliu, T.; Borggrefe, M. & Haghi, D. (2009). Global and regional myocardial function quantification by two dimensional strain in Takotsubo cardiomyopathy. *European Journal of Echocardiography*, Vol.10, No.6, pp. 760-764, ISSN 1532-2114

Heusch, G. & Schulz, R. (1996). Hibernating myocardium: a review. *Journal of Molecular and Cellular Cardiology*, Vol.28, No.12, pp. 2359-2372, ISSN 0022-2828

Iga, K.; Gen, H.; Tomonaga, G.; Matsumura, T. & Hori, K. (1989). Reversible left ventricular wall motion impairment caused by pheochromocytoa - a case report. *Japan Circulation Journal*, Vol.53, No.7, pp. 813-818, ISSN 0047-1828

Jim, M. H.; Chan, A. O.; Tsui, P. T.; Lau, S. T.; Siu, C. W.; Chow, W. H. & Lau, C. P. (2009). A new ECG criterion to identify takotsubo cardiomyopathy from anterior myocardial infarction: role of inferior leads. *Heart Vessels*, Vol.24, No.2, pp. 124-130, ISSN 0910-8327

Kono, T.; Morita, H.; Kuroiwa, T.; Onaka, H.; Takatsuka, H. & Fujiwara, A. (1994). Left ventricular wall motion abnormalities in patients with subarachnoid hemorrhage: neurogenic stunned myocardium. *Journal of the American College of Cardiology*, Vol.24, No.3, pp. 636-640, ISSN 0735-1097

Kurisu, S.; Inoue, I.; Kawagoe, T.; Ishihara, M.; Shimatani, Y.; Nakamura, S.; Yoshida, M.; Mitsuba, N.; Hata, T. & Sato, H. (2004). Time course of electrocardiographic changes in patients with Tako-Tsubo syndrome: comparison with acute myocardial infarction with minimal enzymatic release. *Circulation Journal*, Vol.68, No.1, pp. 77-81, ISSN 1346-9843

Lee, J. W.; Kim, J. Y.; Youn, Y. J.; Sung, J. K.; Lee, N. S.; Lee, K. H.; Yoo, B. S.; Lee, S. H.; Yoon, J. & Choe, K. H. (2010). Clinical characteristics and prognostic factors of stress-induced cardiomyopathy. *Korean Circulation Journal*, Vol.40, No.6, pp. 277-282, ISSN 1738-5520

Lee, J. W. & Kim, J. Y. (2011). Stress-induced cardiomyopathy: the role of echocardiography. *Journal of Cardiovascular Ultrasound*, Vol.19, No.1, pp. 7-12, ISSN 1975-4612

Lee, P. H.; Song, J. K.; Sun, B. J.; Choi, H.O.; Seo, J. S.; Na, J. O.; Kim, D. H.; Song, J. M.; Kang, D. H.; Kim, J. J. & Park, S. W. (2010). Outcomes of patients with stress-induced cardiomyopathy diagnosed by echocardiography in a tertiary referral hospital. *Journal of the American Society of Echocardiography*, Vol.23, No.7, pp. 766-771, ISSN 0894-7317

Leibel, R. L. & Hirsch, J. (1987). Site- and Sex-related differences in adrenoreceptor status of human adipose tissue. *The Journal of Clinical Endocrinology & Metabolism*, Vol.64, No.6, pp. 1205-1210, ISSN 0021-972X

Lyon, A. R.; Rees, P. S.; Prasad, S.; Poole-Wilson, P. A. & Harding, S. E. (2008). Stress (Takotsubo) cardiomyopathy - a novel pathophysiological hypothesis to explain catecholamine-induced acute myocardial stunning. *Natural Clinical Practice Cardiovascular Medicine*, Vol.5, No.1, pp. 22-29, ISSN 1743-4297

Madhavan, M.; Borlaug, B. A.; Lerman, A.; Rihal, C. S. & Prasad, A. (2009). Stress hormone and circulating biomarker profile of apical ballooning syndrome (Takotsubo cardiomyopathy): insights into the clinical significance of B-type natriuretic peptide and troponin levels. *Heart*, Vol.95, No.17, pp. 1436-1441, ISSN 1355-6037

Madhavan, M.; Rihal, C. S.; Lerman, A. & Prasad, A. (2011). Acute heart failure in apical ballooning syndrome (TakoTsubo/stress cardiomyopathy): clinical correlates and

Mayo Clinic risk score. *Journal of the American College of Cardiology*, Vol.57, No.12, pp. 1400-1401, ISSN 0735-1097

Manfredini, R.; Citro, R.; Previtali, M.; Vriz, O.; Ciampi, Q.; Pascotto, M.; Tagliamonte, E.; Provenza, G. & Manfredini, F. (2010). Monday preference in onset of takotsubo cardiomyopathy. *American Journal of Emergency Medicine*, Vol.28, No.6, pp. 715-719, ISSN 0735-6757

Martin, E. A.; Prasad, A.; Rihal, C. S.; Lerman, L. O. & Lerman A. (2010). Endothelial function and vascular response to mental stress are impaired in patients with apical ballooning syndrome. *Journal of the American College of Cardiology*, Vol.56, No.22, pp. 1840-1846, ISSN 0735-1097

Matsuoka, K.; Okubo, S.; Fujii, E.; Uchida, F.; Kasai, A.; Aoki, T.; Makino, K. Omichi, C.; Fujimoto, N.; Ohta, S.; Sawai, T. & Nakano, T. (2003). Evaluation of the arrhythmogenecity of stress-induced "Takotsubo cardiomyopathy" from the time course of the 12-lead surface electrocardiogram. *American Journal of Cardiology*, Vol.92, No.2, pp. 230-233, ISSN 0002-9149

Mendelsohn, M. E. (2002). Protective effects of estrogen on the cardiovascular system. *American Journal of Cardiology*, Vol.89, No.12A, pp. 12E-17E, ISSN 0002-9149

Monté, C. P.; Arends, J. B.; Tan, I. Y.; Aldenkamp, A. P.; Limburg, M. & de, Krom, M. C. (2007). Sudden unexpected death in epilepsy patients: Risk factors. A systematic review. *Seizure*, Vol.16, No.1, pp. 1-7, ISSN 1059-1311

Morel, O.; Sauer, F.; Imperiale, A.; Cimarelli, S.; Blondet, C.; Jesel, L; Trinh, A.; De, Poli, F.; Ohlmann, P.; Constantinesco, A. & Bareiss, P. (2009). Importance of inflammation and neurohumoral activation in Takotsubo cardiomyopathy. *Journal of Cardiac Failure*, Vol.15, No.3, pp. 206-213, ISSN 1071-9164

Nef, H. M.; Mollmann, H.; Akashi, Y. J. & Hamm, C. W. (2010). Mechanisms of stress (Takotsubo) cardiomyopathy. *Nature Reviews Cardiology*, Vol.7, No.4, pp. 187-193, ISSN 1759-5002

Padayachee, L. (2007). Levosimendan: the inotrope of choice in cardiogenic shock secondary to takotsubo cardiomyopathy? *Heart, Lung and Circulation*, Vol.16, pp. S65-S70, ISSN 1443-9506

Park, J. H.; Kang, S. J.; Song, J. K.; Kim, H. K.; Chae, M. L.; Kang, D. H. & Koh, Y. (2005). Left ventricular apical ballooning due to severe physical stress in patients admitted to the medical ICU. *Chest*, Vol.128, No.1, pp. 296-302, ISSN 0012-3692

Park, J. T.; Kim, J. Y.; Kim, Y. W.; Choi, K. H.; Park, B. H. & Lim, H. K. (2010). Stress-induced cardiomyopathy after general anesthesia for total gastrectomy - a case report. *Korean Journal of Anesthesiology*, Vol.58, No.3, pp. 299-303, ISSN 2005-6419

Parodi, G.; Del, Pace, S.; Salvadori, C.; Carrabba, N.; Olivotto, I.; Gensini, G. F. & Tuscany Registry of Tako-Tsubo Cardiomyopathy. (2007). Left ventricular apical ballooning syndromes as a novel cause of acute mitral regurgitation. *Journal of the American College of Cardiology*, Vol.50, No.7, pp. 647-649, ISSN 0735-1097

Pirzer, R.; Elmas, E.; Haghi, D.; Lippert, C.; Kralev, S.; Lang, S.; Borggrefe, M. & Kälsch, T. (2011). Platelet and monocyte activity markers and mediators of inflammation in Takotsubo cardiomyopathy. *Heart Vessels*, DOI 10.1007/s00380-011-0132-6, ISSN 0910-8327

Prasad, A.; Lerman, A. & Rihal, C. S. (2008). Apical ballooning syndrome (Tako-Tsubo or stress cardiomyopathy): a mimic of acute myocardial infarction. *American Heart Journal*, Vol.155, No.3, pp. 408-417, ISSN 0002-8703

Pollick, C.; Cujec, B.; Parker, S. & Tator, C. (1988). Left ventricular wall motion abnormalities in subarachnoid hemorrhage: an echocardiographic study. *Journal of the American College of Cardiology*, Vol.12, No.3, pp. 600-605, ISSN 0735-1097

Rona, G.; Boutet, M. & Huttner, I. (1975). Membrane permeability alterations as manifestation of early cardiac muscle cell injury. *Recent Advances in Studies on Cardiac Structure and Metabolism*, Vol.6, pp. 439-451, ISSN 0363-5872

Rosenbaum, D. M.; Rasmussen, S. G. & Kobilka, B. K. (2009). The structure and function of G-protein-coupled receptors. *Nature*, Vol.459, No.7245, pp. 356-363, ISSN 0028-0836

Sharkey, S. W.; Windenburg, D. C.; Lesser, J. R.; Maron, M. S.; Hause, R. G.; Lesser, J. N.; Haas, T. S.; Hodges, J. S. & Maron, B. J. (2010). Natural history and expansive clinical profile of stress (Tako-tsubo) cardiomyopathy. *Journal of the American College of Cardiology*, Vol.26, No.4, pp. 333-341, ISSN 0735-1097

Scott, I. U. & Gutterman D. D. (1995). Pheochromocytoma with reversible focal cardiac dysfunction. *American Heart Journal*, Vol.130, No.4, pp. 909-911, ISSN 0002-8703

Schmalfuss, C. (2011). Tako-tsubo cardiomyopathy and cardiac magnetic resonance imaging, *Clinical Cardiology*, Vol.34, No.3, pp. 145-146, ISSN 0160-9289

Skovgaard, D.; Holmvang, L.; Bang, L. E.; Lønborg, J. & Hasbak, P. (2010). Imaging of Takotsubo Cardiomyopathy. *Clinical Nuclear Medicine*, Vol.35, No.12, pp. 967-971, ISSN 0363-9762

Silventoinen, K.; Kaprio, J.; Lahelma, E.; Viken, R. J. & Rose, R. J. (2001). Sex differences in genetic and environmental factors contributing to body-height. *Twin Research*, Vol.4, No.1, pp. 25-29, ISSN 1369-0523

Soufer, R.; Arrighi, J. A. & Burg, M. M. (2002). Brain, behavior, mental stress, and the neurocardiac interaction. *Journal of Nuclear Cardiology*, Vol. 9, No.6, pp. 650-662, ISSN 1071-3581

Stöllberger, C.; Finsterer, J. (2011). Why does Takotsubo ("broken heart syndrome") affect more females than males? *International Journal of Cardiology*, Vol.147, No.1, pp. 175-176, ISSN 0167-5273

Sugimoto, K.; Watanabe, E.; Yamada, A.; Iwase, M.; Sano, H.; Hishida, H. & Ozaki, Y. (2008). Prognostic implications of left ventricular wall motion abnormalities associated with subarachnoid hemorrhage. *International Heart Journal*. Vol.49, No.1, pp. 75-85, ISSN 1349-2365

Tappia, P. S.; Hata, T.; Hozaima, L.; Sandhu, M. S.; Panagia, V. & Dhalla, N. S. (2001). Role of oxidative stress in catecholamine-induced changes in cardiac sarcolemmal Ca^{2+} transport. *Archieves of Biochemistry and Biophysics*, Vol.387, No.1, pp. 85-92, ISSN 0003-9861

Uchida, Y.; Egami, H.; Uchida, Y.; Sakurai, T.; Kanai, M.; Shirai, S.; Nakagawa, O. & Oshima, T. (2010). Possible participation of endothelial cell apoptosis of coronary microvessels in the genesis of Takotsubo cardiomyopathy. *Clinical Cardiology*, Vol. 33, No.6, pp. 371-377, ISSN 0160-9289

Ueyama, T.; Ishikura, F.; Matsuda, A.; Asanuma, T.; Ueda, K.; Ichinose, M.; Kasamatsu, K.;Hano, T.; Akasaka, T.; Tsuruo, Y.; Morimoto, K. & Beppu, S. (2007). Chronic estrogen supplementation following ovariectomy improves the emotional stress-induced cardiovascular responses by indirect action on the nervous system and by direct action on the heart. *Circulation Journal*, Vol.71, No.4, pp. 565-573, ISSN 1346-9843

Winchester, D. E.; Ragosta, M.; Taylor, A. M. (2008). Concurrence of angiographic coronary artery disease in patients with apical ballooning syndrome (tako-tsubo cardiomyopathy). *Catheterization and Cardiovascular Interventions*, Vol.72, No.5, pp. 612-616, ISSN 1522-1946

Wittstein, I. S.; Thiemann, D. R.; Lima, J. A.; Baughman, K. L.; Schulman, S. P.; Gerstenblith, G.; Wu, K. C.; Rade, J. J.; Bivalacqua, T. J. & Champion, H. C. (2005). Neurohumoral features of myocardial stunning due to sudden emotional stress. *New England Journal of Medicine*, Vol.10, No.6, pp. 539-548, ISSN 0028-4793

Xiao, R. P. (2001). Beta-adrenergic signaling in the heart: dual coupling of the beta2-adrenergic receptor to G(s) and G(i) proteins. *Science Signaling: the Signal Transduction Knowledge Environment*, Vol.2001, No.104, pp. re15, ISSN 1525-8882

Zeb, M.; Sambu, N.; Scott, P. & Curzen, N. (2011). Takotsubo cardiomyopathy: a diagnostic challenge. *Postgraduate Medical Journal*, Vol.87, No.1023, pp. 51-59, ISSN 0032-5473

14

Torsades de Pointes in Takotsubo Cardiomyopathy with QT Prolongation

Hiroaki Kawano
Department of Cardiovascular Medicine, Nagasaki University
Japan

1. Introduction

Takotsubo cardiomyopathy, or stress-induced cardiomyopathy, is characterized by reversible left ventricular apical ballooning associated with emotional or physiologic stress, mimicking acute myocardial infarction in the absence of significant coronary artery disease at angiography. Although the prognosis for patients with Takotsubo cardiomyopathy is relatively good, it is reported to be associated with long QT syndrome and torsades de pointes (TdP) which is a fatal polymorphic ventricular tachyarrhythmia.

However, only QT prolongation abnormalities is not enough to induce TdP, and other factors associated with Takotsubo cardiomyopathy seem to be needed for the induction of TdP. In this chapter, the mechanism of TdP in Takotsubo cardiomyopathy with QT prolongation is discussed.

2. Takotsubo cardiomyopathy

Takotsubo cardiomyopathy, or stress-induced cardiomyopathy, is a disease exhibiting an acute left ventricular apical ballooning of unknown cause (Kawai et al., 2007). Many cases with takotsubo cardiomyopathy are associated with preceded emotional or physiologic stress. In this disease, the left ventricle takes on the appearance of a Japanese octopus fishing pot called a takotsubo. In takotsubo cardiomyopathy, left ventricular dysfunction is reversible, i.e., it recovers within a few weeks (Figure 1). Other signs include ECG changes, including ST-segment elevation, abnormal Q wave, and T-wave inversions (Figure 2), which mimicks acute myocardial infarction but there is no significant coronary artery disease at angiography (Kawai et al., 2007, Tsuchihashi et al., 2001, Kurisu et al. , 2002).

Several pathophysiological mechanisms have been proposed to explain the features of this syndrome, such as multivessel coronary vasospasm, abnormalities in coronary microvascular function, and catecholamine-mediated cardiotoxicity (Akashi et al, 2002, Kurisu et al, 2003, Sansen V & Holvoet G., 2007). Studies on 123I-metaiodybenzylguanidine suggested the existence of cardiac autonomic damage and/or accelerated cardiac sympathetic nervous function in patients with Takotsubo cardiomyopathy (Akashi et al, 2004, Burgdorf et al, 2008). Nef, et al (Nef et al, 2007) reported that there were contraction bands, increase in fibrosis, and the regional accumulation of inflammatory cells in biopsied specimen of myocardium in acute phase of Takotsubo cardiomyopathy, and they suggested that these findings were similar to those associated with catecholamine cardiotoxicity. These data suggest that catecholamine-mediated cardiotoxicity may be the most plausible cause of Takotsubo cardiomyopathy although the precise aetiology and pathophysiology of this syndrome remain unknown.

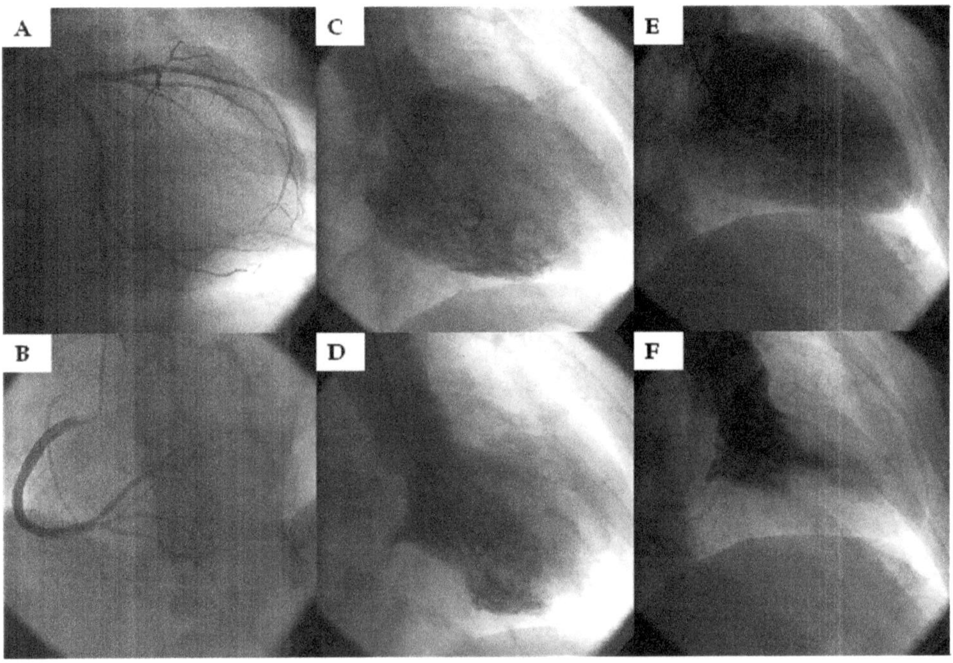

Coronary angiography showed no significant coronary stenosis of the left (A) and right (B)coronary arteries. Left ventriculography demonstrated akinesis of apex of the left ventricle on admission (C, end-diastolic phase; D, end-systolic phase) and showed recovered apical wall motion of the left ventricle about three weeks after admission(C, end-diastolic phase; D, end-systolic phase).

Fig. 1. Coronary angiography and left ventriculography on admission and about three weeks after the admission

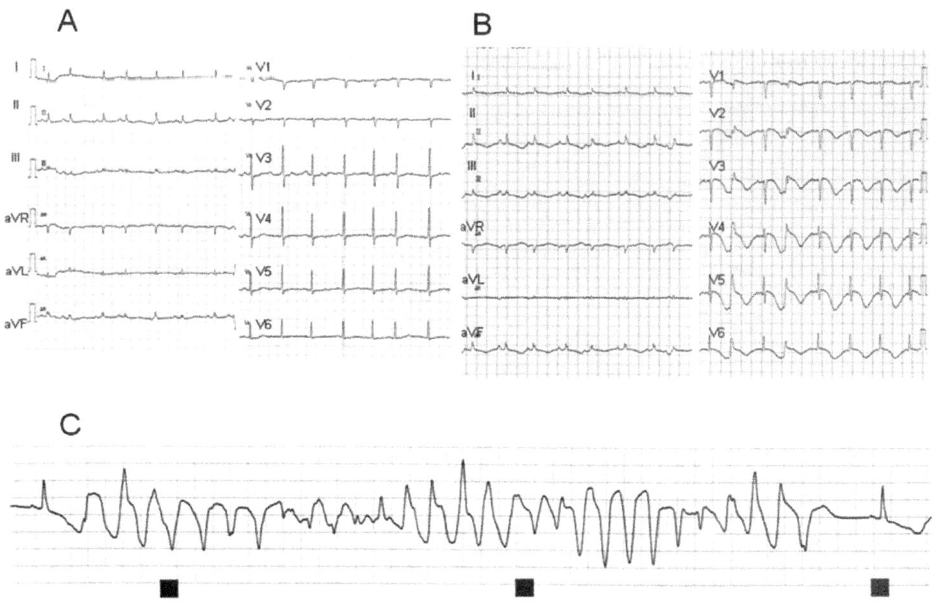

A, ECG showed sinus rhythm, and flat T waves. B, ECG showed sinus rhythm, poor R wave progression in leads V1 to V3, and QT prolongation with a corrected QT interval of 800 msec. C, ECG monitor demonstrated torsades de pointes.

Fig. 2. Electrocardiography (ECG) before (A) and just after (B) the occurrence of Takotsubo Cardiomyopathy, and ECG monitor of torsades de pointes(C)

Takotsubo cardiomyopathy occurs most frequently in women over 50 years of age. The reason for the much more common occurrence in post-menopausal women is unclear. Several explanations have been proposed. Sex hormones may exert important influences on the sympathetic neurohormonal axis (Hinojosa-Laborde et al, 1999) and on coronary vasoreactivity (Sader & Celermajer, 2002). Women appear also to be more vulnerable to sympathetically mediated myocardial stunning (Lambert et al, 2002), and post-menopausal alteration of endothelial function in response to reduced estrogen levels has been advocated as a possible alternative explanation (Taddei et al, 1996).

3. Long QT syndrome (QT prolongation) and torsades de pointes

The Long QT syndrome (LQTS) is originally a hereditary disorder in which most affected family members have delayed ventricular repolarization manifest on the electrocardiogram (ECG) as QT prolongation (Moss et al, 1985). The disorder is associated with an increased propensity to arrhythmogenic syncope, polymorphic ventricular tachycardia (torsades de pointes), and sudden arrhythmic death. LQTS is due to mutations involving principally the myocyte ion-channels, and this monogenetic disorder has an autosomal-dominant inheritance pattern. Since the 3 genes were identified for the 3 major genotypes, a total of 13 forms of LQTS have been reported (Shimizu W & Horie M.).

Recently, mutations in the caveolin-3 gene (*CAV3*) have been linked with the congenital long QT syndrome (LQT9), and mutations in caveolar-localized ion channels may contribute to other inherited arrhythmias. Caveolin-3 is the essential scaffolding protein of caveolae which are specialized membrane microdomains enriched in cholesterol and sphingolipids which are present in multiple cell types including cardiomyocytes. Along with the essential scaffolding protein caveolin-3, a number of different ion channels and transporters have been localized to caveolae in the heart. Mutations in caveolar-localized ion channels may contribute to other inherited arrhythmias, and changes in the caveolar microdomain in acquired heart disease may also lead to dysregulation and dysfunction of ion channels, altering the risk of arrhythmias in conditions such as heart failure (Balijepalli & Kamp, 2008). This indicate that abnormality or damage of structural elements of cardiomyocyte may also induce QT prolongation and arrhythmia.

Long QT syndrome can be also divided into idiopathic (congenital) and acquired forms. QT intervals vary according to age, sex, and heart rate, and acquired long QT syndrome describes pathologic QT interval prolongation. Acquired long QT syndrome can arise in response to various drugs, electrolyte abnormalities (e.g., hypokalemia, hypomagnesemia) and significant bradyarrhythmias. It also becomes a risk of arrhythmogenic syncope, polymorphic ventricular tachycardia (torsades de pointes), and sudden arrhythmic death.

Torsade de pointes (TdP) is a life-threatening arrhythmia that develops as a consequence of a reduction in the repolarization reserve of cardiac cells leading to amplification of electrical heterogeneities in the ventricular myocardium as well as to the development of early after depolarization-induced triggered activity.

Autonomic nervous system may have important role in the initiation of Tdp (Coumel, 1993). The level of adrenergic drive is required for the occurrence of Tdp, and it also produces a sinus tachycardia that would prevent QT prolongation. Autonimic tone influences the QT interval directly by affecting the action potential duration and indirectly by modulating the RR interval. These indicate that the interactions between heart rate and sympathetic nervous activity are complex. Fujiki et al (Fujiki et al, 2001) suggested that the sympathovagal imbalance may have an important role in the dynamic change in the QT interval and initiation of Tdp in patients with long QT syndrome. In patients with acquired long-QT syndrome, Locati et al (Locati et al, 1995) reported that both adrenergic- and pause-dependent mechanisms may have a synergistic role in the genesis of Tdp.

Women are more prone to develop TdP than men either congenital or acquired LQTS, and it is similar to the sex difference of occurrence of Takotsubo cardiomyopathy. Although the precise mechanism has not been clarified, female hormone may exert the influence on cardiac repolarization process (Kurokawa et al, 2009).

4. Torsades de pointes in takotsubo cardiomyopathy with QT prolongation

The presence of QT interval prolongation has been discussed in patients with Takotsubo cardiomyopathy (Abe et al., 2003 , Desmet et al., 2003, Matsuoka et al., 2003), and there have been 17 reported cases of QT interval prolongation and torsades de pointes (TdP) associated with Takotsubo cardiomyopathy (Denney et al., 2005, Sasaki et al., 2006, Okada T, et al., 2007 [in Japanese], Nault et al., 2007, Boulouffe et al., 2007, Patel et al., 2007, Kurisu et al., 2008, Furushima et al., 2008, Hirose et al., 2008, Ghosh et al., 2009, Mahida et al., 2009, Inoue et al., 2009, Kawano et al., 2010, Purvis et al., 2009, Yamada et al., 2011) (Figure 2) (Table 1). Considering the 17 previous cases reported in the literature, QT prolongation in Takotsubo cardiomyopathy has been attributed to hypokalemia (n= 3), bradycardia associated with atrioventricular (AV) block (n=4), idiopathic long QT syndrome (n=2), hypokalemia plus antiarrhythmic therapy (n=1), and hypokalemia plus idiopathic long QT syndrome (n=1), hypokalemia and hypomagnesemia (n=1), hyponagnesemia (n=1), and antibiotic (n=1) in 14 cases, and there was no specific factor associated with QT prolongation in 3 cases. The vasospasm provocation test was performed in only 3 cases, and vasospasm was not induced in any of these cases.

Hypokalemia or hypomagnesemia is one of the most important risk factor because it is present in 7 of 17 (41%) case. Badycardia associated with AV block is also one of the important factor because its presence in 4 of 17 (24%) cases. These observations suggest that electrolyte imbalances and bradycardia are a risk factor for the development of torsades de pointes in patients with Takotsubo cardiomyopathy.

However, only QT prolongation is not enough to induce TdP. Oscillations of the RR interval or the short-long-short (or the long-short) sequence precede the initiation of TdP in patients with acquired prolongation of repolarization (Locati et al., 1995). In most cases of TdP, frequent premature ventricular contraction (PVC)s create long-short sequence, i.e., a VPC generates a post-extrasystolic pause, the following regular beat shows marked QT prolongation from which a subsequent PVC arise, and this beat initiates TdP. Triggered activity originating from early after-depolarization or phase 2 reentry has been suggested as the cause of the PVC which induces long-short initiating sequence and can be the first beat of TdP. However, there is another unique pattern of the initiating of TdP in Takotsubo cardiomyopathy (Kawano et al., 2010,). It seems that premature atrial contraction (PAC) followed by QRS on T wave can also induced reentrant ventricular tachycardia directly (Figure 3). The peak of T wave is known as the vulnerable period of the ventricle. Depolarization at this phase may easily induce unstable reentrant mechanism especially in the case with prominently increased dispersion of repolarization such as long QT syndrome. This mechanism of TdP is also very rare in long QT syndrome. Moreover, that case had already had mild QT prolongation with hypokalemia and PAC before the occurrence of Takotsubo cardiomyopathy. This suggests that other factors associated with Takotsubo cardiomyopathy is needed for the induction of TdP.

Prolongation of action potential duration (APD) due to abnormal ion channel current causes QT prolongation. Dispersion of APD or repolarizaion is thought to be one of the mechanisms of occurrence of Tdp, and Furushima et al. (Furushima et al., 2008) reported abnormal LV reporlarization gradient in a patient with Takotsubo cardiomyopathy. Taken together, dispersion of APD or repolarization in Takotsubo cardiomyopathy as well as QT prolongation may be important in the occurrence of TdP. Adrenergic stimulation may be also related to TdP in Takotsbo cardiomyopathy because catecholamine excess and neurogenic myocardial stunning are thought to be one of the the most plausible causes of Takotsubo cardiomyopathy.

On the other hands, TdP may be one of the trigger of Takotsubo cardiomyopathy in long QT syndrome. Although it occurs most frequently in women over 50 years of age, recent study demonstrated that men with Takotsubo cardiomyopathy-associated QT interval prolongation are at risk for TdP, and that most patients with Takotsubo cardiomyopathy-associated TdP have risk factors for TdP other than the female sex and systolic dysfunction (Samuelov-Kinori, 2009).

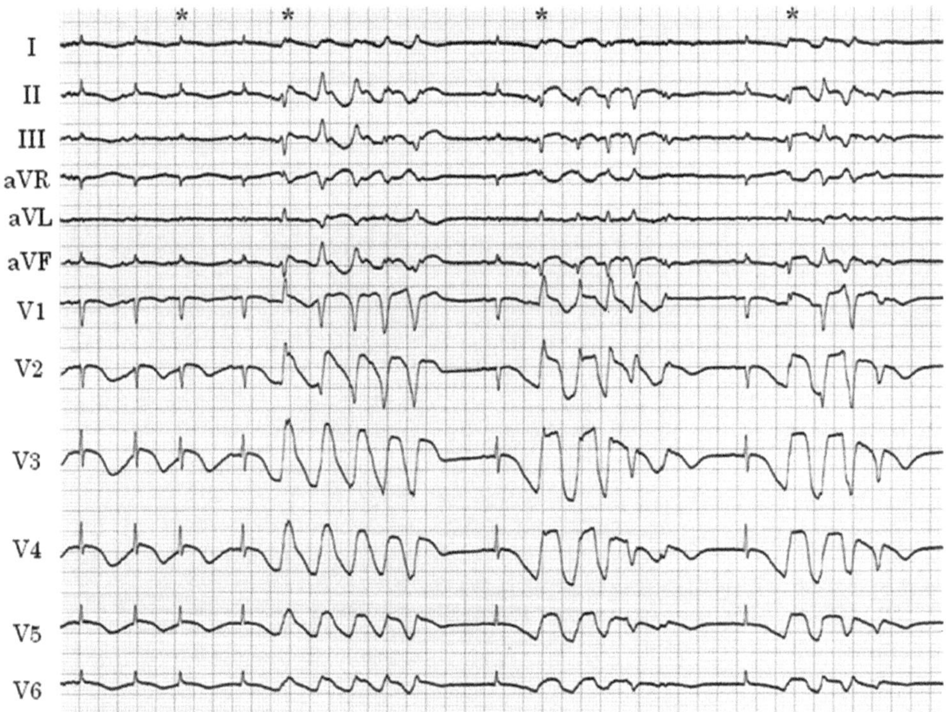

Fig. 3. ECG showed that PACs (*) induced long-short sequence and initiated TdP.

	Age	Sex	Diseases	serum K(mEq/L)	QTc (msec)
1	32	M	migrane, BA, allergic rhinitis	normal	467
2	22	F	LQTS	2.8	730
3	77	M	pneumonia	3.7	730
4	76	F	rhabdomyolysis	3.3	786
5	68	F	none	not determined	prolongation
6	72	F	HT, COPD	not determined	674
7	87	F	AV block	not determined	735
8	78	M	AV block	not determined	735
9	61	F	LQTS	not determined	590
10	63	F	Myasthenia gravis	2.8	549
11	59	F	HT, alcoholic	3.2	669
12	55	F	LQTS	normal	510
13	82	F	AV block	4	630
14	80	M	BA, HT, alcoholic	2.6	800
15	67	F	Depression	3.9	524
16	89	F	AV block	4.6	580
17	81	F	atrial fibrillation	4.3	620

M male, F female, BA bronchial asthma, LQTS idiopathic long QT syndrome, HT hypertension

Table 1. Reports of Takotsubo Cardiomyopathy with Torsades de Pointes

5. Conclusion

We usually pay attention to ventricular arrhythmia in other cardiomyopathy, i.e., hypertrophic cardiomyopathy and dilated cardiomyopathy. And we have to also consider the importance of PAC as well as VPC as the initiator of TdP, the life-threatening arrhythmia in Takotsubo cardiomyopathy .

6. Acknowledgment

I thank editors of Internal Medicine for their excellent advice to discuss the mechanisms of torsasede de pointes in Takotsubo cardiomyopathy.

7. References

Abe Y, Kondo M, Matsuoka R, Araki M, Dohyama K, Tanio H. Assessment of clinical features in transient left ventricular apical ballooning. J Am Coll Cardiol 41: 737-742, 2003

Akashi YJ, Nakazawa K, Sakakibara M, Miyake F, Sasaka K. Reversible left ventricular dysfunction "takotsubo" cardiomyopathy related to catecholamine cardiotoxicity. J Electrocardiol 35: 351-6, 2002

Akashi YJ, Nakazawa K, Sakakibara M, Miyake F, Musha H, Sasaka K. 123I-MIBG myocardial scintigraphy in patients with "takotsubo" cardiomyopathy. J Nucl Med 45:1121-7, 2004

Balijepalli RC& Kamp TJ.Caveolae, ion channels and cardiac arrhythmias. Prog Biophys Mol Biol 98:149-60, 2009

Boulouffe C, Vanpee D, Gabriel L. Stress-induced cardiomyopathy: Takotsubo left ventricular dysfunction. Am J Emerg Med 25: 243-244, 2007

Burgdorf C, von Hof K, Schunkert H, Kurowski V. Regional alterations in myocardial sympathetic innervation in patients with transient left-ventricular apical ballooning (Tako-Tsubo cardiomyopathy). J Nucl Cardiol 15 :65-72, 2008

Coumel P. Cardiac arrhythmia and the autonomic nervous system. J Cardiovasc Electrophysiol 1993; 4: 338-355

Denney SD, Lakkireddy DR, Khan IA. Long QT syndrome and torsade de pointes in transient left ventricular apical ballooning syndrome. Int J Cardiol 100:499-501, 2005

Desmet WJ, Adriaenssens BF, Dens JA. Apial ballooning of the left ventricle: first series in white patients. Heart 89: 1027-1031, 2003

Fujiki A, Nishida K, Mizumaki K, Nagasawa H, Shimono M, Inoue H. Spontaneous onset of torsade de pointes in long-QT syndrome and the role of sympathovagal imbalance. Circ J 65: 1087-1090, 2001

Furushima H, Chinushi M, Sanada A, Aizawa Y. Ventricular repolarization gradients in a patient with takotsubo cardiomyopathy. Europace 10: 1112-1115, 2008

Ghosh S, Apte P, Maroz N, Broor A, Zeineh N, Khan IA. Takotsubo cardiomyopathy as a potential cause of long QT syndrome and torsades de pointes. Int J Cardiol 136: 225-227, 2009

Hinojosa-Laborde C, Chapa I, Lange D, Haywood JR. Gender differences in sympathetic nervous system regulation. Clin Exp Pharmacol Physiol 26:122-126, 1999

Hirose K, Yamaguchi H, Oshima Y, Choraku M, Hirono A, Takamori N, Tamura K. Severe respiratory failure and torsades de pointes induced by disopyramide in a patient with myasthenia gravis. Intern Med 47: 1703-1708, 2008

Inoue M, Kanaya H, Matsubara T, Uno Y, Yasuda T, Miwa K. Complete atrioventricular block associated with takotsubo cardiomyopathy. Circ J 73: 589-592, 2009

Kawai S, Kitabatake A, Tomoike H; Takotsubo Cardiomyopathy Group. Guidelines for diagnosis of takotsubo (ampulla) cardiomyopathy. Circ J.71:990-2, 2007

Kawano H, Matsumoto Y, Arakawa S, Satoh O, Hayano M. Premature atrial contraction induces torsades de pointes in a patient of Takotsubo cardiomyopathy with QT prolongation.Intern Med. 49:1767-73, 2010

Kurisu S, Sato H, Kawagoe T, Ishihara M, Shimatani Y, Nishioka K, Kano Y, Umemura T, Nakamura S. Tako-tsubo-like left ventricular dysfunction with ST-segment elevation: a novel cardiac syndrome mimicking acute myocardial infarction。 Am Heart J 143: 448-455, 2002

Left ventricular apical thrombus formation in a patient with suspected tako-tsubo-like left ventricular dysfunction.

Kurisu S, Inoue I, Kawagoe T, Ishihara M, Shimatani Y, Nishioka K, Umemura T, Nakamura S, Yoshida M, Sato H. Circ J 67: 556-558, 2003

Kurisu S, Inoue I, Kawagoe T, Ishihara M, Shimatani Y, Nakama Y, Ohkawa K, Maruhashi T, Kagawa E, Dai K, Aoyagi T. Torsade de pointes associated with bradycardia and takotsubo cardiomyopathy. Can J Cardiol 24:640-642, 2008

Kurokawa J, Suzuki T, Furukawa T.New aspects for the treatment of cardiac diseases based on the diversity of functional controls on cardiac muscles: acute effects of female hormones on cardiac ion channels and cardiac repolarization. J Pharmacol Sci 109:334-340, 2009

Lambert G, Naredi S, Edén E, Rydenhag B, Friberg P. Monoamine metabolism and sympathetic nervous activation following subarachnoid haemorrhage: influence of gender and hydrocephalus.Brain Res Bull 58:77-82, 2002

Locati EH, Maison-Blanche P, Dejode P, Cauchemez B, Coumel P. Spontaneous sequences of onset of torsade de pointes in patients with acquired prolonged repolarization: quantitative analysis of Holter recordings. J Am Coll Cardiol 25 :1564-75, 1995

Mahida S, Dalageorgou C, Behr ER. Long-QT syndrome and torsades de pointes in a patient with Takotsubo cardiomyopathy: an unusual case. Europace 11: 376-378, 2009

Matsuoka K, Okubo S, Fujii E, Uchida F, Kasai A, Aoki T, Makino K, Omichi C, Fujimoto N, Ohta S, Sawai T, Nakano T. Evaluation of the arrhythmogenicity of stress-induced "Takotsubo cardiomyopathy" from the time course of the 12-lead surface electrocardiogram. Am J Cardiol 92:230-233, 2003

Moss AJ, Schwartz PJ, Crampton RS, Locati E, Carleen E. The long QT syndrome: a prospective international study, Circulation 71: 17–21, 1985

Nault MA, Baranchuk A, simpson CS, Redfearn DP. Takotsubo cardiomyopathy: a novel "proarrhythmic" disease-case report. Anadolu Kardiyol Derg 7(suppl 1): 101-103, 2007

Nef HM, Möllmann H, Kostin S, Troidl C, Voss S, Weber M, Dill T, Rolf A, Brandt R, Hamm CW, Elsässer A.Tako-Tsubo cardiomyopathy: intraindividual structural analysis in the acute phase and after functional recovery. Eur Heart J 28: 2456-2464, 2007

Okada T, Miyata S, Hashimoto K, Maie K, Mochizuki S. Takotsubo cardiomyopathy associated with torsades de pointes and long QT interval: a case report . J Cardiol 50 :83-88, 2007 [in Japanese]

Patel HM, Kantharia BK, Morris DL, Yazdanfar S. Takotsubo syndrome in African-American women with atypical presentatiosn: a single-center exerience. Clin Cardiol 30: 14-18, 2007

Purvis JA, Cunningham EL, McGlinchey PG, Barr SH.Drugs, electrolytes and tako-tsubo cardiomyopathy: triple aetiology of acquired long QT syndrome and torsades de pointes. Ulster Med J. 2009 Sep;78(3):188-9.

Sader MA, Celermajer DS. Endothelial function, vascular reactivity and gender differences in the cardiovascular system. Cardiovasc Res 53:597-604, 2002

Samuelov-Kinori L, Kinori M, Kogan Y, Swartzon M, Shalev H, Guy D, Ferenidou F, Mashav N, Sadeh B, Atzmony L, Kliuk-Ben-Basat O, Steinvil A, Justo D. Takotsubo cardiomyopathy and QT interval prolongation: who are the patients at risk for torsades de pointes? J Electrocardiol. 42:353-357, 2009

Sansen V, Holvoet G. Takotsubo cardiomyopathy presenting as multivessel coronary spasm syndrome: case report and review of the literature. Acta Cardiol 62:507-11, 2007

Sasaki O, Nishioka T, Akima T, Tabata H, Okamoto Y, Akanuma M, Uehata A, Takase B, Katsushika S, Isojima K, Ohtomi S, Yoshimoto N. Association of takotsubo cardiomyopathy and long QT syndrome. Circ J 70:1220-2, 2006

Taddei S, Virdis A, Ghiadoni L, Mattei P, Sudano I, Bernini G, Pinto S, Salvetti A. Menopause is associated with endothelial dysfunction in women. Hypertension 28:576-582, 1996

Tsuchihashi K, Ueshima K, Uchida T, Oh-mura N, Kimura K, Owa M, Yoshimura M, Miyazaki S, Haze K, Ogawa H, Honda T, Hase M, Kai R, Morii I; Angina Pectoris-Myocardial Infarction Investigation in Japan. Transient left ventricular apical ballooning without coronary artery stenosis: a novel heart syndrome mimicking acute myocardial infarction. Angina Pectoris-Myocardial Infarction Investigations in Japan . J Am Coll Cardiol 38: 11-18, 2001

Yamada Y, Tani T, Homma M, Saito S. Two cases of torsades de pointes associated with takotsubo cardiomyopathy as the second insult. J Electrocardiol. 2011 [Epub ahead of print]

15

Torsades de Pointes Associated with Takotsubo Cardiomyopathy: Is It Preventable?

Dan Justo, Arie Steinvil and Itzhak Shapira
Departments of Geriatrics and Cardiology, Tel-Aviv Sourasky Medical Center, Affiliated to Sackler School of Medicine, Tel-Aviv University, Tel-Aviv, Israel

1. Introduction

Takotsubo cardiomyopathy is characterized by transient left ventricular systolic dysfunction and apical dyskinesis (ballooning) in the absence of significant obstructive coronary artery disease. Most patients with Takotsubo cardiomyopathy are females. An emotional stress is believed to be the main trigger of Takotsubo cardiomyopathy (Bybee & Prasad, 2008). Electrocardiographic features of Takotsubo cardiomyopathy might include: ST elevation, T wave inversion, and QT interval prolongation (Thakar et al., 2011).

QT interval prolongation might precede Torsades de Pointes - a potentially deadly polymorphic ventricular tachycardia. Female gender, left ventricular systolic dysfunction, recent conversion of atrial fibrillation to sinus rhythm, administering QT interval prolonging agents, hypokalemia, hypocalcemia, severe hypomagnesemia, and high-degree atrioventricular block, are all risk factors for acquired QT interval prolongation and Torsades de Pointes (Antzelevitch, 2007; Roden, 2004).

The incidence of QT interval prolongation among patient with Takotsubo cardiomyopathy is higher than 50% (Abe et al., 2003; Cangella et al., 2007; Fang et al., 2008; Wittstein et al., 2005), but the incidence Takotsubo cardiomyopathy-associated Torsades de Pointes is probably much lower. It is of great importance to study the clinical circumstances leading to Torsades de Pointes in patients with Takotsubo cardiomyopathy-associated QT interval prolongation since Torsades de Pointes might be fatal, while the prognosis of Takotsubo cardiomyopathy is usually good (Bybee & Prasad, 2008).

Takotsubo cardiomyopathy-associated Torsades de Pointes has been reported in 2005 for the first time (Denney et al., 2005). We have reviewed this case report and additional 14 reports (Akashi et al., 2003; Boulouffe et al., 2007; Finsterer et al., 2007; Furushima et al., 2008; Ghosh et al., 2009; Hirose et al., 2008; Inoue et al., 2009; Kurisu et al., 2008; Mahida et al., 2009; Nault et al., 2007; Okada et al., 2007; Patel et al., 2007; Sasaki et al., 2006) concerning Takotsubo cardiomyopathy-associated Torsades de Pointes in 2009, and we have concluded that males with Takotsubo cardiomyopathy-associated QT interval prolongation are at risk for Takotsubo cardiomyopathy-associated Torsades de Pointes although most patients with Takotsubo cardiomyopathy are females. There has been a trend in the mean maximal QT interval being longer among patients with Takotsubo cardiomyopathy-associated Torsades de Pointes relative to patients with Takotsubo cardiomyopathy-associated QT interval prolongation. Moreover, most patients with Takotsubo cardiomyopathy-associated Torsades de Pointes have had risk factors for Torsades de Pointes other than female gender and left ventricular systolic dysfunction (Samuelov-Kinori et al., 2009). Additional 12 patients with Takotsubo cardiomyopathy-associated Torsades de Pointes have been reported since then (Ahn et al., 2011; Gotyo et al., 2009; Grilo et al., 2010; Kawano et al., 2010; Micallef et al., 2010; Pacha et al., 2010; Peters & Klein, 2011; Purvis et al., 2009; Rotondi et al., 2010; Wedekind et al., 2009; Yamada et al., 2011). We have currently examined whether our previous conclusions are true in face of these new publications. Moreover, we have studied if Torsades de Pointes has been possibly preventable in patients with Takotsubo cardiomyopathy-associated Torsades de Pointes.

2. Material and methods

2.1 Retrieval of reports

We performed a literature search by using the following keywords: "Apical ballooning", "Arrhythmia", "Stress cardiomyopathy", "Sudden death", "Syncope", "Takotsubo", and "Torsades de Pointes". The references in each report were further reviewed for additional publications. Only full-length reports were reviewed. The study group included all patients with Takotsubo cardiomyopathy-associated Torsades de Pointes that had been reported until July 2011. The control group included patients with Takotsubo cardiomyopathy-associated QT interval prolongation that had been reviewed previously (Samuelov-Kinori et al., 2009).

2.2 Risk factors for Torsades de Pointes

Each case report was analyzed for the presence of risk factors for Torsades de Pointes other than female gender and left ventricular systolic dysfunction: recent conversion of atrial fibrillation to sinus rhythm, administering QT interval prolonging agents, hypokalemia (<3.5 mmol/L), hypocalcemia (<8.5 mg/dL), severe hypomagnesaemia (<1 mg/dL), and high-degree atrioventricular block (Antzelevitch, 2007; Roden, 2004). Since genetic analysis was not available for all patients, suspicion of congenital long QT syndrome was also considered a risk factor for Torsades de Pointes, and was defined as QT interval prolongation in the baseline ECG recorded before Takotsubo cardiomyopathy appearance or following its resolution. QT interval prolongation was defined as QTc >430 msec for male patients and QTc >450 msec for female patients according to the Bazett's formula (Bazett, 1920). We used the QTc that was mentioned in the text of each case report by the authors. In few cases we measured the QT interval length in lead II and calculated the QTc according to the ECG strip enclosed.

2.3 Preventable Torsades de Pointes

Each case report of Takotsubo cardiomyopathy-associated Torsades de Pointes was analyzed for the presence or the absence of treatment and prevention measures taken once QT interval prolongation had been noticed and prior to Torsades de Pointes appearance in face of the above-mentioned risk factors for Torsades de Pointes - regardless of whether Takotsubo cardiomyopathy diagnosis had already been made.

2.4 Statistical analysis

Continuous variables were expressed as mean ± standard error. Student t-test was used to compare between mean values of continuous variables with parametric distributions. Mann-Whitney test was used to compare between mean values of continuous variables with non-parametric distributions. Fisher's exact test was used to compare between incidence and prevalence of categorical variables. Two-tailed $p<0.05$ was considered statistically significant. Version 17.0 of the SPSS statistical package was used for all statistical analyses (SPSS Inc., Chicago, IL, USA).

3. Results

Reports concerning 113 patients were reviewed. The study group included 27 patients with Takotsubo cardiomyopathy-associated Torsades de Pointes. The control group included 86 patients with Takotsubo cardiomyopathy-associated QT interval prolongation. Mean age of all patients was 65.1±1.2 years. Most patients were females (n=102; 90.3%). All patients with Takotsubo cardiomyopathy-associated Torsades de Pointes survived, although one patient died of other complications more than two months following Torsades de Pointes (Hirose et al., 2008).

Although most patients were females, the prevalence of male gender was significantly higher among patients with Takotsubo cardiomyopathy-associated Torsades de Pointes relative to patients with Takotsubo cardiomyopathy-associated QT interval prolongation (odds ratio 4.6; 95%Cofidence Interval 1.3-16.7). Mean maximal QTc interval was significantly higher among patients with Takotsubo cardiomyopathy-associated Torsades de Pointes relative to patients with Takotsubo cardiomyopathy-associated QT interval prolongation even prior to Torsades de Pointes appearance. There were no statistical differences between patients with Takotsubo cardiomyopathy-associated Torsades de Pointes and patients with Takotsubo cardiomyopathy-associated QT interval prolongation in terms of mean age, mean lowest ejection fraction, and mean peak Troponin levels (table 1).

		Takotsubo-associated QT interval prolongation (n=86)	Takotsubo-associated Torsades de Pointes (n=27)	p value
Male gender	n (%)	5 (5.8%)	6 (22.2%)	0.021
Age (years)	n available Mean±SE	86 64.7±1.2	27 66.2±3.2	0.680
Maximal QTc interval (msec)	n available Mean±SE	58 555.9±8.4	25 670.2±37.1	0.006
Maximal QTc interval prior to Torsades de Pointes (msec)	n available Mean±SE	58 555.9±8.4	16 676.8±49.7	0.029
Lowest ejection fraction (%)	n available Mean±SE	50 36.5±1.4	11 37.2±4.0	0.850
Peak Troponin levels (ng/mL)	n available Mean±SE	39 5.6±2.5	13 1.7±0.8	0.383

Table 1. Clinical characteristics of reported patients

Overall, 17 (62.9%) patients with Takotsubo cardiomyopathy-associated Torsades de Pointes had one or more risk factors for Torsades de Pointes other than female gender and left ventricular systolic dysfunction, while only two (2.3%) patients with Takotsubo cardiomyopathy-associated QT interval prolongation had risk factors for Torsades de Pointes (odds ratio 71.4; 95%Confidence Interval 14.3-355.5; $p<0.0001$). Electrolyte depletion, i.e., hypokalemia and/or severe hypomagnesemia (n=7; 25.9%), and high-degree atrioventricular block (n=5; 18.5%), were the most prevalent risk factors for Torsades de Pointes and the last triggers for Torsades de Pointes. Four (14.8%) patients were also taking QT interval prolonging agents, although initiation of these agents was not the last trigger for Torsades de Pointes in any case (table 2).

Among patients with Takotsubo cardiomyopathy-associated Torsades de Pointes, the arrhythmia was diagnosed prior to Takotsubo cardiomyopathy most of the times (n=19; 70.4%), and in seven (25.9%) patients Torsades de Pointes was diagnosed upon admission to the emergency department. Nevertheless, Torsades de Pointes was possibly preventable in seven (25.9%) patients: In four patients with QT interval prolongation and apparent electrolyte depletion, hypokalemia and/or severe hypomagnesemia were corrected only following Torsades de Pointes appearance; in three patients with QT interval prolongation and high-degree atrioventricular block, pacemaker was implanted only following Torsades de Pointes appearance (table 2). In other patients, risk factors for Torsades de Pointes were diagnosed only following Torsades de Pointes appearance, or they were addressed too late.

4. Discussion

We have studied reports concerning patients with Takotsubo cardiomyopathy-associated QT interval prolongation and reports concerning patients with Takotsubo cardiomyopathy-associated Torsades de Pointes in order to characterize the clinical circumstances leading to Torsades de Pointes in patients with Takotsubo cardiomyopathy. We have done this before in 2009 (Samuelov-Kinori et al., 2009), but reports concerning patients with Takotsubo cardiomyopathy-associated Torsades de Pointes have almost doubled since then, and it is time to examine if our previous conclusions are still true in face of these new publications. Moreover, we have studied if Torsades de Pointes has been possibly preventable in patients with Takotsubo cardiomyopathy-associated Torsades de Pointes.

Consistent with our previous observation (Samuelov-Kinori et al., 2009), male patients with Takotsubo cardiomyopathy-associated QT interval prolongation are at higher risk for Torsades de Pointes compared with female patients with Takotsubo cardiomyopathy-associated QT interval prolongation, although most patients with Takotsubo cardiomyopathy are females (Bybee & Prasad, 2008). This finding is coherent with a recognized paradox which is still unexplained: women have longer QT interval compared with men but lower incidence of sudden death (Larsen & Kadish, 1998).

In our previous review there has been a trend in the mean maximal QT interval being longer among patients with Takotsubo cardiomyopathy-associated Torsades de Pointes relative to patients with Takotsubo cardiomyopathy-associated QT interval prolongation, although most of the times QT interval prolongation has been noticed only following Torsades de Pointes appearance (Samuelov-Kinori et al., 2009). In face of the new reports concerning patients with Takotsubo cardiomyopathy-associated QT interval prolongation, the trend has become statistically significant: mean maximal QTc interval is significantly higher among

First author	Age	Sex	Diagnosed first	Risk factors for QT interval prolongation and Torsades de Pointes other than female gender and left ventricular systolic dysfunction	Was Torsades de Pointes preventable?
Denney	32	M	Torsades	None	No
Kurisu	78	M	Torsades	Atrioventricular Block	Possibly
Kurisu	87	F	Torsades	Atrioventricular Block	Possibly
Nault	76	M	Torsades	HypoK	Possibly
Okada	77	M	Takotsubo	None	No
Akashi	67	F	Torsades	None	No
Boulouffe	68	F	Takotsubo	None	No
Finsterer	75	F	Torsades	Recent A.Fib conversion	No
Furushima	61	F	Torsades	QT interval prolongation at baseline ECG	No
Ghosh	59	F	Takotsubo	HypoK	Possibly
Patel	72	F	Torsades*	None	No
Sasaki	22	F	Torsades*	HypoK	No
Hirose	63	F	Takotsubo	HypoK + recent A.Fib conversion	No
Inoue	82	F	Torsades*	Atrioventricular Block	No
Mahida	55	F	Torsades	None	No
Micallef	58	F	Takotsubo	None	No
Pacha	64	F	Takotsubo	Recent A.Fib conversion + Amiodarone + HypoCa	No
Grilo	37	F	Torsades	Congenital long QT syndrome + Ketoconazole	No
Rotondi	57	F	Takotsubo	HypoK + HypoMg + HypoCa	Possibly
Wedekind	81	F	Torsades*	None	No
Gotyo	70	M	Torsades	None	No
Purvis	67	F	Torsades	HypoMg + Fluoxetine	Possibly
Kawano	80	M	Torsades	HypoK	No
Yamada	89	F	Torsades*	Atrioventricular Block	No
Yamada	81	F	Torsades	Clarythromycin	No
Peters	50	F	Torsades*	None	No
Ahn	78	F	Takotsubo	Atrioventricular Block	Possibly

Table 2. Clinical characteristics of patients with Takotsubo cardiomyopathy-associated Torsades de Pointes

patients with Takotsubo cardiomyopathy-associated Torsades de Pointes relative to patients with Takotsubo cardiomyopathy-associated QT interval prolongation even prior to Torsades de Pointes appearance. This finding is of great clinical significance beyond statistical significance: mean maximal QTc interval is remarkably high (676.8 msec) in patients with Takotsubo cardiomyopathy-associated Torsades de Pointes prior to Torsades de Pointes appearance - more than 120 msec higher relative to mean maximal QTc interval in patients with Takotsubo cardiomyopathy-associated QT interval prolongation without Torsades de Pointes appearance. This large difference in QT interval prolongation should urge physicians to start treatment and to take prevention measures as soon as possible prior to Torsades de Pointes appearance.

As with our previous review (Samuelov-Kinori et al., 2009), most patients with Takotsubo cardiomyopathy-associated Torsades de Pointes have one or more risk factors for Torsades de Pointes other than female gender and left ventricular systolic dysfunction. Electrolyte depletion and high degree atrioventricular block are the most prevalent risk factors and last triggers for Torsades de Pointes. But this time we have also shown that Torsades de Pointes is possibly preventable in one quarter of the patients should electrolyte depletion and high degree atrioventricular block have been addressed earlier.

4.1 Limitations

Our study is based on a small number of published case reports. Accordingly, the above-mentioned findings are suggestive rather than conclusive. We assume that there are more incidents of Torsades de Pointes in patients with Takotsubo cardiomyopathy that have not been published; for example, when physicians are reluctant to report their deceased patients. Indeed, in all the above-mentioned reports patients have survived Torsades de Pointes. Accordingly; we believe that our findings are more likely an underestimation of the true prevalence of the clinical circumstances that might lead to Torsades de Pointes in Takotsubo cardiomyopathy patients.

4.2 Clinical implications

This study defines four risk factors for Torsades de Pointes in patients with Takotsubo cardiomyopathy whom already have QT interval prolongation to begin with: male gander, marked QT interval prolongation, electrolyte depletion, and high degree atrioventricular block. Electrolyte depletion and high degree atrioventricular block are also last triggers for Torsades de Pointes in patients with Takotsubo cardiomyopathy. Accordingly, we believe electrolyte depletion and high degree atrioventricular block should be addressed as soon as possible in patients with Takotsubo cardiomyopathy in general, and in patients with marked QT interval prolongation in particular.

5. Conclusion

Men with Takotsubo cardiomyopathy-associated QT interval prolongation are at risk for Torsades de Pointes. Most patients with Takotsubo cardiomyopathy-associated Torsades de Pointes have risk factors for Torsades de Pointes other than female gender and left ventricular systolic dysfunction. Electrolyte depletion and high degree atrioventricular block are the most prevalent risk factors and last triggers for Torsades de Pointes. We wish to raise the awareness of risk factors for Torsades de Pointes in patients with Takotsubo cardiomyopathy-associated QT interval prolongation.

6. References

Abe, Y.; Kondo, M.; Matsuoka, R.; Araki, M.; Dohyama, K. & Tanio, H. (2003). Assessment of clinical features in transient left ventricular apical ballooning. *Journal of the American College of Cardiology*, Vol.41, No.5, (March 2003), pp.737-742, ISSN 0735-1097

Ahn, JH.; Park, SH.; Shin, WY.; Lee, SW.; Lee, SJ.; Jin, DK.; Lee, HM. & Eun, JY. (2011). Long QT Syndrome and Torsade de Pointes Associated with Takotsubo Cardiomyopathy. *Journal of Korean medical science*, Vol.26, No.7, (July 2011), pp.959-961, ISSN 1011-8934

Akashi, YJ.; Nakazawa, K.; Kida, K.; Ryu, S.; Takagi, A.; Kishi, R.; Kunishima, T.; Sakakibara, M. & Miyake, F. (2003). Reversible ventricular dysfunction (takotsubo cardiomyopathy) following polymorphic ventricular tachycardia. *Canadian Journal of Cardiology*, Vol.19, No.4, (March 2003), pp.449-451, ISSN 0828-282X

Antzelevitch, C. Ionic, molecular, and cellular bases of QT-interval prolongation and torsade de pointes. *Europace*, Vol.9, Suppl.No.4, (September 2007), pp.iv4-15, ISSN 1099-5129

Bazett, HC. (1920). An analysis of the time-relations of electrocardiograms. *Heart*, Vol.7, (1920), pp.353–370, ISSN 1355-6037

Boulouffe, C.; Vanpee, D. & Gabriel, L. (2007). Stress-induced cardiomyopathy: takotsubo left ventricular dysfunction. *American Journal of Emergency Medicine*, Vol.25, No.2, (February 2007), pp.243-244, ISSN 0735-6757

Bybee, KA. & Prasad, A. (2008). Stress-Related Cardiomyopathy Syndromes. *Circulation*, Vol.118, No.4, (July 2008), pp.397-409, ISSN 0009-7322

Cangella, F.; Medolla, A.; De Fazio, G.; Iuliano, C.; Curcio, N.; Salemme, L.; Mottola, G. & Agrusta, M. (2007). Stress induced cardiomyopathy presenting as acute coronary syndrome: Tako-Tsubo in Mercogliano, Southern Italy. *Cardiovascular Ultrasound*, Vol.5, (October 2007), pp.36, ISSN 1476-7120

Denney, SD.; Lakkireddy, DR. & Khan, IA. (2005). Long QT syndrome and torsade de pointes in transient left ventricular apical ballooning syndrome. *International Journal of Cardiology*, Vol.100, No.3, (April 2005), pp.499-501, ISSN 0167-5273

Fang, CC.; Jao, YT.; Yi, C.; Yu, CL.; Chen, CL. & Wang, SP. (2008). Transient left ventricular apical ballooning syndrome: the first series in Taiwanese patients. *Angiology*, Vol.59, No.2, (April-May 2008), pp.185-192, ISSN 0003-3197

Finsterer, J.; Stöllberger, C.; Sehnal, E.; Valentin, A.; Huber, J. & Schmiedel, J. (2007). Apical ballooning (Takotsubo syndrome) in mitochondrial disorder during mechanical ventilation. *Journal of cardiovascular medicine (Hagerstown, Md.)*, Vol.8, No.10, (October 2007), pp.859-863, ISSN 1558-2027

Furushima, H.; Chinushi, M.; Sanada, A. & Aizawa, Y. (2008). Ventricular repolarization gradients in a patient with takotsubo cardiomyopathy. *Europace*, Vol.10, No.9, (September 2008), pp.1112-1115, ISSN 1099-5129

Ghosh, S.; Apte, P.; Maroz, N.; Broor, A.; Zeineh, N. & Khan, IA. (2009). Takotsubo cardiomyopathy as a potential cause of long QT syndrome and torsades de pointes. *International Journal of Cardiology,* Vol.136, No.2, (August 2009), pp.225-227, ISSN 0167-5273

Gotyo, N.; Kida, M.; Horiuchi, T. & Hirata, Y. (2009). Torsade de pointes associated with recurrent ampulla cardiomyopathy in a patient with idiopathic ACTH deficiency. *Endocrine journal,* Vol.56, No.6, (June 2009), pp.807-815, ISSN 0918-8959

Grilo, LS.; Pruvot, E.; Grobéty, M.; Castella, V.; Fellmann, F. & Abriel, H. (2010). Takotsubo cardiomyopathy and congenital long QT syndrome in a patient with a novel duplication in the Per-Arnt-Sim (PAS) domain of hERG1. *Heart Rhythm,* Vol.7, No.2, (September 2010), pp.260-265, ISSN 1547-5271

Hirose, K.; Yamaguchi, H.; Oshima, Y.; Choraku, M.; Hirono, A.; Takamori, N. & Tamura, K. (2008). Severe respiratory failure and torsades de pointes induced by disopyramide in a patient with myasthenia gravis. *Internal Medicine,* Vol.47, No.19, (October 2008), pp.1703-1708, ISSN 1349-7235

Inoue, M.; Kanaya, H.; Matsubara, T.; Uno, Y.; Yasuda, T. & Miwa, K. (2009). Complete Atrioventricular Block Associated With Takotsubo Cardiomyopathy. *Circulation Journal,* Vol.73, No.3, (March 2009), pp.589-592, ISSN 1346-9843

Kawano, H.; Matsumoto, Y.; Arakawa, S.; Satoh, O. & Hayano, M. (2010). Premature atrial contraction induces torsades de pointes in a patient of Takotsubo cardiomyopathy with QT prolongation. *Internal Medicine,* Vol.49, No.16, (August 2010), pp.1767-1773, ISSN 1349-7235

Kurisu, S.; Inoue, I.; Kawagoe, T.; Ishihara, M.; Shimatani, Y.; Nakama, Y.; Ohkawa, K.; Maruhashi, T.; Kagawa, E.; Dai, K. & Aokage, T. (2008). Torsade de pointes associated with bradycardia and takotsubo cardiomyopathy. *Canadian Journal of Cardiology,* Vol.24, No.8, (August 2008), pp.640-642, ISSN 0828-282X

Larsen, JA. & Kadish, AH. (1998). Effects of gender on cardiac arrhythmias. *Journal of Cardiovascular Electrophysiology,* Vol.9, No.6, (June 1998), pp.655-664, ISSN 1045-3873

Mahida, S.; Dalageorgou, C. & Behr, ER. (2009). Long-QT syndrome and torsades de pointes in a patient with Takotsubo cardiomyopathy: an unusual case. *Europace,* Vol.11, No.3, (March 2009), pp.376-378, ISSN 1099-5129

Micallef, T.; Gruppetta, M.; Cassar, A. & Fava, S. (2010). Takotsubo cardiomyopathy in a patient with severe hypothyroidism: a case report. *Journal of cardiovascular medicine (Hagerstown, Md.),* doi: 10.2459/JCM.0b013e3283403454, ISSN 1558-2027

Nault, MA.; Baranchuk, A.; Simpson, CS. & Redfearn, DP. (2007). Takotsubo cardiomyopathy: a novel "proarrhythmic" disease. *Anadolu Kardiyoloji Dergisi,* Vol.7, Supp.No.l, (July 2007), pp.101-103, ISSN 1302-8723

Okada, T.; Miyata, S.; Hashimoto, K.; Maie, K. & Mochizuki, S. (2007). Takotsubo cardiomyopathy associated with torsades de pointes and long QT interval: a case report. *Journal of Cardiology,* Vol.50, No.1, (July 2007), pp.83-88, ISSN 0914-5087

Pacha, O.; Kadikoy, H.; Amro, M.; Haque, W. & Abdellatif, A. (2010). Torsades de pointes and prolonged QT syndrome in Takotsubo cardiomyopathy. *Journal of cardiovascular medicine (Hagerstown, Md.)*, doi: 10.2459/JCM.0b013e328336b4a6, ISSN 1558-2027

Patel, HM.; Kantharia, BK.; Morris, DL. & Yazdanfar, S. (2007). Takotsubo syndrome in African-American women with atypical presentations: a single-center experience. *Clinical Cardiology*, Vol.30, No.1, (January 2007), pp.14-18, ISSN 1932-8737

Peters, S. & Klein, HU. (2011). WCD LifeVest: Risk stratification in a case of tako-tsubo cardiomyopathy with QT interval prolongation. *Herz*, doi: 10.1007/s00059-011-3440-9, ISSN 0946-1299

Purvis, JA.; Cunningham, EL.; McGlinchey, PG. & Barr, SH. (2009). Drugs, electrolytes and tako-tsubo cardiomyopathy: triple aetiology of acquired long QT syndrome and torsades de pointes. *The Ulster medical journal Ulster*, Vol.78, No.3, (September 2009), pp.188-189, ISSN 0041-6193

Roden, DM. (2004). Drug-induced prolongation of the QT interval. *The New England Journal of Medicine*, Vol.350, No.10, (March 2004), pp.1013-22, ISSN 0028-4793

Rotondi, F.; Manganelli, F.; Lanzillo, T.; Candelmo, F.; Lorenzo, ED.; Marino, L. & Stanco, G. (2010). Tako-tsubo cardiomyopathy complicated by recurrent torsade de pointes in a patient with anorexia nervosa. *Internal Medicine*, Vol.49, No. 12, (June 2010), pp.1133-1137, ISSN 1349-7235

Samuelov-Kinori, L.; Kinori, M.; Kogan, Y.; Swartzon, M.; Shalev, H.; Guy, D.; Ferenidou, F.; Mashav, N.; Sadeh, B.; Atzmony, L.; Kliuk-Ben-Basat, O.; Steinvil, A. & Justo, D. (2009). Takotsubo cardiomyopathy and QT interval prolongation: who are the patients at risk for torsades de pointes? *Journal of electrocardiology*, Vol.42, No.4, (July-August 2009); pp.353-357, ISSN 0022-0736

Sasaki, O.; Nishioka, T.; Akima, T.; Tabata, H.; Okamoto, Y.; Akanuma, M.; Uehata, A.; Takase, B.; Katsushika, S.; Isojima, K.; Ohtomi, S. & Yoshimoto, N. (2006). Association of takotsubo cardiomyopathy and long QT syndrome. *Circulation Journal*, Vol.70, No.9, (September 2006), pp.1220-1222, ISSN 1346-9843

Thakar, S.; Chandra, P.; Hollander, G. & Lichstein, E. (2011). Electrocardiographic Changes in Takotsubo Cardiomyopathy. *Pacing and Clinical Electrophysiology*, doi: 10.1111/j.1540-8159.2011.03151, ISSN 1540-8159

Wedekind, H.; Müller, JG.; Ribbing, M.; Skurzewski, P.; Bozzetti, C.; Meyer-Krahmer, HJ. & Böcker, D. (2009). A fatal combination in an old lady: Tako-Tsubo cardiomyopathy, long QT syndrome, and cardiac hypertrophy. *Europace*, Vol.11, No.6, (June 2009), pp.820-822, ISSN 1099-5129

Wittstein, IS.; Thiemann, DR.; Lima, JA.; Baughman, KL.; Schulman, SP.; Gerstenblith, G.; Wu, KC.; Rade, JJ.; Bivalacqua, TJ. & Champion, HC. (2005). Neurohumoral features of myocardial stunning due to sudden emotional stress. *The New England Journal of Medicine*, Vol.352, No.6, (February 2005), pp.539-548, ISSN 0028-4793

Yamada, Y.; Tani, T.; Homma, M. & Saito, S. (2011). Two cases of torsades de pointes associated with takotsubo cardiomyopathy as the second insult. *Journal of electrocardiology,* doi.org/10.1016/j.jelectrocard.2011.03.002, ISSN 0022-0736

Part 4

Chagas Heart Disease

16

Chagasic Cardiomyopathy

Fernando Rosas[1], Nubia Roa[2], Zulma M. Cucunubá[3], Adriana Cuéllar[4], John Mario Gonzalez[5] and Concepción J. Puerta[6]
[1]*Fundación Clínica Abood Shaio,*
[2]*Clínica de Falla Cardiaca y Trasplante, Hospital Universitario San Ignacio, Facultad de Medicina, Pontificia Universidad Javeriana*
[3]*Grupo de Parasitología, Instituto Nacional de Salud,*
[4]*Grupo de Inmunobiología y Biología Celular, Pontificia Universidad Javeriana,*
[5]*Grupo de Ciencias Básicas Médicas, Facultad de Medicina, Universidad de los Andes,*
[6]*Laboratorio de Parasitología Molecular, Departamento de Microbiología, Pontificia Universidad Javeriana,*
Colombia

1. Introduction

Chagas disease is a systemic parasitic infection caused by the protozoan *Trypanosoma cruzi*, which persists as an important public health problem, mainly in Latin America where triatomine vectors are located in three overlapping cycles of transmission: domestic, peridomestic, and sylvatic. Due to human migration from endemic to developed countries, in recent years Chagas disease has become a recognized global problem. This chapter reviews current literature on chagasic cardiomyopathy, its etiology, epidemiology, immunology, and diagnosis, along with etiologic and symptomatic treatment and prognosis.

2. Etiology

One-hundred years after the discovery of *Trypanosoma cruzi* (Family: *Trypanosomatidae*, Order: *Kinetoplastida*) by Carlos Chagas in Brazil, many aspects of its biology and host relationship remain unraveled. The substantial biological, biochemical, and genetic variability of this parasite, as well as the multiclonal *T. cruzi* infection character are some of the factors that have hampered its study. *T. cruzi* is considered to have a clonal structure with some overlapping events of genetic exchange occurring in the past that have brought about the six currently recognized Discrete Typing Units (DTUs) I to VI. Moreover, within each DTU biological and genetic polymorphism is present, especially in DTUs I and III. The scenario is even more complicated. Recent reports showed that multiple genotypes were obtained when isolates from a single wild mammalian reservoir host were cloned (Llewelyn et al., 2011). The authors proposed that this huge diversity is at least, partially driven by the survival in the host. Nonetheless, significant progress has been achieved with the unveiled *T. cruzi* genome and the following OMICS initiatives such as RNAomic and proteomic analyses, which seek to apply translational medicine to Chagas disease in the near future.

2.1 Life cycle

T. cruzi exhibits a complex life cycle involving four well-defined developmental stages that interplay into two hosts, the blood-sucking insect vector, and the mammalian host (humans and animals). After already-infected insects feed on the mammalian host, they eliminate in their feces the **metacyclic trypomastigotes** (parasite infective form), which penetrate the body through the bite-wound, any damaged tissue, or the mucosa from eyes, nose, or even the digestive tract and invade host cells like fibroblasts, macrophages, and epithelial cells at the inoculation site. In the cytoplasm, free-parasites are differentiated into **amastigotes** (Fig.1A), the intracellular stage, which after several replication rounds transforms back into **trypomastigotes** that rupture the host membrane cell, infecting new cells or disseminating into other organs via the bloodstream.

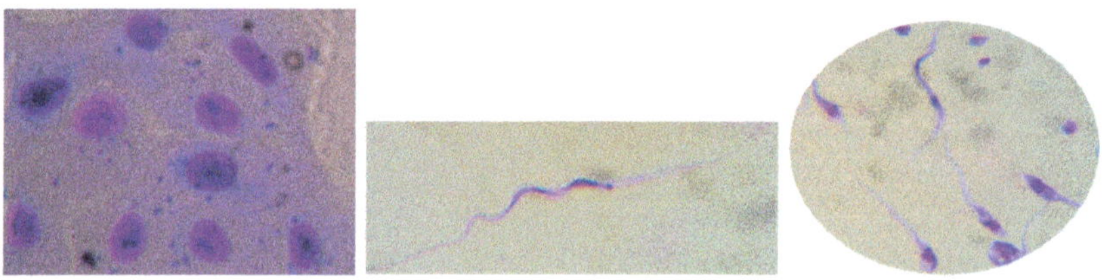

A B C

Fig. 1. (A) Intracellular amastigotes of *T. cruzi*-infecting Vero cells, (B) Trypomastigotes, and (C) Epimastigotes stained with Giemsa. Courtesy of Paola Lasso, and Paula Pavia, Laboratory of Molecular Parasitology, School of Sciences, Pontificia Universidad Javeriana, Bogota D.C., Colombia.

Upon feeding, insects take the **bloodstream trypomastigotes** (Fig. 1B), which once in their digestive tract differentiate into **epimastigotes**, the insect replication stage (Fig. 1C). After reaching the rectum, parasites transform into metacyclic trypomastigotes ready to infect a new mammalian host. From this cycle, it is obvious that the differential expression of parasite genes enable the parasite to accomplish the role played by each of its developmental stages. In this sense, several proteomic studies have been performed to identify molecules participating in cycle-vital processes (Ulrich et al., 2011).

3. Epidemiology and risk factors

3.1 Burden of Chagas disease

An estimated 10-million people are infected worldwide, mostly in Latin America where Chagas disease is endemic. More than 25-million people are at risk of contracting the disease. It is estimated that in 2008 Chagas disease killed >10,000 people. With a latency of 10-30 years, nearly 30% of infected patients develop life-threatening complications, mostly Chagas heart disease (CHD) (WHO, 2010). Direct and indirect costs of *T. cruzi* infection impose an overwhelming load on healthcare systems secondary to hospitalizations and medical and surgical treatments for CHD, gastrointestinal dysfunction, and meningoencephalitis in Latin America (Franco-Paredes et al., 2007). In 1995, the burden of Chagas disease in Latin America was estimated at US$8.156-billion, equivalent to 2.5% of the foreign debt of continental Latin America (Moncayo, 2003). More recent data demonstrate that, globally, Chagas disease is associated with 0.7-million disability-adjusted life years, constituting the sixth most important neglected tropical disease worldwide (Hotez et al., 2006).

3.2 Globalization of Chagas disease

Political and economic situations have stimulated the flow of migration from the 17 Latin American endemic countries to the developed ones (Schmunis & Yadon, 2010). Because of this and parasite transfer by blood contact, intrauterine transfer, laboratory accidents, and organ transplantation; CHD could potentially become a worldwide problem (WHO, 2010) and emerge as a public health issue in non-endemic countries (Field et al., 2010). Currently, in the United States it is estimated that from more than 22 million of immigrants from endemic countries there are approximately 300,000 infected individuals (Bern & Montgomery, 2009). In 15 European countries in 2005, excluding Spain, 2.9% of the 483,074 legal Latin American immigrants were estimated to be infected with *T. cruzi*. By 2008, Spain had received 1,678,711 immigrants from Latin American endemic countries; of these, 5.2% were potentially infected with *T. cruzi* and 17,390 may develop Chagas disease. Likewise, in an analysis of Chagas disease in Spain, most patients were from Bolivia (94.7%) and less from Brazil, Chile, Ecuador, Paraguay, and Honduras (Norman et al., 2010). Other countries outside Europe, where the rates of Latin American immigration are high and present an important prevalence of Chagas disease are Australia, Canada, and Japan (Schmunis & Yadon, 2010).

3.3 Chagas heart disease in endemic countries

Triatomines, the *T. cruzi* vectors, are spread from the south of the United States to the south of Argentina. The rarity of vector-borne transmission in the United States, compared with Latin America, is thought to be the result of better housing conditions and lower efficiency of North American vectors (Bern & Montgomery, 2009). In Latin America, there are more than 125 potential vectors of Chagas disease. However, species with higher vectorial capacity, with domestic habits and with the most geographical distribution belong to *Triatoma*, *Rhodnius*, and *Panstrongylus* genera. For these reasons, there are different targets in control programs of vectors depending on regions. Thus, the Mexico and Central America Initiative (created in 1998) is focused in the control *Rhodnius prolixus*, *Triatoma dimidiata*, *Triatoma barberi*, and *Rhodnius pallescences*; the Initiative of the Andean Countries (created in 1997) is aimed at controlling *R. prolixus*, *T. dimidiata* and *Triatoma maculata*; and finally, the Initiative of the Southern Cone (created in 1991) is aimed at controlling *Triatoma infestans*, *Triatoma brasiliensis*, *Triatoma sordida*, and *Panstrongylus megistus* (Guhl, 2009). The main risk factors for vector-borne transmission are related to previous exposure to poor housing conditions in Latin America (Fig. 3), such as: palm or straw roofs, dirt floors, adobe walls or walls with low quality or incomplete plastering, and the presence of animals inside the bedroom.

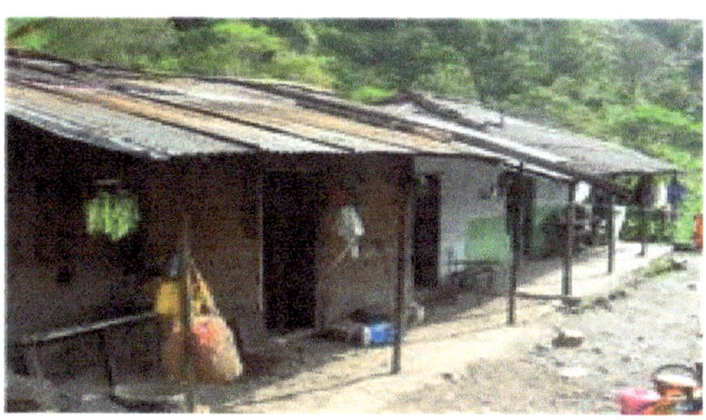

Fig. 2. Typical house in a Chagas disease endemic region, Departamento de Boyacá.
Courtesy of Cielo León, Grupo de Parasitología, Instituto Nacional de Salud, Colombia.

An important change has occurred in trends of Chagas disease in Latin America over recent decades. Such is recognized by several researchers, control policies of vector and blood of *T. cruzi* transmission have shown a positive effect in reducing the incidence of this disease. Thus, since the 1990s until now, an important success in the control of Chagas disease has been observed, especially in Southern Cone countries. So, in 1990, the distribution of Chagas disease in 21 countries was estimated, with more than 45,000 deaths per year and 30-million cases of human infection; while in 2006 the distribution of Chagas disease in 18 countries was estimated, with approximately 12,500 deaths per year and nearly 15-million cases of human infection (Dias et al., 2008). Success in controlling vector transmission in some countries has led to also to focus the attention to other forms of non-vector transmission. Thereby, controlling transmission by transfusion has improved and screening is now obligatory in most endemic countries. Congenital transmission has been detected as an important transmission form, mainly in Bolivia, but other endemic countries have only recently started to approach to this problem. Orally acquired human infection with *T. cruzi* has been known since the 1930s but has the interest in this transmision has increased as a result of the series of outbreaks that have occurred in the Amazon region, which have been associated with the preparation and consumption of some foods, especially in Brazil, Venezuela, and Colombia (Miles, 2010). The rural-to-urban migration movements that have occurred in Latin America since the 1970s and 1980s have changed the traditional epidemiological pattern of Chagas disease as a rural condition and transformed it into an urban infection that can be transmitted via non-vector manners (Moncayo & Silveira, 2009). Moreover, in some countries the vector infestation has occurred in urban areas where vectors have been introduced by passive transportation during migration process, for instance in Cochabamba, Bolivia (Medrano-Mercado et al., 2008), Arequipa, Peru (Bayer et al., 2009), and in Yucatán, Mexico (Guzman-Tapia et al., 2007). On the other hand, adults infected with *T. cruzi* from childhood form a transitional generation, experiencing the simultaneous impact of past infectious exposures and current cardiovascular risk factors, such as sedentary lifestyle, calorie-dense diets, hypertension, and diabetes. Other variables such as longer residence in an endemic province, residence in a rural area and poor housing conditions, male sex, and increased age have been found independent predictors of Chagas cardiomyopathy severity (Hidron et al., 2010).

3.4 Surveillance and health policy

In endemic countries, the tools to interrupt the domestic cycle of *T. cruzi* transmission, such as chemical control, housing improvement, and health education are the most useful methods to prevent Chagas disease (Moncayo & Silveira, 2009). Blood screening is vital to prevent infection through transfusion and organ transplantation and governments should implement policies to promote it (WHO, 2010). In addition, an infrastructure that assures detection and treatment of acute and chronic cases, as well as congenital infection should be developed. In non-endemic countries, screening programs in Latin American pregnant women are increasing and it has been proposed that in some non-endemic countries there is cost-effectiveness to develop it (Sicuri et al., 2011). Regarding strategies to reduce transmission by transfusion in non-endemic countries, there are two different approaches: one is the deferral of individuals at risk of Chagas disease and the second approach is to accept blood donations if specific laboratory assays are negative. This second approach is being introduced in countries where there is a substantial Latin American population, such as the United States, Spain, and France (Castro, 2009). Also, taking into account that knowledge about Chagas disease among doctors in non-endemic countries is very limited (Verani et al., 2010), strategies to improve awareness are very important in order to enhance treatment and follow up of cases.

4. Clinical presentation

4.1 Acute phase

The symptomatic acute phase could be present at any age but it is most common in children under 10 years of age. When the infection is acquired via vector, it takes four to eight weeks for symptoms to develop. In this phase there is an important inflammatory response in the site of contact with bug feces and *T. cruzi* may multiply locally (cutaneous chagoma when it is in the skin). The insect prefers the thinnest skin and that is why the best known sign is Romaña's sign which consists in a unilateral conjunctivitis with periorbital edema, eyelid edema and pre-auricular adenopathy (Biolo et al., 2010). In younger children (under 4 years of age) it is common to found the following symptoms: fever, malaise, muscle pain, anorexia, anemia, sweating, hepatosplenomegaly, heart failure from myocarditis, pericardial effusion, seizures, and somnolence secondary to meningoencephalitis, the more infrequent form of presentation (Gomez et al., 2007). The acute congenital disease should be considered by the medical care system staff in endemic areas; it could be asymptomatic or may be associated to prematurity, low weight, hepatomegaly, splenomegaly, jaundice, anemia, neonatal hepatitis, meningoencephalitis, sepsis, myocarditis, fever, and less frequently megaesophagus, megacolon, megabladder. Without treatment, mortality is 5-10%, the leading causes are encephalomyelitis and heart failure (Prata, 2001). Patients with HIV could reactivate the disease and have meningoencephalitis as a first manifestation (Carod-Artal, 2006). In patients with history of solid organ or bone marrow transplants, 30% reactivate Chagas disease, the acute manifestations could be myocarditis, panniculitis, subcutaneous parasite-containing nodules, and meningoencephalitis (Bern et al., 2007).

4.2 Chronic phase

Once the acute phase is resolved, it begins the chronic phase. This chronic phase could be asymptomatic lifelong or progressive heart and/or gastro esophageal disease. The chronic asymptomatic or indeterminate phase lasts 10 to 30 years. For some authors its definition means epidemiological contact, positive serologic tests, normal physical examination and normal radiological, electrocardiographic and echocardiography studies. Around 30% of these have progressive disease (Higuchi et al., 2003). When Chagas becomes symptomatic, depending on the geographic zone, the disease will have different signs and symptoms. In Central America and northern South America, the heart disease is the common manifestation, but in Brazil and Southern Cone countries it coexists with digestive syndromes (Miles et al., 2003). For the purpose of this review, we will focus on Chagasic cardiomyopathy. The earliest manifestations of heart disease are electrocardiographic abnormalities as the expression of the damage of the conduction system and the symptoms that the patients experience could be related to those abnormalities: atrioventricular block, sinus bradycardia, premature ventricular contractions, atrial fibrillation, and ventricular tachycardia. In 40% of patients with mild heart disease there could be non-sustained ventricular tachycardia, as well as in 90% of patients with heart failure. Sudden death occurs in 38% of patients with chronic disease with or without heart failure, meaning more severe heart disease. The principal cause of sudden death is the malignant ventricular arrhythmia followed by advanced atrioventricular block and cerebral emboli. Non-sustained ventricular tachycardia in Holter monitoring and in stress test, together with low ejection fraction, syncope and pre-syncope, sinus node dysfunction, history of recovery from cardiac arrest, and dyspnea NYHA class III or IV have been recognized of prognostic value in sudden death (Prata, 2001). Symptomatic heart failure occurs in some patients before there is any significant electrocardiography alteration. It could be right or left heart failure; it is very common for patients to have severe structural heart disease and not show symptoms of severe heart failure. It is also common to find severe congestive hepatic disease. Pulmonary and systemic emboli due to dilated chambers of apical aneurism are common clinical manifestations of chronic heart disease (Bern et al., 2007); they have been described in 40% of autopsies (Prata, 2001). A Brazilian study found four predictors of emboli complications: age > 48 years, primary changes in repolarization, apical aneurism, and ejection fraction < 50%, with a 4% annual incidence if all four factors where present (Sousa et al., 2008). Precordial pain is a frequent complaint of patients with Chagas disease. The incidence of this symptom is 15% but other authors report up to 30% (Marin-Neto et al., 2007). The causes of the symptom are not clear; some authors believe that this pain could be caused by microvascular disease.

4.2.1 Classification

A simple classification, published by the Brazilian Consensus on Chagas Diseases, includes functional capacity, electrocardiographic findings, function and size of left ventricle. This classification allowed defining four disease stages with the aim to orientate the patient's therapy (Table 1).

Stage	Electrocardiogram	Echocardiography	Heart failure
A	Altered	Normal	Absent
B1	Altered	Altered LVEF >45%	Absent
B2	Altered	Altered LVEF <45%	Absent
C	Altered	Altered	Compensated
D	Altered	Altered	Refractory

LVEF: left ventricular ejection fraction

Table 1. Classification of cardiac compromise in Chagas chronic cardiomyopathy

5. Pathogenesis of cardiac disease during *T. cruzi* infection

5.1 Host genetic influence

Some works approach the influence of human genetics such as Histocompability Complex Molecules (HLA) or polymorphism in cytokine promoters and their contribution to Chagas disease. So far, association with HLA class II indicated that infected individuals with and without cardiomyopathy had a higher frequency of DRB1*01, DRB1*08, and DQB1*0501 (Fernandez et al., 1998), and the DRB1*01 DQB1*0501 haplotype was more frequent in patients with Chagasic cardiomyopathy (Colorado et al., 2000). Additionally, the HLA-DRB1*1503 allele was associated with genetic susceptibility to cardiac damage (Garcia Borras et al., 2009). All these studies were conducted with small cohorts and with different

Latin American populations. Polymorphisms of cytokine promoters assess the potential pattern of cytokine hypo or hyper secretion in individuals. A study showed the association of transforming growth factor beta (TGFβ1) (Calzada et al., 2009) and lymphotoxin α (LTα) with the risk Chagasic cardiomyopathy progression (Ramasawmy et al., 2007). Tumor necrosis factor (TNFα), a pro-inflammatory agent, is the cytokine with the strongest relationship to cardiac tissue damage in Chagas. There is an association between *T. cruzi* seropositive individuals and the polymorphism in TNF-238A. Indeed, TNFα secretion is higher in non-stimulated and stimulated cells from chronic Chagasic donors (Pissetti et al., 2011) and TNFα serum levels were associated with heart failure (Talvani et al., 2004). In *T. cruzi* experimentally infected rats, the cardiomyopathy ameliorates in animals treated with a TNFα blocking monoclonal antibody (Perez et al., 2009).

5.2 Parasite tropisms

Geographic distribution of an organ-specific chronic disease (cardiac *versus* digestive diseases) and allocation of *T. cruzi* I and II (II to VI in the new classification), supported the hypothesis that disease outcome is linked to the *T. cruzi* genetic variations. Some studies did not show correlations among *T. cruzi* lineages and the clinical forms of Chagas disease (Zafra et al., 2011). Although, the presence of TcI was correlated with higher frequencies of electrocardiogram alterations than individuals infected with TcII, such as ventricular premature beats, first-degree atrioventricular block, sinus bradycardia, abnormal Q-waves, atrial fibrillation, and complex ventricular arrhythmias (Ramirez et al., 2010). In a mouse model infected with two different genetic populations of *T. cruzi,* both parasites were found during the acute infection in several host compartments (blood and organs). However, during chronic infection, a preferential tissue distribution with predominance of certain *T. cruzi* isolates was found (Andrade et al., 1999). Because *T. cruzi* mixed infections in triatomines are found in high rates, a similar phenomenon should take place during human infection.

5.3 Parasite invasion of the host cells

T. cruzi can reach the mammalian host cells via different mucosal tissues (i.e., conjunctiva, oral) or directly into blood (transfusion or congenital). The parasite in vivo can invade a vast range of cells such as monocyte/macrophages, dendritic cells, endothelial cells, fibroblasts, astrocytes, skeletal muscles, enteric nerves, and cardiomyocytes (Epting et al., 2010). Parasite invasion is a multistep process when several *T. cruzi* glycoproteins bind surface molecules on the host cells. Before reaching the target tissues, *T. cruzi* must interact with the endothelial cells to actively penetrate or increase endothelium vasodilatation. Parasite protease can produce inflammations that increase vascular permeability (Epting et al., 2010). Several parasite proteases and glycoprotein expressed by trypomastigotes have been associated with invasion: gp60 (penetrin) gp63, gp35/50, gp82, gp90 a parasite glycosidase, mucins and transialidase such as gp85 or Tc85. The binding of these parasite molecules to host molecules (cytokeratin 18, mucins, heparan sulfates, extracellular matrix proteins such as fibronectin and laminin, and carbohydrates with sialic acid) induce Ca++ mobilization, protein tyrosine phosphorylation and cytoskeleton reorganization in the target cells. Transialidase, glycosylphosphatidylinositol (GPI) anchors surface-bound proteins are in charge of transferring sialic acid residues from the host cell to the parasite glycoproteins. This mechanism seems to be crucial in invasion given that trypomastigotes with no expression of trans-sialidases were poorly invasive to non-phagocytic cells (Epting et al.,

2010). Also, infection by oral route involved other parasite glycoproteins such as mucin-like gp35/50 or gp82 on the surface of the trypomastigotes, resistant to protease digestion. Glycoprotein gp82 binds to the gastric mucin and allows the parasite to invade epithelial cells (Yoshida, 2008).

5.4 Acute and chronic heart involvement in Chagas diseases

5.4.1 Acute myocarditis

Parasite genetic variations, the initial parasite burden, and the host immune response seem to influence the evolution of the Chagas disease. Clinical cardiac involvement is found in nearly 90% of symptomatic patients. Parasite-infected myocardiocytes with intracellular amastigotes (pseudocyst) break up and induce acute inflammation (Coura & Borges-Pereira, 2010). There is massive and diffuse infiltration with predominance of mononuclear cells (Fig. 3A) mainly CD8+ T lymphocytes (LT) up to 60% (Fig. 3B). Whether these LT are *T. cruzi* antigen specific and which chemotactic agents control this migration is unknown. Microarray studies of *T. cruzi* acute infection in mouse cardiomyocytes showed a regulation of 353 genes (111 up regulated and 242 down regulated) associated with inflammation, cytoskeleton, cell interaction, apoptosis, cell cycle, and oxidative stress. Interestingly, early genes up regulated include a vast range of chemokines, which attract mononuclear cells (Manque et al., 2011). In consequence, there is cell destruction (myocytolysis), interstitial edema, hypertrophy of myocardial fibers, and alteration of the cardiac microcirculation with platelet aggregation, production of pro-inflammatory cytokines and expression of vascular adhesion molecules by endothelial cells (Rossi et al., 2010).

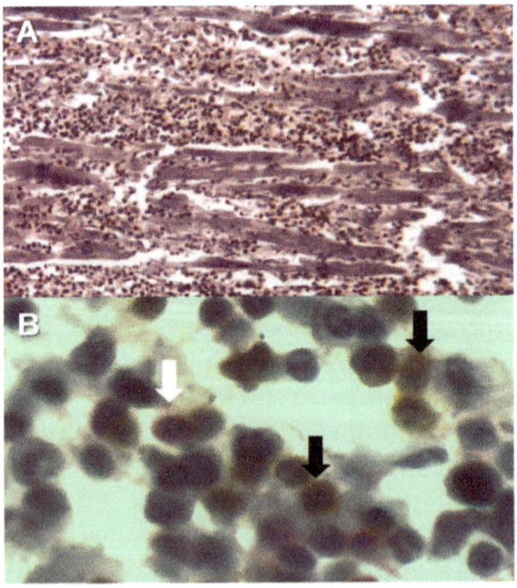

Fig. 3. Immunohistology of a heart with acute Chagas disease showing extensive cellular infiltration 10x (A), and presence of CD8+ (black arrow and brown cells) and CD4+ T cells (white arrow and red cell) with hematoxylin as contra-staining 100x (B). Courtesy of Ana M. Uribe, M.D. Pathology Department, School of Medicine, Pontificia Universidad Javeriana, Bogota D.C., Colombia.

5.4.2 Chronic myocarditis

Contrary to acute infection, in the chronic phase there is scarcity of *T. cruzi* niches; however, there is an extensive, but patchy mononuclear infiltration, with predominance of macrophages and cytotoxic CD8+ T cells (CTL). Myocarditis has a slow progression with changes in the contractile function and dilatation of the heart walls. Increase in metalloproteinase has been described in infected cardiac tissue and associated with remodeling of the extracellular matrix (Gutierrez et al., 2009). Histology analysis shows diffuse myocarditis, myocytolysis, edema, mononuclear cellular infiltration (hallmark of the delayed hypersensitivity), destruction of the conduction system with neuron loss (autonomic denervation), and extensive myocardial fibrosis. Functional studies in Chagasic cardiopathy demonstrated impaired perfusion at the coronary vessels due to microvascular changes (thrombi, inflammation, and spam) (Rossi et al., 2010).

5.5 Mechanisms of tissue damage

5.5.1 Autoimmunity

The autoimmune theory was initially based on the scarcity of parasites found in chronically infected tissue and also on the presence of antibodies and T cells that recognized parasite antigen and cross-reacted with host tissues and molecules. Antibodies against *T. cruzi* bind to human laminin, sulfo-galactosylceramides, cardiac myosin, microtubule-associated proteins, ribosomal proteins, β-adrenergic and muscarinic receptors; heart sarcolemma, blood vessel, neurons, glial cells, myocardium and skeletal muscles (Bonney & Engman, 2008). However, demonstration of the pathological consequences due to autoimmunity in *T. cruzi* infection does not have direct evidence. Most of the auto-antibodies are considered to be natural antibodies that could be induced after tissue injury and exposure of host cell molecules. Also, *T. cruzi* antigens can act as B cell polyclonal stimulators. Against the autoimmunity theory it is known that the immune-suppression exacerbates *T. cruzi* infection and specific anti-parasitic treatment ameliorates the clinical disease (Rossi et al., 2010).

5.5.2 Antigenic persistence and immune response

By using DNA techniques, the presence of *T. cruzi* in tissues during chronic infection has become clear. Antigen persistence triggers inflammation and lymphocyte infiltration. Damage mechanisms are unclear because parasite burden does not explain extensive cell loss. CD8+ T lymphocytes contribute to cytotoxicity probably via perforin and granzyme B, and TGB-β and interleukin-10 (IL-10) secreting macrophages can induce repair and fibrosis through fibroblasts. *T. cruzi* infection also alters microcirculation with the presence of platelets aggregated, microvascular spam, and secretion of vasoconstrictor agents such as tromboxane A2 (TXA2) and platelet activated factors (PAF) by macrophages or endothelin 1 (ET-1) by endothelial cells (Rossi et al., 2010).

6. Human immune response

Innate immune cells such as natural killer cells, macrophages, and dendritic cells detect invading pathogens and alert the immune system through activation cascades. The aim is to elicit innate antimicrobial and inflammatory responses and initiate adaptive immunity to control or eliminate infection. It is accepted that the establishment of chronic infection with *T. cruzi* is a consequence of the inability of the immune response to elicit sterilizing anti-parasite immunity. Therefore, the host innate and adaptive immune response is believed to be the key determinant of the clinical outcome of the disease.

6.1 Innate immunity

Dendritic cells (DCs), natural killer (NK) cells, and monocytes are vital mediators of the innate immune system and promote development of adaptive immune responses. Evidence shows that *T. cruzi* may infect DCs and even proliferate inside them. Consequently, the DC antigen presentation capacity is reduced (Van Overtvelt et al., 2002). In early asymptomatic Chagas disease, higher levels of pro-inflammatory monocytes and expansion of NK cells before the adaptative immunity development has been shown (Vitelli-Avelar, 2006). The role of cytokines such as interleukin (IL)-4, IL-12, TNFα, and interferon (IFN)γ secreted by these cells can be an important element for host resistance during the early stages of infection and also in the genesis of myocarditis (Golgher et al., 2004). It has been shown that two different and independent antigenic stimuli from the parasite induce both an enhancement of IL-10 and a reduction of IL-12 secretion in DCs from Chagasic patients compared to DCs from healthy donors (Cuellar et al., 2008). Although, the innate immune system seems to have a fundamental role in Chagas disease by controlling parasite replication and spread in host tissues, it is not clear if events described here, that mediate inflammatory reaction, can be related to protection or tissue damage in the chronic phase of the disease.

6.2 Humoral immune response

A specific antibody response and B cells in animal models of Chagas disease seem to play an important role for parasite control, especially against the trypomastigotes. In spite of the large number of parasite proteins some molecules have been studied. Indeed, in our previous work, we showed that there is a consistently higher specific IgG response in chronic Chagasic patients against *T. cruzi* kinetoplastid membrane protein-11 (KMP-11), and the *T. cruzi* heat shock protein-70 (HSP-70). The recombinant KMP-11 protein recognition was focused on IgG1 sub-fraction; whereas, the lysate was on IgG3 plus IgG1 in asymptomatic and cardiopathic chronic phases, compared to acute sera from Chagasic patients (Flechas et al., 2009). These data reflect the dynamics of the humoral immune response in Chagas disease and may be an important issue given that IgG1 and IgG3 are the major complement fixing isotypes, which also mediate cooperative function with phagocytes; nevertheless, the role of these specific antibodies in controlling the infection or progressing in disease severity need to be addressed.

6.3 T cells and cytokines

Individuals undergoing chemotherapy generally show protection against viral infections controlled by T cells during lymphopenia, indicating that a small population of T cells can be protective (Turtle et al., 2009). However, reactivation of Chagas disease, defined by a demonstration of trypomastigotes on microscopic examination of blood or the identification of amastigotes on biopsy samples and/or acute clinical manifestations during the chronic phase, can occur among the immunosuppressed patients with heart transplantation (Burgos et al., 2010) or AIDS patients (Almeida et al., 2009). It may be the natural history disease demonstration that T cell response is crucial to control parasite burden and clinical manifestations in a large proportion of patients. Perhaps the most interesting question is how adaptive immune response can contribute to most infected individuals remains asymptomatic whereas an important percentage of these patients develop severe forms of the disease. In humans, it has been shown that CD4+ T cells (Cuellar et al., 2009) and CD8+ T cells (Fiuza et al., 2009) from Chagasic patients specifically produced IFNγ after exposure to *T. cruzi* antigens. Furthermore, chronic Chagasic patients had lower levels of antigen-specific CD8+ T cells secreting IFNγ compared with non-symptomatic individuals (Laucella et al., 2004). Because *T. cruzi* is an intracellular parasite, many groups have focused on the study of CD8+ T cells. Some of them have studied specific CD8+ T cells against peptides derived from cruzipain, FL-160 (Fonseca et al., 2005), KMP-11 (Diez et al., 2006; Lasso et al., 2010), and trans-sialidases (Alvarez et al., 2008) proteins, founding similar frequency of specific CD8+ T cells for these epitopes. Nonetheless, it has been shown that patients with more severe forms of Chagas disease have more differentiated CD8+ T cells which could have lost their functional capacity (Bixby & Tarleton, 2008). One interesting aspect is the control of immune response by regulatory T cells (T_{reg}). Ex vivo, it was shown that children with asymptomatic Chagas disease display a lower frequency of natural T_{reg} CD4+ $CD25^{high}$ compared to non-infected children (Vitelli-Avelar et al., 2006). Interestingly, these cells are in increased levels in peripheral blood of late chronic asymptomatic patients (Vitelli-Avelar et al., 2005). These data suggest that T_{reg} could be important to limiting tissue damage. However, taking into account that additional molecules have been suggested to identify T_{reg}, we used a panel of antibodies for CD4, CD25, FoxP3, and CD127. Our results show higher proportion of T_{reg} in symptomatic chronic Chagasic patients compared to non-infected individuals, indicating that the frequency of T_{reg} can contribute to damage. Fig. 4 despites the CD4+ T_{reg} cells by flow citometry (Lasso et al., 2009).

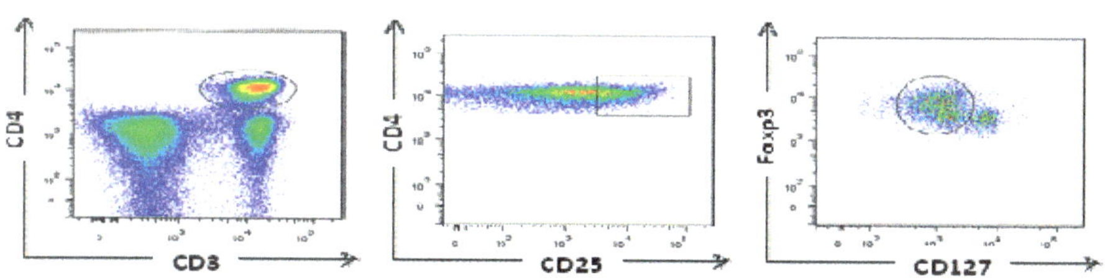

Fig. 4. Regulatory T cells from chronic Chagasic patient identified by high levels of expression of the transcription factor forkhead box transcription factor P3 (FoxP3) and low levels of CD127. Courtesy of Paola Lasso, Pontificia Universidad Javeriana, Bogota D.C., Colombia.

7. Diagnosis

The diagnosis of Chagas disease, as with other infections, is performed on the basis of clinical findings, parasite presence, serological status, and epidemiological data. Furthermore, the disease stage is also an important fact to consider. For instance, as the parasitemia dramatically decreases from acute to chronic phase, in the early phase parasite detection is achieved by parasitological conventional direct tests (see below). Nevertheless, because clinical findings in this stage can be confused with other pathologies, the epidemiological data demonstrating a connection between the patient and the parasite is of special importance (Nicholls et al., 2007). In contrast, in chronic patients, the presence of symptoms or abnormal clinical findings usually correlates with the disease but parasite concentration is low and variable. Bearing in mind that *T. cruzi* infection is life lasting; in the chronic phase serological tests are applied to indirectly demonstrate parasite presence (Enciso et al., 2004). Indeed, the WHO recommends that to diagnose a chronic Chagasic patient; besides having clinical findings compatible with Chagas disease and history of vector contact, there must be at least two positive serological tests with different immunological principles. Finally, chronic asymptomatic patients represent a real challenge for diagnosing inasmuch as there are no clinical findings, and again parasitemia is very low and intermittent. Consequently, the epidemiological patient history is also of most importance (Gil et al., 2007).

7.1 Clinical findings

7.1.1 Electrocardiogram

The most common electrocardiographic manifestations are right bundle branch block (RBBB), anterior fascicular block, premature ventricular contractions, changes in ST segment and T wave, abnormal Q waves, and low voltage of the QRS complex (Fig. 5). The combination of the RBBB and the anterior fascicular block suggest the disease (Garzón et al., 1995). The presence of frequent premature ventricular contractions, including duplets and salvos of non-sustained ventricular tachycardia are a common finding in the Holter monitoring and in the stress test. Premature ventricular contractions correlate with the severity of the ventricular function, but can also occur in patients with preserved ventricular function. Episodes of non-sustained ventricular tachycardia are observed in 40% of the patients with light to moderate ventricular contractibility alterations and in virtually all patients with heart failure, which is more frequent than in other cardiomyopathies. Sustained ventricular tachycardia is another disease marker. This arrhythmia can be produced through programmed ventricular stimulation in nearly 85% of the cases and results from intramyocardial or subepicardial reentrant phenomena, usually located on the inferoposterior and lateral wall of the left ventricle.

7.1.2 X-ray and echocardiography

In patients in the undetermined phase, the cardiac silhouette evaluated in the chest X-ray and the global systolic function in echocardiography are normal. In more advanced stages, the chest X-ray can show cardiomegaly and pulmonary congestion. The disease can cause diffuse damage of the systolic function of the left ventricle. The global systolic function of the left ventricle has prognostic implications. In a cohort of 538 patients grouped into four stages of disease progression, different survival rates were found in the five-year follow up from 98%, 91%, 45% to 13% for those with normal left ventricle function, moderately depressed function, with reversible heart failure, or irreversible heart failure, respectively (Rassi et al., 2010). Some alterations of the segmental contraction of the left ventricle can be detected. The most common is located on the posterior wall with 20% prevalence. The presence of mitral or tricuspid insufficiency is generally associated to ring expansion. The prevalence of aneurysms in the left ventricle varies in the different series, noted on an average of 8.5% in asymptomatic individuals and in patients with severe cardiac damage up to 55%. Through logistic regression analysis, the presence of an apical aneurysm in the left ventricle was an independent predictor of mural Thrombi (Albanesi-Filho et al., 1991). In another work, the finding of an aneurysm was significantly associated to a thrombus and cerebro-vascular accident during a two-year follow up. On some instances, diminished systolic function of the right ventricle can be the only abnormality detected via echocardiography; in general, it is secondary to the severity to the damage of the left ventricle and at high levels of pulmonary pressure. With regards to diastolic function, chronic myocarditis in Chagas disease can diminish ventricular relaxation and diastolic filling. These abnormalities usually precede systolic dysfunction. Reduced compliance of the left ventricle can increase the filling pressure of the left atrium with changes in transmitral and pulmonary venous flow rates. The echocardiography study is recommended as a routine clinical evaluation method in patients with Chagas cardiopathy to determine the stage of the disease, its progression, as well as to estimate survival, dismiss the presence of aneurysms or intracavitary thrombi, and monitor response to treatment.

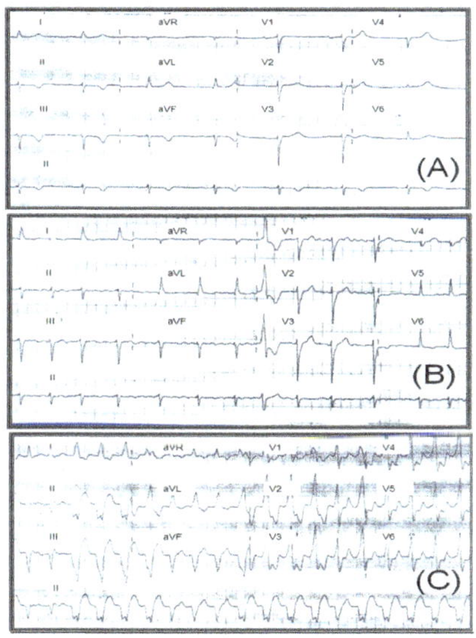

Fig. 5. ECG sequence in a 72-year-old woman diagnosed with Chagas cardiomyopathy and ejection fraction of the left ventricle at 25%. Note sinus bradycardia (A), attrial fibrillation (B), and monomorphic sustained ventricular tachycardia (C). Fundación Clínica Abood Shaio, Bogota D.C., Colombia.

In our experience at Fundación Clínica Abood Sahio (Bogotá, Colombia), from a total of 120 patients evaluated with diagnosis of Chagas cardiomyopathy, 73 women (60%) with mean age of 56.7 +/- 13 years (21-84), clinical manifestations corresponded to dyspnea (42%), palpitations (31%), chest pain (42%), presyncope (24%), syncope (27%), and aborted sudden death (2.5%). Nearly 6.7% of the cases did not present clinical manifestations. The main ECG findings were: right bundle branch block (40%), second and third degree AV block (29.2%), dysfunction of the sinus node (28.3%), ventricular tachycardia (23%), atrial fibrillation (19%), left anterior hemiblock (17.2%), atrial flutter (3.3%), and left bundle branch block (3.3%). In 31% of the cases, the chest X-ray was normal. In 15.8%, severe cardiomegaly was observed. All the patients were subjected to a color Doppler echocardiogram according to internationally recognized norms, finding a mean fraction of the left ventricle of 43.3% (SD +/- 16.5) (10-60) and of the right ventricle at 23.4% (10-40) (Fig. 6). The study was considered normal in 33.6% of the cases. Contractility alterations were documented in 42.4%, with these being globally in 26.5% of the cases, or inferior, apical-inferior and anterior localization. Isolated compromise of the right ventricle was observed in one case (0.8%), suggesting the diagnosis of arrhythmogenic dysplasia of the right ventricle. In 24% of the cases mitral insufficiency was evidenced and 15.2% revealed tricuspid insufficiency. A total of 11 aneurysms (9.7%) were observed, 63.6% of apical localization and 36.3% of inferior localization. Some 8.8% of the patients presented intracavitary thrombi, generally related to aneurysms or global contractility alterations. Holter or electrophysiological study documented ventricular tachycardia (sustained or unsustained) in 19.4% of the cases. Additionally in 10% we observed association to sinus dysfunction and/or AV block with ventricular tachycardia. Anatomic-pathological findings obtained via biopsy or surgery in 10 Chagas patients were: a) hypertrophy and/or b) fibrosis and/or c) chronic inflammatory infiltrate. None of the cases reported parasites in the samples examined by pathology (Rosas et al., 2007).

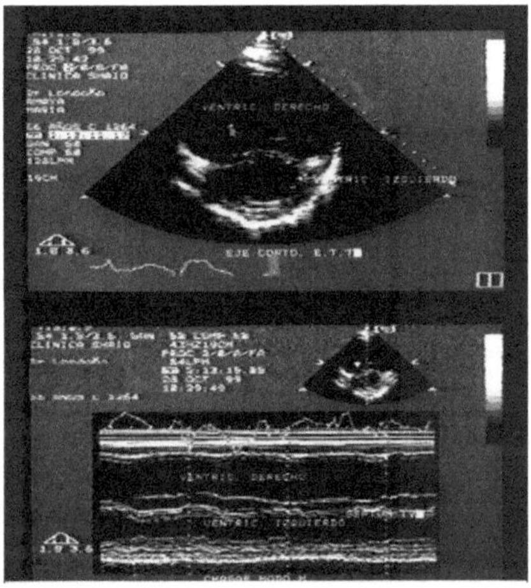

Fig. 6. Echocardiography M mode (A) and bi-dimensional (B) of 54-year-old female with a history of aborted sudden death due to ventricular tachycardia) secondary to Chagasic cardiomyopathy. Note the severe dilatation of right ventricle. Fundación Clínica Abood Shaio, Bogota D.C., Colombia.

7.2 Laboratory tests

7.2.1 Conventional parasitological tests

These can be classified into direct and indirect tests. Direct methods, employed basically in the acute phase, include parasite microscope-observation in blood fresh preparation which permits to observe parasite movement. On the contrary, thin or thick blood smears stained with Giemsa led to a better morphological identification, which is of special importance in areas where *Trypanosoma rangeli* also circulates. Importantly, parasite concentration methods like blood centrifugation, Strout method, and microhematocrit increase the probability of trypomastigote detection. Because of their great time consumption, indirect parasitological methods are generally used to diagnose patients in the chronic phase. They refer to hemoculture and xenodiagnosis (Luquetti, 2007).

7.2.2 Serological tests

There is a broad spectrum of serological tests, whose final goal is to detect anti *T. cruzi* antibodies, usually of the IgG isotype in the chronic phase or IgM in the acute phase. The tests most used, called conventional tests for serological Chagas disease diagnosis, are the indirect immunofluorescence test (IFAT), the enzyme-linked immunoabsorbent assay (ELISA), and the indirect haemaglutination test (IHA). Generally, the antigens used are parasite lysates or mixtures of parasite recombinant proteins. Due to the huge parasite polymorphisms (Rodríguez et al., 2002), it is recommended to use isolates circulating in the specific endemic area or mixture of them.The applied method must be carefully standardized and validated in inter-laboratory international and national tests. Most of the above-mentioned tests can detect the infection in more than 95% of sera. Nevertheless, false-positive reactions can occur in *T. rangeli* or *Lesihmania*-infected patients, as well as false-negative in the case of recently-infected chronic patients or immunosuppressed patients (Gil et al., 2007; Luquetti, 2007).

7.2.3 PCR

PCR tests, because of their power of detection and specificity, constitute a complementary diagnostic method for detecting *T. cruzi* in diverse biological samples. They are of especial interest with chronic patients because of their higher sensitivity compared with conventional parasitological tests. There are several PCR tests available for detecting *T. cruzi*. Their performance varies depending on aspects like type and number of the target amplification, lack of polymorphisms among the parasite DTU-annealing primer target, sample volume, treatment and conservation, DNA extraction method, type of DNA polymerase used, and thermo-cycling program, among variables (Schijman et al., 2011). Some PCR tests show disadvantages like the amplification of polymorphic fragments or of similar-size bands in both *T. cruzi* and *T. rangeli* infections, the deviation of the test towards *T. cruzi* in mixed infections with *T. rangeli*, and the possible integration of the parasite's kDNA in the human genome (Gil et al., 2007; Pavía et al., 2003, 2007). Bearing all this in mind, the Molecular Parasitology Laboratory at Pontificia Universidad Javeriana designed and standardized the TcH2AF-R PCR, specific for *T. cruzi* (Pavia et al., 2003). This PCR amplifies the 16-255 nucleotides of the *T. cruzi* SIRE repetitive element and does not present amplification signal in *T. rangeli*. Assays on triatomine vectors experimentally and naturally infected with *T. cruzi* revealed that TcH2AF-R PCR allows identifying the parasite in all the infected specimens, with performance equal to that of S35/S36 PCR, considered among the most sensitive PCR tests for *T. cruzi* identification (Pavia et al., 2007). Likewise, in blood samples from Chagasic patients, it was observed that of 156 samples, 84 (53.8%) were positive with both TcH2AF-R and S35/S36 PCRs, while 89 (57%) were positive for indirect immunofluorescence (IIF) and enzymatic immunoassay (ELISA) (Gil et al., 2007). A study of the performance of the TcH2AF-R and S35-S36 primers in cardiac tissue of mice infected with *T. cruzi I* showed that by using both pairs of primers it is possible to detect the parasite in the acute and chronic stages of the infection, with performance above that of the micro-hematocrit and eliminate of the histopathological analysis (Barrera et al., 2008). Recently, by combining TcH2AF-R and S35/S36 PCRs, it was possible to follow up a Colombian heart transplant in a Chagasic patient, as well as the first Colombian congenital case (Pavia et al., 2009, 2011). Because of its higher sensitivity, a few real time PCR (qPCR) methods have been developed to monitor drug efficacy and Chagas disease reactivation in transplanted

Chagasic patients. However, international studies to evaluate PCR methods for parasite DNA detection in blood samples as that launched by Shijman et al., (2011) are urgently needed.

7.3 Epidemiological context

Epidemiological data, such as that shown in Table 2, seek to determine if the patient could have been in contact with the parasite.

Epidemiological data	Information included
Born in endemic areas	Housing conditions like thatched roof, dirt floors, adobe walls, etc. Presence of domestic animals. Rural, peri-domestic, or domestic dwellings Time of living in relationship to already performed vector control campaigns in the area (important in congenital transmission)
Living in endemic areas	
Visits to endemic areas	
Vector knowledge	Awareness of vectors circulating in the specific area
Chagasic relatives	Parents, siblings, or any family member infected
Work activity	Important in accidental transmission in both endemic and non-endemic areas
History of blood transfusions	Amount and place
History of organ transplant	Medical and epidemiological history of the donor

Table 2. Epidemiological data supporting risk of *T. cruzi* infection

8. Treatment

8.1 Symptomatic

In the absence of random clinical studies in patients with Chagas disease and heart failure, traditionally the recommendations have been extrapolated from the management guides for heart failure from other causes (Jessup et al., 2009). However, it should be noted that in the physiopathology of the Chagas disease there are clinical and therapeutic peculiarities with important implications. For example, high doses of diuretics are necessary in advanced stages of the disease due to predominance of the systemic congestion manifestations over signs of pulmonary congestion. In patients with Chagas cardiopathy, conduction disturbances are also frequent, which may be aggravated by the use of Digoxin, Amiodarone, and specially Beta-blockers (Marin-Neto et al., 2010). Cardiac re-synchronization is a treatment alternative for patients with heart failure, especially in the presence of left bundle branch block. However, its usefulness in patients with right bundle branch block common in Chagas disease has not been shown as patients with another type of pathology in the presence of this conduction alteration. Other palliative procedures like dynamic cardiomyoplasty and partial left ventriluculotomy are contraindicated because of unsatisfactory results. Heart transplant is an option indicated in patients selected in final stages of cardiac insufficiency. In these cases, it must be highlighted that the immunosuppressant therapy indicated to avoid transplant rejection may induce reactivation of the *T. cruzi* infection (Campos et al., 2008). Under certain circumstances, reducing the dosage of immunosuppression is recommended, as well as starting etiological treatment in cases of reactivation (Fiorelli et al., 2005). The potential benefit of transplanting stem cells in patients with Chagasic cardiopathy is under evaluation (Tura et al., 2007). Because of the high frequency of thrombus-embolic phenomena, anticoagulation is indicated in patients with atrial fibrillation, in the prior embolism, in the presence of aneurysms or thrombi, and in cases of heart failure in advanced stages even in the absence of random controlled studies that prove its efficacy. Some observational data suggest that Amiodarone can improve survival in patients with Chagas disease with risk of sudden death due to malignant arrhythmia (Garguichevich et al., 1995). For this reason, Amiodarone is usually recommended in patients with sustained ventricular tachycardia and in cases of unsustained ventricular tachycardia associated to ventricular systolic dysfunction (Leite et al., 2003). Patients with sustained ventricular tachycardia with hemodynamic instability and in cases of aborted sudden death, the implant of a cardio-defibrillator is recommended (Rassi et al., 2009). Radiofrequency ablation is an alternative in patients with ventricular tachycardia (D´Avila et al., 2002); however, its impact on survival and recurrence of the arrhythmia is yet to be established. The finding of severe bradyarrhythmias like those observed in the complete AV block and in the sinus dysfunction must be treated by implanting a definitive pacemaker as in other cardiac conditions (Epstein et al., 2008). The benefit of the pacemaker implant in patients with Chagasic cardiopathy is mainly based on reports of case series.

8.2 Etiological

The only medications currently used with Chagas disease due to ethical and efficiency reasons are Nifurtimox and Benznidazole (Bern et al., 2007). Based on the literature review, the recommendations of the antitrypanocidal therapy vary according to the phase and form of the Chagas disease, the patient's age, and the severity of the disease. The pharmacological therapy is recommended in all acute and congenital cases, in infection by reactivation, in patients up to 18 years of age, and in children. For adults between 19 and 50 years of age and without advanced cardiopathy, the treatment can be offered (Bern et al., 2007). In individuals above 50 years of age, risk of toxicity from the drug may be higher than in young adults and the treatment is considered optional. Once the diagnosis has been confirmed through corresponding serological tests, patients must be evaluated with a clinical history and a careful physical exam. Additionally, in all cases, an electrocardiogram should be performed. With asymptomatic individuals without electrocardiographic alterations, the prognosis tends to be favorable and it is recommended that these patients be monitored every 12 to 24 months. Patients with electrocardiographic changes consistent with the disease's cardiovascular compromise should be evaluated via thoracic X-ray and echocardiogram that permit defining the ventricular size and function, as well as other types of structural alterations and via 24-h electrocardiographic monitoring or Holter test to detect arrhythmias.

9. Prognosis

The prognosis of some diseases like Chagas has not been easy to establish because of the great differences in their clinical course among the affected countries. Results like the survey by Maguire et al., (1987) showed that from 20-59 years of age, the risk was strongly related to electrocardiography status. Indeed, patients with ventricular conduction defects have higher mortality rates than infected patients without electrocardiographic abnormalities. Also, it was observed that abnormal diastolic function is related to severe myocardial damage (Rocha et al., 2009). Another survey found that there are six prognostic factors of disease development: NYHA class III or IV, cardiomegaly on chest radiography, segmental or global wall motion abnormalities on echocardiography, non-sustained ventricular tachycardia on Holter monitoring, low QRS voltage on electrocardiography, and male sex (Rassi et al., 2006). Recent studies have found that there are four echocardiographic variables associated with the disease outcome: left ventricular ejection fraction, right ventricular function, E/E′ ratio, and left atrium volume (Rocha et al., 2009). Finally, the prognosis of the patient will rest on the good care and follow up of the caregivers. Chagas disease is no longer a disease of the poor; it is now a disease of any country with important socioeconomic impact.

10. Conclusions

Prediction markers for disease development, and progression, immunotherapy and vaccine strategies, new anti-*T. cruzi* drugs, and world-standardized PCR tests, are urgently required to improve early diagnosis and treatment of this worldwide health problem. Government, health organizations, and scientists all over the world need to come together to construct policies and strategies to prevent and control this silent but devastating disease in endemic and non endemic countries.

11. Acknowledgments

The authors express gratitude to the Vicerrectoria Académica at Pontificia Universidad Javeriana for financially supporting this proposal, as well to other agencies funding our research projects, which permit us to achieve this manuscript: Colciencias (projects 1203-493-26159, 1109-04-18231, 1203-333-18692), TWAS (project No. 827), Pontificia Universidad Javeriana (projects No. 609, 784, 1034, 1707, 1767, 2089, 3333), and Universidad de los Andes [associate professor grant (JMG) from the Vicerrectoria de Investigaciones, Universidad de los Andes]. We would also like to thank the patients and the healthy controls who participated in our researches.

12. References

Albanesi-Filho, FM.; Gomes, JB. (1991). O tromboembolismo em pacientes com lesão apical da cardiopatia chagásica crônica. *Revista Portuguesa de Cardiologia*, Vol.10, No. 1, (January 1991), pp.35-42, ISSN 0870-2551

Almeida, E.A.; Silva, E.L.; Guariento, M.E. et al. (2009). Fatal evolution of Chagas'disease/Aids co-infection: diagnostic difficulties between myocarditis reactivation and chronic chagasic myocardiopathy. *Revista da Sociedade Brasileira de Medicina Tropical*, Vol.42, No.2, (March-April 2009), pp. 199-202, ISSN 0037-8682

Alvarez, M.G.; Postan, M.; Weatherly, D.B. et al. (2008). HLA Class I-T cell epitopes from trans-sialidase proteins reveal functionally distinct subsets of CD8+ T cells in chronic Chagas disease. *PLoS Neglected Tropical Diseases*, Vol.2, No.9, (September 2008), e288, ISSN 1935-2735

Andrade, L.O.; Machado, C.R.; Chiari, E. et al. (1999). Differential tissue distribution of diverse clones of *Trypanosoma cruzi* in infected mice. *Molecular and Biochemical Parasitology*, Vol.100, No.2, (May 1999), pp. 163-172, ISNN 1872-9428

Barrera, Y.K.; Guevara, J.M.; Pavía, P.X. et al. (2008).Evaluation of TcH2AF-R and S35-S36 primers in PCR tests for the detection of *Trypanosoma cruzi* in mouse cardiac tissue. *Biomedica*, Vol. 28, No. 4, (December 2008), pp. 616-626, ISSN 0120-4157

Bayer, A.M.; Hunter, G.C. ; Gilman, R.H. et al. (2009). Chagas disease, migration and community settlement patterns in Arequipa, Peru. *PLoS Neglected Tropical Diseases*, Vol. 3, No. 12, (December 2009), pp.e567, ISSN 1935-2735

Bern, C. & Montgomery, S.P. (2009). An estimate of the burden of Chagas disease in the United States. *Clinical Infectious Diseases*, Vol.49, No.5, (September 2009), pp. e52-e54, ISSN 1058-4838

Bern, C.; Montgomery S.P.; Herwaldt B.L. et al. (2007). Evaluation and treatment of Chagas disease in the United States. *Journal of the American Medical Association*, Vol. 298, No. 18, (November 2007), pp. 2171-2181, ISSN 1538-3598

Biolo, A.; Ribeiro A.L. & Clausell, N. (2010). Chagas cardiomyopathy-where do we stand after a hundred years?. *Progress in Cardiovascular Diseases*, Vol.52, (January-February 2010), pp. 300-316, ISSN 1532-8643

Bixby, L.M. & Tarleton, R.L. (2008). Stable CD8+ T cell memory during persistent *Trypanosoma cruzi* infection. *Journal of Immunology*, Vol.181, No.4, (August 2008), pp. 2644-2650, ISSN 1550-6606

Bonney, K.M. & Engman, D.M. (2008). Chagas heart disease pathogenesis: one mechanism or many? *Current Molecular Medicine*, Vol.8, No. 6 (September 2008), pp. 510-518, ISSN 1875-5666

Burgos, J.M.; Diez, M.; Vigliano, C. et al. (2010). Molecular identification of *Trypanosoma cruzi* discrete typing units in end-stage chronic Chagas heart disease and reactivation after heart transplantation. *Clinical Infectious Diseases*, Vol.51, No.5, (September 2010), pp. 485-495, ISSN 1058-4838

Calzada, J.E.; Beraún, Y.; González, C.I. et al. (2009). Transforming growth factor beta 1(TGFbeta1) gene polymorphisms and Chagas disease susceptibility in Peruvian and Colombian patients. *Cytokine*, Vol.45, No.3, (March 2009), pp.149-53, ISSN 1096-0023

Campos, S.V.; Strabelli, T.M.; Amato, N.V. et al. (2008). Risk factors for Chagas' disease reactivation after heart transplantation. *Journal of Heart and Lung Transplantation*, Vol. 27, No. 6, (June 2008), pp. 597-602, ISSN 1557-3117

Carod-Artal, F.J. (2006). Chagas' disease and ischemic stroke. *Neurologia*, Vol. 21, No. 3, (April 2006), pp. 135-149, ISSN 0213-4853

Castro, E. (2009). Chagas' disease: lessons from routine donation testing. *Transfusion Medicine*, Vol.19, No.1. (February 2009), pp.16-23, ISSN 1365-3148

Colorado, I.A.; Acquatella, H.; Catalioti, F. et al. (2000). HLA class II DRB1, DQB1, DPB1polymorphism and cardiomyopathy due to *Trypanosoma cruzi* chronic infection. *Human Immunology,* Vol.61, No. 3 (March 2000), pp. 320-355, ISSN 1879-1166

Coura, J.R. & Borges-Pereira, J. (2010). Chagas disease: 100 years after its discovery. A systemic review. *Acta Tropica,* Vol.115, No.1-2, (July-August 2010), pp.5-13, ISSN 1873-6254

Cuellar, A.; Rojas, F.; Bolanos, N. et al. (2009). Natural CD4+ T-cell responses against *Trypanosoma cruzi* KMP-11 protein in chronic chagasic patients. *Immunology and Cell Biology,* Vol.87, No.2, (February 2009), pp. 149-153, ISSN 0818-9641

Cuellar, A.; Santander, S.P.; Thomas, M.C. et al. (2008). Monocyte-derived dendritic cells from chagasic patients vs healthy donors secrete differential levels of IL-10 and IL-12 when stimulated with a protein fragment of *Trypanosoma cruzi* heat-shock protein-70. *Immunology and Cell Biology,* Vol.86, No.3, (March-April 2008), pp. 255–260, ISSN 0818-9641

D'Avila, A.; Splinter, R.; Svenson, R.H. et al. (2002).New perspectives on catheter-based ablation of ventricular tachycardia complicating Chagas' disease: experimental evidence of the efficacy of near infrared lasers for catheter ablation of Chagas' VT. *Journal of Interventional Cardiac Electrophysiology,* Vol. 7, No.1, (August 2002), pp.23-38, ISSN 1572-8595

Dias, J.C.; Prata, A. & Correia, D. (2008). Problems and perspectives for Chagas disease control: in search of a realistic analysis. *Revista da Sociedade Brasileira de Medicina Tropical,* Vol.41, No.2. (November 2008), pp. 193-196, ISSN 0037-8682

Diez, H.; López, M.C.; Del Carmen Thomas, M.C. et al. (2006). Evaluation of IFN-gamma production by CD8 T lymphocytes in response to the K1 peptide from KMP-11 protein in patients infected with *Trypanosoma cruzi. Parasite Immunology,* Vol.28, No.3, (March 2006), pp. 101-105, ISSN 0141-9838

Enciso, C.; Montilla, M.; Santacruz, M.M. et al. (2004). Comparison of the indirect immunofluorescent (IFAT), ELISA test and the comercial Chagatek test for anti-*Trypanosoma cruzi* antibodies detection. *Biomedica,* Vol. 24, No.1, (March 2004), pp. 104-108, ISSN 0120-4157

Epstein, A.E.; DiMarco, J.P.; Ellenbogen, K.A. et al. (2008). ACC/AHA/HRS 2008 Guidelines for device-based therapy of cardiac rhythm abnormalities. *Journal of the American College of Cardiology,* Vol. 51, No. 21,(May 2008), pp. 1-62, ISSN 0735-1097

Epting, C.L.; Coates, B.M. & Engman, D.M. (2010). Molecular mechanisms of host cell invasion by *Trypanosoma cruzi. Experimental Parasitology,* Vol.126, No.3, (November 2010), pp.283-291, ISSN 1090-2449

Fernandez-Mestre, M.T.; Layrisse, Z.; Montagnani, S. et al. (1998). Influence of the HLA class II polymorphism in chronic Chagas' disease. *Parasite Immunology,* Vol. 20, No. 4, (April 1998), pp.197-203, ISSN 0141-9838

Field, V.; Gautret, P.; Schlagenhauf, P. et al. (2010). Travel and migration associated infectious diseases morbidity in Europe, 2008. *BMC Infectious Diseases,* Vol.10, No.330, (November 2010), pp. e330, ISSN 1471-2334

Fiorelli, AI.; Stolf, NA.; Honorato, R. et al. (2005). Later evolution after cardiac transplantation in Chagas' disease. *Transplantation Proceedings,* Vol.37, No.6, (July-August 2005), pp. 2793–2798, ISSN 0041-1345

Fiuza, J.A.; Fujiwara, R.T.; Gomes, J.A. et al. (2009). Profile of central and effector memory T cells in the progression of chronic human chagas disease. *PLoS Neglected Tropical Diseases*, Vol.3, No.9, (September 2009), pp. e512, ISSN 1935-2735

Flechas, I.D.; Cuellar, A.; Cucunubá, Z.M. et al. (2009). Characterising the KMP-11 and HSP-70 recombinant antigens' humoral immune response profile in chagasic patients. *BMC infectious diseases*, Vol.25, No.9, (November 2009), pp.186, ISSN 1471-2334

Fonseca, S.G.; Moins-Teisserenc, H.; Clave, E. et al. (2005). Identification of multiple HLA-A*0201-restricted cruzipain and FL-160 CD8+ epitopes recognized by T cells from chronically *Trypanosoma cruzi*- infected patients. *Microbes and Infection*, Vol.7, No.4, (April 2005), pp. 688-697, ISSN 1286-4579

Franco-Paredes, C.; Von, A.; Hidron, A. et al. (2007). Chagas disease: an impediment in achieving the millennium development goals in Latin America. *BMC International Health and Human Rights*, Vol.7, No.7, (August 2007), pp. e7, ISSN 1472-698X

García Borrás, S.; Racca, L.; Cotorruelo, C. et al. (2009). Distribution of HLA-DRB1 alleles in Argentinean patients with Chagas' disease cardiomyopathy. *Immunological Investigations*, Vol.38 No.3-4 (2009), pp. 268-275, ISSN 1532-4311

Garguichevich, J.J.; Ramos, J.L.; Gambarte A. et al. (1995). Effect of amiodarone therapy on mortality in patients with left ventricular dysfunction and asymptomatic complex ventricular arrhythmias: Argentine pilot study of sudden death and amiodarone (EPAMSA). *American Heart Journal*, Vol, 130, No.3, (September 1995), pp. 494-500, ISSN 1097-6744

Garzón, S.A.; Lorga, A.M.; Nicolau, J.C. (1995). Electrocardiography in Chagas' heart disease. *Sao Paulo Medical Journal* , Vol. 113, No. 2, (April 1995), pp.802–13, ISNN 1516-3180

Gil, J.; Pavía, P.X.; Montilla, M. et al. (2007). Comparison of a PCR test based on the histone H2A/SIRE genes with classical serological tests for the diagnosis of chronic Chagas disease in Colombian patients. *Biomedica,* Vol.27, Suppl.1, (January 2007), pp.83-91, ISSN 0120-4157

Golgher, D. & Gazzinelli, R.T. (2004). Innate and acquired immunity in the pathogenesis of Chagas disease. *Autoimmunity*, Vol.37, No.5, (August 2004), pp. 399-409, ISSN 0891-6934

Gomez, E.A.; Senior, J.M.; Vélez, S. et al. (2007). Guías colombianas sobre la evaluación y el manejo de la falla cardíaca crónica del adulto. *Revista Colombiana de Cardiología*. Vol. 14, Supl.2, (October 2007), pp.12-50, ISSN 0120-5633

Guhl, F. (2009). Chagas disease: reality and perspectives. *Biomedica*, Vol.20, No.3, (December 2009), pp.228-234, ISSN 0188-493X

Gutierrez, F.R.; Guedes, P.M.; Gazzinelli, R.T. et al. (2009). The role of parasite persistence in pathogenesis of Chagas heart disease. *Parasite Immunology* Vol.31 No.11 (November 2009) pp.673-85, ISSN 1365-3024

Guzmán-Tapia, Y.; Ramírez-Sierra, M.J. & Dumonteil, E. (2007). Urban infestation by *Triatoma dimidiata* in the city of Mérida, Yucatán, México. *Vector Borne and Zoonotic Diseases*, Vol.7, No.4, (December 2007), pp. 597-606, ISSN 1530-3667

Hidron, A.I; Gilman, R.H.; Justiniano, J. et al. (2010). Chagas cardiomyopathy in the context of the chronic disease transition. *PLoS Neglected Tropical Diseases*, Vol.4, No.5, (May 2010), pp. e688, ISSN 1935-2735

Higuchi, Mde L.; Benvenuti, L.A.; Martins Reis, M. et al. (2003). Pathophysiology of the heart in Chagas'disease: current status and new development. *Cardiovascular Research*, Vol. 60, (October 2003), pp. 96-167, ISSN 1755-3245

Hotez, P.J.; Molyneux, D.H.; Fenwick, A. et al. (2006). Incorporating a rapid-impact package for neglected tropical diseases with programs for HIV/AIDS, tuberculosis, and malaria. *PLoS Medicine*, Vol.3, No.5, (January 2006), pp. e102, ISSN 1549-1277

Jessup, M.; Abraham, W.T.; Casey D.E. et al. (2009), focused update: ACCF/AHA Guidelines for the diagnosis and management of heart failure in adults: a report of the American College of Cardiology Foundation/American Heart Association Task Force on Practice Guidelines: developed in collaboration with the International Society for Heart and Lung Transplantation. *Circulation*, Vol.14, No. 119, (April 2009), pp. 1977-2016, ISSN 0009-7332

Lasso, P.; Cuellar, A.; Rosas, F. et al. (2009). Células dendríticas y linfocitos T reguladores naturales en pacientes con enfermedad crónica de Chagas. *Infectio*, Vol.13, No.4, (Diciembre 2009), pp. 246-253, ISSN 0123-9392

Lasso, P.; Mesa, D.; Cuéllar, A. et al. (2010). Frequency of specific CD8+ T cells for a promiscuous epitope derived from *Trypanosoma cruzi* KMP-11 protein in chagasic patients. *Parasite Immunology*, Vol.32, No.7, (July 2010), pp. 494-502, ISSN 0141-9838

Laucella, S.A.; Postan, M.; Martin, D. et al. (2004). Frequency of interferon-gamma-producing T cells specific for *Trypanosoma cruzi* inversely correlates with disease severity in chronic human Chagas disease. *Journal of Infectious Disease*, Vol.189, No.5, (March 2004), pp. 909–918, ISSN 0022-1899

Leite, L.R.; Fenelon, G.; Simoes A., et al. (2003). Clinical usefulness of electrophysiologic testing in patients with ventricular tachycardia and chronic chagasic cardiomyopathy treated with amiodarone or sotalol. *Journal of Cardiovascular electrophysiology*, Vol.14, No.6, (June 2003), pp. 567–573, ISNN 1540-8167

Llewellyn, M.S.; Rivett-Carnac, J.B.; Fitzpatrick, S. et al. (2011). Extraordinary *Trypanosoma cruzi* diversity within single mammalian reservoir hosts implies a mechanism of diversifying selection, *International Journal of Parasitology*, Vol. 41, No.6, (May 2011), pp. 609-614, ISSN 1879-0135

Luquetti, A. (2007). Diagnóstico de la enfermedad de Chagas. In: Enfermedad de Chagas. F. Rosas.; D. Venegas.; M. Cabrales, (Ed.), 25-31, *Sociedad Colombiana de Cardiología y Cirugía Cardiovascular*, Bogotá, Colombia ISBN 978-958-97065-9-6

Maguire, J.H.; Hoff, R.; Sherlock, I. et al. (1987). Cardiac morbidity and mortality due to Chagas' disease: prospective electrocardiographic study of a Brazilian community. *Circulation*, Vol. 75, No. 6, (Jun3 1987), pp. 1140-1145, ISSN 0009-7322

Manque, P.A.; Probst, C de S.; Pereira, M.C. et al. (2011). *Trypanosoma cruzi* infection induces a global host cell response in cardiomyocytes. *Infection and Immunity*, Vol.79, No.5, (February 2011), pp.1855-1862, ISSN 1098-5522

Marin-Neto, J.A.; Cunha-Neto, E.; Maciel, B.C. et al. (2007). Pathogenesis of chronic Chagas heart disease. *Circulation*, Vol. 115, No. 9, (March 2007), pp 1109-1123, ISSN 0009-7332

Marín-Neto, J.A.; Rassi, A Jr.; Maciel, BC., et al. (2010). Chagas heart disease. In: *Evidence-based cardiology*, Yusuf, S.; Cairns, JA.; Camm, AJ.; Fallen, EL.; Gersh, BJ, pp. 823–841, London: BMJ Books, ISBN 978-1-4051-5925-8, London UK

Medrano-Mercado, N.; Ugarte-Fernandez, R.; Butrón, V. et al. (2008).Urban transmission of Chagas disease in Cochabamba, Bolivia. *Memórias do Instituto Oswaldo Cruz*, Vol.103, No.5, (August 2008), pp. 423-430, ISSN 1678-8060

Miles, M.A.; Feliciangeli, M.D. & de Arias, A.R. (2003) American Trypanosomiasis (Chagas' disease) and the role of molecular epidemiology in guiding control strategies. *British Medical Journal*, Vol. 326. pp. 1444-1448, ISSN 09598138

Miles, M.A. (2010). Orally acquired Chagas disease: lessons from an urban school outbreak. *Journal of Infectious Diseases*, Vol.201, No.9, (May 2010), pp. 1282-1284, ISSN 0022-1899

Moncayo, A. (2003). Chagas disease: current epidemiological trends after the interruption of vectorial and transfusional transmission in the Southern Cone countries. *Memórias do Instituto Oswaldo Cruz*, Vol.98, No.5, (July 2003), pp. 577-591, ISSN 1678-8060

Moncayo, A. & Silveira A.C. (2009) Current epidemiological trends for Chagas disease in Latin America and future challenges in epidemiology, surveillance and health policy. *Memórias do Instituto Oswaldo Cruz*, Vol.104, Supl.1, (July 2009), pp. 17-30, ISSN 1678-8060

Nicholls, R.S.; Cucunubá, Z.M.; Knudson, A. et al. (2007).Acute Chagas disease in Colombia: a rarely suspected disease. Report of 10 cases presented during the 2002-2005 period. *Biomedica*, Vol.27, Suppl. 1, (January 2007), pp.8-17. ISSN 0120-4157

Norman, F.F.; Pérez de Ayala, A.; Pérez-Molina, J.A. et al. (2010).Neglected tropical diseases outside the tropics. *PLoS Neglected Tropical Diseases*, Vol.4, No.7, (July 2010), pp. e762, ISSN 1935-2735

Pavía, P.X.; Roa, N.; Uribe, A.M. et al. (2011).Using S35-S36 and TcH2AF-R primer-based PCR tests to follow-up a Chagas' disease patient who had undergone a heart transplant. *Biomédica*, Vol. 31, No.2, ISSN 0120-4157

Pavía, P.X.; Cuervo, C.L.; Montilla, M., et al. (2003). Diseño y estandarización de una prueba de PCR para la detección específica de *Trypanosoma cruzi*. *Infectio*, Vol. 7, No.3, (August 2003), pp.129-136, ISSN 0123-9392

Pavia, P.X.; Montilla, M.; Flórez, C. et al. (2009).The first case of congenital Chagas' disease analyzed by AP-PCR in Colombia. *Biomédica*, Vol. 29, No.4, (December 2009), pp. 513-522, ISSN 0120-4157

Pavía, P.X.; Vallejo, G.A.; Montilla, M. et al. (2007). Detection of *Trypanosoma cruzi* and *Trypanosoma rangeli* infection in triatomine vectors by amplification of the histone H2A/SIRE and the sno-RNA-C11 genes. *Revista do Instituto de Medicina Tropical de São Paulo*, Vol. 49, No.1, (January- February 2007), pp. 23-30, ISSN 0036-4665

Pérez, A.R.; Fontanella, G.H.; Nocito, A.L. et al. (2009). Short treatment with the tumour necrosis factor-alpha blocker infliximab diminishes chronic chagasic myocarditis in rats without evidence of *Trypanosoma cruzi* reactivation. *Clinical and Experimental Immunology*, Vol.157, No.2, (August 2009), pp.291-299. ISSN 1365-2249

Pissetti, C.W.; Correia, D.; De Oliveira, R.F. et al. (2011). Genetic and Functional Role of TNF-alpha in the Development *Trypanosoma cruzi* infection. *PLoS Neglected Tropical Disease*, Vol.5, No.3, (March 2001), pp.976, ISSN 1935-2735

Prata, A. (2001). Clinical and epidemiological aspects of Chagas' disease. *Lancet Infectious Diseases*, Vol. 1, No. 2, (September 2001). pp. 92-100, ISNN 1473-3099

Ramasawmy, R.; Fae, K.C.; Cunha-Neto, E. et al. (2007). Polymorphisms in the gene for lymphotoxin-alpha predispose to chronic Chagas cardiomyopathy. *Journal of Infectious Diseases*, Vol. 196, No.12, (December 2007), pp.1836-1843, ISSN 1537-6613

Ramírez, J.D.; Guhl, F.; Rendón, L.M. et al. (2010).Chagas cardiomyopathy manifestations and *Trypanosoma cruzi* genotypes circulating in chronic Chagasic patients. *PLoS Neglected Tropical Disease*, Vol.4, No.11, (November 2010) pp.e899, ISSN 1935-2735

Rassi, A. Jr.; Rassi, A. & Little, W.C. (2006). Development and validation of a risk score for predicting death in Chagas' heart disease. *New England Journal of Medicine*, Vol. 355, No. 8, (August 2006), pp. 799-808, ISSN 0028-4793

Rassi, A. Jr.; Rassi, A. & Marin-Neto, J.A. (2009). Chagas heart disease: pathophysiologic mechanisms, prognostic factors and risk stratification. *Memorias do Instituto Oswaldo Cruz*, Vol.104, Supl.1, (May 2009), pp. 152-158, ISNN 1678-8060

Rassi, A. Jr.; Rassi, A. & Marin-Neto, J.A. (2010). Chagas Disease. *Lancet*, Vol. 375, No. 9723 (April 2010) pp.1388–1402, ISSN 1474-547X

Rocha, M.O.; Nunes, M.C. & Ribeiro, A.L. (2009). Morbidity and prognostic factors in chronic chagasic cardiopathy. *Memorias do Instituto Oswaldo Cruz*, Vol. 104, Supl. 1, (July 2009), pp.159-166, ISSN 1678-8060

Rodríguez, P.; Escalante, M.; Díez, H. et al. (2002). Variability of 6 Colombian strains of *Trypanosoma cruzi* with restriction fragment length polymorphisms (RFLP) and random amplification of polymorphic DNA (RAPD). *Biomedica*, Vol. 22, No. 3, (September 2002), pp. 263-271, ISSN 0120-4157

Rosas, F. (2007). Cardiomiopatía Chagásica, In: *Enfermedad de Chagas*. F. Rosas.; D. Venegas.; M. Cabrales, (Ed.), pp. 47-62, Sociedad Colombiana de Cardiología y Cirugía Cardiovascular, ISBN 978-958-97065-9-6, Bogotá, Colombia

Rossi, M.A.; Tanowitz, H.B.; Malvestio, L.M. et al. (2010). Coronary microvascular disease in chronic Chagas cardiomyopathy including an overview on history, pathology, and other proposed pathogenic mechanisms. *PLoS Neglected Tropical Disease*, Vol. 4, No.8 (August 2010), pp.e674, ISSN 1935-2735

Schijman, A.G.; Bisio, M.; Orellana, L. et al. (2011). International study to evaluate PCR methods for detection of *Trypanosoma cruzi* DNA in blood samples from Chagas disease patients. *PLoS Neglected Tropical Disease*, Vol.5, No.1, (January 2011), pp.e931, ISSN 1935-2735

Schmunis. G.A. & Yadon, Z.E. (2010). Chagas disease: a Latin American health problem becoming a world health problem. *Acta Trópica*, Vol.115, No.1-2, (July-August 2010), pp.14-21, ISSN 0001-706X

Sicuri, E.; Muñoz, J.; Pinazo, M.J. et al. (2011).Economic evaluation of Chagas disease screening of pregnant Latin American women and of their infants in a non endemic area. *Acta Tropica*, Vol.118, No.2, (May 2011), pp. 110-117, ISSN 1873-6254

Sousa, A.S.; Xavier, S.S.; Freitas, G.R. et al. (2008). Prevention strategies of cardioembolic ischemic stroke in Chagas' disease. *Arquivos Brasileiros de Cardiologia*, Vol.91, No. 5, (November 2008), pp. 306-310, ISSN 0066-782X

Talvani, A.; Rocha, M.O.; Barcelos, L.S. et al. (2004). Elevated concentrations of CCL2 and tumor necrosis factor-alpha in chagasic cardiomyopathy. *Clinical Infectious Diseases*, Vol.38, No.7, (April 2004), pp.943-950, ISSN 1537-6591

Tura, B.R.; Martino, H.F.; Gowdak, L.H. et al. (2007). Multicenter randomized trial of cell therapy in cardiopathies—MiHeart Study. *Trials*, Vol. 8, No.2, (January2007), ISSN 1745-6215

Turtle, C.J.; Swanson, H.M.; Fujii, N. et al. (2009). A distinct subset of self-renewing human memory CD8+ T cells survives cytotoxic chemotherapy. *Immunity*, Vol.31, No.5, (November 2009), pp.834-844, ISSN 1074-7613

Ulrich, P.N.; Jiménez, V.; Park, M. et al. (2011). Identification of Contractile Vacuole Proteins in *Trypanosoma cruzi*. *PLoS One*, Vol. 6, No.3, pp. e18013, ISSN 1932-6203

Van Overtvelt, L.; Andrieu, M.; Verhasselt, V. et al. (2002). *Trypanosoma cruzi* down-regulates lipopolysaccharide-induced MHC class I on human dendritic cells and impairs antigen presentation to specific CD8 (+) T lymphocytes. *International Immunology*, Vol.14, No.10, (October 2002), pp. 1135–1144. ISSN 0953-8178

Verani, J.R.; Montgomery, S.P.; Schulkin, J. et al. (2010). Survey of obstetrician-gynecologists in the United States about Chagas disease. *American Journal of Tropical Medicine and Hygiene*, Vol.83, No.4, (October 2010), pp.891-895, ISSN 0002-9637

Vitelli-Avelar, D.M.; Sathler-Avelar, R.; Dias, J.C. et al. (2005). Chagasic patients with indeterminate clinical form of the disease have high frequencies of circulating CD3+CD16-CD56+ natural killer T cells and CD4+CD25 High regulatory T lymphocytes. *Scandinavian Journal of Immunology*, Vol.62, No.3, (September 2005), pp. 297-308, ISSN 0300-9475

Vitelli-Avelar, D.M.; Sathler-Avelar, R.; Massara, R.L. et al. (2006). Are increased frequency of macrophage-like and natural killer (NK) cells, together with high levels of NKT and CD4+CD25high T cells balancing activated CD8+ T cells, the key to control Chagas' disease morbidity?. *Clinical and Experimental Immunology*, Vol.145, No.1, (July 2006), pp. 81-92, ISSN 0009-9104

WHO. (2010). Chagas disease (American trypanosomiasis) fact sheet. *Weekly Epidemiology Record*, Vol. 85, No.34, (August 2010), pp. 334-336, ISSN 0049-8114

Yoshida, N. (2008). *Trypanosoma cruzi* infection by oral route: how the interplay between parasite and host components modulates infectivity. *Parasitology International*, Vol. 57, No.2, (June 2008), pp.105-109, ISSN 1873-0329

Zafra, G.; Mantilla, J.C.; Jácome, J. et al. (2011). Direct analysis of genetic variability in *Trypanosoma cruzi* populations from tissues of Colombian chagasic patients. *Human Pathology*, doi:10.1016/j.humpath.2010.11.012, (February 2011), ISSN 1532-8392

17

Chagas Heart Disease

Clara Isabel González and Julio César Mantilla
Grupo de Inmunología y Epidemiología Molecular, GIEM,
Facultad de Salud, Universidad Industrial de Santander
Colombia

1. Introduction

Chagas disease (CD) or American trypanosomiasis is a complex zoonosis produced by the infection with the intracellular protozoan parasite *Trypanosoma cruzi*. Although the disease was first described in 1909 by the Brazilian physician Carlos Chagas, this disease affects human beings since antiquity as it was demonstrated by paleoparasitology studies which proved the presence of DNA in mummies dating back to 9000 years old (Aufderheide et al., 2004; Guhl et al., 1999). The parasite *T. cruzi* is a hemoflagellate protozoan belonging to the Mastigophora class, Kinetoplastida order, Trypanosomatidae family, genus Trypanosoma, the group Stercoraria. It was named in honor of Oswaldo Cruz, who was the mentor of Carlos Chagas.

T. cruzi has a complex life cycle involving two hosts, an invertebrate, especially an insect vector and some vertebrates, including man and domestic and wild reservoirs (Tyler & Engman, 2001). The presence of CD in humans is purely accidental, as when the man came into contact with natural foci and caused ecological imbalances causing the adaptation of vectors to human dwellings and new food sources. Thus three overlapping cycles were established: the wild cycle, the peridomestic cycle and the domestic cycle (Coura, 2007). The parasite occurs in a variety of hosts and infects 150 species from 24 families of domestic (e.g., dogs, cats and guinea pigs) and wild animals (e.g., rodents, marsupials, and armadillos) (Rassi, et al., 2010). The vectors involved in the transmission of CD are insects of the Phylum Arthropoda, Class Insecta, Order Hemiptera, Family Reduviidae, belonging to the subfamily Triatominae. There have been reported approximately 130 species of wild and domiciliary triatomines although only a handful is the competent vector for *T. cruzi* (Schofield, 1981). The domestic species mainly colonize rural homes and peri-urban areas and these species are responsible for most human cases of Chagas disease in endemic areas. Sylvatic species are inhabitants of strict wild habitats such as cracks of rocks, bird nests or burrows of mammals and caves, among others. *Rhodnius prolixus* is the main domestic vector in the northern countries of South America and Central America, *Triatoma dimidiata* in Central America and *Triatoma infestans* in countries of the southern of South America (Guhl, 2007), these species are well adapted to human habitation.

T. cruzi presents four different morphological and biological forms: epimastigote, a replicative form located in the mid gut of the insect vector, it is the predominant form in the axenic culture; metacyclic trypomastigote develops in the posterior intestine and rectum of the insect vector and is the infective form; amastigote replicative stage, is located in the cytoplasm of mammalian host cells where it replicates by binary fission; blood trypomastigote comes from amastigote differentiation, leading to disruption of the host cell and releases into the bloodstream, where they are taken again by the blood-sucking vector (Brener, 1971) (Figure 1)

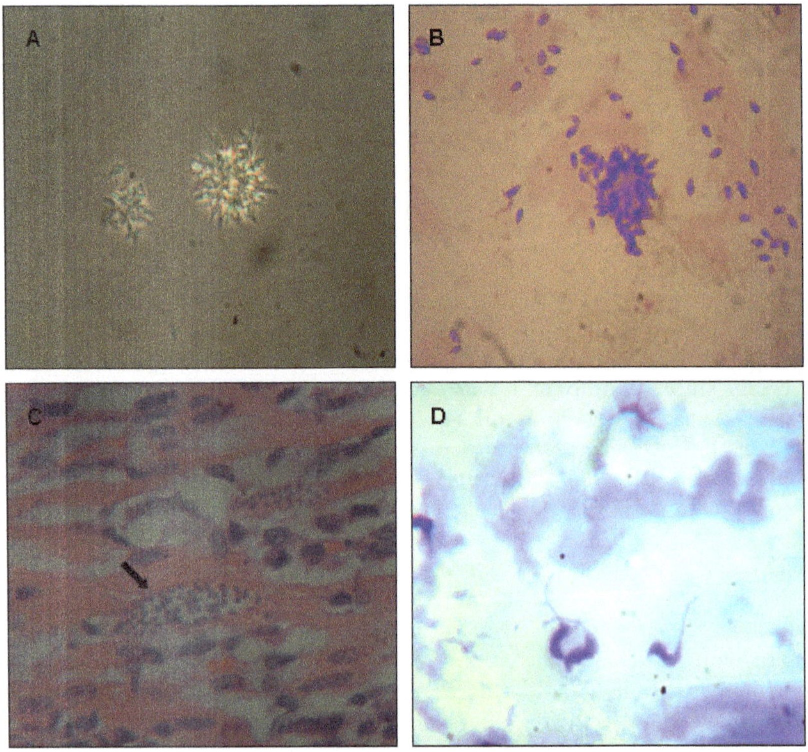

Fig. 1. *Trypanosoma cruzi* different stages. A) Epimastigotes of culture B) Amastigotes in Vero cells C) Nests of amastigotes in cardiac tissue D) Blood trypomastigotes stained with hematoxiylin-eosin.

The classic forms of *T. cruzi* transmission are vectorial, congenital, by transfusion, through organ transplants and labour accident. Vector-borne transmission is the most common and is contaminative by the presence of the infectious form in the faeces of the vector which is released when feeding on the host. The trypomastigotes penetrate through the opening of the bite or loss of continuity due to scratching or active penetration of oral or ocular mucosa. Before screening programs in blood banks, transfusion was the second form of transmission by the presence in donor's blood or blood products infected with parasite forms (Schmunis, 1999). Another important source of transmission is the donation of organs from infected individuals with the development of acute Chagas in the immunosuppressed recipient (Barcan et al., 2005). The passage of the parasite from infected mother to her baby during pregnancy, childbirth or while breast-feeding is high in some endemic regions, specially in Bolivia. The congenital transmission can lead to abortions, premature births or infected babies (Torrico et al., 2004).

2. The impact of Chagas disease

CD is currently is recognized by the World Health Organization (WHO) as one of the tropical neglected diseases and the infection with *T. cruzi* is the third parasitic infection after malaria and schistosomiasis (Schmunis & Yadon, 2010). CD is an important public health problem in 21 countries of South and Central America. The Pan American Health Organization (OPS, 2006) estimates that 7.7 million people are infected with *T. cruzi*, 109 million are at risk of infection and 12,500 deaths occur per year. The number of new annual cases of vector-borne infection is 41,000 and congenital Chagas' is 14,000 (WHO 2008).

Although this disease is considered typical of rural areas and poor suburbs with inadequate housing conditions, in recent decades in many Latin American countries there has been a substantial migration from rural to peri-urban areas. Migration has not only occurred from rural to urban areas in Latin America, but also to developed countries of North America, Europe and Asia. Accordingly, further cases have been detected in non-endemic countries like the USA, Canada, Spain, Japan and Australia due to population migration from endemic countries. In the United States have reported more than 300,000 people infected with *T. cruzi* and in Spain from 40 to 60,000 (Bern & Montgomery, 2009; Gascon et al., 2010).

The migration in endemic countries has led to the passive transport of vectors and the emergence of cases in areas considered of low endemicity. Additionally, the national initiatives for the elimination of the domestic vectors, including not only insecticide spraying but also a rural housing improvement, have led to the elimination of traditional vectors. However, a new transmission pattern is being introduced due to the presence of palms and trees located close to houses and sylvatic vectors that are attracted sporadically by light and feeding conditions. Consequentially, transmission by new vectors has arisen and often these vectors often have high rates of infection. This couple with the presence of wild reservoirs in the peridomestic area presenting high rates of infection has led to an alternate form to vectorial transmission in these areas, such as oral transmission (Briceño-León, 2009). This form of transmission is usually associated with acute and fatal outcomes and it has been increasing especially in the Brazilian Amazon where it is considered an emerging disease (Coura et al., 2002). The first report was given in 1960 in Teutonia with five deaths involved (Valente et al., 2009). Since then 600 new cases of acute Chagas have been reported, 50% associated with oral transmission. There are also reports in Venezuela (Alarcon de Noya et al., 2010), Mexico (Salazar-Schettino et al., 2011) and in the last three years in Colombia has increased, especially in Santander with six outbreaks of acute Chagas and three fatal cases (Díaz et al., 2009).

3. Clinical aspects of Chagas disease

3.1 Phases of Chagas disease

3.1.1 Acute phase

The clinic course of CD could have two phases: acute and chronic. The acute phase is characterized by the presence of *T. cruzi* trypomastigotes in the bloodstream, the parasitaemia generally persists for 4–8 weeks and it resolves spontaneously. In the majority of cases, especially in adults, this phase of infection is asymptomatic, however a small percentage of patients develops the acute disease characterized by important manifestations such as malaise, prolonged high fever, headache, edema, hepatomegaly, splenomegaly and generalized lymphadenopathy (Prata, 2001). In the acute form of CD, the first signs appear

7–10 days after infection. The Romaña's sign is observed when the parasite penetrates the conjunctiva; but when the parasite penetrates through the skin the patient develops the chagoma at the site of inoculation. The adjacent lymph nodes to the site of entry of the parasite are generally compromised, which together with the conjunctival or eyelid lesions constitute the ophthalmo - lymphonodal complex. Aproximately the fifty percent of the patients who develop the acute CD has Romaña's sign, and one-quarter has the inoculation chagoma. The Romaña's sign is characterized by painless, unilateral swelling of the upper and lower eyelid, with rose -violet coloration, congestion and edema of the conjunctiva, the submandibular, preauricular or other near lymphonode are enlarged, but not adhering to deep layers, occasionally may appear palpebral and periorbital cellulitis, sometimes with necrosis and abundant parasites. The inoculation chagoma generally appear on the skin of the face or the extremities, and is a forunculoid lesion, with a rose violet tone. In these patients, the initial electrocardiogram is normal, but after 2-3 weeks might show anomalies such sinus tachycardia, low QRS voltage or first grade atrioventricular block, the chest radiograph is also normal, however it might show cardiomegaly (Dias, 1989; Rassi et al., 2010).

The majority of patients, (90% or more) with acute CD survive the initial infection and remain healthy and asymptomatic, but a few individuals, between 2 -10%, generally infants or immunodepressed patients, or many people like children or adults who acquired the infection due to oral contamination, develop an acute and severe disease with myocarditis and cardiac insufficiency or with meningoencephalitis, clinical conditions that maybe cause death (Nobrega et al., 2009). Regarding to the central nervous system (CNS) involvement in CD, in the initial acute phase, the infection is asymptomatic and only a small percentage of cases develops encephalitis in the acute phase of disease; headache, seizure, focal neurologic signs and progressive decrease in consciousness are the notorious symptoms (Cordova et al., 2007).

3.1.2 Chronic phase

The great majority of patients, who were infected with *T. cruzi*, remain asymptomatic in the chronic phase, without abnormalities in the electrocardiogram and the radiological evaluations of the heart, esophagus and colon. This form of the chronic phase of CD is named indeterminate form, it is present in the half of infected people of endemic areas, and may persist until dead in 40-50% of the cases. All patients with the indeterminate form of CD are positive in serological or parasitological examinations, and do not have symptoms or signs of the disease, but using specialized methods such as ambulatory electrocardiographic monitoring or endomyocardial biopsies, may demonstrate that they have at least some degree of cardiac damage. The morphologic features of the indeterminate form of CD in autopsies performed for us in individuals who died of other causes, include discrete focal infiltration of mononuclear cells with lymphocytes predominance, and mild interstitial fibrosis, these changes are notorious in the subendocardical zone, and near to the cardiac conduction system. The change from the indeterminate form to the determinate cardiac or digestive occurs slowly in a lapse of 10 - 20 years after the initial infection, in a few cases, approximately 2-3% per year. In these patients, the CD adopts a slow and benign course, but others develop dilated cardiomyopathy, heart congestive failure or arrhythmias. In sporadic cases the CD progresses directly from the acute form to determinate chronic form of human CD, and is named the subacute form, that generally affects young adults, these patients develop severe cardiopathy with cardiac failure (Marin-Neto et al., 1999).

In the chronic phase of CD, the fundamental morphological feature in patients with chronic chagasic cardiopathy (CCC) is a mixture of cellular infiltration of lymphocytes and monocytes with few plasma cells, and fibrous tissue, that correlate with diverse clinical symptoms and signs, since asymptomatic to a congestive syndrome with damage of conduction system, arrhythmias, disturbances in the ventricular repolarization and the extrasystoles. Thromboembolic phenomens due to cardiac mural thrombosis are also frequent. In the majority of these patients, in the thorax radiographs, the heart contour appears normal. In some cases the lack of symptoms is surprising, and it does not have correlation with damage of tissue detected under microscopical examination. The symptomatic patients with CCC related palpitations by arrhythmias or fatigue by cardiac failure. In the physical examination, the arrhythmias and the extrasystoles are the most frequent clinical features detected. In these patients, the cardiac failure has a slow and progressive course, generally with features of right failure predominating the legs edema, jugular ingurgitation, ascites, and hepatomegaly. The thromboembolic manifestations due to mural thrombosis are frequent, and in autopsies done by us, the pulmonary thromboembolism is the most common anatomopathological feature, although brain embolism is also recognized in a few cases. After the manifestations of cardiac failure, the patients may recover or die in a later episode to one year after the first symptoms of decompensation. In these patients the periganglionitis with reduction of neuronal bodies especially in the sympathetic system, the sinusal node fibrosis, and destruction of tissues of cardiac conduction system and the myocardial cells are related with the early alterations of autonomous nervous system. The described changes can explain the reduction of the response to cardiovagal reflex in the sinusal node, and the reduction of variability of the heart frecuency. The cardiovagal denervation increased the sympathetic tone and could explain why the arrhythmias, blockades and sudden death are the first clinical manifestations in these patients (Samuel et al., 1983; Rassi et al., 2001).
The digestive form of CD is present almost exclusively in Argentina, Brazil, Chile and Bolivia, although they have reported isolated cases in Colombia, Central America and Mexico. The symptoms are the consequence of achalasia. The dysphagia is the first disturbance that may lead to malnutrition and weight loss. Odynophagia and epigastric pain also occurs in cases of megaesophagus, and chronic constipation, abdominal distension and occasionally intestinal obstruction of large bowel in cases of megacolon (Florez et al., 2010).

3.2 Pathological anatomy

The changes described below are the product of the experience gathered in the practice of autopsies of patients who died of various forms of CD, and reflect the interaction between inflammatory response, cellular damage and alterations of the extracellular matrix, three pathologic processes generated by the parasite in the tissues, particularly in the heart, esophagus, colon and central nervous system.
In the acute phase when the infectious forms of *T. cruzi* penetrate in the cell, such macrophages, fibroblasts, Schwann cells, and myocytes, they transform in amastigotes, subsequently reproduce and form the parasitic nest or pseudocyst, after 3 - 5 days the parasite differentiates to trypomastigote, the pseudocyst enlarges, breaks the cell, releasing intact or degenerate forms of the parasite, which act in the interstitium as a particle that promotes the inflammatory response. In these cases the heart is enlarged, congestive, flaccid

with haemorrhagic foci on the epicardic surface, and at the cut, the cardiac chambers are dilated and the myocardium shows areas of haemorrhage and necrosis (Figure 2 A and B). In the microscopic examination, the extent of the inflammatory response is proportional to the number of pseudocyst and damaged cells. A dense interstitial infiltration of lymphocytes, macrophages, with a few neutrophils and eosinophils around the pseudocyst and damaged cells is observed in the acute severe form of CD (Figure 2 C and D).

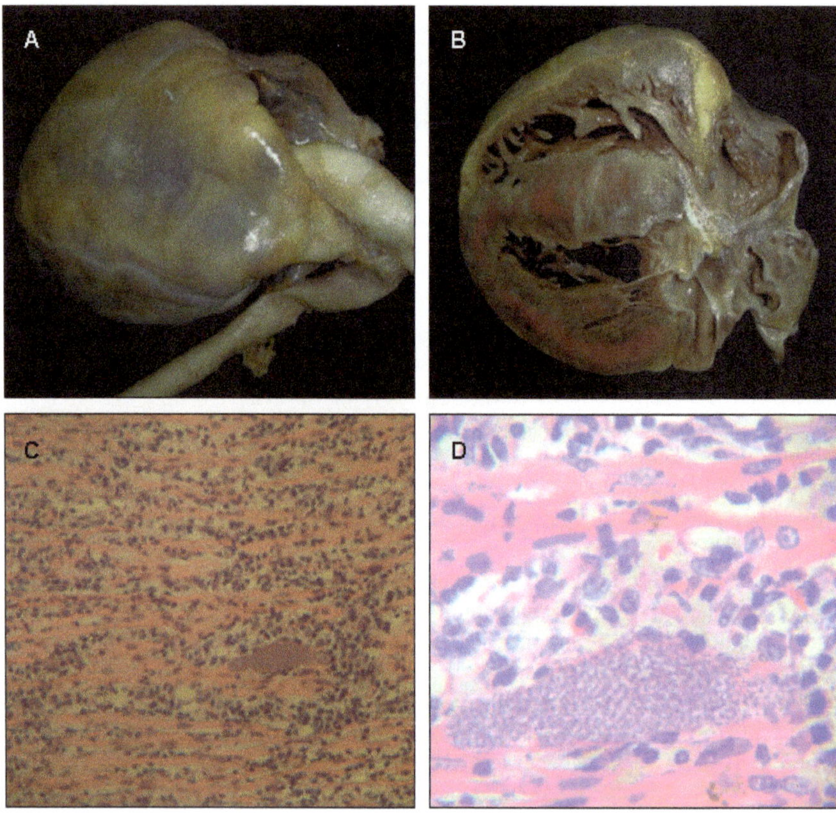

Fig. 2. Acute Chagas heart disease A) Heart enlarged with rounded shape. B) The surface of cut shows dilatation of four chambers, with pale and red areas, which correspond to focus of inflammation, necrosis and haemorrhage C) Nest of *Trypanosoma cruzi*, dense interstitial infiltrate of lymphocytes, plasma cells and monocytes with necrosis of myocardial cells D) Nest of *Trypanosoma cruzi* with rupture of myocardial cell and infiltrate inflammatory of mononuclear cells.

In the chronic phase of CD, the most important feature in chagasic cardiopathy, is the enlarge of heart with dilatation of chambers, mural thrombus (Figure 3A) and the mixture of cellular infiltration of lymphocytes, monocytes with a few plasma cells, and fibrous tissue (Figure 3B). In the adipose tissue of epicardium there are mononuclear cells with predominance of lymphocytes, which are more abundant around the nervous fibers and ganglionar cells (Figure 3C and 3D).

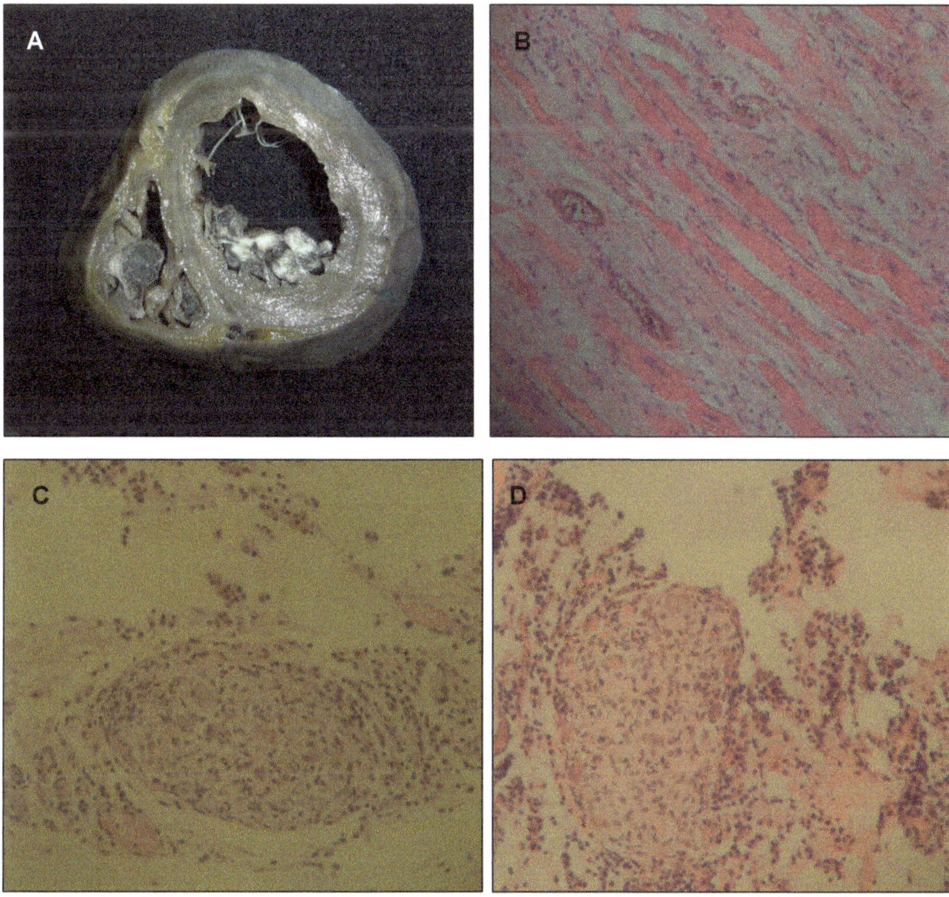

Fig. 3. Chronic Chagas heart disease A) Heart enlarged with dilatation of ventricles and mural thrombus B) Separation of the myocardial fibers, edema, abundant fibroblasts whith extracellular matrix increase, and scarce mononuclear inflammatory cells. C and D) Marked infiltration of lymphocytes and plasma cells around the nervous fibers and ganglionar neurons of cardiac plexus.

In case of oral transmission of the parasite, in the esophagus mucosa there are abundants lymphocytes and histiocytes, but the parasites are scarce or not identified (Zafra et al., 2008; Mantilla et al., 2010). In the digestive form the CD, the megaesophagus and megacolon are the result of destruction of neuronal bodies of intramural autonomic nervous ganglia of Meissner and Auerbach of the digestive tube in these sections.

4. Diagnosis and treatment

4.1 Laboratory diagnosis

The diagnosis of *T. cruzi* infection depends on the phase of infection, in the acute phase the patent parasitemia allows the use of parasitological methods to see or culture the parasite in

the first weeks. The diagnosis is difficult in the chronic phase, mainly due the very low or intermittent parasitemia, therefore, the serological methods are usual. Additionally, CD endemic areas also present endemicity of other parasites especially *Leishmania sp.* and *T. rangeli* (Gomes et al., 2009). This fact leads to the serological methods which present high sensitivity but lack of specificity because of antigenic cross-reactivity. Therefore, the World Health Organization recommends that at least two assays based on different techniques should be used. The serological methods frequently used in the diagnosis of CD are enzyme-linked immunosorbent assays (ELISA), indirect hemagglutination assays (IHA), immunofluorescence indirect assays (IFI), immunoblotting assayss (IB), and immunochromatographic assay. These methods used crude antigens but recombinant proteins and synthetic peptides are being used to improve the specificity (Hernandez et al., 2010; Praast et al., 2011; Umezawa et al., 2001; Umezawa et al., 2004).
On the other hand, molecular methods, in particular amplification by the polymerase chain reaction (PCR), provide an alternative diagnosis of CD (Gomes et al., 1999) specially to confirm diagnosis in case of inconclusive serology; in addition, it has been performed nested-PCR assays (N-PCR) (Marcon et al., 2002), quantitative real-time PCR assays (qRT-PCR) (Piron et al., 2007) and oligochromatography assays (OligoC) (Deborggraeve et al., 2009) to improve the detection of *T. cruzi* DNA.

4.2 Treatment

The treatment of CD is aimed at two main aspects: the removal of the parasite and the symptomatic management of cardiac manifestations. The options for the treatment of CD are restricted to the use of two drugs, the nifurtimox and the benznidazole. These drugs are indicated in the acute phase of infection, congenital forms, reactivation associated with immunosuppression especially in children and young adults with infections transmitted by blood transfusion and organ transplantation. Although the benznidazole have proven to be effective in the early stage of chronic infection its effectiveness at the late stage is limited. Both drugs produce serious complications such as neurological toxicity, depression, anorexia, vomiting and depression in bone marrow. Antitrypanosomal treatment in mild and late stage Chagas disease is under study by the BENEFIT trial (Rassi et al., 2010). The drug resistance is a major problem in the treatment of infectious and tropical diseases. In CD has a strong impact on the increase in the number of therapeutic failure aggravated by the few options of treatment, currently, there are numerous efforts in the search for treatment alternatives.
The amioradone is used in the management of cardiac symptoms especially for patients with sustained ventricular tachycardia, and for those with non-sustained ventricular tachycardia and myocardial dysfunction. Patients haemodynamically unstable, and those resuscitated from sudden death are treated with implantable cardioverter defibrillators (Rassi et al., 2010).

5. Pathogenesis and pathophysiology

The pathogenesis of CD is a process that is not fully understood. Most individuals infected with *T. cruzi* do not develop an acute phase and the injury to the myocardium and nervous system is directly related to tissue parasitism. The rupture of the nests of parasites in the tissues releases antigens of *T. cruzi* sensitizing cardiac and neuronal fibers, leading to the destruction of these cells by anti-*T. cruzi* response mediates by CD8+ and CD4+ lymphocytes (Palomino et al., 2000). For the chronic phase, different mechanisms have been proposed; it is currently accepted that the inflammatory response generated by the parasite, which has not been eliminated by the immune system induces chronic inflammation in some individuals leading to tissue damage (Tarleton, 2003). There are several factors that directly or indirectly contribute to the progression and therefore evolution of the CD in the host. Some of these factors are inherent to the parasite, as the virulence related to their tissue tropism, their genetic and antigenic features, others are related to the host, such as age, race, nutritional status, immune response and genetic constitution (Dutra & Gollob 2008).

5.1 Associated to *T. cruzi*

T. cruzi presents a great heterogeneity both genotypic and phenotypic (Tibayrenc et al., 1993) and consists of different populations which circulate among humans, vectors, domestic animals and wild reservoirs. These populations show different behaviors in terms of parasitaemia, virulence, pathogenicity, interactions with host cells, tissue tropism and sensitivity to drugs. *T. cruzi* has been classified into several groups, initially using biochemical markers (zymodemes) and subsequently molecular markers (esquizodemes, clonets and lineages). The last meeting of experts standardized the nomenclature of *T. cruzi* and accepted the existence of six discrete typing units (DTUs) called TCI-VI (Zingales et al., 2009). The heterogeneity of *T. cruzi* extends to the forms and severity of clinical presentation with a particular geographical distribution. In Brazil, Tc I is present in the sylvatic cycle of transmission with low parasitemia in humans and experimental animals, therefore it is considered non-virulent, except for some reports of the Amazon (Texeira et al., 2006). By contrast, in this country Tc II is involved in the domestic cycle of transmission and causes high parasitemias, human infections and both heart and gastrointestinal diseases (Zingales et al., 1998). The same behavior is observed in other southern countries of South America as Argentina, Chile, Paraguay and Uruguay. By contrast, in the northern countries of South America and Central America predominates Tc I associated with heart disease and involved in both domestic and sylvatic cycle (Higo et al., 2004). Recently, our group reported the presence for both groups for the first time, Tc I and Tc II group in blood of seropositive individuals to antigens of *T. cruzi* associated with chagasic cardiomyopathy (CC) (Zafra et al., 2008, Gonzalez et al., 2010). The two groups were also identified in tissues of deceased patients with CC, with predominance of Tc I (Zafra et al., 2011). One individual presented a mixed infection with Tc I and Tc II, but Tc II was the group associated with cardiac involvement (Mantilla et al., 2009).

5.2 Associated with the host

5.2.1 Innate immune response

In recent years, new data related with interaction between innate immune cells and *T. cruzi* have been presented. This interaction is crucial in controlling parasite replication and removal by the action of phagocytic cells, activation of antigen presenting cells and natural killer cells (NK) in the host tissue. The innate immune cells recognize pathogen associated molecular patterns (PAMPs) through their pattern recognition receptors (PRR). The best characterized PRRs are Toll-like receptors (TLRs), which are expressed in the cell membrane or are located intracellularly. When TLRs recognize microbial components, it induces signals responsible for the activation and production of inflammatory cytokines and chemokines (Akira & Takeda, 2004). In *T. cruzi*, TLR2 was the first receptor identified which recognizes glycosylphosphatidylinositol (GPI)-anchores mucin-like glycoproteins, distributed to the cell surface membrane of *T. cruzi* trypomastigotes (Campos et al., 2001). This receptor also recognizes the *T. cruzi* protein Tc52 and induces dendritic cell activation (Ouaissi et al., 2002). The TLR4-MD2 complex recognizes glycoinositolphospholipids containig ceramide (GIPL) (Bafica et al., 2006) and TLR9 recognizes DNA rich in CpG sequences. The TLR-mediated MyD88 signaling pathway induces pro-inflammatory cytokines as TNF-α and IL-12 and stimulates the production of nitric oxide (NO) involved in parasite clearance (Bafica et al., 2006). Other mechanisms for the TLR- independent recognition of *T. cruzi* have been described and involved the molecule NOD1 that induces type I IFNs (Kayama & Takeda, 2010). Innate immunity in turn acts as an immunomodulatory specific immune response through the generation of the microenvironment of cytokines that regulates the differentiation of effector T cell subpopulations (Bilate & Cunha-Neto, 2008, Dutra et al., 2009).

5.2.2 Adaptative immune response

The role of the adaptative immune response in the pathogenesis of CD has been subject of much controversy, for decades the role of the autoimmune component was accepted as directly responsible for heart damage (Takle & Hudson, 1989). This was supported by the detection of autoantibodies against cardiac antigens, chronicity and difficulty of finding parasites in affected individuals (Cunha-Neto et al., 1995). However, the development of more sensitive molecular tests that allowed detection of low numbers of parasites, the fact that immunosuppressed patients developed acute and severe CD and experimental models showed that the parasite, even in small amounts was essential for the development of the disease (Zhang & Tarleton, 1999; Tarleton, 2003). The presence of autoantibodies may be explained by the release of autoantigens as the result of the immune response against the parasite (Cunha-Neto et al., 1995).

Currently, the role of chronic inflammation and unbalance of the immune response generated by the parasite is accepted as responsible for the damage and tissue regeneration associated with organ dysfunction (Dutra & Gollob 2008). Although heart inflammatory cells contribute to control parasite growth, they are also involved in perpetuating inflammatory infiltrate. In chagasic patients the cellular infiltrate consists mainly of T lymphocytes with a predominance of CD8+ cells but also contains CD4+ cells and macrophages. Both CD8+ cell and CD4+ exhibit characteristics of activated T cells and correlate with the expression of inflammatory cytokines such as TNF-α and INF-γ and a smaller number of regulatory cells producing IL-10 (Araújo et al., 2007). Patients with chronic CC have higher serum levels of TNF-α and CCL2 compared with asymptomatic individuals (Talvani et al., 2004). In this context, cytokines, chemokines, receptors and signaling pathways associated with activation of pro-inflammatory proteins and with low expression of immunoregulatory proteins will be clearly associated with the immunopathogenesis of CD. This coupled with the fact that most infected individuals remain asymptomatic throughout life and only between 15 to 30% of them developed the disease demonstrates the importance of host genetic component. Thus individuals with genetic predisposition to proinflammatory phenotype in the presence of *T. cruzi* would be those that develop chronic and severe forms of the disease.

6. Chagas disease as a complex disease

6.1 Human genome variation

The variation in the human genome sequence plays an important role, yet little known in the etiology of many diseases. The establishment of the association between genotype and phenotype is crucial for understanding biological processes and in the case of disease, pathogenic mechanisms that lead to their development. For monogenic diseases, the methods of genetic linkage and physical maps facilitated the identification of mutations responsible for the phenotype associated with pathology. Thus numerous Mendelian-type diseases were identified. However, most common diseases are complex and multifactorials therefore, are the result of the effect of multiple genetic variants on the phenotype and their interaction with environmental factors. In the case of infectious diseases is known that not only the genotypic and phenotypic differences of the microorganism determine the development of a particular disease, but also the variation in the host genome may have an important role in the development of resistance or susceptibility.

6.2 Single nucleotide polymorphisms (SNP)

SNP type polymorphisms are the most common forms of genetic variation in the human genome, currently the common SNPs estimated density is about 10 to 15 million (The International HapMap Consortium 2007, http://www.hapmap.org). Its usefulness as genetic markers associated with various infectious and noninfectious diseases has been amply demonstrated (Pacheco & Moraes, 2009). The SNPs have been the markers most commonly used for its stability, low mutation rate and are plentiful throughout the genome, being found in exons affecting the protein function, in introns or regulatory regions affecting gene expression and therefore the processing and maturation of the messenger, or many of them have been identified in intergenic regions with effect unknown over gene expression or phenotype (Frazer et al., 2009). Numerous reports using one or more polymorphisms have been published (Pacheco & Moraes, 2009), but most of them only explain less than 5% of the observed contribution of the genetic component to the risk of disease. This fact substantially limits the use of these markers to predict risk and in some cases the results have been controversial. One of the main problems with these studies is that in many cases it is not known a direct effect on the phenotype and in common diseases the effect is modest. Therefore, it is necessary to identify other variables involved and the interaction among them (Feero et al., 2010). Another limitation in this type of study is related to the number of SNPs, which in an individual genome is from 3 to 4 million and in the human genome it is estimated between 10 to 11 million (Frazer et al., 2009). Thus an individual would require testing thousands of polymorphisms to identify genes involved in susceptibility to a particular pathology.

The International HapMap Project (The International HapMap Consortium 2003-2007) has overcome some of the difficulties in mapping SNPs and identification of susceptibility genes in complex diseases. The advances are related with the reduction in the number of SNPs to be genotyped, increased statistical power and the accurate mapping in association studies. This project HapMap anticipates building a database for common haplotypes in different human populations (www.hapmap.org). When the markers are in linkage disequilibrium (LD) in the population, there is redundant information. If two markers are in complete LD, each of the genotypes of a SNP is completely determined by the other, thus the genotyping of one will suffice for the information of the two (Conrad et al., 2006). The selection of non-redundant markers present in an area with high density of markers has been called "haplotype tagging" and the SNPs selected by this method are called "tag-SNPs" or label SNP (de Baker et al., 2006). The main objective of this haplotype tagging is to reduce the number and cost of genotyping, keeping most of the information that they contain (Daly et al., 2001). The technological progress in the last decade, related to the development of high density maps of markers, maps of linkage disequilibrium and haplotypes (Cardon & Abecasis, 2003), the use of microarrays for genotyping of SNPs (Steemers & Gunderson, 2007) and bioinformatics tools have helped overcome some of these difficulties. Based on these developments, in recent years the genome scans (GWAS) have popularized (Cheung et al., 2005; Galvan et al., 2010). In fact, after 5 years of the first GWAS, which identified the association of complement factor H with macular degeneration related to age (Klein et al., 2005) there have been published more than 450 GWAS and associations with more than 2000 SNPs in numerous human diseases such as type 1 and 2 diabetes, Crohn's disease, rheumatoid arthritis, prostate cancer, breast, tuberculosis and visceral leishmaniasis among many others (Manolio 2010; Ku et al., 2010). Many of these studies have identified markers on genes already known for its role in the pathogenesis of the disease, but others have also identified strong associations with genes that apparently have not relation with the characteristic of the disease process (Frazer et al., 2009).

6.3 Human genome variation in Chagas disease

The chronic CD courses in 70% of individuals without symptoms and only between 15-30% of infected individuals have cardiac involvement and/or digestive, with different levels of severity and mortality. This clearly suggests the role of the individual genetic component in disease development, a fact that is reinforced with the identification of strains of mice with different susceptibility phenotypes. The C3H strain develops cardiac lesions similar to human chagasic cardiomyopathy, the A/J phenotype presents different pathology and DBA/2 is totally resistant (Marinho et al., 2004). The association related with genetic susceptibility or resistance to infection with *T. cruzi* in human has been demonstrated in some epidemiological studies related to the molecules of the major histocompatibility complex (MHC) (Llop et al., 1991; Fernández-Mestre et al., 1998; Nieto et al., 2000; Layrisse et al., 2000; Williams-Blangero et al., 2003; Moreno et al., 2004).

The identification of biomarkers to establish an association with the risk of developing the disease is critical because could be used not only in prevention and prognosis but also as a therapeutic target. It is now clearly accepted that the immune response is crucial in the pathogenesis of CD and especially the role of the chronic inflammation in the tissular damage (Dutra & Gollob 2008). The balance between anti-inflammatory and pro-inflammatory cytokines and their receptors is crucial in determining whether *T. cruzi* parasites will be eliminated without causing tissue damage. Thus, the lack of efficient immunoregulation in cardiomyopathic patients could contribute to clinical forms of CD. In this sense, case-control studies have searched association between onset or severity of the disease and the functional polymorphisms of genes known to participate in host inflammatory response.

6.3.1 Variation in pro-inflamatory cytokines

In CD, it has been observed that patients infected with *T. cruzi* display increased levels of plasma TNF-α compared to non-infected individuals, where plasma TNF-α levels were 4-fold higher in asymptomatic and cardiomyopathic patients with left ventricular ejection fraction (LVEF) >50% and 8-fold higher cardiomyopathic patients with LVEF ≤50% than non-infected individuals (Ferreira et al., 2003). In fact, the measurement of TNF-α level has been suggested as a tool to identify patients with heart dysfunction (Talvani et al., 2004).

Some positive associations have been observed in Mexican and Brazilian populations, between polymorphisms of regulatory region of *TNFA* gene and CC (Rodríguez-Pérez et al., 2005; Drigo et al., 2006; Pissetti et al., 2011). The most studied allelic form (*TNFA* -308) has functional implication because it affects the TNF-α level. However, discrepancies have been observed with Peruvian and Brazilian populations in which the frequencies of genetic variants were similar in asymptomatic individuals and CC patients (Beraún et al., 1998; Drigo et al., 2007). These differences could be affected by some factors. Among the most important factors would be: sample size, genetic differences between populations, criteria for the selection of controls (study design), linkage disequilibrium with HLA genes and influence of other polymorphisms present in the same region. Some polymorphisms of *TNFA* gene show a high level of LD, and the haplotypes formed by these variants could be affecting levels of protein expression (Figure 4). In Colombian population of highly endemic area we also found associations with genetic variants in *TNFA* and *TNFR2* genes (Criado et al., publication process). Unlike other chronic inflammatory diseases such as rheumatoid arthritis in which the blocking of TNF-α has been used successfully in treatment, in CD the experimental evidence using animal models showed that TNF-α blockade enhances left ventricular dysfunction (Bilate et al., 2007). Therefore, it is necessary to understand the regulation of the expression of TNF-α and its receptors and the effect of host polymorphisms for the use of therapeutic strategies with target TNF-α.

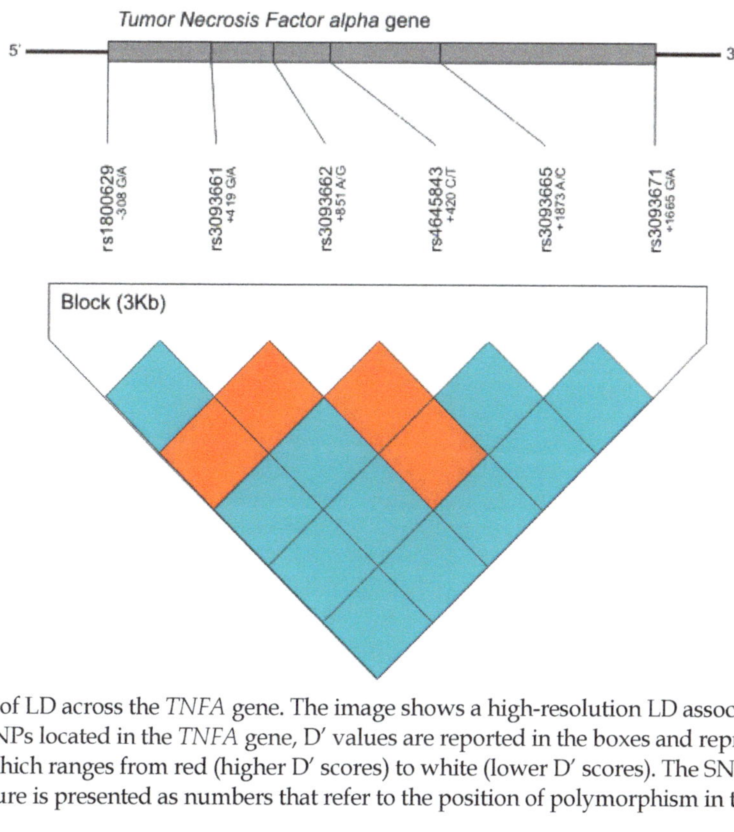

Fig. 4. Plot of LD across the *TNFA* gene. The image shows a high-resolution LD association plot between SNPs located in the *TNFA* gene, D′ values are reported in the boxes and represented by color, which ranges from red (higher D′ scores) to white (lower D′ scores). The SNP nomenclature is presented as numbers that refer to the position of polymorphism in the gene.

In our study population we also found associations of functional polymorphisms present in other pro-inflammatory cytokine genes such as *IL1B* (Flórez et al., 2006), *IL12B* (Zafra et al., 2007), *IFNG* (Torres et al., 2010), and lack of association with *IL6* (Torres et al., 2010) (Table 1).

6.3.2 Variation in chemokines and chemokine receptors

The inflammatory infiltrate of mononuclear cell is driven by a set of specific chemokines that determine the type of cells present in the tissue. Chemokines and chemokine receptors play an important role in mediating the extravasation and accumulation of specific effector and memory cells in chronic inflammatory processes in several diseases. In CD there is experimental evidence in patients with CC and models of *T. cruzi* infection that show that chemokines and chemokine receptors may be relevant mediators of leukocyte influx, which is involved in the pathogenesis of the disease (Teixeira et al., 2002; Marino et al., 2004; Talvani et al., 2004; Machado et al., 2005; Gomes et al., 2005; Guedes et al., 2010; Manque et al., 2011). Genetic variants in genes of chemokine receptors as *CCR5* have been also studied in Peruvian and Venezuelan populations with the identification of a protection marker (Calzada et al., 2001; Fernandez-Mestre et al., 2004). *CCR5* gene polymorphisms had been extensively studied in HIV and have been defined haplogroups which are affecting the transcriptional activity (Gonzalez et al., 1999). These haplogroups are composed by different combinations of *CCR2* and *CCR5* SNPs (Figure 5). Analyzing individual polymorphisms we found association between *CCR5*-2733 polymorphism and CC and also in four variants present in haplogroup HHE (*CCR2* +190, *CCR5* -2733, -2554 and -1835).

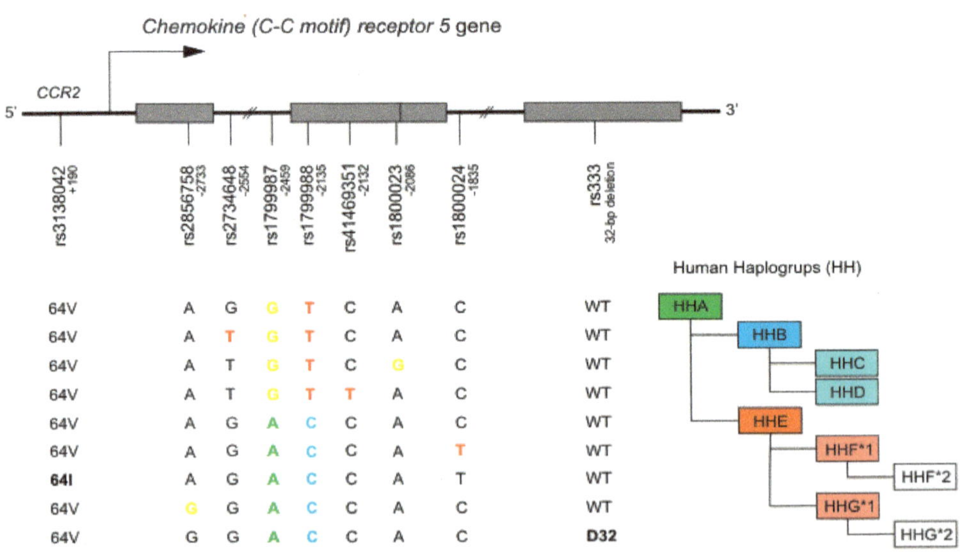

Fig. 5. Human haplogroups of *CCR2* and *CCR5* polymorphisms.

No association was observed with polymorphisms analysed in the chemokines *CCL5* and *CXCL8* genes (Flórez et al., publication process). The genetic variant -2518 in the chemokine *CCL2/MCPI* promotor gene was associated with CC in Brazilian population (Ramasawmy et al., 2009).

6.3.3 Variation in anti-inflammatory cytokines

Monocytes of patients with the indeterminate form, but not patients with CC showed high expression of interleukin 10, suggesting a lack of immunoregulation in these patients (Costa el al., 2009; D'Avila et al., 2009). The anti-inflammatory cytokines, such as interleukin 4 and IL-10, promote Th2 differentiation and limit Th1 response (Jankovic et al., 2001). This polarization favors the permanence of the parasite in the myocardium but keeps the inflammatory response under control, which appears to be important for avoiding the development of CC (Higuchi et al., 2003; Cunha-Neto et al., 2005). Different groups have found markers associated with decreased production of anti-inflammatory cytokines in patients with CC (Costa et al., 2009). We have analyzed other genes of regulatory proteins, such as *TGFB1* (Calzada et al., 2009), *MIF* (Torres et al., 2009), *IL4, IL4RA* and *IL10* (Florez et al., 2011) which are associatted with CC. However, in the latter gene we were unable to demonstrate association between *IL10* gene polymorphism and CD. Other pro-inflammatory and anti-inflammatory genes have been analyzed, such as *BAT1* and *IKBL/NFKBIL1, MAL/TIRAP* (Ramasawmy et al., 2006 and 2009), *PTPN22* (Robledo et al., 2007), *CTLA4* (Fernandez-Mestre et al, 2009) (Table 1).
There are few reports of genome mapping applied to the study of CD in murine models which showed a possible region of susceptibility to the disease directly related with survival to infection in the murine H-2 locus, which corresponds to the human Major Histocompatibility Complex (MHC) located in chromosome 17 (Wrightsman et al., 1984). In a more recent study, the entire genome of mice strains susceptible and resistant were mapping at intervals of 10-15 cM with microsatellite. The regions with marked influence in the severity of CD, are mainly located on chromosome 17 on the murine MHC, but were also identified as candidate regions on chromosomes 5 and 13 (Graefe et al., 2003, 2006). In humans, chromosomal mapping studies on CD have not been reported. All this evidence showing the association of multiple genes and the development of CD, as in other infectious and noninfectious diseases, suggests that susceptibility/resistance to develop CD would be determined by variations in a large number of polymorphic genes. In fact, a single SNP can not fully explain the susceptibility or resistance to a complex disease. Therefore, the genetic susceptibility to *T. cruzi* infection and the development of cardiomyopathy is complex and heterogeneous and likely to involve multiple genes, each with a modest contribution on the pathogenesis of the disease. The availability of high throughput methods enabling of genotyping individual DNA samples at 500,000 or more loci using SNP chip have led to genome wide association studies (GWAS) of more than 40 diseases and human phenotypes (Manolio, 2010). Despite the current limitations and the adjustments of bioinformatic tools for analyzing this vast amount of information, these studies of genomic medicine would allow in a near future obtain the individual genetic profiles and define the genes underlying the phenotype associated with the disease and its severity.

Genes	SNP	Population	Association	Reference
Innate immunity				
TLR 2	R753Q	Colombian	negative	Zafra
TLR4, TLR9	D299G, -1237	Colombian	negative	Zafra
TLR 1,2,4,9	I602S, R753Q, D299G, R392stop codon, -1237, -1486	Brazilian	negative	Ramasawmy
MAL/TIRAP	S180L	Brazilian	CC	Ramasawmy
Pro-inflamatory genes				
NOS	microsatélite	Peruvian	negative	Calzada
NRAMP	-236	Peruvian	negative	Calzada
TNFA	-308	Peruvian	negative	Beraún
		Mexican	CC	Rodriguez-Pérez
		Brazilian	negative	Drigo
		Brazilian	negative	Pissetti
		Colombian	CC	Criado
	-238	Peruvian	negative	Beraún
		Mexican	negative	Rodriguez-Pérez
		Brazilian	negative	Drigo
		Brazilian	CC	Pissetti
	-1031	Colombian	negative	Criado
TNFR2	+676 (M196R)	Colombian	monomorphic	Criado
LTA	+80, +252	Brazilian		Ramasawmy
IL1B	+5810	Colombian	CC	Flórez
	-31,-511, +3954	Colombian	negative	Flórez
		Mexican		Cruz-Robles
IL1RN	+8006, +8061, +11100	Colombian	negative	Flórez
		Mexican		Cruz-Robles
IL1A	-889, +4845	Colombian	negative	Flórez
IL12B	+1188	Colombian	CC	Zafra
IFGN	+874	Colombian	CC	Torres
IL6	-174	Colombian, Peruvian	negative	Torres
CCR5	59029, Δ32	Peruvian	negative	Calzada
	59029, Δ32	Venezuelan	negative	Fernández-Mestre
	-2733, -2554	Colombian	CC	Flórez
CCL2/MCPI	-2518	Brazilian	CC	Ramasawmy
Anti-inflamatory genes				
BAT1	-22, 348	Brazilian	CC	Ramasawmy
IKBL/NFKBIL1	-62, -262	Brazilian	CC	Ramasawmy
IL10	-1082	Brazilian	CC	Costa
	-1082, -819, -592	Colombian	negative	Flórez
PTPN22	1858	Colombian, Peruvian	negative	Robledo
MIF	-173	Colombian, Peruvian	CC	Torres
TGFB	-988, -800, -509, +263	Colombian, Peruvian	negative	Torres
	+10	Colombian, Peruvian	CC	Torres
CTLA4	+49	Venezuelan	negative	Fernández-Mestre
IL4	-590	Colombian	negative	Flórez
IL4RA	+148	Colombian	CC	Flórez
	1124, 1218, 1902	Colombian	negative	Flórez

Table 1. Polymorphisms of immune response genes studied in Chagas Disease

6.4 Host-parasite interaction, changes in gene expression by the infectious process

The infection process involves changes in host cell gene expression caused by the parasite. Therefore, transcriptional profiling is frequently used as a genome-wide tool to screen for the impact of pathogens on host cell functions (Costales et al., 2009). This approach that analyzes the differential expression to identify genes or proteins related with the pathogenesis is widely used in different pathologies. Taking advantages of microarray expression platform comparisons are made between healthy and sick individuals or between strains of susceptible or resistant animal models or between infected and uninfected cells. Currently, two approachs have been integrated so that data from microarrays can be analyzed in the context of the Quantitative Trait Loci (QTLs), a strategy called genetic genomics (Jansen & Nap 2001; Nica et al., 2010). Genetics Genomics is a powerful tool to elucidate the basis of complex traits and disease susceptibility that integrates genotype and phenotype information (Pérez-Enciso et al., 2007).

In CD studies using different cell lines infected with *T. cruzi* or tissues from diseased individuals compared to healthy tissue have been realized. This allowed to identify an increased number of over-expressed genes associated with immune response, such as growth factors, immunoglobulins, cytokines and genes related with cell membrane, lipid metabolism and oxidative phosphorylation (Graefe et al., 2006; Mukherjee et al., 2003; Mukherjee et al., 2006). More recently in several human cell lines was observed overexpression of cytokines with higher overexpression of interferon-stimulated genes and also independent genes of cytokines (Costales, 2009). An analysis of gene expression in heart tissue of five patients with CC and seven with dilated cardiomyopathy suggests that genes of immune response, lipid metabolism and mitochondrial oxidative phosphorylation could be involved in the development of heart failure (Cunha-Neto, 2005). In mice models, myocarditis was associated with immune-inflammatory responses (chemokines, adhesion molecules, cathepsins, and MHC molecules), and fibrosis was associated with extracellular matrix components, lysyl oxidase, and tissue inhibitor of metalloproteinase (Soares et al., 2010). With this approach, our group performed a study for determining differential expression patterns in T lymphocytes of individuals with or without CC. Using the Gen Ontology (GO) tool we could establish the biological pathways associated with over-expression in immune response genes, cell signaling and structure of cardiac tissue. Therefore, genetic genomic strategy could allow establish and identify the risk genotype and phenotype of the patient. In addition would make it possible to identify gene interaction networks responsible for the development of CD.

7. Perspectives

For the control of CD should be used not only the traditional approachs of public health with campaigns to eradicate the domiciled vector, control of transmission in blood banks, and now oral transmission, but implement and promote the use of new developments in genomics, proteomics and pharmacogenomics. The association studies and genetic genomic can provide information to identify genes related with disease development and so develop not only prevention and control programs but identify potential targets for treatment and vaccine design.

8. References

Akira, S., & Takeda, K. (2004).Toll-like receptor signalling. *Nat Rev Immunol*, Vol.4, No.7, (July 2004), pp. 499-511, ISSN 1474-1733

Alarcon de Noya, B.; Diaz-Bello, Z.; Colmenares, C., et al. (2010). Large urban outbreak of orally acquired acute Chagas disease at a school in Caracas, Venezuela.*J Infect Dis*, Vol.201, No.9, (March 2010), pp. 1308-1315, ISSN 1537-6613

Araujo, F.F.; Gomes, J.A.; Rocha, M.O., et al. (2007). Potential role of CD4+CD25HIGH regulatory T cells in morbidity in Chagas disease. *Front Biosci*, Vol.12, (May 2007), pp. 2797-2806, ISSN 1093-4715

Aufderheide, A.C.; Salo, W.; Madden, M., et al. (2004). A 9,000-year record of Chagas' disease.*Proc Natl Acad Sci U S A*, Vol.101, No.7, (February 2004), pp. 2034-2039, ISSN 0027-8424

Bafica, A.; Santiago, H.C.; Goldszmid, R., et al. (2006). Cutting edge: TLR9 and TLR2 signaling together account for MyD88-dependent control of parasitemia in Trypanosoma cruzi infection. *J Immunol*, Vol.177, No.6, (September 2006), pp. 3515-3519, ISSN 0022-1767

Barcan, L.; Luna, C.; Clara, L., et al. (2005). Transmission of T. cruzi infection via liver transplantation to a nonreactive recipient for Chagas' disease. *Liver Transpl*, Vol.11, No.9, (Augusts 2005), pp. 1112-1116, ISSN 1527-6465

Beraun, Y.; Nieto, A.; Collado, M.D., et al. (1998). Polymorphisms at tumor necrosis factor (TNF) loci are not associated with Chagas' disease. *Tissue Antigens*, Vol.52, No.1, (August 1998), pp. 81-83, ISSN 0001-2815

Bern, C., & Montgomery, S.P. (2009). An estimate of the burden of Chagas disease in the United States.*Clin Infect Dis*, Vol.49, No.5, (July 2009), pp. e52-54, ISSN 1537-6591

Bilate, A.M., & Cunha-Neto, E. (2008). Chagas disease cardiomyopathy: current concepts of an old disease. *Rev Inst Med Trop Sao Paulo*, Vol.50, No.2, (May 2008), pp. 67-74, ISSN 0036-4665

Brener, Z. (1971). Life cycle of Trypanosoma cruzi.*Rev Inst Med Trop Sao Paulo*, Vol.13, No.3, (May 1971), pp. 171-178, ISSN 0036-4665

Briceno-Leon, R. (2009). Chagas disease in the Americas: an ecohealth perspective. *Cad Saude Publica*, Vol.25 Suppl 1, (March 2009), pp. S71-82, ISSN 1678-4464

Calzada, J.E.; Beraun, Y.; Gonzalez, C.I., et al. (2009). Transforming growth factor beta 1 (TGFbeta1) gene polymorphisms and Chagas disease susceptibility in Peruvian and Colombian patients. *Cytokine*, Vol.45, No.3, (January 2009), pp. 149-153, ISSN 1096-0023

Calzada, J.E.; Nieto, A.; Beraun, Y., et al. (2001). Chemokine receptor CCR5 polymorphisms and Chagas' disease cardiomyopathy.*Tissue Antigens*, Vol.58, No.3, (November 2001), pp. 154-158, ISSN 0001-2815

Campos, M.A.; Almeida, I.C.; Takeuchi, O., et al. (2001). Activation of Toll-like receptor-2 by glycosylphosphatidylinositol anchors from a protozoan parasite. *J Immunol*, Vol.167, No.1, (June 2001), pp. 416-423, ISSN 0022-1767

Cardon, L.R., &Abecasis, G.R. (2003). Using haplotype blocks to map human complex trait loci. *Trends Genet*, Vol.19, No.3, (March 2003), pp. 135-140, ISSN 0168-9525

Conrad, D.F.; Jakobsson, M.; Coop, G., et al. (2006).A worldwide survey of haplotype variation and linkage disequilibrium in the human genome. *Nat Genet*, Vol.38, No.11, (October 2006), pp. 1251-1260, ISSN 1061-4036

Cordova, E.; Boschi, A.; Ambrosioni, J., et al. (2008). Reactivation of Chagas disease with central nervous system involvement in HIV-infected patients in Argentina, 1992-2007.*Int J Infect Dis*, Vol.12, No.6, (March 2008), pp. 587-592, ISSN 1878-3511

Costa, G.C.; da Costa Rocha, M.O.; Moreira, P.R., et al. (2009). Functional IL-10 gene polymorphism is associated with Chagas disease cardiomyopathy. *J Infect Dis*, Vol.199, No.3, (December 2008), pp. 451-454, ISSN 0022-1899

Costales, J.A.; Daily, J.P., &Burleigh, B.A. (2009). Cytokine-dependent and-independent gene expression changes and cell cycle block revealed in Trypanosoma cruzi-infected host cells by comparative mRNA profiling. *BMC Genomics*, Vol.10, (June 2009), pp. 252, ISSN 1471-2164

Coura, J.R. (2007). Chagas disease: what is known and what is needed--a background article. *Mem Inst Oswaldo Cruz*, Vol.102 Suppl 1, (December 2007), pp. 113-122, ISSN 0074-0276

Coura, J.R.; Junqueira, A.C.; Fernandes, O., et al. (2002). Emerging Chagas disease in Amazonian Brazil. *Trends Parasitol*, Vol.18, No.4, (May 2002), pp. 171-176, ISSN 1471-4922

Cunha-Neto, E.;Duranti, M.; Gruber, A., et al. (1995). Autoimmunity in Chagas disease cardiopathy: biological relevance of a cardiac myosin-specific epitope crossreactive to an immunodominantTrypanosomacruzi antigen. *Proc Natl Acad Sci U S A*, Vol.92, No.8, (April 1995), pp. 3541-3545, ISSN 0027-8424

Cunha-Neto, E.; Dzau, V.J.; Allen, P.D., et al. (2005). Cardiac gene expression profiling provides evidence for cytokinopathy as a molecular mechanism in Chagas' disease cardiomyopathy. *Am J Pathol*, Vol.167, No.2, (July 2005), pp. 305-313, ISSN 0002-9440

Cheung, V.G.; Spielman, R.S.; Ewens, K.G., et al. (2005). Mapping determinants of human gene expression by regional and genome-wide association. *Nature*, Vol.437, No.7063, (October 2005), pp. 1365-1369, ISSN 1476-4687

D'Avila, D.A.; Guedes, P.M.; Castro, A.M., et al. (2009). Immunological imbalance between IFN-gamma and IL-10 levels in the sera of patients with the cardiac form of Chagas disease.*Mem Inst Oswaldo Cruz*, Vol.104, No.1, (March 2009), pp. 100-105, ISSN 1678-8060

Daly, M.J.; Rioux, J.D.; Schaffner, S.F., et al. (2001). High-resolution haplotype structure in the human genome.*Nat Genet*, Vol.29, No.2, (October 2001), pp. 229-232, ISSN 1061-4036

de Bakker, P.I.; Burtt, N.P.; Graham, R.R., et al. (2006). Transferability of tag SNPs in genetic association studies in multiple populations. *Nat Genet*, Vol.38, No.11, (October 2006), pp. 1298-1303, ISSN 1061-4036

Deborggraeve, S.; Coronado, X.; Solari, A., et al. (2009). T. cruziOligoC-TesT: a simplified and standardized polymerase chain reaction format for diagnosis of Chagas disease. *PloS Negl Trop Dis*, Vol.3, No.6, (June 2009), pp. e450, ISSN 1935-2735

Díaz, M.L.; Flórez, O.; Mantilla, J.C.; Ramírez, A.N.; Hernández, L.M. Gualdrón, L.; García, C. & González, C.I. (2009). Brote de Chagas agudo en Santander: casos fatales asociados con probable transmision oral. *Biomédica*, Vol.29, (Supl1), pp. 210-211, ISSN 0120-4157

Dias, J.C. (1989). The indeterminate form of human chronic Chagas' disease A clinical epidemiological review. *Rev Soc Bras Med Trop*, Vol.22, No.3, (July 1989), pp. 147-156, ISSN 0037-8682

Drigo, S.A.; Cunha-Neto, E.;Ianni, B., et al. (2006). TNF gene polymorphisms are associated with reduced survival in severe Chagas' disease cardiomyopathy patients. *Microbes Infect*, Vol.8, No.3, (January 2006), pp. 598-603, ISSN 1286-4579

Drigo, S.A.; Cunha-Neto, E.;Ianni, B., et al. (2007). Lack of association of tumor necrosis factor-alpha polymorphisms with Chagas disease in Brazilian patients. *Immunol Lett*, Vol.108, No.1, (December 2006), pp. 109-111, ISSN 0165-2478

Dutra, W.O., &Gollob, K.J. (2008). Current concepts in immunoregulation and pathology of human Chagas disease.*Curr Opin Infect Dis*, Vol.21, No.3, (May 2008), pp. 287-292, ISSN 0951-7375

Dutra, W.O.; Menezes, C.A.; Villani, F.N., et al. (2009). Cellular and genetic mechanisms involved in the generation of protective and pathogenic immune responses in human Chagas disease. *Mem Inst Oswaldo Cruz*, Vol.104 Suppl 1, (September 2009), pp. 208-218, ISSN 1678-8060

Feero, W.G.; Guttmacher, A.E., & Collins, F.S. (2010). Genomic medicine--an updated primer.*N Engl J Med*, Vol.362, No.21, (May 2010), pp. 2001-2011, ISSN 1533-4406

Fernandez-Mestre, M.T.; Layrisse, Z.; Montagnani, S., et al. (1998). Influence of the HLA class II polymorphism in chronic Chagas' disease. *Parasite Immunol*, Vol.20, No.4, (June 1998), pp. 197-203, ISSN 0141-9838

Fernandez-Mestre, M.T.; Montagnani, S., &Layrisse, Z. (2004). Is the CCR5-59029-G/G genotype a protective factor for cardiomyopathy in Chagas disease? *Hum Immunol*, Vol.65, No.7, (August 2004), pp. 725-728, ISSN 0198-8859

Fernandez-Mestre, M.; Sanchez, K.;Balbas, O., et al. (2009). Influenceof CTLA-4 gene polymorphism in autoimmune and infectious diseases. *Hum Immunol*, Vol.70, No.7, (April 2009), pp. 532-535, ISSN 1879-1166

Ferreira, R.C.; Ianni, B.M.; Abel, L.C., et al. (2003). Increased plasma levels of tumor necrosis factor-alpha in asymptomatic/"indeterminate" and Chagas disease cardiomyopathy patients. *Mem Inst Oswaldo Cruz*, Vol.98, No.3, (July 2003), pp. 407-411, ISSN 0074-0276

Florez, O.; Zafra, G.; Morillo, C., et al. (2006). Interleukin-1 gene cluster polymorphism in chagas disease in a Colombian case-control study. *Hum Immunol*, Vol.67, No.9, (September 2006), pp. 741-748, ISSN 0198-8859

Florez, O.; Martin, J., & Gonzalez, C.I. (2011). Interleukin 4, interleukin 4 receptor-alpha and interleukin 10 gene polymorphisms in Chagas disease.*Parasite Immunol*, Vol.(July 2011), pp. 1-6, ISSN 1365-3024

Frazer, K.A.; Murray, S.S.; Schork, N.J., et al. (2009).Human genetic variation and its contribution to complex traits. *Nat Rev Genet*, Vol.10, No.4, (March 2009), pp. 241-251, ISSN 1471-0064

Galvan, A.; Falvella, F.S.; Frullanti, E., et al. (2010). Genome-wide association study in discordant sibships identifies multiple inherited susceptibility alleles linked to lung cancer. *Carcinogenesis*, Vol.31, No.3, (December 2009), pp. 462-465, ISSN 1460-2180

Gascon, J.; Bern, C., & Pinazo, M.J. (2010). Chagas disease in Spain, the United States and other non-endemic countries.*Acta Trop*, Vol.115, No.1-2, (August 2009), pp. 22-27, ISSN 1873-6254

Gomes, J.A.; Bahia-Oliveira, L.M.; Rocha, M.O., et al. (2005). Type 1 chemokine receptor expression in Chagas' disease correlates with morbidity in cardiac patients. *Infect Immun*, Vol.73, No.12, (November 2005), pp. 7960-7966, ISSN 0019-9567

Gomes, M.L.; Galvao, L.M.; Macedo, A.M., et al. (1999). Chagas' disease diagnosis: comparative analysis of parasitologic, molecular, and serologic methods. *Am J Trop Med Hyg*, Vol.60, No.2, (March 1999), pp. 205-210, ISSN 0002-9637

Gomes, Y.M.; Lorena, V.M., &Luquetti, A.O. (2009). Diagnosis of Chagas disease: what has been achieved? What remains to be done with regard to diagnosis and follow up studies? *Mem Inst Oswaldo Cruz*, Vol.104 Suppl 1, (September 2009), pp. 115-121, ISSN 1678-8060

Gonzalez, C.I.; Ortiz, S., & Solari, A. (2010).Colombian Trypanosoma cruzi major genotypes circulating in patients: minicircle homologies by cross-hybridization analysis. *Int J Parasitol*, Vol.40, No.14, (August 2010), pp. 1685-1692, ISSN 1879-0135

Gonzalez, E.; Bamshad, M.; Sato, N., et al. (1999). Race-specific HIV-1 disease-modifying effects associated with CCR5 haplotypes. *Proc Natl Acad Sci U S A*, Vol.96, No.21, (October 1999), pp. 12004-12009, ISSN 0027-8424

Graefe, S.E.; Meyer, B.S.; Muller-Myhsok, B., et al. (2003). Murine susceptibility to Chagas' disease maps to chromosomes 5 and 17. *Genes Immun*, Vol.4, No.5, (July 2003), pp. 321-325, ISSN 1466-4879

Graefe, S.E.; Streichert, T.; Budde, B.S., et al. (2006). Genes from Chagas susceptibility loci that are differentially expressed in T. cruzi-resistant mice are candidates accounting for impaired immunity. *PLoS One*, Vol.1, (December 2006), pp. e57, 1932-6203

Guedes, P.M.; Veloso, V.M.; Talvani, A., et al. (2010). Increased type 1 chemokine expression in experimental Chagas disease correlates with cardiac pathology in beagle dogs. *Vet Immunol Immunopathol*, Vol.138, No.1-2, (July 2010), pp. 106-113, ISSN 1873-2534

Guhl, F. (2007).Chagas disease in Andean countries.*Mem.Inst.Oswaldo Cruz*, Vol.102 Suppl 1, (September 2007), pp. 29-38, ISSN 0074-0276

Guhl, F.; Jaramillo, C.; Vallejo, G.A., et al. (1999). Isolation of Trypanosoma cruzi DNA in 4,000-year-old mummified human tissue from northern Chile. *Am J Phys Anthropol*, Vol.108, No.4, (May 1999) pp. 401-407, ISSN 0002-9483

Hernandez, P.; Heimann, M.; Riera, C., et al. (2010).Highly effective serodiagnosis for Chagas' disease.*Clin Vaccine Immunol*, Vol.17, No.10, (July 2010), pp. 1598-1604, ISSN 1556-679X

Higo, H.; Miura, S.; Horio, M., et al. (2004). Genotypic variation among lineages of Trypanosoma cruzi and its geographic aspects. *Parasitol Int*, Vol.53, No.4, (July 2004), pp. 337-344, ISSN 1383-5769

Higuchi Mde, L.; Benvenuti, L.A.; Martins Reis, M., et al. (2003). Pathophysiology of the heart in Chagas' disease: current status and new developments. *Cardiovasc Res*, Vol.60, No.1, (October 2003), pp. 96-107, ISSN 0008-6363

Jankovic, D.; Sher, A., & Yap, G. (2001). Th1/Th2 effector choice in parasitic infection: decision making by committee. *Curr Opin Immunol*, Vol.13, No.4, (August 2001), pp. 403-409, ISSN 0952-7915

Jansen, R.C., & Nap, J.P. (2001). Genetical genomics: the added value from segregation. *Trends Genet*, Vol.17, No.7, (June 2001), pp. 388-391, ISSN 0168-9525

Kayama, H., & Takeda, K. (2010).The innate immune response to Trypanosoma cruzi infection.*Microbes Infect*, Vol.12, No.7, (March 2010), pp. 511-517, ISSN 1769-714X

Klein, R.J.; Zeiss, C.; Chew, E.Y., et al. (2005). Complement factor H polymorphism in age-related macular degeneration. *Science*, Vol.308, No.5720, (March 2005), pp. 385-389, ISSN 1095-9203

Ku, C.S.; Loy, E.Y.; Pawitan, Y., et al. (2010). The pursuit of genome-wide association studies: where are we now? *J Hum Genet*, Vol.55, No.4, (March 2010), pp. 195-206, ISSN 1435-232X

Layrisse, Z.; Fernandez, M.T.; Montagnani, S., et al. (2000). HLA-C(*)03 is a risk factor for cardiomyopathy in Chagas disease. *Hum Immunol*, Vol.61, No.9, (September 2000), pp. 925-929, ISSN 0198-8859

Llop, E.; Rothhammer, F.; Acuna, M., et al. (1991). HLA antigens in Chagas cardiomyopathy: new evidence based on a case-control study. *Rev Med Chil*, Vol.119, No.6, (June 1991), pp. 633-636, ISSN 0034-9887

Machado, F.S.; Koyama, N.S.; Carregaro, V., et al. (2005). CCR5 plays a critical role in the development of myocarditis and host protection in mice infected with Trypanosoma cruzi. *J Infect Dis*, Vol.191, No.4, (January 2005), pp. 627-636, ISSN 0022-1899

Manolio, T.A. (2010). Genomewide association studies and assessment of the risk of disease.*N Engl J Med*, Vol.363, No.2, (July 2010), pp. 166-176, ISSN 1533-4406

Manque, P.A.; Probst, C.; Pereira, M.C., et al. (2011). Trypanosoma cruzi infection induces a global host cell response in cardiomyocytes. *Infect Immun*, Vol.79, No.5, (February 2011), pp. 1855-1862, ISSN 1098-5522

Mantilla, J.C.; Zafra, G.A.; Macedo, A.M., et al. (2010). Mixed infection of Trypanosoma cruzi I and II in a Colombian cardiomyopathic patient. *Hum Pathol*, Vol.41, No.4, (February 2010), pp. 610-613, ISSN 1532-8392

Marcon, G.E.; Andrade, P.D.; de Albuquerque, D.M., et al. (2002). Use of a nested polymerase chain reaction (N-PCR) to detect Trypanosoma cruzi in blood samples from chronic chagasic patients and patients with doubtful serologies. *Diagn Microbiol Infect Dis*, Vol.43, No.1, (June 2002), pp. 39-43, ISSN 0732-8893

Marino, A.P.; da Silva, A.; dos Santos, P., et al. (2004). Regulated on activation, normal T cell expressed and secreted (RANTES) antagonist (Met-RANTES) controls the early phase of Trypanosoma cruzi-elicited myocarditis. *Circulation*, Vol.110, No.11, (September 2004), pp. 1443-1449, ISSN 1524-4539

Marin Neto, J.A.; Simoes, M.V., &Sarabanda, A.V. (1999). Chagas' heart disease. *Arq Bras Cardiol*, Vol.72, No.3, (October 1999), pp. 247-280, ISSN 0066-782X

Moreno, M.; Silva, E.L.; Ramirez, L.E., et al. (2004).Chagas' disease susceptibility/resistance: linkage disequilibrium analysis suggests epistasis between major histocompatibility complex and interleukin-10. *Tissue Antigens*, Vol.64, No.1, (June 2004), pp. 18-24, ISSN 0001-2815

Mukherjee, S.; Belbin, T.J.; Spray, D.C., et al. (2003). Microarray analysis of changes in gene expression in a murine model of chronic chagasic cardiomyopathy.*Parasitol Res*, Vol.91, No.3, (August 2003), pp. 187-196, ISSN 0932-0113

Mukherjee, S.; Belbin, T.J.; Spray, D.C., et al. (2006). Microarray technology in the investigation of diseases of myocardium with special reference to infection. *Front Biosci*, Vol.11, (December 2005), pp. 1802-1813, ISSN 1093-4715

Mukherjee, S.; Nagajyothi, F.; Mukhopadhyay, A., et al. (2008). Alterations in myocardial gene expression associated with experimental Trypanosoma cruzi infection. *Genomics*, Vol.91, No.5, (March 2008), pp. 423-432, ISSN 1089-8646

Nica, A.C.; Montgomery, S.B.; Dimas, A.S., et al. (2010). Candidate causal regulatory effects by integration of expression QTLs with complex trait genetic associations.*PloS Genet*, Vol.6, No.4, (April 2010), pp. e1000895, ISSN 1553-7404

Nieto, A.; Beraun, Y.; Collado, M.D., et al. (2000). HLA haplotypes are associated with differential susceptibility to Trypanosoma cruzi infection. *Tissue Antigens*, Vol.55, No.3, (April 2000), pp. 195-198, ISSN 0001-2815

Nobrega, A.A.; Garcia, M.H.; Tatto, E., et al. (2009). Oral transmission of Chagas disease by consumption of acai palm fruit, Brazil. *Emerg Infec tDis*, Vol.15, No.4, (April 2009), pp. 653-655, ISSN 1080-6059

Organización Panamericana de la Salud. (2006). Estimación cuantitativa de la enfermedad d Chagas en las Americas. Montevideo, Uruguay: OPS.

Ouaissi, A.; Guilvard, E.; Delneste, Y., et al. (2002). The Trypanosoma cruzi Tc52-released protein induces human dendritic cell maturation, signals via Toll-like receptor 2, and confers protection against lethal infection. *J Immunol*, Vol.168, No.12, (June 2002), pp. 6366-6374, ISSN 0022-1767

Pacheco, A.G., &Moraes, M.O. (2009). Genetic polymorphisms of infectious diseases in case-control studies.*Dis Markers*, Vol.27, No.3, (November 2009), pp. 173-186, ISSN 1875-8630

Palomino, S.A.; Aiello, V.D., & Higuchi, M.L. (2000). Systematic mapping of hearts from chronic chagasic patients: the association between the occurrence of histopathological lesions and Trypanosoma cruzi antigens. *Ann Trop Med Parasitol*, Vol.94, No.6, (November 2000), pp. 571-579, ISSN 0003-4983

Perez-Enciso, M.; Quevedo, J.R., &Bahamonde, A. (2007). Genetical genomics: use all data. *BMC Genomics*, Vol.8, (March 2007), pp. 69, ISSN 1471-2164

Piron, M.; Fisa, R.; Casamitjana, N., et al. (2007). Development of a real-time PCR assay for Trypanosoma cruzi detection in blood samples. *Acta Trop*, Vol.103, No.3, (July 2007), pp. 195-200, ISSN 0001-706X

Pissetti, C.W.; Correia, D.; de Oliveira, R.F., et al. (2011). Genetic and functional role of TNF-alpha in the development Trypanosoma cruzi infection.*PloS Negl Trop Dis*, Vol.5, No.3, (March 2011), pp. e976, ISSN 1935-2735

Praast, G.; Herzogenrath, J.; Bernhardt, S., et al. (2011). Evaluation of the Abbott ARCHITECT Chagas prototype assay. *Diagn Microbiol Infect Dis*, Vol.69, No.1, (December 2010), pp. 74-81, ISSN 1879-0070

Prata, A. (2001). Clinical and epidemiological aspects of Chagas disease. *Lancet Infect Dis*, Vol.1, No.2, (March 2002), pp. 92-100, ISSN 1473-3099

Ramasawmy, R.; Cunha-Neto, E.; Fae, K.C., et al. (2009). Heterozygosity for the S180L variant of MAL/TIRAP, a gene expressing an adaptor protein in the Toll-like receptor pathway, is associated with lower risk of developing chronic Chagas cardiomyopathy. *J Infect Dis*, Vol.199, No.12, (May 2009), pp. 1838-1845, ISSN 0022-1899

Ramasawmy, R.; Fae, K.C.; Cunha-Neto, E., et al. (2008). Variants in the promoter region of IKBL/NFKBIL1 gene may mark susceptibility to the development of chronic

Chagas' cardiomyopathy among Trypanosoma cruzi-infected individuals. *Mol Immunol*, Vol.45, No.1, (June 2007), pp. 283-288, ISSN 0161-5890

Ramasawmy, R.; Fae, K.C.; Cunha-Neto, E., et al. (2007). Polymorphisms in the gene for lymphotoxin-alpha predispose to chronic Chagas cardiomyopathy. *J Infect Dis*, Vol.196, No.12, (January 2008), pp. 1836-1843, ISSN 0022-1899

Ramasawmy, R.; Cunha-Neto, E.; Fae, K.C., et al. (2006).The monocyte chemoattractant protein-1 gene polymorphism is associated with cardiomyopathy in human Chagas disease. *Clin Infect Dis*, Vol.43, No.3, (June 2006), pp. 305-311, ISSN 1537-6591

Ramasawmy, R.; Cunha-Neto, E.; Fae, K.C., et al. (2006). BAT1, a putative anti-inflammatory gene, is associated with chronic Chagas cardiomyopathy. *J Infect Dis*, Vol.193, No.10, (April 2006), pp. 1394-1399, ISSN 0022-1899

Rassi, A., Jr.; Rassi, A., & Marin-Neto, J.A. (2010). Chagas disease. *Lancet*, Vol.375, No.9723, (April 2010), pp. 1388-1402, ISSN 1474-547X

Rassi, A., Jr.; Rassi, S.G., & Rassi, A. (2001). Sudden death in Chagas' disease. *Arq Bras Cardiol*, Vol.76, No.1, (February 2001), pp. 75-96, ISSN 0066-782X

Robledo, G.; Gonzalez, C.I.; Morillo, C., et al. (2007). Association study of PTPN22 C1858T polymorphism in Trypanosoma cruzi infection.*Tissue Antigens*, Vol.69, No.3, (May 2007), pp. 261-264, ISSN 0001-2815

Rodriguez-Perez, J.M.; Cruz-Robles, D.; Hernandez-Pacheco, G., et al. (2005). Tumor necrosis factor-alpha promoter polymorphism in Mexican patients with Chagas' disease.*Immunol Lett*, Vol.98, No.1, (March 2005), pp. 97-102, ISSN 0165-2478

Salazar Schettino, P.M.; Bucio Torres, M.; Cabrera Bravo, M., et al. (2011). Chagas disease in Mexico.Report of two acute cases.*Gac Med Mex*, Vol.147, No.1, (March 2011), pp. 63-69, ISSN 0016-3813

Samuel, J.; Oliveira, M.; Correa De Araujo, R.R., et al. (1983). Cardiac thrombosis and thromboembolism in chronic Chagas' heart disease. *Am J Cardiol*, Vol.52, No.1, (July 1983), pp. 147-151, ISSN 0002-9149

Schmunis, G.A. (1999). Prevention of transfusional Trypanosoma cruzi infection in Latin America. *Mem Inst Oswaldo Cruz*, Vol.94 Suppl 1, (June 2000), pp. 93-101, ISSN 0074-0276

Schmunis, G.A., & Yadon, Z.E. (2010). Chagas disease: a Latin American health problem becoming a world health problem. *Acta Trop*, Vol.115, No.1-2, (November 2009), pp. 14-21, ISSN 1873-6254

Schofield, C.J. (1981). Chagas disease, triatomine bugs, and bloodloss. *Lancet*, Vol.1, No.8233, (June 1981), pp. 1316, ISSN 0140-6736

Soares, M.B.; de Lima, R.S.; Rocha, L.L., et al. (2010). Gene expression changes associated with myocarditis and fibrosis in hearts of mice with chronic chagasic cardiomyopathy. *J Infect Dis*, Vol.202, No.3, (June 2010), pp. 416-426, ISSN 1537-6613

Steemers, F.J., & Gunderson, K.L. (2007).Whole genome genotyping technologies on the BeadArray platform. *Biotechnol J*, Vol.2, No.1, (January 2007), pp. 41-49, ISSN 1860-7314

Takle, G.B., & Hudson, L. (1989).Autoimmunity and Chagas' disease.*Curr Top Microbiol Immunol*, Vol.145, (January 1989), pp. 79-92, ISSN 0070-217X

Talvani, A.; Rocha, M.O.; Barcelos, L.S., et al. (2004a). Elevated concentrations of CCL2 and tumor necrosis factor-alpha in chagasic cardiomyopathy.*Clin Infect Dis*, Vol.38, No.7, (March 2004), pp. 943-950, ISSN 1537-6591

Talvani, A.; Rocha, M.O.; Ribeiro, A.L., et al. (2004b). Chemokine receptor expression on the surface of peripheral blood mononuclear cells in Chagas disease.*J Infect Dis*, Vol.189, No.2, (January 2004), pp. 214-220, ISSN 0022-1899

Tarleton, R.L. (2003). Chagas disease: a role for autoimmunity? *Trends Parasitol*, Vol.19, No.10, (October 2003), pp. 447-451, ISSN 1471-4922

Teixeira, M.M.; da Silva, F.M.; Marcili, A., et al. (2006). Short communication: Trypanosoma cruzi lineage I in endomyocardial biopsy from a north-eastern Brazilian patient at end-stage chronic Chagasic cardiomyopathy. *Trop Med Int Health*, Vol.11, No.3, (March 2006), pp. 294-298, ISSN 1360-2276

Teixeira, M.M.; Gazzinelli, R.T., & Silva, J.S. (2002).Chemokines, inflammation and Trypanosoma cruzi infection. *Trends Parasitol*, Vol.18, No.6, (May 2002), pp. 262-265, ISSN 1471-4922

Tibayrenc, M.; Neubauer, K.; Barnabe, C., et al. (1993). Genetic characterization of six parasitic protozoa: parity between random-primer DNA typing and multilocus enzyme electrophoresis. *Proc Natl Acad Sci U S A*, Vol.90, No.4, (February 1993), pp. 1335-1339, ISSN 0027-8424

Torres, O.A.; Calzada, J.E.; Beraun, Y., et al. (2010a). Lack of association between IL-6-174G/C gene polymorphism and Chagas disease.*Tissue Antigens*, Vol.76, No.2, (March 2010), pp. 131-134, ISSN 1399-0039

Torres, O.A.; Calzada, J.E.; Beraun, Y., et al. (2010b). Role of the IFNG +874T/A polymorphism in Chagas disease in a Colombian population.*Infect Genet Evol*, Vol.10, No.5, (April 2010), pp. 682-685, ISSN 1567-7257

Torres, O.A.; Calzada, J.E.; Beraun, Y., et al. (2009). Association of the macrophage migration inhibitory factor -173G/C polymorphism with Chagas disease. *Hum Immunol*, Vol.70, No.7, (April 2009), pp. 543-546, ISSN 1879-1166

Torrico, F.; Alonso-Vega, C.; Suarez, E., et al. (2004). Maternal Trypanosoma cruzi infection, pregnancy outcome, morbidity, and mortality of congenitally infected and non-infected newborns in Bolivia.*Am J Trop Med Hyg*, Vol.70, No.2, (March 2004), pp. 201-209, ISSN 0002-9637

Tyler, K.M., & Engman, D.M. (2001). The life cycle of Trypanosoma cruzi revisited. *Int J Parasitol*, Vol.31, No.5-6, (May 2001), pp. 472-481, ISSN 0020-7519

Umezawa, E.S.; Luquetti, A.O.; Levitus, G., et al. (2004).Serodiagnosis of chronic and acute Chagas' disease with Trypanosoma cruzi recombinant proteins: results of a collaborative study in six Latin American countries. *J Clin Microbiol*, Vol.42, No.1, (January 2004), pp. 449-452, ISSN 0095-1137

Umezawa, E.S.; Nascimento, M.S., &Stolf, A.M. (2001). Enzyme-linked immunosorbent assay with Trypanosoma cruzi excreted-secreted antigens (TESA-ELISA) for serodiagnosis of acute and chronic Chagas' disease. *Diagn Microbiol Infect Dis*, Vol.39, No.3, (May 2001), pp. 169-176, ISSN 0732-8893

Valente, S.A.; da Costa Valente, V.; das Neves Pinto, A.Y., et al. (2009). Analysis of an acute Chagas disease outbreak in the Brazilian Amazon: human cases, triatomines, reservoir mammals and parasites. *Trans R Soc Trop Med Hyg*, Vol.103, No.3, (January 2009), pp. 291-297, ISSN 1878-3503

Williams-Blangero, S.; VandeBerg, J.L.; Blangero, J., et al. (2003).Genetic epidemiology of Trypanosoma cruzi infection and Chagas' disease. *Front Biosci*, Vol.8, (April 2003), pp. e337-345, ISSN 1093-4715

World Health Organization Chagas disease (2008) WHO: control and elimination. Report of the Secretariat, executive board EB124/17. 124th Session 27 Provisional agenda item 4.14. November 2008.

Wrightsman, R.A.; Krassner, S.M.; Watson, J.D., et al. (1984).Role of the H-2s haplotype in survival of mice after infection with Trypanosoma cruzi. *Infect Immun*, Vol.44, No.2, (May 1984), pp. 351-354, ISSN 0019-9567

Zafra, G.; Mantilla, J.C.; Jacome, J., et al. (2011). Direct analysis of genetic variability in Trypanosomacruzi populations from tissues of Colombian chagasic patients. *Hum Pathol*, Vol.42, No.8, (August 2011), pp. 1159-1168, ISSN 1532-8392

Zafra, G.; Mantilla, J.C.; Valadares, H.M., et al. (2008). Evidence of Trypanosoma cruzi II infection in Colombian chagasic patients.*Parasitol Res*, Vol.103, No.3, (June 2008), pp. 731-734, ISSN 0932-0113

Zafra, G.; Morillo, C.; Martin, J., et al. (2007). Polymorphism in the 3' UTR of the IL12B gene is associated with Chagas' disease cardiomyopathy. *Microbes Infect*, Vol.9, No.9, (July 2007), pp. 1049-1052, ISSN 1286-4579

Zhang, L., & Tarleton, R.L. (1999). Parasite persistence correlates with disease severity and localization in chronic Chagas' disease. *J Infect Dis*, Vol.180, No.2, (July 1999), pp. 480-486, ISSN 0022-1899

Zingales, B.; Andrade, S.G.; Briones, M.R., et al. (2009). A new consensus for Trypanosoma cruzi intraspecific nomenclature: second revision meeting recommends TcI to TcVI. *Mem Inst Oswaldo Cruz*, Vol.104, No.7, (December 2009), pp. 1051-1054, 1678-8060

Zingales, B.; Souto, R.P.; Mangia, R.H., et al. (1998). Molecular epidemiology of American trypanosomiasis in Brazil based on dimorphisms of rRNA and mini-exon gene sequences. *Int J Parasitol*, Vol.28, No.1, (March 1998), pp. 105-112, ISSN 0020-7519

Permissions

The contributors of this book come from diverse backgrounds, making this book a truly international effort. This book will bring forth new frontiers with its revolutionizing research information and detailed analysis of the nascent developments around the world.

We would like to thank Josef Veselka, MD, PhD, for lending his expertise to make the book truly unique. He has played a crucial role in the development of this book. Without his invaluable contribution this book wouldn't have been possible. He has made vital efforts to compile up to date information on the varied aspects of this subject to make this book a valuable addition to the collection of many professionals and students.

This book was conceptualized with the vision of imparting up-to-date information and advanced data in this field. To ensure the same, a matchless editorial board was set up. Every individual on the board went through rigorous rounds of assessment to prove their worth. After which they invested a large part of their time researching and compiling the most relevant data for our readers. Conferences and sessions were held from time to time between the editorial board and the contributing authors to present the data in the most comprehensible form. The editorial team has worked tirelessly to provide valuable and valid information to help people across the globe.

Every chapter published in this book has been scrutinized by our experts. Their significance has been extensively debated. The topics covered herein carry significant findings which will fuel the growth of the discipline. They may even be implemented as practical applications or may be referred to as a beginning point for another development. Chapters in this book were first published by InTech; hereby published with permission under the Creative Commons Attribution License or equivalent.

The editorial board has been involved in producing this book since its inception. They have spent rigorous hours researching and exploring the diverse topics which have resulted in the successful publishing of this book. They have passed on their knowledge of decades through this book. To expedite this challenging task, the publisher supported the team at every step. A small team of assistant editors was also appointed to further simplify the editing procedure and attain best results for the readers.

Our editorial team has been hand-picked from every corner of the world. Their multi-ethnicity adds dynamic inputs to the discussions which result in innovative outcomes. These outcomes are then further discussed with the researchers and contributors who give their valuable feedback and opinion regarding the same. The feedback is then collaborated with the researches and they are edited in a comprehensive manner to aid the understanding of the subject.

Apart from the editorial board, the designing team has also invested a significant amount of their time in understanding the subject and creating the most relevant covers. They scrutinized every image to scout for the most suitable representation of the subject and create an appropriate cover for the book.

The publishing team has been involved in this book since its early stages. They were actively engaged in every process, be it collecting the data, connecting with the contributors or procuring relevant information. The team has been an ardent support to the editorial, designing and production team. Their endless efforts to recruit the best for this project, has resulted in the accomplishment of this book. They are a veteran in the field of academics and their pool of knowledge is as vast as their experience in printing. Their expertise and guidance has proved useful at every step. Their uncompromising quality standards have made this book an exceptional effort. Their encouragement from time to time has been an inspiration for everyone.

The publisher and the editorial board hope that this book will prove to be a valuable piece of knowledge for researchers, students, practitioners and scholars across the globe.

List of Contributors

Oliver Strohm
University of Calgary, Canada
Center for Cardiology and Pediatric Cardiology Baden-Baden, Germany

Abdullah Shehab
UAE University, United Arab Emirates

Anwer Qureshi
Tawam Hospital, Al Ain, United Arab Emirates

Marlon A.G.M. Olimulder, Michel A. Galjee, Jan van Es, Lodewijk J. Wagenaar and Clemens von Birgelen
Medisch Spectrum Twente, the Netherlands

Michael F. Hill
Department of Medicine, Division of Cardiovascular Medicine, Vanderbilt University Medical Center, Nashville, Tennessee, United States of America

Chaitanya Dutt, Vijay Chauthaiwale, Anookh Mohanan, KumarPrafull Chandra, Shitalkumar Zambad, Ram Gupta and Siralee Parikh
Torrent Pharmaceuticals Limited, India

Jiung-Pang Huang and Li-Man Hung
Department and Graduate Institute of Biomedical Sciences and Healthy Aging Research Center, College of Medicine, Chang Gung University, Tao-Yuan, Taiwan

Alina Yu. Babenko, Alekber A. Bairamov, Elena N. Grineva and Eugenia O. Ulupova
Almazov Federal Heart, Blood and Endocrinology Centre, St. Petersburg, Russia

Takashi Ito and Junichi Azuma
Hyogo University of Health Sciences, Japan

Jan Klimas
Department of Pharmacology and Toxicology, Faculty of Pharmacy, Comenius University in Bratislava, Slovak Republic

Giuseppe Visani and Alessandro Isidori
Hematology and Stem Cell Transplant Center, Marche Nord Hospital, Via Lombroso, Pesaro, Italy

Giorgio Minotti
Center for Integrated Research and Drug Sciences, Campus Bio-Medico University, Via Alvaro Del Portillo, Rome, Italy

Sandeep Vetteth, Deepak Malhotra and Joseph I. Shapiro
University of Toledo, United States of America

Abdul Moiz Hafiz
Winthrop-University Hospital, Mineola, New York, USA

M. Fuad Jan, Timothy E. Paterick,Suhail Allaqaband and A. Jamil Tajik
Aurora Cardiovascular Services, Aurora Sinai/Aurora St. Luke's Medical Centers, University of Wisconsin School of Medicine and Public Health, Milwaukee, Wisconsin, USA

Sachio Kawai
Department of Cardiology, Juntendo University School of Medicine, Tokyo, Japan

Jun-Won Lee and Jang-Young Kim
Division of Cardiology, Department of Internal Medicine, Korea

Hyun-Kyo Lim
Department of Anesthesiology and Pain Medicine, Yonsei University Wonju College of Medicine, Wonju, Korea

Sungwoo Ryoo
Division of Biology, Kangwon National University, Chuncheon, Korea

Hiroaki Kawano
Department of Cardiovascular Medicine, Nagasaki University, Japan

Dan Justo, Arie Steinvil and Itzhak Shapira
Departments of Geriatrics and Cardiology, Tel-Aviv Sourasky Medical Center, Affiliated to Sackler School of Medicine, Tel-Aviv University, Tel-Aviv, Israel

Fernando Rosas
Fundación Clínica Abood Shaio, Colombia

Nubia Roa
Clínica de Falla Cardiaca y Trasplante, Hospital Universitario San Ignacio, Facultad de Medicina, Pontificia Universidad Javeriana, Colombia

Zulma M. Cucunubá
Grupo de Parasitología, Instituto Nacional de Salud, Colombia

Adriana Cuéllar
Grupo de Inmunobiología y Biología Celular, Pontificia Universidad Javeriana, Colombia

John Mario Gonzalez
Grupo de Ciencias Básicas Médicas, Facultad de Medicina, Universidad de los Andes, Colombia

Concepción J. Puerta
Laboratorio de Parasitología Molecular, Departamento de Microbiología, Pontificia Universidad Javeriana, Colombia

Clara Isabel González and Julio César Mantilla
Grupo de Inmunología y Epidemiología Molecular, GIEM, Facultad de Salud, Universidad Industrial de Santander, Colombia